USMLE™ Step 2 CK Qbook
Fifth Edition

OTHER BOOKS BY KAPLAN MEDICAL

USMLE™ Step 2 CK Qbook
Fifth Edition

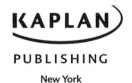

KAPLAN

PUBLISHING

New York

USMLE™ is a joint program of the Federation of State Medical Boards of the United States, Inc. and the National Board of Medical Examiners.

Published by Kaplan Publishing, a division of Kaplan, Inc.
395 Hudson Street, 4th floor
New York, NY 10014

Printed in the United States of America

10 9 8 7 6 5 4 3 2

ISBN-13: 978-1-60978-226-9

Test-Taking and Study Strategies Guide

Author

Steven R. Daugherty, PhD
Director of Education and Testing
Kaplan Medical
Rush Medical College
Chicago, IL

Contributor

Judy A. Schwenker, MS
Director of Study Skills
Kaplan Medical

Contributing Editors

Mary Tyler Lloyd, MD, MPH
Director of Medical Curriculum
Kaplan Medical

Sonia Reichert, MD
Medical Curriculum Consultant
Brooklyn, NY

USMLE Step 2 CK Qbook

Editors

Michael S. Manley, MD
Director, Medical Curriculum
Kaplan Medical
Department of Neurosciences
University of California–San Diego

Leslie D. Manley, PhD
Director, Medical Curriculum
Kaplan Medical
Departments of Neurosciences and Pharmacology
University of California–San Diego

Contributors

Monica Asnani, MD
Paveljit S. Bindra, MD
Dragana Bugarski-Kirola, MD
Jason A. Campagna, MD, PhD
Judith U. Cope, MD, MPH
Michelle DeWolf, DO
Pier Luigi Di Patre, MD, PhD
Michael D. Greicius, MD, MPH
Anusha H. Hemachandra, MD, MPH
Keith Herr, MD
Alfred N. Krauss, MD
Justin Lee, MD
Carlos Pestana, MD, PhD
Reed Pitre, MD
Elizabeth S. Severson, MD
Nancy Standler, MD, PhD
Adam C. Urato, MD

Contributing Editors

Elissa Levy, MD
New York, NY

Sonia Reichert, MD
Medical Curriculum Coordinator
Brooklyn, NY

Executive Vice President, Kaplan Test prep and Admissions

Rochelle Rothstein, MD

Executive Director of Curriculum

Richard Friedland, DPM

AVAILABLE ONLINE

Free Additional Practice

kaptest.com/booksonline

As owner of this guide, you are entitled to get more practice online. Log on to kaptest.com/booksonline to access a selection of USMLE™ workshops and practice questions.

Access to this selection of online USMLE™ practice material is free of charge to purchasers of this book. When you log on, you'll be asked to input the book's ISBN number (see the bar code on the back cover). And you'll be asked for a specific password derived from the text in this book, so have your book handy when you log on.

For any Test Changes or Late-Breaking Developments

kaptest.com/publishing

The material in this book is up-to-date at the time of publication. However, the Federation of State Medical Boards (FSMB) and the National Board of Medical Examiners (NBME) may have instituted changes in the test after this book was published. Be sure to carefully read the materials you receive when you register for the test. If there are any important late-breaking developments—or any changes or corrections to the Kaplan test preparation materials in this book—we will post that information online at kaptest.com/publishing.

Feedback and Comments

kaplansurveys.com/books

We'd love to hear your comments and suggestions about this book. We invite you to fill out our online survey form at kaplansurveys.com/books. Your feedback is extremely helpful as we continue to develop high-quality resources to meet your needs.

Contents

Preface

Preparing for and doing well on the USMLE Step 2 CK are essential requirements on the road to becoming a practicing physician. The skills needed for preparation and execution on multiple-choice tests have little to do with the day-to-day practice of medicine but are necessary hurdles that you must overcome to advance in your medical career. Take heart—this task is not insurmountable; there have been many ahead of you. It only requires some knowledge of techniques, a little planning, a dash of impertinence, and, above all, patience. This Qbook is intended to help you with this process.

- The first chapter, titled "Inside the USMLE Step 2 Exam," within the *Test-Taking and Study Strategies Guide* section was developed to help you gain a better understanding of the exam. It includes a thorough analysis of the question subtypes. In addition, it describes the overall purpose of the exam, as well as its structure and design (including the USMLE's FRED™ software interface), and offers crucial insights to help you do your best on test day.

- The last three chapters of the *Test-Taking and Study Strategies Guide* section offer practical suggestions to help you make the most of your preparation time and to avoid common pitfalls in the exam itself. These chapters summarize the key study and test strategies that have helped thousands of students achieve their maximum score. Use these strategies and approaches as you work through the tests in this Qbook. Also, reread the final chapters of this guide as your exam approaches to get great advice on what to do during the weeks leading up to the exam, as well as on test day itself.

- The *Qbook Practice Tests* contain a total of 850 Step 2 CK–style questions divided into blocks of 50 questions each. These blocks are designed to give you a sense of how the actual exam is constructed. Each test is followed by comprehensive explanations of both the correct and incorrect answer choices. We recommend that you wait until you complete your review of a subject area before taking an exam, that you take each exam in the allotted one-hour time frame, and that you do not look at the answers until you have completed an exam in its entirety. Following each test, review why each answer is correct and why each distractor is wrong. This will provide you with the information needed to answer other similar questions on the same topic. There are two exams each in Obstetrics/Gynecology, Psychiatry, and Surgery; three in Pediatrics; and eight in Internal Medicine. A list of standard lab values can be found for easy reference on pages 525 and 526.

Best of luck on your Step 2 CK exam.

Kaplan Medical

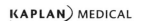

Chapter One:
Inside the USMLE Step 2 Exam

ABOUT THE USMLE

The United States Medical Licensing Examination (USMLE) consists of three steps designed to assess a physician's ability to apply a broad spectrum of knowledge, concepts, and principles and to evaluate the physician's basic patient-centered skills.

Step 1 (multiple-choice exam)—This exam is designed to test how well the examinee understands and applies concepts integral to the basic and clinical sciences.

Step 2 (two separate exams)—The Step 2 Clinical Knowledge (CK) is a multiple-choice exam designed to determine whether the examinee possesses the medical knowledge and understanding of clinical science considered essential for the provision of patient care under supervision. The Step 2 Clinical Skills (CS) is a separate, "hands-on" exam that tests the examinee's clinical and communication skills through his/her ability to gather information from standardized patients, perform a physical examination, communicate the findings to the patient, and write a patient note.

Step 3 (multiple-choice exam)—This exam assesses the examinee's ability to apply medical knowledge and the understanding of biomedical and clinical science essential for the unsupervised practice of medicine, with emphasis on patient management in ambulatory settings.

The results of the USMLE are reported to medical licensing authorities in the United States and its territories ("state boards") for use in granting the initial license to practice medicine. The examination serves to provide a common basis for evaluation of all candidates for licensure. The USMLE is sponsored by the Federation of State Medical Boards (FSMB) and the National Board of Medical Examiners (NBME).

DESCRIPTION OF THE STEP 2 CK EXAM

USMLE Step 2 CK is a nine-hour, computerized examination that serves as the clinical science exam of the licensing pathway. Its purpose is to determine whether an examinee possesses the medical knowledge and understanding of clinical science considered essential for the provision of patient care under supervision. As the complement to the Clinical Skills Step 2 CS exam, Step 2 CK consists of multiple-choice questions that will test you on the principles of clinical science that are important to the practice of medicine in postgraduate training.

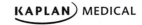

What Is Tested on the Step 2 CK Exam

Step 2 CK tests primary care medicine. Subjects covered on the USMLE Step 2 CK include but are not limited to:

- Internal medicine
- Obstetrics and gynecology
- Pediatrics
- Preventive medicine and public health
- Psychiatry
- Emergency medicine
- Dermatology
- Neurology
- Geriatrics
- Surgery

For a detailed description of examination content areas, see the USMLE website (www.usmle. org). Note that the diseases listed in the outline do *not* represent an all-inclusive list. Questions are generally, *but not exclusively*, focused on the listed disorders. In addition, not all listed topics are included on each examination. Remember also that categorizations and content coverage are subject to change.

Examination Structure

The nine-hour Step 2 CK exam consists of approximately 350 questions, divided into eight blocks of one hour each. Each of the eight blocks contains approximately 44 questions from the full range of topics covered on the exam. You will be able to skip back and forth among test questions, but only within a block of questions. Once the hour is up, you will be unable to return to that block of questions. When you start the testing session, your session clock will begin counting down from nine hours. When the nine hours are up, the test will shut off completely.

Within your nine-hour session time, you will have to complete eight, one-hour sections.

Strategy Tip

View the computer tutorial at home and skip the computer tutorial on test day for an additional 15 minutes of break time.

Step 2 CK at a Glance

Examination Length: Eight 60-minute blocks administered in one 9-hour testing session; computer tutorial: 15 minutes; breaks: 45 minutes, self-scheduled

Number of Questions: Approximately 350; 44 questions per 1-hour block

Question Types: Two types of multiple-choice question: single best answer and matching set

The additional hour can be used to view the tutorial (up to 15 minutes) and to take breaks, including lunch. If you skip the tutorial (which you should because you can review it on the USMLE website), you will have a full hour of break time.

Whenever you begin a new block, the section clock will count down from 60 minutes (the session clock will continue to count down from the original nine hours). When you complete a section (block), you'll get information about how many sections you have left, as well as your remaining session time. If you complete a section early, you can add those minutes to your rest time. You can never add minutes to your test time.

Question Order

The questions on the Step 2 CK exam are presented in a random, interdisciplinary sequence—there are no "content-specific" sections. This makes the exam quite challenging, as you are required to possess the mental agility to jump back and forth among many topic areas. Test questions focus on topics that are relevant to the practice of medicine. All the questions are presented in multiple-choice format.

Question Length

The question stems on the Step 2 CK exam tend to be considerably longer than those on Step 1, almost always including a case history and laboratory data. Interpretation of physical signs and symptoms, clinical and personal histories, tables, imaging studies, and the results of other diagnostic studies are frequently required.

MULTIPLE-CHOICE QUESTION FORMATS

There are two basic question formats on the Step 2 CK exam: one single best answer and extended matching. You will encounter both types throughout the *USMLE Step 2 CK Qbook*, which is designed to simulate actual exam questions.

Approximately 75–80 percent of the questions on the exam are in the one-best-answer format. These questions will be the first ones in each block. You will be presented with a statement or question followed by a list of 3 to 26 options from which you are required to select the one best answer. (Five choices is by far the most common.)

The final questions (20–25 percent) in each block are in the extended matching set format. Each of these sets consists of a list of lettered choices usually related to a common subject (e.g., renal diseases or neurologic disorders). You must choose the single answer that best corresponds to each numbered question. There can be up to 26 answer choices (although 10 is most common). There are usually about two or three questions corresponding to each matching set. A small number of matching questions in each block will require you to pick more than one correct answer.

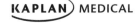

Note

The Step 2 CK exam does not feature negatively phrased questions (i.e., questions with the words NOT, EXCEPT, or LEAST in the stem).

UNDERSTANDING DISTRACTORS

Getting a question correct means selecting the best answer. Incorrect options are called distractors. Their purpose is to distract, that is, to get you to pick them rather than the best answer. Each distractor will be selected by some examinees, or it would not be included as an option. Every option fools somebody. Your job is to not be misled.

In general, distractors will seem plausible and few will stand out as obviously incorrect. Distractors may be partially right answers but not the best answer. Common misconceptions, incomplete knowledge, and faulty reasoning will cause you to select a distractor.

The question writers are told that their distractors must follow these five rules:

- They must be homogeneous. For example, they will be all laboratory tests or all therapies, not a mix of the two.
- They must be incorrect or definitely inferior to the correct answer. There will be enough of a difference between the right answer and the distractors to allow a distinction. For example, if estimating the percentage of a population with a disease, the options will differ by more than five percent.
- They must not contain any hints to the right answer. Distractors are meant to induce you to make an incorrect choice, not give you clues to the correct one.
- They must seem plausible and attractive to the uninformed. If you are not sufficiently familiar with a topic, you may well find that all of the options look good.
- They must be similar to the correct answer in construction and length. Thus, trying to "psych out" the question by looking for flaws in its construction is not a useful strategy.

Answer choices that do not adhere to these rules are not used on the exam. All options are meant to distract you, but often one of the distractors will seem better than the others, the so-called "preferred distractor." This is the wrong answer chosen most often. Preferred distractors are why you can often get yourself down to two choices: the correct answer versus the preferred distractor.

Selecting the correct answer is not a matter of splitting hairs. The correct answer will be clearly correct. If you think two answers are so close that you cannot reasonably choose between them, then the odds are that neither one is correct; you need to look carefully at a different option.

Reading the Question

The examiners know that the thing you least want to do on a long clinical case question is read the question. However, questions are constructed so that if you do not read them, you're likely to get them wrong.

A sophisticated question writer can take advantage of this tendency. If students are likely to stop reading the question part way down, the question writer can include key information in the last part of the question, knowing that many students will never get there. If you stop reading halfway through the question, you will often miss important, if not crucial, information.

So how should students approach long clinical case questions? Start with the notion that you are going to read the question. Stop trying to find a way around reading the question and just do it. Time spent reading the question is time well spent.

If you find yourself confused by the question or if you are short on time, try these strategies:

Think as You Read

Many students read the question and then try to figure out what is going on. By then it's too late. You should be figuring out the question as you read it initially. This means stop at every period and tell yourself what is going on. Summarize the question to that point and decide what issues seem most important. Create an ongoing hypothesis that you can confirm or disconfirm as you move through the question.

Read the Last Line to Set Up Reading the Question

If you do this right, this can be a very effective strategy. But be careful: If you read the question first and then read through the entire case, that's a great approach. However, many people read the question instead of reading the case and then go skim through the case looking for one crucial piece of information to answer the question. Invariably, they come across a red herring, and they choose the wrong answer.

If You Find Yourself Short on Time, Use the "Rule of Three"

Here's the rule: Never pick an answer on the basis of one piece of information. You must have three pieces of supporting information to be sure that you are on target. If you do find three pieces of information telling you the same thing, then you can feel very confident that you now understand what's going on.

THE COMPUTER-BASED TEST

Although you'll receive a tutorial on using the computer on test day, be sure you're comfortable with this format by running the tutorial and sample materials on the USMLE website to become familiar with it prior to your test date. Experiment with taking the test in blocks and know the screen and all the test features well. A normal laboratory values table, including Standard International conversions, will be available as an online reference when you take the examination. Other computer interface features include clickable icons for marking questions to be reviewed, automated review of marked and incomplete questions, a clock indicating the time remaining, and a help application.

During the defined time to complete the items in each block, you may answer the items in any order, review your responses, and change answers. After you exit the block, or when time expires, you can no longer review test items or change answers.

UNDERSTANDING FRED™: HOW TO USE THE USMLE™ SOFTWARE

The FRED™ software provides:

1) a window that shows answers within a block
2) the ability to highlight and/or strike out
3) the ability to annotate a question
4) categorization within the display of normal laboratory values to make them easier to access

Note

You *do not* have to use the new FRED™ features. If you discover that they are distracting you, then the right solution is simple: Ignore the new features and place your concentration where it belongs—on the exam question.

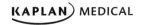

Show Answers Window

In the older NBME software, students could review their answer choices within a given block by clicking on the ITEM REVIEW button at the bottom of the screen. In the FRED™ software, the ITEM REVIEW button is gone. In its place is a window down the left-hand side of the screen that lists the question number and any answer given to each question in the block. This enables students to track where they are in the block and provides an easy way to make sure they have answered every question in the block.

Highlight/Strikeout Options

One of the most consistent complaints from students when the USMLE moved from the paper-and-pencil mode to a computer-based presentation was the loss of the ability to underline key words within the question stem and to cross out answer choices that were decided to be incorrect. The FRED™ software gives both of these abilities back to students. The key to these functions is a button at the top of the screen that allows student to select HIGHLIGHT, STRIKEOUT, or neither.

Highlighting feature

When HIGHLIGHT is turned on, you can use your mouse to highlight in yellow a section of text. This yellow highlighting will remain even after you move your mouse onto something else.

Used appropriately, highlighting can also keep you engaged and make sure you are actually taking content out of the question rather than just reading without retention. Highlighting can help to draw you into the details and avoid the mental mistake of skimming over the question without focusing on the presented details.

Strikeout feature

When STRIKEOUT is turned on, text in options that you click on with your mouse will be faded from black to a grayish color. This moves them to the background (while not completely removing it from view) and provides a clear visual indication that you have ruled out that option as a choice. If you can read the options and select the best answer directly, you will not need to use the strikeout feature. If one answer looks best, pick it and move on.

Annotation Window

FRED™ provides a window in which you can write question-specific comments. You can use this annotation feature to create a symptom list or to remind yourself of something if you desire to revisit the question.

Categorized Lab Values

As with the NBME software, FRED™ gives you the ability to look up the reference ranges for standard laboratory values, which may be presented as a part of your question stem. Previously, these lab values were presented as a long list that blocked out much of the screen. FRED™ groups the lab values into categories such as blood, cerebrospinal, hematologic, and sweat and urine. When you click on each category, you will be shown the lab values and reference ranges only for that category. This reduces the size of the list you have to scan and makes a particular value easier to find.

Although the categorization of the lab value reference ranges is an improvement to the previous presentation, looking up lab values still takes time. Every time you click on the LAB VALUES button, you are pulling yourself away from your focus on the question. Our advice, therefore, is what it

Note

Highlighting can be very useful when creating a symptom list in a long clinical case item or for making sure that some significant feature of the presented information is remembered at the end of the question.

Note

Don't use the strikeout feature on every question, but only on the questions where you are trying to improve your odds by eliminating options.

Note

The annotation window is probably more trouble than it's worth. It takes time to write a note. Your best approach is always to deal with each question as you come to it and then move on. Look forward, not backward.

always has been: Learn your normal lab values so you do not have to look them up. You should know these already before you walk into the exam. If you forget a reference range, the LAB VALUES button is there to help you. But consider this button a safety net. It is there to bail you out if you need it.

Other Minor Changes

In addition to these major changes, FRED™ repositions important buttons and information on your screen. The exam clock has been moved from the upper right to the upper left corner of the screen. All navigation buttons have now been consolidated at the top center of the screen. This includes the buttons for moving forward to the next question, back to the previous question, lab values, as well as the new highlight/strikeout and annotation features.

Putting all the buttons in the same place and at the top of the screen makes the FRED™ interface a bit more intuitive and easier to use. And because the exam questions are at the top of the screen, moving all key buttons to the top of the screen allows the student to focus on one portion of the screen rather than having to look for the necessary buttons at the periphery. This narrowing of focus tends to help with concentration.

SCORE REPORTING

The USMLE program recommends a minimum passing score for each Step. Currently, the passing score as set by the USMLE program is 189 for Step 2 CK. This corresponds to answering 60 to 70 percent of the items correctly. The mean score for first-time examinees from accredited medical schools in the United States is in the range of 200 to 220, and the standard deviation is approximately 20. Your score report will include the mean and standard deviation for recent administrations of the exam.

There will also be a two-digit score on your score report. This two-digit score is derived from the three-digit score and is used to meet requirements of some medical licensing authorities that the passing score be reported as 75.

The graphical profiles which appear on the back of your individual Step 2 CK score report are provided as an assessment tool for your benefit and will not be reported or verified to any third party. The profiles summarize relative areas of strength and weakness to aid in self-assessment. Percentiles are not provided in connection with USMLE scores.

ELIGIBILITY

To be eligible to take the Step 2 CK, you must be in one of the following categories at the time of application and on test day:

- A medical student officially enrolled in, or a graduate of, a U.S. or Canadian medical school program leading to the MD degree that is accredited by the Liaison Committee on Medical Education (LCME)
- A medical student officially enrolled in, or a graduate of, a U.S. medical school program, leading to the DO degree that is accredited by the American Osteopathic Association (AOA)
- A medical student officially enrolled in, or a graduate of, a medical school outside the U.S. and Canada and eligible for examination by the Educational Commission for Foreign Medical Graduates for its certificate

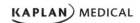

- Fifteen minutes is allotted to complete the tutorial and 45 minutes for break time. The 45 minutes for breaks can be divided in any manner, according to your preference. For example, you can take a short break at your seat after you complete a block, or you can take a longer break for a meal outside the test center after you complete a few blocks.

- Once you begin a block of the test, no breaks are provided during the block. Each block lasts approximately 60 minutes. During blocks, the clock continues to run even if you leave the testing room for a personal emergency. Each block ends when its time expires or when you exit from it.

- As you progress through the blocks of the test, you should monitor how many blocks are remaining and how much break time is remaining. If you take too much break time and exceed the allocated or accumulated break time, your time to complete the last block(s) in the testing session will be reduced.

- The test session ends when you have started and exited all sections or the total time for the test expires.

EXAMINEES WITH DISABILITIES

Reasonable accommodations will be made for USMLE examinees with disabilities who are covered under the Americans with Disabilities Act (ADA). If you wish to apply for test accommodations, you must send your official request and documentation at the same time that you apply for the exam. See the USMLE website for more information.

FOR MORE INFORMATION

- See the USMLE *Bulletin of Information* and the USMLE website at www.usmle.org. Changes can occur after the *Bulletin* is released, so monitor the USMLE website for the most current information about the test.

- Refer to the website of your registration entity: ECFMG for students and graduates of international medical schools; the NBME for students and graduates of U.S. and Canadian medical schools.

- Run the sample Step 2 CK test materials and tutorials provided at the USMLE website.

Chapter Two: **Study Techniques**

ACTIVE LEARNING

Active use of material increases retention and facilitates recall. Repetition makes memories. Each instance of recall produces a new memory trace, linking it to another moment of life and increasing the chance for recall in the future. Memory is dynamic. Recall actually changes neuronal structures. To be truly useful, a piece of information needs to be triangulated, connected to a number of other concepts or, better yet, experiences. For the USMLE Step 2 CK exam, meaning, not mere information, is your goal.

Rereading textbooks from cover to cover and underlining—yet again, in a different color—every line on every page is not an efficient way to learn. You need to focus on the material most likely to be on the examination. Studying that material through active application is the best way to enhance your understanding and retention of the information.

The following study techniques will help you develop better ways to prepare for the exam, but remember, learning for retention and use requires active involvement.

Remember

Active use of the study material is the key to successful studying.

CHOOSING WHAT TO STUDY (AND WHAT TO IGNORE)

How can you possibly know what is likely to be on your examination? There are a number of approaches.

1. Talk to medical school faculty. They often have seen past exams or have reviewed an item analysis and can tell you the topics most likely to appear on the examination. They should be able to direct you to what is essential knowledge in their field and what is less important.
2. Talk to students and colleagues who took the examination in past years. Do they remember some topics being particularly "hard hit"? Was there a "flavor" to the exam? For example, did there seem to be a lot of Pathology?
3. Students who took the exam in the past cannot tell you what will be on the exam that you will take, but they can direct you to the high-yield content areas that you must make sure to master. It's highly recommended to talk with people who have taken the exam. However, be cautious. Candidates typically overestimate how much of their weakest area was on the exam. They are most likely to recall tested content that they got wrong.
4. Take advantage of the questions that can be downloaded from the USMLE's website (www. usmle.org). These practice questions will help indicate the content structure of the exam. Every year new topics are added to the content outline, and some older ones are eliminated. These changes are likely to indicate new questions that you will not hear about from any other source, so be sure to check out these sources. The good news is that this USMLE book contains a general outline of everything that can be tested on the exam. The less good news is that as you peruse the outline, you will soon realize that there is more content indicated than any one person can possibly master in detail.

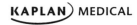

5. Certain topics are standard; others appear as trends. In general, topics begin to appear on the exam two to three years after they reach prominence in the scientific/lay community. Any interesting medical topic that appeared in the literature at least two years ago is a candidate for inclusion on the exam.

6. Beware of the trap of "studying for the last exam"—exam content differs from year to year. This year's exams will be different from last year's. And within any given year, your exam will be different from that of others. This is especially true because the exam is computerized.

CHOOSING HOW TO STUDY

Mastering the material you must learn for this exam is a three-stage process. These stages parallel the functional organization of memory.

Basic Terms and Definitions

You must learn basic terms and definitions. This provides the core vocabulary to understand the content being tested. This stage is a matter of simple recognition and memorization. Terms and definitions are learned by the use of associational memory. This is the level where mnemonics can be useful.

Central Concepts

You must learn central concepts for each of the seven subject areas. This is a matter of being able to explain the meaning of concepts, how they are used, and how they connect with other concepts. Understanding the cross-linkages within subjects and across subjects will serve you well over the course of the exam.

Your basic mental task here is that of reconstructive memory, learning to recall concepts in terms of how things fit together. At this stage, the practice of recalling one concept facilitates the recall of other related ideas. Patterns begin to emerge. This is the level at which diagrams, tables, and pictures can be most helpful.

Application

You must be able to apply the concepts in presented clinical settings and recognize what concepts are most important in minicase presentations. This is the hardest stage of preparation, and the one that most students neglect. Achieving your best possible score depends on knowing not only what concepts mean, but also how they are applied in a given medical situation.

The task at this level is that of reasoning, understanding the implications of presented information, and being able to choose the appropriate action from the available options. At this level, study/discussion groups and doing practice questions can be most helpful.

Your method of study and your study schedule should be arranged to allow you to master each of these stages in turn. As you make your decisions about how you will study, the following suggestions may be helpful:

- Be organized. Set up an organized study schedule and adhere to it. The biggest danger when preparing for the exam is spending too much time on one area or ignoring one subject altogether. Decide how much time you will study each day and put your time in like it is a job. Schedule regular breaks and keep them.

- Decide what your weak areas are by taking pretests, a diagnostic exam, using information from your coursework, or using the questions in each book. Begin your study plan with your weak areas and plan to cover those at least twice before the exam.

- Do not entirely neglect your strong areas, but allocate less time to them. This can be difficult. Research suggests that, left on their own, most students study what they know best and give less time to subjects that make them uncomfortable. Reverse this process and spend the most time on the subjects that make you the most uncomfortable.

- Emphasize integration by reviewing subjects together and/or by organ system. This will greatly aid your preparation for Step 2 CK, which emphasizes the integration of basic sciences. This type of review is best conducted in a group with other people. Other people may look at the same material differently than you and help you expand your perspective and understanding.

- Review materials in related clusters. For example, take the anemias and review how each might present, the basic epidemiology, what lab tests would differentiate, the underlying mechanisms, and initial therapies for each. Using this strategy allows you to "preview" questions and anticipate both the correct answer and the most likely distractors.

- Keep your sessions short; no more than an hour to an hour and a half with at least a 15-minute break. Your concentration declines significantly after an hour or so. Sitting longer will provide only minimal extra return. In addition, the break time allows the short-term memory to be consolidated into long-term memory.

- Do not reread textbooks. Use review books that consolidate the information for you.

- Limit the number of information sources from which you study. Select one main review book for each subject. If you have several books, use one as your primary study material and the others as back-up to clarify points as needed. Too many study sources creates overload, and overload stifles comprehension.

HIGHLY EFFECTIVE STUDY METHODS

Each person has his or her own preferred way of studying. You will have to decide what will work best for you. High-yield study methods all have one feature in common: The more active you are with the material, the more content you will ultimately retain. Remember, your goal in studying is not just to put in the most time, but to be efficient. Many of the best students make use of the following techniques:

Ask Yourself Questions

One of the best study techniques is to pose questions to yourself as you review material. Perhaps you'll want to jot them down on index cards to share with others and to practice later. By asking yourself questions, you are framing the material, challenging yourself to focus on key areas, and preparing for questions you may well see on the examination. Your goal is not to learn knowledge for general use, but to be able to answer multiple-choice exam questions.

This strategy will move you from thinking like a student answering questions to thinking like a faculty member who is writing questions. By this process, you "get into" the head of the question writers and begin to understand what makes a good question and the basic science issues likely to be at the core of presented questions.

Note

It is easy to discover your weak areas by watching your own reaction to each subject. Whatever subject or subject areas you like the least are probably the ones in which you are the weakest.

Remember

Do not entirely neglect your strong areas, but pay less attention to them when studying, leaving them later for review.

Study Tip

The key is not how long you spend studying, but getting the most out of the time.

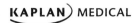

Use Graphs and Charts

Many common graphs and charts appear repeatedly on the exam. Practice reading graphs, charts, and tables. Try abstracting the salient facts quickly from a graph or chart. This may be expedited by using a plain sheet of paper to cover unneeded information and to focus your attention on selected information.

Drawing the graph yourself seems to help you remember it more than just looking at it multiple times. Drawing a graph from memory will give you the confidence that you've truly mastered the material. Again, the more active you are with the material, the more likely you are to both remember it and understand important nuances.

Paraphrase

Practice paraphrasing material to highlight important information. Paraphrasing means processing the material you have read; telling yourself what is important and unimportant as you read through it; and summarizing the key content in your own words.

Pretend that you are the teacher who is in charge of presenting the content. What would you choose to emphasize? What would you leave out if you were short on time? How would you explain the concept to someone new to the field? Remember, if you can say it in your own words, then you really know it.

The art of paraphrasing will allow you to answer questions with extensive information in the stem, such as case histories, much more efficiently. Many students say the most difficult part of the exams is getting through the large volume of reading required for each question. When you are paraphrasing, do not treat every piece of information with the same emphasis, but decide what is important and what is not. Developing this skill will also be helpful as you progress through your medical career.

Summary Notes

Creating summary notes is a great study technique and will reinforce your paraphrasing skills. Summary notes are your personal representation of key points in the material written in a way that makes sense to you. Summary notes should run parallel to your primary study material and should serve to annotate, illustrate, and amplify the key points of that material. The physical action of simply writing the notes tends to reinforce learning and aid long-term retention. Once completed, summary notes provide a ready guide for those times when you review the material.

Study Groups

Study with friends or colleagues in groups of four or five. The best groups comprise people with a range of expertise. Try to form a group where each person's weakness is complemented by someone else's strengths.

The goal of these study groups is not to show your colleagues how much you know. Rather, it's to find the holes in your knowledge while you still have time to correct those gaps. Don't be afraid to tackle the tough topics. With the aid of your study group, things will make sense much sooner than they will on your own. Challenge each other. Pose hypothetical situations and seek agreement as to the best answers.

THE KAPLAN MEDICAL METHOD: THREE TRIES FOR AN ANSWER

You have three chances to get each question right. If you cannot get a clear answer using these three attempts, you do not know the answer. Mark your favorite letter and move on to the next question. The key to this strategy is that you always know what you are going to do next. This helps you feel in control and reduces anxiety.

Step 1: Read the Question.

This may seem trivial, but studies have shown that most students look at the answers first. Questions cause anxiety and answers provide the solution, so many people go right for the solution. However, you cannot pick the correct answer until you know what you are being asked.

Superior students generally spend about 45 seconds reading the question and about 15 to 20 seconds choosing from the given options. Poorer students tend to reverse this time allocation, spending less time on the question and more on the options. Time reading the question is time well spent. More time on the question means more time spent thinking.

- Read the question and pick out key words. Key words are diagnostic information, abnormal values, indications of gender or race, and any qualifying terms.
- Read carefully enough so that you only have to read the question once. Going back over the question takes time. Read for comprehension the first time.

Paraphrasing is the key to effective reading. Superior test takers continuously summarize the key information in a brief fashion while reading the question. This allows you to look to the options with a sharp focus on the key elements and lessens the need to go back to reread it while examining the choices. Look at the following question to see how this is done.

Remember

You can't give a correct answer to a question that you haven't read.

> A 75-year-old smoker and alcohol abuser is hospitalized for evaluation of a squamous cell carcinoma of the larynx. On his second hospital day, he complains of sweating, tremors, and vague gastrointestinal distress. On physical examination, he is anxious and has a temperature of 101° F, heart rate of 104/min, BP of 150/100 mm Hg, and a respiratory rate of 22 breaths per minute. Later that day, he has three generalized tonic-clonic seizures. Which of the following is the most likely cause of his seizures?
>
> (A) Alcohol withdrawal
> (B) Brain metastasis
> (C) Febrile seizure
> (D) Hypocalcemia
> (E) Subdural hematoma
>
> *(Answer: A)*

The mental paraphrasing for this question might be as follows:

An old man with laryngeal cancer who smokes and drinks too much has sweats, tremor, anxiety, and some GI problems—he has three seizures a few days after admission. What's causing the seizures?

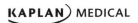

Paraphrasing is the mental equivalent of underlining. It helps you select what's important and keep those key facts in mind while you are evaluating possible answers. Like most test-taking skills, it also takes practice. If you practice paraphrasing material when you study, you will find that you have developed the basics to answer questions. Paraphrase each time you work with questions to gain skill and confidence.

Step 2: The Prediction Pass.

After reading the question, stop. Before looking at the options, try to come up with an answer. We call this the prediction pass because you are trying to think like the question writer and predict the correct answer. By the USMLE's own rules, questions are written so that any expert in the field can come up with the correct answer without having any options present.

With the correct answer in mind, you are less likely to be led astray by distractors. Remember, they are supposed to distract you and convince you to pick the wrong answer. If you see the answer you thought of, scan the other answers to be sure that it is the best. Then pick it and move on to the next question.

Step 3: The Selection Pass.

After reading the question, look down through all of the distractors, in order (A, B, C, D, E, F, G, etc.). If you see a correct answer, pick it. This is the selection pass. If the answer seems obvious and direct, good. Do not trick yourself into thinking the question must be tricky or more difficult.

Most answers will be clearly correct. If you find yourself making up a long story why one option is better than another, stop yourself. You are probably wrong. *The correct answer should be clearly correct.* If two answers seem to be almost the same, then neither one is correct. Once you have identified what looks like the best answer, choose it and move on to the next question.

Step 4: The Final Pass.

If, after reading through the options, you are still not sure of the answer, you have one final try: the final pass. At this stage, rather than trying for a correct answer, you are eliminating those you know to be incorrect. Using this strategy, you can usually eliminate all but two of the options.

When you have narrowed your choices down to only two options, you have now arrived at the most crucial moment of the exam. The correct action at this point is to pick one of the two answers and move on to the next question. If you are really unsure of the correct answer, which one you pick does not matter. With two options to choose from, you have a 50 percent chance of getting the question correct, rather than the 20 percent chance you started with.

Make a choice. Many people waste time at this point by not choosing. Some people, when they have eliminated all but two answers, go back and reread the question in hopes of finding some information that will help them choose between the two options. Time spent talking with students and watching their thought processes during the exam suggests that this is the wrong strategy. When students reread a question at this point, they tend to add to it or pick out single features that help them feel better about choosing one of the answers. However, it does not help them pick the right answer. By adding assumptions to the question, students may feel more confident, but they are really mentally rewriting the question to be one that they feel more comfortable answering. The answer they pick is then the right answer to the question that they envision, but not for the actual question presented.

If after these three passes (1. Prediction Pass, 2. Selection Pass, 3. Final Pass) you still are not sure of the answer, your best option is to guess. At this point, mark any letter and move on to the next question. No answer counts the same as a wrong answer.

Questions with a large number of options should be handled the same way as all one-best-answer questions. The only difference is that you should not do a Final Pass because it would eat up too much time. That means these questions usually take less time to handle if done correctly.

Remember, the key to doing well on this exam is to train yourself to make choices. If you do not know an answer, admit it, make your best guess, and move on to the next question.

TIPS FOR THE WEEK BEFORE THE EXAM

During the last few days before the exam, you should be tapering off your studying and getting into mental and physical shape.

1. This is not the time for cramming in new material, but time to organize and integrate what you already know. Work on making what you know more accessible.

2. Review keywords, phrases, and concepts. Look over your summary notes one more time. This is the time to drill yourself on essential information. The key is to practice recall, not simply read over the material again. What you need to know is probably already in your head. Your task now is to train yourself to access the information when you need it. Doing practice questions is a good way to reinforce your recall skills. Remember, practice questions are often harder than the questions on the real exam, so do not panic if you do not get them right. Use them to clarify your understanding of key details.

3. Have an honest conversation with yourself and decide what you do not know. No one can know everything that is asked on this exam. Be honest with yourself about what you do and do not know. Knowing that you do not know something gives you more of a sense of control on the exam and makes you less likely to panic when you encounter the material and/or waste time on questions you are not likely to get correct. When you come to a question that you know that you do not know, simply mark your favorite letter and move on!

4. Get yourself onto the right time schedule. Wake up every day at the same time you will need to on the day of the exam. This will get your circadian rhythm coordinated with the exam schedule. Do not nap between 8:00 A.M. and 5:00 P.M. Otherwise, you will accustom your body to shutting down during critical exam hours.

5. You should be getting a sufficient amount of sleep. For most people that means at least six to seven hours a night. Sleep is an essential time for your brain to consolidate what you have learned. You need sleep; it makes you a more efficient learner when you are awake.

6. Take some time each day to relax. Have a good meal. Take a walk in the fresh air. Find time for exercise. The change of pace will refresh you and the physical activity will help you relax and sleep at night.

7. Consider the impact of your personal relationships on your preparation. Family responsibilities and obligations can be very distracting. The week before the exam you should avoid family confrontations and any stressful relationships. Your focus should be on the exam and nothing else. The other parts of your life can wait.

8. If you haven't done so already, visit the Prometric Center where you will be taking the exam. It will be indicated on your exam entry ticket. This will ensure you know how to get there and how much time you should allow for the commute. You can see where you should park, and see what the computer setup is like.

9. If you have not yet done so, review the tutorial. Become familiar with the interface, the location of key information on the screen, and how to navigate between screens. If you walk into the exam familiar with the exam, you will not have to use any of your valuable break time to do this on test day.

Remember

Use the time before the exam for review, not for trying to learn new material.

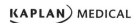

THE DAY BEFORE THE EXAM

1. Take the day off from all studying. This is your day to relax and gather your strength before the main event. Get out of bed at the same time you will have to get up the next day, and then treat this day as a vacation day to reward yourself for all your hard work. If you must study, limit yourself to reviewing your own notes and flashcards.

2. Have some fun. Go for a walk. Listen to your favorite music. Go see a good comedy or an action movie that will allow cathartic release. Go shopping. Spend time with a significant other. Do whatever you like. You have worked hard and deserve it.

3. Make sure that you have checked out the basics for the exam:

    *   Have you worked through the USMLE tutorial?

    *   Do you know where the exam is being given and how to get there?

    *   Do you have alternative transportation if, for example, your car does not start?

    *   Do you trust your alarm clock to wake you up in time? If not, make arrangements with friends as a backup. You want to be sure to wake up rested, refreshed, and on time.

4. Lay out what you'll need for your exam before you go to sleep. This includes your photo identification, scheduling permit, and confirmation number, as well as any personal items like eyeglasses. While you're at it, don't forget to pack a lunch!

5. Call your friends and classmates and make some plans to celebrate after the exam is over. You'll need to blow off some steam anyhow, and talking with colleagues will remind you that you are not in this by yourself.

6. Be sure to do some physical activity. Just taking a walk for an hour will help relax you.

7. Get a good night's sleep. To help you sleep, consider a hot bath or warm milk. Avoid taking sleeping medication as it may leave you groggy in the morning.

THE DAY OF THE EXAM

This is not the most important day of your career, but just another hurdle on your way to becoming a licensed physician. Keep it in perspective. Treat the exam like what it is, a routine mechanical exercise. You are not a doctor for this day, but an assembly line worker. Rather than making cars or toasters, you are answering questions. Deal with each question as you come to it, make your choice, and then move on.

No matter how well prepared you are for the USMLE Step 2 CK exam, you will get many questions wrong. This is not an exam where you should expect to know every answer. Remember, 70 percent correct puts you well over the mean! Knowing this, your test-taking strategy should be somewhat different than it may be when you take other exams.

Doing well on this exam means spending your time on those questions you are most likely to get correct, and not wasting time on questions you are likely to get wrong. Two minutes spent on a question that you get wrong is two minutes wasted. Approach every question assuming that you will be able to answer it correctly. If you discover that you can not arrive at a clear answer, admit it, make a choice, and move on to the next question. The core idea is a simple one. You know you will get some questions wrong. Therefore, admit which ones they are and spend your time on those questions for which your probability of a correct answer is higher.

TEST-TAKING TIPS

Try to arrive 30 minutes early to the Prometric Center so you are not rushed and have time to get organized. You will be given a locker to store your personal items and then assigned a computer station. Remember that you have a total of 8 hours to complete 352 questions in 44-question blocks. You will have one hour for each block of questions, and a total of one hour to be used throughout the day for breaks and lunch. You will be required to sign out when taking breaks.

To cope with fatigue, you will need to schedule breaks. Our recommended schedule for the exam is:

Question Block	Break Time at End of Block
Block 1	No break
Block 2	5-minute break
Block 3	5-minute break
Block 4	30-minute lunch break
Block 5	No break
Block 6	10-minute break
Block 7	Done!

This allows you ten minutes extra to use as needed. You should also be aware that if you leave the exam room during a block, it will be marked as an irregularity in your testing session. So consider after each block whether you want to take a bathroom break during your break time.

Chapter Four: **Summary Pointers**

SUMMARY POINTERS

The USMLE Step 2 CK is an all-day exam. The day can seem long and tiring. You need to have a clear goal in mind and a clear plan for reaching that goal. You need to be in good mental and physical shape for the exam.

REMEMBER

1. Not every question counts (although you can't tell which ones do and which ones do not).

2. You need to be prepared in all of the seven core subjects: Anatomy, Behavioral Sciences, Biochemistry, Microbiology/Immunology, Pathology, Pharmacology, and Physiology. A question in one subject counts just as much as one in another.

3. Become familiar with the basic single best answer question types: positively worded, two-step, bait and switch, true/false, clinical case, and conjunction questions.

4. You must be able to answer questions regarding material presented as either basic knowledge or as applied to clinical tasks. Increasingly, for this exam, application of knowledge is the key.

5. Spend some time becoming familiar with what is likely to be tested, but be careful of the mistake of "studying for last year's exam."

6. Be organized and plan your study time. Kaplan has a variety of resources ranging from home study materials to live lecture review courses that you may find useful in this regard. Make a study plan and stick to it!

7. Strongly consider forming a study group and helping each other review information. Presenting to each other is one of the best ways to learn to use the material you have studied.

8. Practice questions only after mastering the underlying material. Always do questions in clusters and within a time limit.

9. Taper off your preparation before the exam to give yourself a chance to rest up mentally and physically.

10. During the exam, read each question and answer them in order. Never change an answer. Segment your time to be sure you are not squeezed at the end of the exam.

11. Do not linger over questions you do not know. Move on and use the time to answer questions you do know.

12. You have three chances to get every question right: prediction, selection, and final passes. If you can't get a good answer after these three tries, guess and move on.

13. Consider using any of the time-tested behavioral strategies, especially taking a "time out" for coping with anxiety and distracting negative thoughts during the exam.

14. Take care of yourself. Suffering doesn't help anyone.

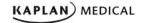

THE USMLE STEP 2 CK EXAMINATION: DOS AND DON'TS

DOs

DO remember the content of the computer-based test (CBT) will be similar to previous exams, as will the amount of time per question (just over one minute).

DO be organized. Set up an organized study schedule and adhere to it.

DO be sure to make up questions while you study (use index cards) and form a study group to review important content.

DO use graphs and charts in texts to speed up your comprehension of the material. A picture is worth a thousand words, and the exam will test you using similar images.

DO practice questions under a time limit similar to the actual exam. In general, your rule should be one minute per question.

DO understand that there is material tested that you will either be unfamiliar with or never really fully understood. Don't panic! Guess and move on.

DO know that you are not required to pass each subsection (physio, biochem, etc.) of the exam separately, but only to answer enough questions correctly to attain an overall passing score.

DO understand that you will only need to get about 70 percent of the questions right to receive a passing score.

DO realize you'll probably see more pictures than in past exams. They are only intended to test you on core basic science content.

DO know that not all of the questions on the exam will count. Anywhere from 30 to 35 questions on the exam are included so they can be pretested and evaluated for use in later exams. In addition, as many as 10 to 15 other questions may be eliminated from the scored pool after the exam results are reviewed.

DO make sure your selected answer matches *all* the information presented in the question. All answers are somewhat likely; you want to pick the one *most* likely.

DO be prepared for two-step questions, where you will need to make two correct decisions to arrive at the correct answer (e.g., come up with a diagnosis, then decide what the treatment should be).

DO remember when you have the question down to two choices, you need to pick one and move on. Lingering over the question tends to result in making the wrong choice.

DON'Ts

DON'T just practice questions without preparatory studying. Review material first until you feel you know it, and then use questions to test yourself.

DON'T do practice questions individually. Do them in clusters with five to ten as a minimum to get yourself used to moving from question to question, and **DON'T** look up answers after each question.

DON'T get into the habit of lingering over a question or thinking about it for an extended period of time. You **DON'T** have this luxury on the real exam.

DON'T just memorize material! Learn and understand how to apply the content in presented scenarios. Very little of the exam will test rote memory for basic facts, and that's not enough to pass.

DON'T reread your textbooks from cover to cover. You need to focus on the material most likely to be on the examination. Talk to others who have taken the exam to see how they prepared. Talk to faculty. Download the Step 2 CK Content Description and Sample Test Materials document.

DON'T assume commercial review books and practice exams are current. A good rule of thumb is that whatever appears in most of the review books is probably important, and whatever appears in just one book is most likely peripheral.

DON'T be afraid to face your weak or least-liked areas. Take pretests and/or diagnostic exams to help you narrow down strengths and weaknesses. Begin your study plan with your weak areas and plan to cover those at least twice before the exam. **DON'T** entirely neglect your strong areas, but leave them for a time closer to the examination.

DON'T expect traditional exam "tricks," short cuts, or buzz words to point you to the correct answer. The USMLE has put great effort into eliminating these cues from the exam.

DON'T get caught by distractors. They may be partially right answers, but not the best answer. Common misconceptions, incomplete knowledge, and faulty reasoning will cause you to select a distractor.

DON'T substitute reading the last line of the question for reading the whole question. This can cause you to miss important information or point you to distractors intended to confuse the issue.

DON'T skip any questions. If you don't know it when you come to it, you are not likely to know it later. Deal with each question as you come to it, answer it as best you can, and move on to the next question.

DON'T change an answer. Your odds of changing a correct answer to a wrong one are so much higher than the reverse that it is simply not worth the risk.

MENTAL/EMOTIONAL PREPARATION

People differ tremendously in their reaction to test situations. Some appear to sail through—confident and calm—whereas others experience mental and physiologic symptoms of test anxiety such as insomnia, nausea, muscle twitching, or increasing inability to concentrate. If you have serious concerns about test anxiety, don't wait until the day before to seek help. Deal with the problem so anxiety doesn't increase as exam day approaches and your options for dealing with it decrease to zero. This is a situational problem, and effective treatment is available.

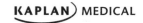

Here are some suggestions for how to deal with test anxiety and some exercises that may help you to cope.

1. **Avoid negative thoughts and feelings.** Negative self talk such as, "There is no way I can pass this exam" can be distracting and produce more anxiety about the test. Focusing on avoiding failure is a recipe for failure. Focus instead on achieving success.

2. **Make anxiety your friend.** A degree of anxiety on the day of the examination is not only natural, but also beneficial. How often have you heard of people responding well beyond their daily abilities when pushed to the limits psychologically? However, there is no need for you to push yourself to the limits, you simply need to be a little tense and anticipatory on exam day. Incapacitating anxiety will destroy your ability to pass. We have heard many individuals say, "I knew everything, I even taught my peers, but I didn't pass. I don't understand it." Anxiety may do this to you!

3. **Seek help if necessary.** If you find that your studying is being overwhelmed by your anxiety, the most useful thing you can do may be to seek counseling. Talking to someone about your anxiety is not a waste of time if your study time is unproductive due to that anxiety. Get help to be more productive.

4. **Be aware of obsessive thoughts.** If you find yourself focusing on your inability to answer questions, the volume of material, or doubts about your ability to pass the exam, try giving yourself something else to think about. Keeping your mind focused on a small task at hand, such as the information you are currently studying, will help you avoid letting obsessive thoughts distract you.

5. **Make a study schedule.** Purchase a calendar and write out which subjects you will study and a time frame for each. Leave room for breaks and "free time." This helps you gain control over your life and your studying. Following a schedule gives you structure, which makes you more efficient and reduces stress.

6. **Improve your attention control.** Awareness is like a searchlight. Whatever you direct your attention to is pretty clear, but other things and events tend to fade into the periphery. Try directing your attention separately to sights, sounds, the feelings in your hands, feet, etc. Your awareness can shift very quickly from one focus to another; however, you can only be fully aware of whatever is in your realm of focus at one particular moment. Use this fact to redirect your wandering thoughts and feelings by focusing your attention. In time this will allow you to quickly de-emphasize extraneous thoughts by redirecting them to simple bodily functions. Keep in mind how attention works:

   - You can attend to only one thing at a time.
   - Attention is voluntary and immediate, focusing on the *now*. The future has no role to play.
   - You can monitor your own attention.
   - Attention can be redirected.
   - Focusing on other things that are more relevant can redirect irrelevant attention.
   - You cannot pay attention continuously to one thing without breaks.

7. **Use visualization.** Spend a few moments thinking back to a crisis situation that you handled beautifully. Perhaps it was a medical emergency or a family quarrel where you intervened and helped solve the issue. It can be any type of crisis in which you took charge successfully. Recall how strong and in control you felt, how effectively you controlled a bad scene, even what the setting was like. Reflect on the event to recall it in as much detail as you can. Each day while you are studying, spend five to ten minutes revisiting this past event until you are able to bring it back in your mind with great clarity and detail. Now, when you feel an anxious feeling welling up, take a mental time out and revisit this scene. When you do, all the emotions of that day will also return and replace those anxious feelings.

8. **Use an Affirmation Card.** Take 30 minutes or so to write a series of statements on an index card. The statements should describe what you believe are your greatest personal strengths, character traits, and talents. You might state that you are a deeply empathetic person, or that you are very good at solving problems. It doesn't matter what you write down, as long as you believe each statement is true and that you are proud of that skill, personality aspect, or talent. Once you have created the card, keep it with you as you study and practice with test questions. When anxious feelings begin to intrude, take out the card and read through it slowly, realizing the truth of what you have written. With practice, this process will help focus you and lessen negative thoughts.

9. **Take a mental "time out."** If anxious or angry thoughts interfere while you are practicing with questions, try this exercise. Close your eyes, take some slow, deep breaths, and flex, then relax first the muscles in your neck, then your shoulders, then your lower limbs. Use a 1-2-3 count for each inhaled and exhaled breath to keep your breathing deep and even. The whole process will only take a few minutes and will help you reduce the physical symptoms of anxiety and allow you to return to the test with a calm, focused state of mind.

10. **Learn and practice deep breathing techniques.** It can be difficult to focus your attention when you are anxious, but deep breathing can help. With enough practice during stressful events, this technique will become second nature during the exam.

11. **Use "time out" during the exam.** If necessary, to break the anxiety loop during the exam, back away from the mouse and keyboard and take a few deep breaths. Thirty seconds of rest will seem like 30 minutes in the middle of the exam. Try timing yourself and see how long it feels. By taking very little time away, you get a lot of mental rest. When the exam becomes too much, the best strategy is not to push yourself to concentrate harder, but to back off and rest for a few moments. You will find that when you return to the exam, your anxiety will be reduced, and the questions will make more sense.

A FINAL COMMENT

This is not a test of your intelligence or even of how good a doctor you will be. This is a test of your capacity to identify and apply core principles within the constraints of the multiple-choice format. Planning, preparation, practice, perseverance, and patience will lead you to your best score. Good luck, and remember, we're here to help!

| SECTION TWO |

Qbook Practice Tests

Internal Medicine:

1. A 23-year-old woman comes to the physician for a health maintenance examination. She is in good health and exercises regularly. Her height is 172 cm (68 in) and weight is 66 kg (145 lb). Her blood pressure is 120/80 mm Hg, pulse is 74/min, and respirations are 12/min. Physical examination is unremarkable except for heart auscultation, which reveals an isolated midsystolic click. Which of the following is the most common cause of this auscultatory finding?

   (A) Bicuspid aortic valve

   (B) Congenital pulmonary stenosis

   (C) Mitral valve prolapse

   (D) Ruptured papillary muscle

   (E) Tricuspid regurgitation

2. A 50-year-old man comes to the physician because of gingival bleeding, epistaxis, and fever for two days. He appears acutely ill. His temperature is 39° C (102° F), blood pressure is 120/70 mm Hg, pulse is 120/min, and respirations are 22/min. Bilateral rhonchi are heard on chest examination. He is admitted for further evaluation. Chest x-ray shows bibasilar infiltrates consistent with bronchopneumonia. Blood tests show 12,000 leukocytes/mm^3 with numerous myeloid blasts. Platelet count is 15,000/mm^3. A bone marrow biopsy demonstrates hypercellular marrow, with 35% blasts. Elongated cytoplasmic inclusions consistent with Auer rods are appreciated in peripheral and marrow blasts. Which of the following is the most likely diagnosis?

   (A) Acute lymphocytic leukemia (ALL)

   (B) Acute myelogenous leukemia (AML)

   (C) Chronic myelogenous leukemia (CML)

   (D) Leukemoid reaction

   (E) Myelodysplastic syndrome

3. A 48-year-old man comes to the physician because of a two-day history of severe low back pain. He states that he has had periodic low back pain for years, but this is more severe than usual and radiates to the buttock and down the right leg. His temperature is 36.8° C (98.2° F). Examination shows some rigidity of the lumbar spine. The pain is exacerbated by applying pressure on the paravertebral region in the lower lumbar spine and by passively raising the leg at 45 degrees while the patient lies supine. A reduced Achilles tendon reflex is noted. Which of the following is the most appropriate next step in management?

   (A) MRI examination of vertebral column

   (B) Nonsteroidal anti-inflammatory drugs (NSAIDs) and two days of bed rest

   (C) Plain x-ray examination of the lumbosacral spine

   (D) Radionuclide bone scanning

   (E) Surgical consultation

4. A previously healthy 30-year-old man is injured in an automobile accident. He is taken to the emergency department, where he is noted to have multiple lacerations of his extremities, some of which are bleeding profusely. His blood pressure is 70/palpable mm Hg. The decision is made to transfuse two units of blood after rapid cross-matching. No reactions are detected in the blood bank. Ten minutes after the transfusion, the patient develops a severe case of hives. The development of hives in this setting would most likely be seen in a patient with which of the following syndromes?

   (A) Adenosine deaminase deficiency

   (B) Ataxia telangiectasia

   (C) DiGeorge syndrome

   (D) Selective IgA deficiency

   (E) Wiskott-Aldrich syndrome

A 71-year-old man presents complaining of dyspnea for the past week. The patient has a history of diabetes and hypertension and was recently diagnosed with cancer. He is currently on multiple drug therapy. On examination, temperature is 37.2° C (99.0° F), his blood pressure is 140/90 mm Hg, pulse is 90/min, and respirations are 22/min. His lungs have a few crackles at the bases with no wheezing. A chest x-ray film shows bilateral diffuse interstitial markings. Which of the following medications is likely responsible for the patient's dyspnea?

(A) Bleomycin

(B) Cisplatin

(C) Mithramycin

(D) Verapamil

(E) Vincristine

6. A 30-year-old woman complains of fatigue and dyspnea for the past two months. She reports that she has also lost 15 pounds during this time. She has been previously healthy and is not taking any medications. She is pale and thin and has a flow murmur on her cardiac examination. She also has mildly enlarged supraclavicular lymph nodes. Laboratory results are notable for a hematocrit of 30%, mean corpuscular volume (MCV) of 78 μm^3, decreased transferrin iron binding capacity (TIBC), and increased ferritin. A screening erythrocyte protoporphyrin level is <35 $\mu g/dL$, and a blood smear shows microcytic red cells. Which of the following is the most likely diagnosis?

(A) Anemia of chronic disease

(B) Aplastic anemia

(C) Lead poisoning

(D) Pyridoxine deficiency

(E) Spherocytosis

(F) Thiamine deficiency

7. A 50-year-old man comes to the physician because of an unusual appearing mole on his upper back. He says that his wife has noted a recent change in its color and shape. The lesion measures 0.7 cm and has ill-defined margins and irregular pigmentation. The patient is otherwise healthy and takes no medication. Which of the following is the most appropriate next step in management?

(A) Follow-up examination in six months

(B) Topical application of *Podophyllum* resin

(C) Cryotherapy with liquid nitrogen

(D) Shave biopsy

(E) Incisional biopsy

(F) Excisional biopsy

8. A 52-year-old man with a history of chronic low back pain complains of three days of a cough productive of purulent sputum, fever, and left-sided subcostal pain worsened by breathing. A single episode of shaking chills accompanied the onset of the illness. He has no gastrointestinal complaints. His temperature is 40° C (104° F), blood pressure is 160/80 mm Hg, pulse is 100/min, and respirations are 38/min with nasal flaring and splinting. The cardiac and abdominal examinations are within normal limits. There are moist crackles and egophony at the left lung base. A chest x-ray film shows a left lower lobe infiltrate. Gram stain of the sputum shows multiple polymorphonuclear leukocytes and occasional epithelial cells. Which of the following is the most likely pathogen?

(A) Gram-negative diplococci

(B) Gram-negative rods

(C) Gram-positive cocci in clusters

(D) Gram-positive diplococci in chains

(E) Gram-positive rods

9. A 38-year-old man who works as a reporter for a travel magazine comes to his physician because of the acute onset of jaundice, malaise, and fever to 38.5° C (101° F). He had returned from Burma two weeks ago, where he spent four weeks. He says that he abstains from alcohol beverages and does not take any medications. Laboratory studies show elevated serum aminotransferases, high bilirubin (both total and direct), and negative serology for hepatitis A virus (HAV) and C virus (HCV) infection. He was vaccinated for hepatitis B virus (HBV) three years ago and is now positive for anti-HBsAg antibodies. Which of the following serologic markers should be tested as the most appropriate next step in diagnosis?

    (A) Anti-HCV IgG antibodies by RIBA
    (B) Anti-HDV IgG antibodies
    (C) Anti-HEV IgM antibodies
    (D) Anti-HGV IgG antibodies
    (E) HBsAg

10. A 50-year-old man returns to his home in Minnesota after a diving trip to Belize (Central America). The day after his return, he comes to the physician because of diarrhea, abdominal cramps, and nausea. His temperature is 37° C (98.6° F). His stools do not contain mucus or blood. Microscopic examination of a stool sample reveals no leukocytes. Which of the following is the most likely pathogen?

    (A) *Bacillus cereus*
    (B) *Clostridium perfringens*
    (C) *Escherichia coli*
    (D) Rotavirus
    (E) *Staphylococcus aureus*

11. A 65-year-old man with a history of peripheral vascular disease develops thromboembolic disease in his left leg accompanied by dry gangrene. Laboratory tests show elevated serum lactic acid, and his arterial pH is 7.27. An ECG in this patient is most likely to show which of the following?

    (A) Peaked T waves
    (B) QT prolongation
    (C) ST depression
    (D) T wave inversion
    (E) U waves

12. A 35-year-old man has had nocturnal attacks of severe periorbital headache for the past five days. Each episode awakens him at night within two hours of falling asleep, lasts for less than an hour, and is associated with ipsilateral rhinorrhea and lacrimation. There is no family history of similar headaches. Careful evaluation does not reveal any objective evidence of neurologic dysfunction. The pupils are equal and normally reactive to light. His temperature is 37° C (98.6° F), blood pressure is 125/75 mm Hg, and pulse is 72/min. Which of the following is the most likely diagnosis?

    (A) Cluster headache
    (B) Depression headache
    (C) Giant cell arteritis
    (D) Migraine
    (E) Tension headache
    (F) Trigeminal neuralgia

13. A 32-year-old African American woman complains of mild fevers and fatigue for the past month. She has no significant past medical history. Her temperature is 38.1° C (100.6° F), blood pressure is 115/70 mm Hg, pulse is 75/min, and respirations are 18/min. Nontender, mobile cervical and axillary lymph nodes are noted. Auscultation of the lungs reveals fine crackles bilaterally. A chest x-ray film shows hilar lymphadenopathy and diffuse interstitial infiltrates. Lymph node biopsy shows noncaseating granulomas. Which of the following is the most appropriate therapy?

    (A) Allopurinol

    (B) Angiotensin converting enzyme (ACE) inhibitor

    (C) Cyclosporine

    (D) Glucocorticoids

    (E) Isoniazid

14. A 20-year-old man comes to the physician because he has noticed blood in his urine on several occasions over the past year. Each episode of hematuria occurred in association with an upper respiratory tract infection or a flulike illness. Physical examination is unremarkable. A urine dipstick test shows mild proteinuria and microhematuria. Serum levels of electrolytes, creatinine, and blood urea nitrogen are within normal limits. Serum levels of IgA are elevated. Which of the following is the most likely diagnosis?

    (A) Berger disease

    (B) Goodpasture syndrome

    (C) Henoch-Schönlein purpura

    (D) Minimal change disease

    (E) Postinfectious glomerulonephritis

    (F) Wegener granulomatosis

15. A 60-year-old woman presents to a physician complaining of a swelling in her neck. Her past medical history is significant for rheumatoid arthritis and Sjögren syndrome. Physical examination reveals a mildly nodular, firm, rubbery goiter. Total serum thyroxine (T_4) is 10 mg/dL, and third-generation thyroid-stimulating hormone (TSH) testing shows a level of 1.2 mIU/mL. Antithyroid peroxidase antibody titers are high. Which of the following is the most likely diagnosis?

    (A) Euthyroid sick syndrome

    (B) Graves disease

    (C) Hashimoto thyroiditis

    (D) Silent lymphocytic thyroiditis

    (E) Subacute thyroiditis

16. A 22-year-old man comes to the physician because he has developed patches of hair loss in his scalp and beard over several months. The patient's medical history is unremarkable, but his family history is significant for Addison disease in a sister and vitiligo in his mother. Physical examination shows two sharply demarcated areas of alopecia in the scalp and one in the right cheek. The skin in these areas is perfectly smooth and covered only by sparse short hair shafts. In addition, pitting of nail plates is noted. A biopsy of affected skin demonstrates lymphocytic infiltrates around hair follicles. Which of the following is the most appropriate next step in management?

    (A) Psychiatric consultation

    (B) Topical application of minoxidil

    (C) Oral administration of iron sulfate

    (D) Topical injections of corticosteroids

    (E) Systemic corticosteroids

17. A 75-year-old white man complains to a physician of abdominal pain. His temperature is 37° C (98.6° F), blood pressure is 110/65 mm Hg, pulse is 63/min, and respirations are 16/min. The abdomen is soft, with focal tenderness in the left lower quadrant. His erythrocyte count is 4.5 million/mm³, leukocyte count is 9000/mm³ with 60% neutrophils and 5% bands, and platelet count is 250,000/mm³. Serum chemistries show:

Sodium	140 mEq/L
Potassium	5 mEq/L
Chloride	102 mEq/L
Creatinine	1.1 mg/dL
Urea nitrogen	12 mg/dL

Which of the following is the most appropriate next step in diagnosis?

(A) Barium enema

(B) Colonoscopy

(C) CT of abdomen

(D) Plain film of abdomen

(E) Trial therapy of a liquid diet

18. A 38-year-old man comes to the physician because of slowly progressive visual impairment that makes him "bump into objects" on both sides. He also reports that, while driving, he has trouble switching lanes because he needs to turn his head all the way backward to look for other cars. Ocular examination shows bitemporal field vision loss with preserved visual acuity. Examination of the fundus is unremarkable. Which of the following is the most likely diagnosis?

(A) Pituitary adenoma

(B) Occipital lobe meningioma

(C) Optic glioma

(D) Optic nerve atrophy

(E) Optic neuritis

(F) Retinal detachment

19. An 18-year-old woman complains of myalgias, a sore throat, and painful mouth sores for three days' duration. Her temperature is 38.2° C (100.8° F), blood pressure is 110/80 mm Hg, pulse is 84/min, respirations are 15/min. Her gingiva are edematous and erythematous, and there are vesicles on her right upper and lower lips. Her pharynx is mildly erythematous without exudate, and there is tender mobile cervical lymphadenopathy. Her breath is not fetid, and the dentition is normal. Which of the following is the most likely causal agent?

(A) *Actinomyces israelii*

(B) Coxsackie virus

(C) Herpes simplex virus 1

(D) *Nocardia asteroides*

(E) *Streptococcus pyogenes*

20. A 35-year-old man complains of chronic vague gastric pain of several years' duration. The pain is sometimes relieved by food. Serum immunoglobulin studies for IgG and IgA antibodies directed against *Helicobacter pylori* are strongly positive. Endoscopy with gastric antral biopsy demonstrates gastritis but no ulcerative lesions. *H. pylori* organisms are seen with special stains on the biopsy fragments. The patient is treated with a 1-week course of omeprazole (20 mg bid), plus clarithromycin and metronidazole (500 mg bid each). Which of the following is the most appropriate noninvasive test to determine whether the *H. pylori* has been eradicated?

(A) Culture of gastric biopsy

(B) Rapid urease test

(C) Repeat qualitative IgA and IgG antibodies against *H. pylori*

(D) Repeat quantitative IgA and IgG antibodies against *H. pylori*

(E) Urea breath test

21. A 52-year-old man comes to the physician because of slowly progressive weakness in his legs. He also complains of clumsiness with his right hand, which creates difficulties with buttons or turning keys. Examination reveals mild bilateral footdrop and leg weakness. Fasciculation and mild wasting are observed in the calf muscles. There is no spasticity or impaired sensation. The speech is normal, but fasciculation of the tongue is appreciated. Respiration, pulse, and temperature are normal. A muscle biopsy shows evidence of denervation with reinnervation. Which of the following is the most likely diagnosis?

    (A) Amyotrophic lateral sclerosis (ALS)

    (B) Charcot-Marie-Tooth disease

    (C) Guillain-Barré syndrome

    (D) Myasthenia gravis

    (E) Spinal muscular atrophy

22. An 18-year-old man is referred for evaluation of hypertension. On examination, he appears in no apparent discomfort and states that he has never had any health problems. His height is 175 cm (69 in), and his weight is 70 kg (154 lb). There is no pitting edema in the lower legs or jugular vein distention. The lungs are clear to auscultation. Blood pressure is 162/80 mm Hg in the upper extremities and 115/77 mm Hg in the lower extremities. Femoral pulses are weaker than radial pulses. A systolic murmur is appreciated at the base of the heart and is particularly intense in the back. The ECG shows changes consistent with left ventricular hypertrophy, and a chest x-ray film reveals notching of the inferior margins of the ribs. Which of the following is the most likely diagnosis?

    (A) Atrial septal defect (ASD)

    (B) Coarctation of the aorta

    (C) Congenital aortic stenosis

    (D) Congenital pulmonary stenosis

    (E) Patent ductus arteriosus

    (F) Tetralogy of Fallot

    (G) Ventricular septal defect (VSD)

23. A 50-year-old alcoholic man with chronic hepatitis C infection is brought to the emergency department by the police, because he has blisters and crusted lesions on sun-exposed skin of his face and lower arms. Plasma porphyrins are elevated, and follow-up studies demonstrate elevated uroporphyrin I in urine and iso-coproporphyrin in feces. A biopsy of one of the lesions reveals subepidermal blisters with minimal inflammation, thickening of vessel walls in the papillary dermis, marked solar elastosis, and "caterpillar bodies" in the roof of the blister. Which of the following is the most likely diagnosis?

    (A) Acute intermittent porphyria

    (B) Delta-aminolevulinic acid dehydratase deficiency

    (C) Erythropoietic protoporphyria

    (D) Hereditary coproporphyria

    (E) Porphyria cutanea tarda

24. A 40-year-old woman is admitted to the hospital because of fever, headache, confusion, and jaundice for one week. She underwent hysterectomy two months ago and began estrogen replacement therapy with ethinyl estradiol and a progestin. On admission, her temperature is 38.7° C (102° F), blood pressure is 140/90 mm Hg, pulse is 98/min, and respirations are 20/min. She is disoriented to time and place. Physical examination reveals jaundiced sclerae and skin, purpura on the trunk, and bleeding gums. A stool guaiac test is positive for occult blood. Blood and urine cultures are negative, but urinalysis reveals hemoglobinuria. Blood studies show:

Hematocrit	28%
Red blood cells	2.5 million/mm^3
Leukocytes	10,000/mm^3
Platelets	15,000/mm^3
Serum	
BUN	40 mg/dL
Creatinine	2.8 mg/dL
LDH	800 U/L
Bilirubin	
Total	4.0 mg/dL
Direct	0.8 mg/dL

Coagulation tests are within normal limits; fibrin-split products and Coombs test are negative. A peripheral blood smear shows schistocytes, helmet cells, and triangle cells. Which of the following is the most likely diagnosis?

(A) Disseminated intravascular coagulation (DIC)

(B) Evans syndrome

(C) Hemolytic-uremic syndrome (HUS)

(D) Idiopathic (autoimmune) thrombocytopenic purpura (ITP)

(E) Malignant hypertension

(F) Thrombotic thrombocytopenic purpura (TTP)

25. A 30-year-old woman is seen in the emergency department because of severe abdominal pain. The pain has progressively worsened for the past day and is accompanied by nausea, vomiting, and diarrhea. The patient has had several similar episodes in the past that developed over the course of hours to days and lasted for a week or more. She has had surgeries for suspected appendicitis and suspected biliary tract disease, neither of which was confirmed once the abdomen was entered. Her temperature is 37° C (98.6° F), blood pressure is 140/100 mm Hg, pulse is 120/min, and respirations are 16/min. Abdominal examination demonstrates minimal abdominal tenderness and no rebound tenderness. Measurement of which of the following will most likely confirm the diagnosis?

(A) Erythrocyte porphyrins

(B) Fecal porphyrins

(C) Plasma porphyrins

(D) Urine porphobilinogen

(E) Urine porphyrins

26. An otherwise healthy 15-year-old boy undergoes evaluation for a newly diagnosed ventricular septal defect (VSD). The boy is at the 50th percentile for height and 45th percentile for weight. He plays soccer regularly with his school team and has never had any significant health problems. His blood pressure is 120/76 mm Hg, pulse is 72/min, and respirations are 11/min. An ECG is unremarkable, but echocardiography demonstrates a defect in the upper interventricular septum with cardiac chambers of normal size. Doppler ultrasound and radionuclide flow studies reveal a small left-to-right shunt with a pulmonary-to-systemic flow ratio of less than 1.5. Which of the following is the most significant complication of this patient's condition?

(A) Arrhythmia

(B) Infective endocarditis

(C) Pulmonary hypertension

(D) Right-sided heart failure

(E) Shunt reversal

27. A 33-year-old man presents with recurrent pain and swelling of the right knee. These symptoms started four years ago and are often precipitated by minor trauma. The joint fluid has been tested during acute episodes, and although clearly inflammatory, there has been no evidence of urate crystals, bacteria, or blood. Clinical examination reveals a moderately swollen and tender joint. A complete blood count (CBC), prothrombin time (PT), partial thromboplastin time (PTT), and serum chemistries are normal. X-ray films show speckling of the articular cartilage and increased joint space without marginal erosions. Which of the following is the most likely diagnosis?

    (A) Hemophiliac arthritis

    (B) Lyme arthritis

    (C) Monarticular rheumatoid arthritis

    (D) Osteoarthritis

    (E) Pseudogout

    (F) Psoriatic arthritis

28. A 25-year-old man with a 7-year history of ulcerative colitis consults a physician because of insidious onset of progressive fatigue, pruritus, and jaundice. Laboratory studies are notable for elevation of serum alkaline phosphatase that is not accompanied by significant elevations of aspartate aminotransferase (AST) or alanine aminotransferase (ALT). An antimitochondrial antibody test is negative. Endoscopic retrograde cholangiography demonstrates multiple short strictures and saccular dilations of the biliary tree, both in extrahepatic and intrahepatic sites. Liver biopsy demonstrates bile duct proliferation, periductal fibrosis, inflammation, and loss of bile ducts. Which of the following is the most likely explanation for these findings?

    (A) Bile duct tumor

    (B) Choledocholithiasis

    (C) Congenital polycystic liver

    (D) Primary biliary cirrhosis

    (E) Primary sclerosing cholangitis

29. One day after sustaining a laceration of the right hand at work, a 28-year-old man comes to the emergency department because of fever, chills, and painful swelling of the right arm. His temperature is 39.4° C (103° F), blood pressure is 110/65 mm Hg, pulse is 110/min, and respirations are 20/min. His right arm is swollen and extremely tender from the elbow up to the shoulder. The skin shows a diffuse dusky erythema. Sensation to touch and pain is reduced in the forearm and hand. A blood sample is immediately taken for cultures. Which of the following is the most appropriate next step in management?

    (A) Supportive measures until culture results are available

    (B) Treatment with clindamycin

    (C) Treatment with penicillin V

    (D) Parenteral treatment with penicillin G

    (E) Parenteral treatment with vancomycin

    (F) Surgical exploration and debridement

30. Over a two-month period, a 50-year-old woman with a history of polycythemia vera develops abdominal pain and gross ascites. Physical examination demonstrates smooth hepatomegaly and mild jaundice. Pressure applied over the liver fails to distend the jugular veins. The abdomen is grossly edematous and the abdominal wall shows a tortuous venous pattern. Edema of the legs is prominent. Which of the following is the most likely diagnosis?

    (A) Budd-Chiari syndrome

    (B) Hepatic cirrhosis

    (C) Hepatocellular carcinoma

    (D) Primary sclerosing cholangitis

    (E) Steatosis

31. A previously healthy, 48-year-old woman presents with easy fatigability, anorexia, and a 5-kg (11-lb) weight loss for 2 months. She also reports night sweats and occasional temperatures to 38° C (100° F). On examination, the spleen is palpable 4 cm below the left costal arch. Blood tests reveal a hemoglobin of 16 g/dL, 500,000 platelets/mm^3, and 170,000 leukocytes/mm^3. The differential count shows a left shift, with predominance of mature granulocytes, bands, and metamyelocytes; blasts are 3%. Serum chemistry is remarkable for low leukocyte alkaline phosphatase and high uric acid. Cytogenetic studies demonstrate the presence of the Philadelphia chromosome in white blood cells. Which of the following is the most likely diagnosis?

    (A) Acute myelogenous leukemia (AML)

    (B) Chronic lymphocytic leukemia (CLL)

    (C) Chronic myelogenous leukemia (CML)

    (D) Leukemoid reaction

    (E) Myelofibrosis

32. A 60-year-old alcoholic man is brought to the emergency department with hematemesis. His pulse is 110/min, blood pressure is 100/60 mm Hg, and respirations are 19/min. He has multiple spider angiomata on his back and chest, and bilateral gynecomastia. Abdominal examination is significant for hepatosplenomegaly, and a distended abdomen which is tympanic on percussion. His testicles are small, and a rectal examination produces guaiac-negative stool. His hematocrit is 23%. After placement of a nasogastric tube, 400 mL of bright red blood is evacuated. After initial fluid resuscitation, which of the following is the most appropriate next step in management?

    (A) Barium swallow

    (B) Esophageal balloon tamponade

    (C) Esophagogastroscopy

    (D) Exploratory celiotomy

    (E) Selective angiography

    (F) Transjugular intrahepatic portosystemic shunt

33. A 72-year-old man with a history of peripheral vascular disease and recurrent chest pain underwent cardiac catheterization three hours ago. Angiography showed 80% occlusion of the left main coronary artery. He now complains of diarrhea and severe constant mid-abdominal pain. On examination, his temperature is 37.2° C (99° F), blood pressure is 170/90 mm Hg, pulse is 102/min, and respirations are 22/min. The lungs are clear, and the abdomen is soft and nondistended without focal tenderness. Bowel sounds are hypoactive, and no masses are palpable. Rectal examination reveals occult blood in the stool. Which of the following is the most likely diagnosis?

    (A) Gastric ulcer

    (B) Mesenteric ischemia

    (C) Pancreatitis

    (D) Perforated duodenal ulcer

    (E) Staphylococcal gastroenteritis

34. A 22-year-old man presents with a six-month history of nonbloody diarrhea, malaise, recurrent abdominal cramps, and temperatures to 38.5° C (101.3° F). At this time, he is afebrile. Examination reveals a palpable, ill-defined mass in the right lower quadrant of the abdomen. Palpation causes local tenderness without guarding. Oral ulcers are also noted. Laboratory studies show:

Hemoglobin	11.5 g/dL
Leukocyte count	12,800/mm^3
Albumin	2.8 g/dL
Sedimentation rate	45 mm/h

An upper gastrointestinal series with small bowel follow-through reveals a sharply demarcated stenotic segment in the terminal ileum. The patient undergoes laparotomy, and the involved segment of ileum is resected. Which of the following is the most likely diagnosis?

    (A) Carcinoma

    (B) Celiac disease

    (C) Chronic appendicitis

    (D) Crohn disease

    (E) Pseudomembranous colitis

    (F) Ulcerative colitis

35. A 55-year-old male smoker with diabetes and hypertension presents with complaints of chest pain on exertion. Exercise stress testing shows reversible ischemia in the anteroseptal portion of the heart after exercising for four minutes. Cardiac catheterization reveals an 80% stenosis of the left main coronary artery. Which of the following is the most appropriate intervention?

    (A) Re-examination in six months or sooner if symptoms worsen

    (B) Beta blocker

    (C) Sublingual nitroglycerin as needed

    (D) Percutaneous balloon angioplasty

    (E) Coronary artery bypass grafting

36. A 55-year-old woman with a history of rheumatoid arthritis since age 28 presents with new symptoms of recent onset. She complains of persistent fatigue, weight loss, diarrhea, and leg swelling. Furthermore, she has had pain in her wrists with a tingling sensation at the tips of her thumbs and first two digits, which bothers her especially at night. Examination reveals waxy skin plaques in the axillary folds, macroglossia, hepatosplenomegaly, pitting edema of the legs, and peripheral neuropathy. The stool guaiac test is positive. Serum chemistry studies show only mild hypoalbuminemia. On urinalysis, proteinuria in the nephrotic range is found without hematuria. Which of the following is the most appropriate next step in diagnosis?

    (A) Electrophoresis of serum proteins

    (B) X-rays of vertebral column and skull

    (C) Biopsy of skin, rectal mucosa, or abdominal fat

    (D) Renal biopsy

    (E) Endomyocardial biopsy

37. A 68-year-old woman complains of numbness and difficulty walking. Family members mention that her behavior has also become erratic over the past several months. She has a past medical history of Crohn disease, for which she underwent ileal resection ten years ago. Laboratory results indicate a hematocrit of 20% and a mean corpuscular volume (MCV) of 110 μm^3. Blood smear shows large red cells with hypersegmented neutrophils. Which of the following is the most likely cause of these findings?

    (A) Ferrochelatase deficiency

    (B) Folate deficiency

    (C) Hydroxymethylbilane synthase deficiency

    (D) Intrinsic factor deficiency

    (E) Iron deficiency anemia

    (F) Vitamin malabsorption

38. A 60-year-old man consults a physician because of intense forefoot pain on one side that is triggered by exercise. One week earlier, he ran a 25-km marathon, and the pain started midway through the race. He continued to run anyway, as he wished to finish the race, and the pain disappeared within seconds of finishing. He rested the next day, and then began to run the following day. The pain started much more quickly this time, and he stopped running when it did. The pain persisted for a few minutes and then stopped. He then rested for three days, to give his foot time to heal. When he began to run again, his forefoot began to hurt almost immediately, and he decided to consult a physician. Which of the following is the most likely diagnosis?

    (A) Achilles tendinitis

    (B) Epiphysitis of the calcaneus

    (C) Fracture of the posterolateral talar tubercle

    (D) Metatarsal stress fracture

    (E) Posterior Achilles tendon bursitis

39. A 44-year-old man is admitted for treatment of an infection with *Staphylococcus aureus*. His course is complicated by the development of dry gangrene on his right toe. His blood pressure drops to 85/48 mm Hg, and he is bleeding from multiple sites. A peripheral blood smear shows multiple schistocytes. Laboratory evaluation of prothrombin time (PT), partial thromboplastin time (PTT), and platelets would most likely show which of the following?

    (A) Elevated PT, elevated PTT, decreased platelets

    (B) Elevated PT, elevated PTT, elevated platelets

    (C) Elevated PT, normal PTT, decreased platelets

    (D) Normal PT, elevated PTT, decreased platelets

    (E) Normal PT, normal PTT, decreased platelets

40. A 75-year-old African American man is transferred from a nursing home to the emergency department. For the past two hours, the man has had acute, left-sided abdominal pain that started in the left iliac fossa. While waiting to be seen, he suddenly passes stool mixed with dark blood clots. His temperature is 38.1° C (100.6° F), blood pressure is 110/85 mm Hg, pulse is 120/min, and respirations are 18/min. Abdominal examination demonstrates localized tenderness along the descending colon. An x-ray film taken after barium enema excludes intra-abdominal free air. The colon lumen is decreased and irregular, with mucosal thickening, and there is gas in the wall of the colon. Which of the following is the most likely diagnosis?

    (A) Appendicitis

    (B) Colon cancer

    (C) Crohn disease

    (D) Ischemic colitis

    (E) Ulcerative colitis

41. A 37-year-old woman comes to medical attention with a three-month history of recurrent episodes of hemoptysis and low-grade fever. Her temperature is 37.6° C (100° F), blood pressure is 123/82 mm Hg, pulse is 74/min, and respirations are 14/min. A chest x-ray film demonstrates bilateral perihilar infiltrates. In addition to mild anemia and leukocytosis, laboratory analysis shows:

    Blood, serum

BUN	23 mg/dL
Creatinine	2.2 mg/dL
Erythrocyte sedimentation rate	50/min
Complement levels	Normal
Antinuclear antibodies	Negative
Antineutrophil cytoplasmic antibodies (ANCA)	Positive, c-ANCA pattern

    Urinalysis

Protein	2+
Red blood cells	10/hpf

    A renal biopsy shows granulomas with necrotizing vasculitis and scattered mesangial deposits of immunoglobulin and complement. Which of the following is the most likely diagnosis?

    (A) Churg-Strauss syndrome

    (B) Goodpasture syndrome

    (C) Polyarteritis nodosa

    (D) Tuberculosis

    (E) Wegener granulomatosis

42. A 65-year-old African American man presents with dull, persistent abdominal pain with radiation to the back. He has lost 20 lb over the past three months. His appetite is markedly decreased, with associated nausea and vomiting. Laboratory analysis reveals a blood glucose of 280 mg/dL. Physical examination is remarkable for mid-epigastric tenderness and a positive Homans sign in the left calf. He has no significant past medical history. Which of the following is the most likely diagnosis?

    (A) Chronic pancreatitis

    (B) Gastric cancer

    (C) Hepatic cancer

    (D) Pancreatic cancer

    (E) Type 2 diabetes mellitus

43. A 56-year-old man with a 5-year history of hypertension treated with diuretics and enalapril comes to medical attention because of right flank pain. His temperature is 37° C (98.6° F) and blood pressure is 145/95 mm Hg. Physical examination shows tenderness in the right costovertebral angle and bilaterally enlarged kidneys. A urine dipstick test reveals microhematuria. Which of the following is the most appropriate next step in diagnosis?

    (A) Cytologic examination of urine

    (B) Ultrasonography

    (C) CT scan of the abdomen

    (D) Intravenous pyelography (IVP)

    (E) Renal biopsy

44. A 54-year-old man comes to the physician because of right leg pain for four months. He describes it as a deep pain in the calf muscles that occurs intermittently after walking for a given distance and subsides after resting for a few minutes. He has been smoking 20-30 cigarettes a day for the past 25 years and drinks alcohol occasionally. His temperature is 36.8° C (98.2° F), blood pressure is 154/93 mm Hg, pulse is 74/min, and respirations are 13/min. Examination shows thinning of the right calf compared with the left, as well as hair loss on the right leg. Reflexes and sensation are normal. Femoral pulses are normal on both sides, but the right popliteal and pedal pulses are barely detectable. Which of the following is the most likely diagnosis?

    (A) Atherosclerotic stenosis of the common iliac artery

    (B) Atherosclerotic stenosis of the distal superficial femoral artery

    (C) Peripheral polyneuropathy

    (D) Prolapse of intervertebral disk in the lumbar spine

    (E) Thromboangiitis obliterans

45. A 60-year-old woman presents with a gradual increase in abdominal girth for the past two months. She denies any history of alcohol use and had a positive PPD test many years ago. Physical examination reveals ascites and dullness to percussion at her right lung base. She has no spider angiomata, caput medusae, palmar erythema, or lower extremity edema. A chest x-ray film shows a right pleural effusion. Laboratory studies reveal the following:

Aspartate aminotransferase (AST)	12 U/L
Alanine aminotransferase (ALT)	11 U/L
Alkaline phosphatase	80 U/L
Total bilirubin	0.5 mg/dL
Direct bilirubin	0.1 mg/dL
HBsAg	Negative
HBsAb	Positive
HBcAb	Positive
HCAb	Negative

An abdominal paracentesis reveals a transudative fluid with 50 white blood cells and few mononuclear cells. Cytology of the fluid is negative for malignant cells and acid-fast bacilli. Which of the following is the most likely diagnosis?

    (A) Alcoholic cirrhosis

    (B) Hepatitis B cirrhosis

    (C) Hepatitis C cirrhosis

    (D) Meigs syndrome

    (E) Peritoneal tuberculosis

46. A 56-year-old man presents to the emergency department with fever and abdominal pain. His past medical history is significant for hypertension, constipation, and diverticulosis. Two days ago, he began to experience profound left lower quadrant pain and, over the next 48 hours, he had high fevers and nausea. His temperature is 38.3° C (101° F), and his abdomen is diffusely tender with marked tenderness in the left lower quadrant. Laboratory analysis shows a leukocyte count of 18,300/μm^3, with 91% polymorphonuclear cells and 6% band forms. Which of the following procedures would be most likely to confirm the likely diagnosis?

    (A) Abdominal CT scan

    (B) Abdominal ultrasound

    (C) Flat and upright abdominal radiographs

    (D) Barium enema

    (E) Exploratory laparotomy

47. A 58-year-old woman comes to the physician because of persistent joint aches affecting hands and hips in an asymmetric distribution. The pain has slow onset and is aggravated by activity. She reports a brief (less than 30 minutes) phase of morning stiffness relieved by heat and movement. She denies fever or weight loss. On the contrary, she has gained approximately 5% of her baseline weight in the past 6 months. Her temperature is 37° C (98.6° F), blood pressure is 130/80 mm Hg, pulse is 74/min, and respirations are 12/min. Examination reveals nodular thickening of the distal interphalangeal joints without redness. Mild limitation in joint motion is appreciated bilaterally in the hand joints and in the right hip joint. The patient's walking is characterized by a slightly shortened length of stride on the right side. Cardiac and respiratory examination reveals no abnormalities. At this time, which of the following is the most appropriate next step in diagnosis?

    (A) No further evaluation necessary
    (B) Complete blood count and erythrocyte sedimentation rate
    (C) Blood test for rheumatoid factor
    (D) Blood test for antinuclear antibodies
    (E) X-ray studies
    (F) Bone densitometry
    (G) Diagnostic arthrocentesis

48. A 55-year-old man has been known for many years to have liver cirrhosis secondary to hepatitis C. His clinical condition had been stable until approximately three months ago, when he seemed to decompensate. He has developed worsening jaundice, increased ascites, and mild encephalopathy. For the past three weeks he has also complained of vague, constant, right upper quadrant abdominal pain. Physical examination shows a nodular liver, but it is no different than it had been in the past. CT scan demonstrates the presence of a solid tumor mass near the dome of the right lobe, where it could not be felt by palpation. The mass is approximately 8 cm in diameter, and it was not seen on a CT scan that had been done a year earlier. Because of the location of the mass, the radiologist is reluctant to attempt a needle biopsy. Which of the following is an additional useful diagnostic test in this patient?

    (A) Alpha-fetoprotein (AFP)
    (B) Carcinoembryogenic agent (CEA)
    (C) 5-hydroxyindoleacetic acid (5-HIAA)
    (D) Hepatitis C titers
    (E) Portal vein angiogram

The response options for items 49-50 are the same. You will be required to select one answer for each item in the set.

(A) Coyote bite

(B) Exposure to cows or sheep

(C) Exposure to ticks

(D) History of contact with rabbits or other rodents

(E) History of recent travel to tropical countries

(F) Ingestion of home-canned food

(G) Ingestion of inadequately cooked pork

(H) Ingestion of inadequately cooked salmon

(I) Ingestion of unpasteurized milk products

(J) Prior transfusion of blood or blood products

(K) Raccoon bite

(L) Recent admission to a hospital

(M) Recent exposure to a child with chickenpox

(N) Unprotected sexual intercourse

(O) Use of IV drugs

(P) Working in a hemodialysis center

(Q) Working in an aviary

For each patient with an infectious illness, select the most likely mode of transmission.

49. A 28-year-old G2P1 woman comes to the physician at 30 weeks gestation with abdominal pain, cramps, and passage of clear vaginal fluid. The patient undergoes premature labor and delivers a stillborn child. Her only recent history is a flu-like illness with fever, myalgias, and mild diarrhea.

50. A 45-year-old man comes to the physician four days after developing a pruritic papule on his right forearm. This lesion transformed into a vesicle and then a black eschar within 36 hours of onset. On examination, the eschar is surrounded by extensive edema and erythema and four to five peripheral vesicles. He has been afebrile all this time, but now his temperature is 39.0° C (102.2° F). Smears of the skin lesion reveal gram-positive encapsulated rods.

Internal Medicine Test One:
Answers and Explanations

ANSWER KEY

1. C	26. B
2. B	27. E
3. B	28. E
4. D	29. F
5. A	30. A
6. A	31. C
7. F	32. C
8. D	33. B
9. C	34. D
10. C	35. E
11. A	36. C
12. A	37. F
13. D	38. D
14. A	39. A
15. C	40. D
16. D	41. E
17. E	42. D
18. A	43. B
19. C	44. B
20. E	45. D
21. A	46. A
22. B	47. A
23. E	48. A
24. F	49. I
25. D	50. B

1. **The correct answer is C.** The most characteristic manifestation of a mitral valve prolapse is a midsystolic click. This frequently asymptomatic condition may be associated with chest pain, dyspnea, palpitations, and other nonspecific symptoms. Patients with a midsystolic click as the only sign are usually asymptomatic; however, those with a systolic murmur may have hemodynamically significant mitral valve regurgitation. In addition, mitral valve prolapse is associated with an increased incidence of infective endocarditis, arrhythmias, sudden death, and cerebral embolism.

Bicuspid aortic valve (**choice A**) is the most frequent type of congenital defect of the aortic valve. It may manifest with valvular stenosis, giving rise to a systolic murmur sometimes associated with an opening click.

Congenital pulmonary stenosis (**choice B**) is a rare condition that gives auscultatory signs similar to aortic stenosis (i.e., a harsh systolic murmur sometimes associated with an opening click).

A ruptured papillary muscle (**choice D**) may develop as a complication of infective endocarditis or myocardial infarction. It may lead to mitral or tricuspid regurgitation and thus manifest with a systolic murmur not associated with clicks.

Tricuspid regurgitation (**choice E**) manifests with a harsh systolic murmur that increases in intensity during inspiration. The most common cause is right ventricular overload; less common causes are infective endocarditis and right ventricular myocardial infarction.

2. **The correct answer is B.** The clinical manifestations are consistent with acute myelogenous leukemia (AML). This disease of middle-aged people (median age at presentation is 50 years) is due to neoplastic transformation of a bone marrow stem cell that is incapable of differentiating into mature leukocytes. A large number of blasts invade the bone marrow and the peripheral blood. AML is subdivided into seven types with different prognostic and therapeutic implications. These types are determined on the basis of the degree of maturation of blasts, their morphology, and coexisting cytogenetic abnormalities. Leukocytosis may be mild or even absent ("aleukemic leukemia"). However, most of the circulating leukocytes are blasts or immature myeloid forms. Signs and symptoms result from neutropenia, anemia, and thrombocytopenia. Auer rods consist of eosinophilic, needle-like inclusions in myeloid cells and are pathognomonic of AML.

In contrast to AML, acute lymphocytic leukemia (ALL; **choice A**) is a disease of children, with a peak of incidence from three to seven years. ALL represents 80% of all cases of acute leukemia in children. The clinical presentation is similar to that of AML. The lymphocytic nature of blasts is confirmed by demonstrating lymphocytic markers, such as *terminal deoxynucleotide transferase (TdT)*.

Chronic myelogenous leukemia (CML; **choice C**) is also a disorder of middle-aged persons. Neoplastic bone marrow precursors in this condition are still capable of differentiating along myeloid lines, so that most circulating leukemic cells appear as mature white blood cells. CML is a myeloproliferative disorder, so the platelet count and erythrocyte count are usually normal or even increased. Leukocytosis in CML is usually striking, often higher than 500,000/mm^3. The Philadelphia chromosome, the result of a balanced translocation between 9q and 22q, is present in 95% of cases.

A leukemoid reaction (**choice D**) is defined as an abnormal elevation of the white cell count in response to infections. Circulating leukocytes, however, are normal in morphology and never exceed 50,000/mm^3. Leukocyte alkaline phosphatase is useful in differentiating leukemoid reaction from myeloid leukemia. The enzyme is elevated in leukemoid reaction but low in leukemia.

Myelodysplastic syndromes (**choice E**) constitute a complex set of bone marrow disorders, in which at least two cell lines are affected. These conditions are characterized by cytopenias (anemia, thrombocytopenia, and/or neutropenia) associated with hypercellular bone marrow. Cytopenias are due to ineffective hematopoiesis. The progression is usually indolent, but transformation to acute leukemia occurs in some cases.

3. **The correct answer is B.** The clinical picture strongly suggests herniation of an intervertebral disc causing compression of a spinal root (S1, considering radiation of the pain and reflex alterations). Supporting this diagnosis is also the positive straight leg-raising test (Lasegue sign). When the history and physical examination support a diagnosis of disc herniation, conservative management is all that is needed. Current recommendations include treatment with NSAIDs and bed rest of short duration (no longer than two days). Longer periods of bed rest do not provide any additional benefit.

MRI examination of vertebral column (**choice A**) is certainly the diagnostic procedure of choice to visualize soft tissue structures of the vertebral column. MRI is reserved for cases in which more detailed imaging information would change the therapeutic approach.

Plain x-ray examination of the lumbosacral spine (**choice C**) provides nonspecific information. Almost any person older than 40 has some signs of degenerative joint disease of the lumbar column. Plain radiographs should be performed when the clinical symptomatology suggests diseases other than disc herniation, such as tumors or infections.

Radionuclide bone scanning (**choice D**) is useful in detecting foci of osteomyelitis or bone metastases, but not disc disease.

Surgical consultation (**choice E**) should be sought if the patient does not respond to appropriate treatment or if there are severe or evolving neurologic deficits. Percutaneous lumbar discectomy may be performed under local anesthesia as an alternative to laminectomy.

4. **The correct answer is D.** Selective IgA deficiency is a relatively common condition (1 in 700 incidence in Caucasians), in which patients are genetically unable to synthesize IgA for either serum or bodily secretions. The underlying defect is a failure of B cells to differentiate into IgA-producing plasma cells. Most individuals with selective IgA deficiency are asymptomatic; about 5% have recurrent respiratory tract infections. The condition becomes clinically significant when blood transfusion is required, since they may develop anaphylaxis when exposed to blood products containing IgA. This can happen even on the first transfusion, presumably because they have been exposed to IgA in animal products that they have eaten. The condition can be confirmed with serum electrophoresis studies, which show an absence of IgA. Once diagnosed, the individuals (and families) need to be taught to tell their physicians about the IgA deficiency, so that only IgA free transfusions will be used.

Adenosine deaminase deficiency (**choice A**) is a cause of severe combined immunodeficiency.

Ataxia telangiectasia (**choice B**) is characterized by cerebellar ataxia, telangiectasias, and immunodeficiency.

DiGeorge syndrome (**choice C**) is characterized by hypoparathyroidism, thymic aplasia, and deficient T cell function.

Wiskott-Aldrich syndrome (**choice E**) is characterized by thrombocytopenia, lymphopenia, and atopic eczema.

5. **The correct answer is A.** Bleomycin can cause pneumonitis, which progresses to pulmonary fibrosis. Cough and shortness of breath are indications of the development of this complication. The pulmonary toxicity is usually age- and dose-related, although an allergic form of pneumonitis has been reported.

Cisplatin (**choice B**) produces tinnitus, hearing loss, and nephrotoxicity.

Mithramycin (**choice C**) is associated with hemolytic uremic syndrome, thrombocytopenia, hepatotoxicity, and nephrotoxicity.

Calcium-channel blockers, such as verapamil (**choice D**), cause headache, dizziness, and nausea. They may increase the extent of heart block and worsen congestive heart failure.

Vincristine (**choice E**) causes neuropathy rather than pulmonary symptoms.

6. **The correct answer is A.** This is anemia of chronic disease. In contrast to iron deficiency anemia, the TIBC is decreased, but ferritin is increased. The microcytosis can be the same as in iron deficiency. This patient may have an infection or an occult malignancy and needs further workup for the loss of weight.

Aplastic anemia (**choice B**) can be the result of exposure to drugs, such as chloramphenicol, that can lead to the suppression of erythrocyte production. A low reticulocyte count, which is an indication of immature red cells, can be helpful in diagnosis of this illness. Bone marrow biopsy may show hypocellularity of the marrow.

Lead poisoning (**choice C**) occurs following the inhalation of lead dust or fumes or following the ingestion of lead. Presentation in these patients ranges from abdominal discomfort, myalgia, headache, and weight loss to peripheral neuropathy and encephalopathy. Laboratory studies show a normal serum iron, a normal TIBC, microcytosis, and basophilic stippling on peripheral blood smear. A screening erythrocyte protoporphyrin level is >35 µg/dL, indicating the need for blood lead testing.

Pyridoxine is a cofactor for the manufacture of porphyrins, which are needed for the manufacture of hemoglobin. Therefore, pyridoxine deficiency (**choice D**) may cause a microcytic hypochromic anemia, but the laboratory panel above is characteristic of anemia of chronic disease.

Hereditary spherocytosis (**choice E**) is a genetic defect arising from mutations in red cell cytoskeletal proteins. This leads to a cell wall defect, which in turn leads to removal of excess cell wall in the spleen. Surface tension causes these cells to become spheres.

Thiamine deficiency (**choice F**) has been implicated in a rare megaloblastic anemia in children. It is also seen in malnourished alcoholics, and intramuscular repletion is often required.

7. **The correct answer is F.** The gross appearance of the lesion, along with its recent changes over a presumably short period, is highly suggestive of malignant melanoma. The proportion of melanomas that arise from pre-existing benign nevocellular nevi is not known. In the *dysplastic nevus syndrome*, however, a dysplastic nevus-melanoma sequence is well established. Nevertheless, an excisional biopsy should be carried out for any pigmented skin lesion that shows one or more of the following features: asymmetric or fuzzy border, irregular or variegated color, and diameter greater than 0.6 cm. According to the American Cancer Society, the mnemonic ABCD may serve to recall the most important suspicious signs:

Asymmetry, Border irregularity, Color variegation, and Diameter >0.6 cm. Bleeding and ulcerations are malignant signs, albeit far less frequent. Melanoma is the most common cause of death due to skin malignancies. Physicians can play a crucial role in prevention by referring patients who have moles with such suspicious features to dermatologists. The initial approach to a suspicious mole or clinically obvious melanoma consists of total excision (excisional biopsy) with a small margin. If a diagnosis of melanoma is confirmed pathologically, wider margins are excised on a second operation.

Follow-up examination in 6 months (**choice A**) would result in a dangerous delay in diagnosis and treatment.

Topical application of *Podophyllum* resin (**choice B**) and cryotherapy with liquid nitrogen (**choice C**) are treatments used for genital warts, as well as for other common benign lesions, such as seborrheic keratosis. These methods should never be used on pigmented lesions.

Shave biopsy (**choice D**) is applicable to many types of superficial skin lesions, including basal cell carcinomas, but is inappropriate for melanomas. Proper diagnosis and evaluation of depth of invasion in melanomas can be achieved only on full-thickness biopsies.

Incisional biopsy (i.e., partial sampling; **choice E**) is not appropriate unless the lesion is too extensive (such as giant congenital nevi or lentigo maligna). There is no evidence for the belief that incisional biopsy facilitates cancer spread.

8. **The correct answer is D.** This patient is demonstrating the classic picture of pneumococcal pneumonia. *Streptococcus pneumoniae* is the most common cause of community-acquired pneumonia in this age group. The usual presentation is sudden onset of shaking chills, with rigors, high fever, and difficulty breathing. Pleuritic chest pain is often present and signifies bacterial infection. A white blood cell count, not provided in this case, most often is significantly elevated with a left shift (predominantly bands and polymorphonuclear cells). Chest x-ray films usually reveal a lobar distribution of the pneumonia. Pleural effusions are present in up to 30% of the cases. Gram stain of the sputum commonly reveals gram-positive diplococci in chains.

Gram-negative diplococci (**choice A**) would be present in pneumonia due to *Moraxella catarrhalis* (formerly *Branhamella catarrhalis*). This pathogen may produce acute pneumonia and usually occurs in the elderly or in those with a history of chronic bronchitis or obstructive lung disease.

Gram-negative rods (**choice B**) are not a usual cause of pneumonia in this population of patients. Gram-negative rods causing pneumonia include *Klebsiella*, *Enterobacter*, *Serratia*, and *Proteus*, which occur more commonly in patients who are debilitated, alcoholics, or residing in nursing homes or similar institutions. These bacteria are often responsible for nosocomial pneumonias and, infrequently, community-acquired pneumonia.

Gram-positive cocci in clusters (**choice C**) that cause pneumonia are usually *Staphylococcus aureus*. *S. aureus* is an uncommon cause of community-acquired pneumonia. When it does cause disease, it is usually during or just following an epidemic of viral influenza. *S. aureus* may be seen year-round in the hospital, because it is a common cause of nosocomial pneumonia.

Gram-positive rods (**choice E**) would likely be *Corynebacterium diphtheriae* (diphtheria). This patient presents with pneumonia, not diphtheria (an infection that occurs in the pharynx, middle ear, larynx, skin, or bronchi).

9. **The correct answer is C.** Hepatitis E virus (HEV) is rare in the U.S., but outbreaks of acute hepatitis E occur in some countries, namely Mexico, India, Afghanistan, and Burma. The infectious agent is transmitted by the oral-fecal route, usually from infected water. HEV is generally self-limited, but it is important to note that it carries a 10% to 20% mortality rate in pregnant women. Similar to HAV, HEV infection does not cause chronic hepatitis or a carrier state. The onset of IgM antibodies to HEV is concomitant with the appearance of clinical symptomatology, whereas IgG will become detectable after the acute phase.

RIBA (recombinant immunoblot assay) for anti-HCV antibodies (**choice A**) is used to confirm a diagnosis of hepatitis C in patients with positive anti-HCV antibodies by the more conventional enzyme immunoassay test. The latter has a 50% specificity, and false positive results are likely in patients with hypergammaglobulinemia. Occasionally, HCV RIBA is also used when the enzyme immunoassay is negative, but there are strong clinical grounds to suspect that the patient has HCV hepatitis. There is no reason to suspect HCV hepatitis in this case.

Anti-HDV antibodies (**choice B**) are found in association with hepatitis D virus infection. HDV is a "defective" RNA virus that causes hepatitis only in the presence of the surface antigen of HBV (HBsAg). In the U.S., HDV is usually associated with IV drug abuse. HDV may coinfect or superinfect patients with HBV. Superinfection is associated with increased risk for fulminant hepatitis or rapid progression to cirrhosis.

Anti-HGV antibodies (**choice D**) are found in 50% of IV drug abusers and 30% of patients receiving hemodialysis. HGV is a flavivirus transmitted by the parenteral route. The infection is followed by viremia lasting for at least 10 years. The pathogenic role of HGV is still uncertain.

HBsAg (**choice E**) detection implies ongoing HBV replication in the organism. HBsAg appears first in the blood before HBV infection becomes clinically evident. Persistence of HBsAg is associated with infectivity. HBV infection would be unlikely in this case, since the patient developed anti-HBV antibodies after vaccination.

10. **The correct answer is C.** Traveling abroad often entails abrupt changes in diet and climate, as well as exposure to conditions of poor sanitation, all of which results in a high incidence of diarrhea. This is self-limiting and manifests with watery diarrhea and dehydration, but no fever or other signs of systemic infection. The most frequent cause of *traveler's diarrhea* is enterotoxigenic *Escherichia coli*.

The remaining infectious agents listed here are all potential causes of noninflammatory diarrhea, which is not associated with blood and mucus in the stool, fever, systemic signs of infection, or fecal leukocytes.

Bacillus cereus (**choice A**), *Clostridium perfringens* (**choice B**), and *Staphylococcus aureus* (**choice E**), along with enterotoxigenic *E. coli*, are the most common agents associated with food poisoning due to production of toxins. All these pathogens produce a similar clinical picture of watery diarrhea, sometimes with nausea and vomiting, but no fever.

Rotavirus (**choice D**) is one of the most important infectious causes of diarrhea in infants and young children in developing countries. It may also cause diarrhea in adults exposed to infected children.

11. **The correct answer is A.** Peaked T waves are associated with significant hyperkalemia that may lead to arrhythmia. In this patient, the primary mechanism of hyperkalemia is acidosis. As a result of the lowered pH, the extracellular concentration of protons increases, thereby increasing the H^+/K^+ antiports on the cell surface, driving protons into the cells and potassium into the extracellular space. ECG changes indicate an increased risk for cardiac arrhythmia and therefore the hyperkalemia should be immediately corrected. Calcium gluconate should be administered to decrease membrane excitability.

Hypocalcemia causes prolonged QT intervals (**choice B**). The QT interval is the time difference between ventricular depolarization and repolarization. Since the QT interval depends on the heart rate, the corrected QT interval (QTc) is often used. The correction factor incorporates the interval between consecutive P waves.

ST depression (**choice C**) would be seen in an ischemic event. It is important to compare the new ECG with an old one to determine whether the depression is new. If this is the case, the patient with such ECG changes should at least be placed on aspirin and observed for an ischemic event.

T wave inversion (**choice D**) is another indication that the patient may be undergoing an ischemic event. Once again, it is important to compare the new ECG with an old one. Furthermore, if the new ECG shows upright T waves, but the old one shows inverted T waves, this denotes "pseudonormalization" and once again indicates an ischemic event.

U waves (**choice E**) are seen in hypokalemia. If an ECG shows these changes, the risk of an arrhythmia is significant, and the hypokalemia must be corrected immediately. This can usually be achieved by administering oral potassium, but occasionally IV potassium may be required.

12. **The correct answer is A.** The clinical presentation is characteristic of cluster headache. In its classic form, cluster headache manifests as nocturnal attacks that last between 30 minutes and 2 hours. These are often precipitated by alcohol consumption and recur daily for up to eight weeks. Each "cluster" is then followed by a pain-free interval lasting for one year on average. The pathogenesis is probably related to disturbances of the serotoninergic pathways originating from the raphe nuclei. Acute attacks may be shortened by oxygen, sumatriptan, and ergotamine preparations; several prophylactic agents are available to prevent clusters.

Depression headache (**choice B**) is often worse in the morning and is frequently associated with other manifestations of depression.

The headache due to giant cell arteritis (**choice C**) usually manifests in elderly patients and is associated with scalp tenderness over the affected superficial temporal artery. Systemic signs and symptoms can be present, including myalgia, weight loss, and malaise. The erythrocyte sedimentation rate is elevated.

Classic cases of migraine (**choice D**) begin in early adulthood and manifest as episodic unilateral throbbing headache, often associated with nausea, photophobia, and visual symptoms.

Tension headache (**choice E**) has a diffuse, band-like character and feels worse in the back of the head. Pain slowly increases and may last for many hours or even days.

Trigeminal neuralgia (**choice F**) is a disorder of the sensory nucleus of CN V that produces episodic, severe, and lancinating pain in the distribution of one or more divisions of the trigeminal nerve. Pain is often precipitated by well defined trigger zones (e.g., washing or shaving) and is not associated with Horner syndrome or rhinorrhea.

13. **The correct answer is D.** This patient has pulmonary sarcoidosis. The peak age group for sarcoidosis is 20-40 years, and the disease seems to be more common in blacks. Noncaseating granulomas can occur in the lungs, heart, kidneys, skin, liver, or other organs. Most characteristically, the patients are asymptomatic and the disease is detected by an abnormal chest x-ray film, which usually shows bilateral symmetric hilar adenopathy often associated with paratracheal adenopathy and/or parenchymal infiltrates. Patients may have uveitis, peripheral arthritis, skin involvement with granulomas, or erythema nodosum. The lungs are the most frequently involved organ; pulmonary symptoms, when present, include dyspnea on exertion, nonproductive cough, and wheezing. Radiologic abnormalities are graded 0-3. Grade 0 is associated with a normal x-ray. Grade 1 is associated with lymph node enlargement without pulmonary parenchymal abnormalities. Grade 2A is a combination of lymph node and diffuse pulmonary parenchymal disease. Grade 2B is a diffuse parenchymal disease without lymph node enlargement. Grade 3 is associated with radiographic changes indicating more chronic disease with pulmonary fibrosis ("honey-combing"). Many patients show spontaneous total remission of disease for a period up to three years. Prednisone is usually the drug of choice for treatment, with a starting dose of 30-40 mg/day.

Neither allopurinol (**choice A**) nor cyclosporine (**choice C**), an immune modulator, has been proven to be of benefit in sarcoidosis.

Levels of ACE may be elevated in patients with active sarcoidosis but are also elevated in many other diseases. ACE is produced by the epitheliod cells of granulomas and, thus, may be elevated in the serum of sarcoid patients. There is no evidence that ACE inhibitors (**choice B**) have any therapeutic value in treatment of sarcoidosis.

At one point in history, some theorized that sarcoidosis was caused by a type of mycobacterium, related to tuberculosis. However, this has not been definitively proven. Furthermore, isoniazid (**choice E**) has not been shown to be beneficial.

14. **The correct answer is A.** The clinical presentation is consistent with Berger disease or IgA *nephropathy*, the most frequent form of glomerulonephritis in the U.S. (and probably worldwide). Often, microhematuria or mild proteinuria occurs as an incidental finding or as recurring episodes following upper respiratory or intestinal infections. IgA deposition in the mesangium is the most characteristic morphologic abnormality, and serum IgA is increased in 50% of patients (hence the designation). Up to 50% of patients will eventually progress to chronic renal failure.

Goodpasture syndrome (**choice B**) typically involves both the lungs and kidneys. Hemoptysis and nephritic syndrome are the clinical manifestations. Linear deposition of anticollagen antibodies along the glomerular and pulmonary basement membranes is the pathognomonic finding on biopsy. This is a severe condition that requires aggressive immunosuppressive treatment.

The renal changes of Henoch-Schönlein purpura (**choice C**) are very similar to those of Berger disease. These conditions, in fact, are thought to represent different manifestations of a common spectrum of diseases, in which autoimmune damage is mediated by IgA. In Henoch-Schönlein purpura, nephritic syndrome is associated with palpable purpura of the lower extremity, arthralgias, and abdominal pain. The disorder usually affects children.

Minimal change disease (**choice D**) is characterized by edema, albuminuria, and changes in blood lipids and proteins. It is usually seen in children, and it doesn't present with episodic hematuria. Proteinuria is of the nephrotic range.

Postinfectious glomerulonephritis (**choice E**) commonly occurs one to two weeks after an infection by group A *Streptococcus* (pharyngitis or impetigo) and manifests with nephritic syndrome. Hematuria developing in the setting of Berger disease, instead, is concomitant with an upper respiratory infection (so-called sympharyngitic hematuria).

Wegener granulomatosis (**choice F**) is a necrotizing granulomatous vasculitis involving the upper respiratory system and the kidneys. Systemic symptoms are present, with fever, weight loss, and malaise. Aggressive immunosuppression is the mainstay of therapy.

15. **The correct answer is C.** Hashimoto disease is a chronic, destructive lymphocytic infiltration of the thyroid glands. It is probably the most common cause of primary hypothyroidism in the U.S. It has an 8:1 female predominance and increases in incidence with age. Many patients also have other autoimmune diseases. The description of the goiter in the question stem is typical of that produced by Hashimoto disease; the physical signs and symptoms of hypothyroidism are also present in longer-standing cases. Early in the disease, as in this case, T4 and TSH levels may be normal. Antithyroid peroxidase antibodies (against the specific antigen formerly detected with antimicrosomal antibodies) are observed in almost all patients with Hashimoto disease, but can also sometimes be detected in patients with Graves disease and silent lymphocytic thyroiditis.

Euthyroid sick syndrome (**choice A**) occurs in patients with severe systemic illness who are clinically euthyroid but have abnormal thyroid function tests.

Graves disease (**choice B**) causes a diffuse toxic goiter and would exhibit both the signs and laboratory findings of hyperthyroidism.

Silent lymphocytic thyroiditis (**choice D**) usually occurs in postpartum women and may be a mild, usually spontaneously reversible, variant of Hashimoto disease.

Subacute thyroiditis (**choice E**) is a virally caused acute inflammatory disease that causes thyroid tenderness and pain.

16. **The correct answer is D.** The skin condition described is *alopecia areata*, a form of baldness that may affect any region of the body. Its pathogenesis is probably immune-related, considering the frequent association with autoimmune disorders, such as Hashimoto thyroiditis, pernicious anemia, and Addison disease. The finding of perifollicular lymphocytic infiltration in affected areas seems to support an autoimmune origin. The patches of hair loss in alopecia areata are rather haphazardly distributed but sharply demarcated. An important feature is the presence of "exclamation hairs" (tiny hair shafts) in the zone of active shedding. In 80% of cases, the hair regrows spontaneously, but permanent loss is observed in the other 20%. Local injection of triamcinolone or application of anthralin ointment has been beneficial in hastening recovery.

Psychiatric consultation (**choice A**) may be appropriate for *trichotillomania*, a compulsive habit of pulling one's own hair out. In this disorder, the patches of hair loss are often unilateral (on the right side if the patient is right-handed, and vice versa), have irregular borders, and show hairs of varying lengths.

Topical application of minoxidil (**choice B**) is widely used for treatment of the most common form of alopecia, namely *androgenetic baldness*, which is related to androgenic hormonal influences. The pattern of androgenetic baldness is characteristic and well known. Minoxidil treatment results in temporary hair regrowth, especially in patients younger than 50 and those with less extensive areas of hair loss.

Oral administration of iron sulfate (**choice C**) may be beneficial in another form of alopecia, named *telogen effluvium*. In this condition, an increased number of hairs are lost daily on combing or shampooing. It is due to an increase in the percentage of hairs in telogen (resting) phase and occurs in association with severe malnutrition, termination of pregnancy, stress from surgery or infection, and oral contraceptives. However, some studies have indicated that iron deficiency may play an important causative role in telogen effluvium.

Systemic corticosteroids (**choice E**) have not been shown to have any advantage over local injection in cases of alopecia areata.

17. **The correct answer is E.** The probable diagnosis is diverticulitis. The relatively mild symptoms, normal vital signs, and normal laboratory values in this patient indicate that he is not very ill. This means that he can be treated at home with rest, a liquid diet, and oral antibiotics, such as cephalexin. In this setting, the response to the therapeutic trial itself serves as a confirmatory test. In most cases, the symptoms will resolve rapidly on this regimen, and the diet can be gradually advanced to a soft, low-roughage diet supplemented with daily psyllium seed extract. At approximately one month, a high-roughage diet is resumed. Seriously ill patients with diverticulitis are usually treated in the hospital and may require IV antibiotics. Surgery will be needed in only about 20% of these patients.

Barium enema studies (**choice A**), typically with air contrast, can be performed if necessary at two weeks to confirm the presence of diverticula.

Colonoscopy (**choice B**) can be used alternatively to barium enema after two weeks to identify diverticula and rule out other conditions, such as proctitis or colon cancer, which would not be as likely in this patient with mild symptoms. Colonoscopy should not be performed during acute infection as there is an increased risk for perforation when the colon is inflamed.

CT of the abdomen (**choice C**) is used in severe cases when the differential diagnosis includes pelvic abscess and appendicitis.

Plain film of the abdomen (**choice D**) is of limited utility in this setting but may show increased gas in the bowel if the diverticulitis has lowered intestinal motility.

18. **The correct answer is A.** The visual deficit present in this patient is described as bilateral temporal hemianopia and is due to chiasmatic lesions that compromise the crossing fibers originating from the temporal retina. A large pituitary adenoma (*macroadenoma*) that extends beyond the sella turcica into the suprasellar region is the most common cause of temporal hemianopia. Craniopharyngioma and meningioma are other causes.

Occipital lobe meningioma (**choice B**) may push on the visual cortex and produce visual symptoms that are referred to the contralateral half of the visual field (*homonymous hemianopia*).

Optic glioma (**choice C**) is a tumor of glial origin, usually an astrocytoma, that develops within the optic nerve. Visual symptoms develop slowly and are of the ipsilateral eye.

Optic nerve atrophy (**choice D**) involves damage to the nerve from ischemia, inflammation, glaucoma, toxic substances, and trauma. Symptoms include diminished visual acuity, reduced visual fields, abnormal color vision, and poor pupillary response to light. The optic disc appears pale or white on ophthalmoscopy.

Optic neuritis (**choice E**) will result in unilateral visual loss that develops rapidly. Multiple sclerosis is an important cause of optic neuritis.

Retinal detachment (**choice F**) results in blurring of vision that affects only one eye. Myopia and cataract extraction are the two most common predisposing factors.

19. **The correct answer is C.** Gingivostomatitis and pharyngitis are the most frequent clinical manifestations of primary herpes simplex virus 1 (HSV-1) infection, and are most commonly seen in children and young adults. Clinical signs and symptoms include fever, malaise, myalgias, and cervical adenopathy. Common lesions may involve the hard and soft palate, gingiva, tongue, lips, and facial area. The lesions are classically vesicular with an erythematous base.

Actinomyces israelii (**choice A**) causes an indolent suppurative infection. These anaerobic actinomycetes are commensals of the gastrointestinal tract and mouth. The organism may invade via a break in the oral mucosa or via aspiration into the lung. Poor dental hygiene and dental abscesses predispose to cervicofacial lesions. Infection presents as a chronic suppurative lesion with adjacent tissue showing inflammation with fibrosis and draining sinuses. Myalgias and low-grade fevers are rare with facial actinomycetes.

Coxsackie virus (**choice B**) infection may result in herpangina, an exanthematous disease characterized by acute onset of fever and sore throat. Small vesicular lesions and white papules (lymph nodules) surrounded by a red halo are typically seen over the posterior half of the palate, pharynx, and tonsillar areas. Lip and facial lesions are rare.

Nocardia asteroides (**choice D**) are aerobic actinomycetes that cause disease most often in the lung, but also at any site of tissue trauma. Lesions produced by *Nocardia* show suppuration, necrosis, and abscess formation with sinus tracts draining purulent material.

Streptococcus pyogenes (**choice E**) causes streptococcal pharyngitis, with the highest incidence in children aged 5-15 years. Patients usually present with the sudden onset of sore throat, particularly with pain on swallowing. Associated symptoms include fever, malaise, headache, and anorexia. On examination, there is diffuse edema and erythema of the posterior pharynx. The tonsils, if present, are enlarged and erythematous with an exudate. The cervical nodes are tender and enlarged. Oral lesions are limited to the posterior pharynx.

20. **The correct answer is E.** *Helicobacter pylori* is a small, gram-negative bacterium that lives in and locally destroys the mucus coating that lines the stomach. The organism has been linked to a wide variety of problems, including gastritis, peptic ulcer disease, gastric cancer, and gastric lymphoma. Because of these associations, physicians have become more aggressive about therapy. *H. pylori* is a hardy organism and requires concurrent therapy with multiple agents for eradication. The original regimen combined bismuth subsalicylate (Pepto-Bismol), tetracycline, and metronidazole, and had only an 80% cure rate in compliant patients who followed the regimen for two weeks. The schedule listed in the question stem is a more modern one; it is both easier to follow and has a better cure rate. Alternative regimens may substitute amoxicillin (1 g bid) for metronidazole, or may substitute lansoprazole (30 mg bid) for omeprazole. These more effective regimens have caused a problem in determining whether eradication has occurred, however, because the course is so short that IgG and IgA antibodies against *H. pylori* have not had time to decrease by the end of therapy. The urea breath test is a relatively new test in which the patient is given oral urea that has been labeled with 13C or 14C. The *H. pylori* bacteria contain the enzyme urease and are able to metabolize the urea, producing radioactively labeled CO_2, which can be measured in breath samples taken 20-30 minutes after ingestion. It is recommended that this test be delayed until four weeks after the end of the regimen, since recent antibiotic use may have decreased the number of organisms enough to produce a negative test, without having achieved true eradication.

Culture of gastric biopsy (**choice A**) is highly specific but requires both endoscopic biopsy and fastidious culture technique. Therefore, this method is not often used clinically for follow-up studies.

The rapid urease test (**choice B**) is performed on gastric tissue. It is rapid, specific, and sensitive, but requires endoscopy to obtain the biopsy fragment.

Qualitative assays of antibodies against *H. pylori* (**choice C**) may be positive for up to three years after eradication of the infection.

Quantitative assays of antibodies against *H. pylori* (**choice D**) drop slowly for up to a three years after eradication of the infection.

21. **The correct answer is A.** Flaccid paresis involving the lower extremities, footdrop, hand clumsiness, muscle wasting, and especially fasciculation in a middle-aged person are highly suggestive of amyotrophic lateral scle-

rosis (ALS). This results from degeneration of the motor neurons in the spinal cord (lower motor neuron) and leads to denervation of skeletal muscle. His tongue fasciculations result from degeneration of motor neurons of cranial nerve nuclei (XII). Continued bulbar involvement will likely eventually affect pharyngeal and facial musculature, leading to progressive dysarthia and dysphasia. Surviving neurons may reinnervate denervated myofibers by sprouting of their axons. The finding of denervation/reinnervation in a muscle biopsy is confirmatory of the clinical diagnosis. The patient will later develop evidence of corticospinal and cortico-bulbar (upper motor neuron) degeneration as his disease progresses.

Charcot-Marie-Tooth disease (**choice B**) is an autosomal recessive demyelinating disease of peripheral nerves that manifests in children or young adults with marked atrophy of the calf muscles and distal muscle weakness. For this reason, the disorder is also known as *peroneal muscular atrophy*.

Guillain-Barré syndrome (**choice C**) manifests with ascending paralysis (first the lower, then the upper extremities are involved) and results from a chronic inflammatory response leading to demyelination of peripheral nerves. It is often preceded by an upper respiratory tract infection.

Myasthenia gravis (**choice D**) is characterized by fluctuating muscle weakness that usually begins in the ocular muscles, resulting in diplopia and ptosis. Since the disorder is due to impaired cholinergic transmission at the neuromuscular junction, skeletal muscle biopsy is within normal limits at the light microscopic level.

Spinal muscular atrophy (SMA; **choice E**) is the infantile counterpart of ALS. SMA is a group of hereditary disorders, the most frequent form of which is Werdnig-Hoffmann disease (SMA type 1), which leads to death by the third year of life.

22. **The correct answer is B.** The specific signs that suggest the correct diagnosis include the wide discrepancy between the blood pressure in the upper extremities and lower extremities, the systolic murmur heard on the back, and the notching of the ribs appreciated on x-ray. Coarctation of the aorta, in its most frequent (adult) type, consists of a stenotic aortic segment just distal to the origin of the left subclavian artery. Hypertension develops in the branches proximal to the stenosis, and hypotension in the aorta distal to it. In the most severe forms, the patients may develop left ventricular failure in infancy, but the most common presenting picture is that of a young adult with hypertension, which may lead to left ventricular hypertrophy or cerebral hemorrhage.

Atrial septal defect (ASD; **choice A**) is generally asymptomatic. A large ASD usually leads to right ventricular

failure in middle age. A systolic murmur is heard at the pulmonary area, and S2 is widely split.

Congenital aortic stenosis (**choice C**) gives rise to a harsh systolic murmur heard along the left sternal border and radiating to the neck. It is due to congenitally abnormal, usually bicuspid, aortic valves.

Congenital pulmonary stenosis (**choice D**) is a rare form of congenital valvular disease. Mild-to-moderate stenosis is usually asymptomatic, but severe cases result in right-sided heart failure or sudden death. A systolic murmur is heard at the second left intercostal space, often preceded by an ejection click.

Individuals with a small or medium-size patent ductus arteriosus (**choice E**) are usually asymptomatic until middle age. This anomaly is associated with a characteristic continuous "machinery-like" murmur, which is maximal at the pulmonary area and often accompanied by a thrill.

Tetralogy of Fallot (**choice F**) is the most common form of *cyanotic* congenital heart disease. The four features include subpulmonary stenosis, ventricular septal defect, overriding aorta, and right ventricular hypertrophy. The degree of subpulmonary stenosis is the single most important determinant of the clinical severity and symptomatology. Most infants present with early cyanosis.

Ventricular septal defect (VSD; **choice G**) is the most frequent congenital cardiac anomaly. Most cases are asymptomatic. Large VSDs lead to right ventricular overload and are associated with a harsh pansystolic murmur along the left sternal border associated with a thrill.

23. **The correct answer is E.** Porphyria cutanea tarda is the most common of all of the porphyrias, and is consequently a likely target on the USMLE. It causes chronic blistering and crusting lesions on sun-exposed skin. The defective enzyme in heme synthesis is uroporphyrinogen decarboxylase. Precipitating factors include iron (even in normal amounts in some cases), estrogen use, alcohol use, and chronic hepatitis C infection. Skin biopsy can be helpful but is usually not completely specific (the "caterpillar bodies" in the question stem are clumps of basement membrane material). Porphyrin analyses demonstrate the findings in the question stem.

Acute intermittent porphyria (**choice A**) is one of the more common forms of porphyria and typically presents with severe abdominal pain.

Delta-aminolevulinic acid dehydratase deficiency (**choice B**) is a rare form of porphyria that can cause abdominal pain and hemolysis.

Erythropoietic porphyria (**choice C**) is one of the more common forms of porphyria and typically presents in childhood or infancy with acute, rather than chronic, photosensitivity with pain and swelling after sunlight exposure.

Hereditary coproporphyria (**choice D**) is a rare porphyria than presents with abdominal pain.

24. **The correct answer is F.** The key data to make a correct diagnosis include the following: severe thrombocytopenia, which results in a bleeding diathesis; elevated indirect bilirubin and high LDH with schistocytes in the blood smear, indicating microangiopathic hemolytic anemia; renal dysfunction (high creatinine); and neurologic and systemic symptoms (headache, confusion, and fever). Negative findings important to rule out similar conditions include a negative Coombs test and absence of fibrin split products. Thrombotic thrombocytopenic purpura (TTP) is a disorder of unclear pathogenesis, perhaps related to circulating platelet-agglutinating factors. It presents with a characteristic combination of microangiopathic hemolytic anemia, fever without infection, neurologic symptoms, bleeding diathesis secondary to thrombocytopenia, and renal impairment. This condition may be precipitated by pregnancy or use of estrogens.

Disseminated intravascular coagulation (DIC; **choice A**) can be differentiated from TTP because of abnormal coagulation tests. In DIC, microangiopathic hemolysis is also present, but prothrombin time (PT) is prolonged, fibrinogen levels are reduced, and fibrin split products are elevated.

Evans syndrome (**choice B**) refers to coexistence of autoimmune hemolytic anemia (positive Coombs test), and autoimmune thrombocytopenic purpura (see **choice D**).

Hemolytic-uremic syndrome (HUS; **choice C**) is not significantly different from TTP. The two conditions, in fact, are considered manifestations of the same pathogenetic spectrum. However, the vascular bed of the CNS is not involved in HUS; thus, mental status changes are not part of the clinical picture.

Idiopathic (autoimmune) thrombocytopenic purpura (ITP; **choice D**) is an immune disorder caused by autoantibodies to platelet antigens. Systemic illness is not present in ITP, which is characterized by isolated thrombocytopenia without other hematologic abnormalities. Ten percent of cases will manifest in association with autoimmune hemolytic anemia (*Evans syndrome*).

Malignant hypertension (**choice E**) may cause microangiopathic hemolytic anemia. However, blood pressure values would be extremely elevated.

25. **The correct answer is D.** The porphyrias are due to metabolic defects in heme synthesis. Although they occur in a variety of forms, the most common are acute intermittent porphyria (which this patient has), erythro-

poietic protoporphyria (which presents with painful skin and acute swelling), and porphyria cutanea tarda (which presents with chronic blistering skin lesions). Acute intermittent porphyria characteristically presents with neurovisceral symptoms, which may mimic an acute abdomen. The abdominal pain produced is a nerve problem rather than an inflammation, which is why exploratory surgery in these patients is usually unrewarding. Patients with long-standing cases may have demonstrable damage to motor nerves as well, which typically begins as weakness in the shoulders and arms. The condition is relatively rare (although it is the most common acute porphyria); therefore, it is suspected more often than it is confirmed. The combination of complaints of severe pain, distraught behavior, and absence of physical findings may lead clinician to suspect the patient either is abusing drugs or has psychiatric problems. Failure to make the diagnosis also raises the risk of potentially dangerous complications because of drug interactions with the disease (barbiturates are a notorious offender). The biochemical defect in acute intermittent porphyria is a block in porphobilinogen deaminase. Determination of urinary porphobilinogen levels, which are best measured in a 24-hour urine collected during the period when the patient is symptomatic, is the most important screening test for acute intermittent porphyria. Aminolevulinic acid (ALA), which is an early precursor in heme synthesis, is also elevated in the urine. IV heme can be given for therapy.

Erythrocyte porphyrins (**choice A**) can be used to screen for erythropoietic protoporphyria.

Fecal porphyrins (**choice B**) are a second-line choice for screening for porphyria cutanea tarda.

Plasma porphyrins (**choice C**) can be used to screen for either porphyria cutanea tarda or erythropoietic porphyria.

Urine porphyrins (**choice E**) can be used to screen for porphyria cutanea tarda.

26. **The correct answer is B.** A small ventricular septal defect (VSD) is usually asymptomatic, manifesting with a systolic murmur sometimes associated with a thrill along the left sternal border. Patients with the typical murmur as the only manifestation have a normal life expectancy but are more prone to develop infective endocarditis. Thus, antibiotic prophylaxis is mandatory before dental procedures or other procedures that might produce bacteremia.

Arrhythmias (**choice A**) do not constitute a particular risk for patients with VSD.

A large VSD leads to a significant left-to-right shunt, which increases the right ventricular load and results in pulmonary hypertension (**choice C**) and right ventricular hypertrophy. The long-term effect of these hemodynamic alterations is right-sided heart failure (**choice D**). A shunt associated with a pulmonary-to-systemic flow ratio of less than 1.5 is hemodynamically inconsequential and should not be repaired surgically. Large shunts should be repaired to prevent late-onset pulmonary hypertension and heart failure.

Shunt reversal (**choice E**) develops when the right ventricular pressure exceeds that in the left ventricle and the shunt becomes right-to-left. This is a long-term complication of unrepaired large VSDs.

27. **The correct answer is E.** Recurrent episodes of inflammatory arthritis, absence of urate crystals, and speckling (due to calcification) of the articular cartilage are virtually diagnostic of pseudogout. The knee is the most common joint involved. Identification of calcium pyrophosphate crystals in joint aspirates is diagnostic (weakly birefringent on polarized microscopy). It may be hereditary, may develop 24-28 hours after surgery, or may be associated with metabolic diseases, such as hyperparathyroidism, hemachromatosis, hypomagnesemia, acromegaly, Wilson disease, hypothyroidism, and gout.

Recurrent hemorrhages into joints, especially the knees, are characteristic of poorly treated hemophilia (**choice A**). Minor or unappreciated trauma may precipitate individual events. Healing is associated with inflammation and proliferation of the synovial membrane, and can lead to significant joint destruction. Widening of the intercondylar notch of the femur is characteristic. Other clinical features of hemophilia are invariably present.

Chronic monarticular or oligoarticular involvement, especially of the knee, is a feature of Lyme disease (**choice B**). The primary stage of the disease may be unrecognized. Calcification or erosions of the articular cartilage do not occur.

Rheumatoid arthritis (**choice C**) is uncommonly monarticular but enters the differential diagnosis. Rheumatoid factor in the joint fluid may be positive, even when the serum rheumatoid factor is not. The pattern of presentation is chronic, rather than recurrent acute, monarticular arthritis.

Osteoarthritis (**choice D**) at age 33, in the absence of prior major trauma, would be rare. Crystal arthropathy may coexist with degenerative arthritis, and the latter can progress more rapidly in the presence of crystal-induced damage. Acute exacerbation of stable osteoarthritis should be evaluated for coexistent crystal arthritis, as the management strategy may be altered.

Psoriatic arthritis (**choice F**) classically involves distal interphalangeal joints and also has characteristic changes in the nails (pitting, transverse ridging, onycholysis). In the majority of cases, characteristic skin lesions are present before joint lesions appear. On x-ray, there are gross destructive changes in isolated small joints with associated erosions, ankylosis, and a "pencil-in-cup" appearance.

28. **The correct answer is E.** Primary sclerosing cholangitis is a condition in which fibrosing inflammation of the intrahepatic and extrahepatic bile duct systems eventually lead to the obliteration of the bile ducts and development of cirrhosis. The underlying etiology of the damage is unclear, although toxic, infectious, and/or autoimmune mechanisms have been postulated. The clinical presentation illustrated in the question stem is typical. The association with inflammatory bowel disease, particularly ulcerative colitis, may provide a helpful clue. In some patients, AST and ALT may be mildly increased. The liver biopsy may be similar in primary sclerosing cholangitis and the related condition, primary biliary cirrhosis. The antimitochondrial antibody test can be helpful, because it is negative in primary sclerosing cholangitis and positive in roughly 95% of cases of primary biliary sclerosis. The most definitive study is endoscopic retrograde cholangiography, which establishes that the bile duct lesions extend outside the liver.

Although a bile duct tumor (**choice A**) can cause a localized dilatation of the bile duct system proximal to the lesion, it would not produce the characteristic pattern of alternating saccular dilations and strictures seen in this patient with endoscopic retrograde cholangiography.

Choledocholithiasis (**choice B**) is a stone in the extrahepatic bile duct system and would be seen on endoscopic retrograde cholangiography as a blockage to the flow of contrast dye.

Congenital polycystic liver (**choice C**) is a rare condition that can produce massive hepatomegaly but usually causes surprisingly few medical problems.

Primary biliary cirrhosis (**choice D**) can have a very similar biopsy appearance to primary sclerosing cholangitis. However, it does not have extrahepatic bile duct disease and usually is positive for antimitochondrial antibodies.

29. **The correct answer is F.** The acute symptomatology is consistent with necrotizing fasciitis, a severe infection of the subcutaneous tissue and fascia caused by group A streptococci. The bacteria gain entry into the subcutaneous tissue through a skin lesion and produce rapidly spreading cellulitis, combined with systemic signs and symptoms of toxemia. Anesthesia/hypoesthesia is a particularly important clue to the diagnosis. As soon as necrotizing fasciitis is suspected, surgical exploration and debridement is mandatory.

Limiting care to supportive measures until culture results are available (**choice A**) may lead to rapid necrosis of the affected limb and death due to septic shock.

Treatment with clindamycin (**choice B**) or penicillin V (**choice C**) is appropriate for patients with streptococcal skin infections that are not sufficiently severe to warrant parenteral treatment.

Parenteral treatment with vancomycin (**choice E**) or penicillin G (**choice D**) is used for skin infections (especially erysipelas) due to streptococci. Penicillin remains the drug of choice for the treatment of streptococcal infections, but vancomycin may be used in severely penicillin-allergic patients. Erysipelas is not associated with such severe systemic signs of infection and usually involves the face.

30. **The correct answer is A.** Budd-Chiari syndrome is a disorder in which hepatic venous outflow is obstructed because of thrombosis of the major hepatic veins. The blood clots may extend into the inferior vena cava, causing the abdominal wall signs and edema of the legs illustrated in the question stem. The condition is rare and typically occurs in the setting of a coagulopathy due to hematologic disease (myeloproliferative disorders, polycythemia vera, sickle cell disease, paroxysmal nocturnal hemoglobinuria) or in disorders of the coagulation (defects in normal inhibitors, such as antithrombin III, protein C, protein S, factor V Leiden; antiphospholipid antibodies; and possibly high estrogen states, such as oral contraceptive use or pregnancy). The disorder either presents with acute hepatic failure or, more commonly, progresses over several months. Early recognition of the syndrome is important so that thrombolytics and long-term anticoagulation can be given. Some patients respond to medical management, whereas others with fulminant or end-stage disease may require liver transplantation.

Hepatic cirrhosis (**choice B**) develops slowly and produces a nodular liver.

Hepatocellular carcinoma (**choice C**) would produce a liver mass. Ascites is a late finding and usually develops slowly.

Primary sclerosing cholangitis (**choice D**) is an inflammation of the bile ducts that does not usually produce ascites unless it has progressed to cirrhosis.

Steatosis (**choice E**), or fatty liver, does not produce ascites.

31. **The correct answer is C.** Chronic myelogenous leukemia (CML) is a myeloproliferative disorder developing from neoplastic transformation of a bone marrow stem cell that still retains the capacity to differentiate along erythrocytic, megakaryocytic, granulocytic, or monocytic lines. Thus, the peripheral blood in CML is characterized by striking leukocytosis, with myeloid cells present at different degrees of differentiation and in direct proportion to their degree of maturation. Therefore, immature cells—blasts and promyelocytes—are less numerous than mature granulocytes or monocytes. Blasts are usually less than 5%. CML is characterized by the presence of the Philadelphia chromosome, arising from a balanced translocation involving chromosomes 9q and 22q. This results in the formation of a bcr/abl fusion gene encoding a protein with tyrosine kinase activity. The presence of the Philadelphia chromosome is definitive evidence for CML.

Acute myelogenous leukemia (AML; **choice A**) results from neoplastic transformation of a stem cell that has lost the capacity to differentiate fully into mature blood cells. Thus, large numbers of blasts are present in peripheral blood and bone marrow. The Philadelphia chromosome is absent in most cases. There are seven subtypes of AML, defined by the morphology of the leukemic cells and their cytogenetic abnormalities. The most frequent form (with full myeloid maturation), is associated with t(8;21).

Chronic lymphocytic leukemia (CLL; **choice B**) and its lymphomatous counterpart—small lymphocytic lymphoma—derive from neoplastic proliferation of small, well-differentiated lymphocytes. CLL is associated with marked lymphocytosis (up to 200,000/mm^3) in peripheral blood. Patients present with fatigue and lymphadenopathy, but often lymphocytosis is discovered incidentally.

A leukemoid reaction (**choice D**) is an exuberant form of leukocytosis (with leukocyte counts up to 50,000/mm^3) that may follow infections. Sometimes it is difficult to distinguish between true leukemia and a leukemoid reaction, but presence of the Philadelphia chromosome rules out the latter. Leukocyte alkaline phosphatase is elevated in leukemoid reaction, low in CML.

Myelofibrosis (**choice E**) is a chronic myeloproliferative disorder characterized by marrow fibrosis and widespread extramedullary hematopoiesis, resulting in massive splenomegaly. The Philadelphia chromosome is absent. Teardrop erythrocytes are characteristically present in peripheral blood smears.

32. **The correct answer is C.** The patient has a history of alcohol abuse and signs of chronic liver disease, and now presents with an upper gastrointestinal bleed (UGIB). The sudden onset of hematemesis in the absence of abdominal pain in a patient with chronic liver disease is consistent with hemorrhage from esophageal varices. However, one-half to two-thirds of patients with cirrhosis who present with a UGIB have a nonvariceal source, and many have more than one source. Therefore, prompt identification of the origin of bleeding is crucial to guiding therapy.

Esophagogastroscopy is the appropriate first step in identifying, and in many cases treating, the source of bleeding.

Barium swallow (**choice A**) has no role in the diagnosis of a UGIB.

Esophageal balloon tamponade (**choice B**) is used in patients with a confirmed diagnosis of variceal hemorrhage who continue to bleed despite endoscopic treatment.

Emergent celiotomy (**choice D**) is reserved for patients who continue to bleed despite endoscopic therapy.

Angiography (**choice E**) is used only when esophagogastroscopy has failed to reveal a bleeding source.

A transjugular intrahepatic portosystemic shunt (TIPS; **choice F**) is a percutaneous connection within the liver, between the portal and systemic circulations. TIPS placement diverts portal blood flow into the hepatic vein and thus decreases the pressure gradient in patients with portal venous hypertension. TIPS is indicated in acute variceal bleeding that cannot be successfully controlled with medical treatment. Therefore, it would not be used in this patient until other measures have been attempted.

33. **The correct answer is B.** This patient has mesenteric arterial occlusion with ischemia as a complication of an angiographic procedure. This is a typical case of iatrogenic occlusion. This patient is very susceptible to this complication because of his history of peripheral vascular disease, coronary artery disease, and severe atherosclerotic disease. Iatrogenic mesenteric ischemia occurs most commonly after angiographic procedures or operations on the aorta. Angiography may cause intestinal ischemia by dislodging of atheromata from a diseased vessel wall, by dissection of the vessel, or by formation of the intimal flap. Mesenteric ischemia is accompanied by sudden severe epigastric and mid-abdominal pain. Forceful vomiting and evacuation of stool commonly follow the onset of pain. Early after embolization, physical examination of the abdomen may be entirely unremarkable. Later, a classic presentation is severe abdominal pain out of proportion to physical findings. Abdominal distention, guarding, and absence of bowel sounds are associated with intestinal infarction and imply disease progression. Stool may be positive for occult blood. No laboratory tests are pathognomonic for mesenteric embolism or visceral ischemia.

Pain from a gastric ulcer (**choice A**) would not occur suddenly. In addition, if this patient had a perforated gastric ulcer, he would have some local signs of peritonitis, and the abdominal examination would correlate more closely with the degree of abdominal pain, unlike the situation with mesenteric ischemia.

Pancreatitis (**choice C**) does not occur as a result of cardiac catheterization. It can occur after endoscopic retrograde cholangiopancreatography (ERCP) with dye injection into the pancreatic duct. In addition, pancreatitis does not lead to occult blood in the stool.

Abdominal examination of a patient with a perforated duodenal ulcer (**choice D**) would reveal some local signs of peritonitis, and the patient's symptoms would not be so "out of proportion" to the abdominal examination.

Staphylococcal food poisoning/gastroenteritis (**choice E**) usually occurs three to six hours after ingestion of contaminated food. However, this patient had a cardiac catheterization; he did not eat a tuna sandwich with contaminated mayonnaise. Furthermore, vomiting is usually the prominent symptom with staphylococcal food poisoning.

34. **The correct answer is D.** The clinical picture is consistent with Crohn disease (CD). Nonbloody diarrhea, abdominal pain and cramps, malaise, and low-grade fever are the most common, but rather nonspecific, presenting symptoms. CD affects the terminal ileum most frequently (hence the old designation of terminal ileitis), so that tenderness and a mass can often be detected on palpation in the lower left quadrant of the abdomen. The most characteristic signs of CD include sharp demarcation of affected segments from adjacent noninvolved loops and presence of nonnecrotizing granulomas in biopsies. Strictures resulting in bowel obstruction may necessitate surgical resection, as in this case.

Carcinoma (**choice A**) is highly unlikely, considering the clinical picture, location of lesion (small bowel cancer is rare), and young age of the patient.

Celiac disease (**choice B**) is a chronic diarrheal disease that is characterized by intestinal malabsorption and precipitated by indigestion of gluten-containing foods. The disease also presents with nonbloody diarrhea, cramps, and abdominal distension due to fluid- and gas-filled intestinal loops. Distinguishing features on small bowel series are flocculation of barium, small bowel dilatation, and flattening of normal mucosal fold pattern. Occasionally, ulceration and strictures may occur.

Chronic appendicitis (**choice C**) is a rather controversial entity. Repeated bouts of acute appendicitis, especially when incompletely controlled with antibiotic therapy, may rarely result in periappendiceal and pericolic adhesions.

Pseudomembranous colitis (**choice E**) is due to the toxins produced by *Clostridium difficile*. This condition develops as a complication of broad-spectrum antibiotic treatment, particularly in hospitalized patients. It affects the colon (not the ileum) and manifests with greenish, foul-smelling diarrhea. Endoscopic and pathologic examination reveal the characteristic yellow-green plaques adherent to the mucosa.

Ulcerative colitis (UC) (**choice F**) shares many clinical and pathologic features of CD, so that an "umbrella" designation of *inflammatory bowel disease* is used to refer to both conditions when a specific diagnosis is not yet made. Features not consistent with UC (thus favoring CD) include involvement of ileum (which is exceptional in UC), sharp demarcation of the affected bowel segment, and presence of granulomas on histologic examination.

35. **The correct answer is E.** This patient has exertional angina, an abnormal stress test, and occlusive atherosclerotic disease of the left main coronary artery. He is at high risk for adverse cardiac events, including myocardial infarction and death, and should receive treatment. The treatment of choice is coronary artery bypass grafting, which has been shown to decrease symptoms and mortality in patients with left main coronary artery disease.

   The patient needs immediate treatment, so instructing the patient to return in six months (**choice A**) is unwise.

   Beta blockers (**choice B**) decrease anginal symptoms and mortality from coronary artery disease, but are not a replacement for definitive revascularization procedures. Furthermore, their use may be contraindicated in diabetics, as these agents can intensify hypoglycemia while masking hypoglycemic symptoms.

   Sublingual nitroglycerin (**choice C**) is helpful in managing the anginal pain of coronary artery disease but does nothing to alter the course of the disease or decrease mortality.

   Angioplasty (**choice D**) is not an option in the therapy of left main disease, since inflating the balloon completely occludes the lumen of the artery and transiently interrupts all blood flow to the myocardium.

36. **The correct answer is C.** Long-standing rheumatoid arthritis is currently one of the most common causes of systemic *amyloidosis*. This may give rise to a complex clinical picture resulting from amyloid deposition in the skin, kidneys, tongue, gastrointestinal tract, or peripheral nerves, for example. Carpal tunnel syndrome, skin plaques in the axillary region, nephrotic syndrome, hepatosplenomegaly, and macroglossia are among the most common manifestations. Chronic diarrhea with malabsorption and occult bleeding are frequent as well. Biopsies of the skin, rectal mucosa, abdominal fat pad, or gingiva are the most helpful to confirm the clinical diagnosis.

   Electrophoresis of serum proteins (**choice A**) is useful in demonstrating monoclonal gammopathy, which is usually associated with plasma cell neoplasia or dyscrasia. Multiple myeloma is a frequent cause of amyloidosis, but this condition is accompanied by osteolytic bone lesions, bone pains, spontaneous fractures, anemia, and propensity for infections.

X-rays of vertebral column and skull (**choice B**) should be considered when there is clinical evidence suggesting multiple myeloma as the underlying cause of amyloidosis. The clinical history in this case suggests rheumatoid arthritis as the most likely underlying etiology.

Renal biopsy (**choice D**) and endomyocardial biopsy (**choice E**) may also be used to demonstrate amyloid deposition in the myocardium or kidney, but these should be used only when other, less invasive procedures have been ineffective.

37. **The correct answer is F.** The ileal resection indicates that this patient is not absorbing the vitamin B_{12}-intrinsic factor complex, leading to vitamin B_{12} deficiency. This deficiency can result in dorsal column degeneration, causing the observed neurologic symptoms. Vitamin B_{12} deficiency will also cause macrocytic anemia and lead to the development of hypersegmented neutrophils.

   Ferrochelatase deficiency (**choice A**) would lead to erythropoietic protoporphyria, which is inherited as an autosomal dominant trait. Skin photosensitivity begins in childhood. The CNS is spared. It is similar to sideroblastic anemia in its hematologic manifestation.

   Folate deficiency (**choice B**) should not produce the neurologic symptoms observed, although it would certainly cause macrocytic anemia.

   Hydroxymethylbilane synthase (HMB-synthase) deficiency (**choice C**) causes acute intermittent porphyria. It is inherited in an autosomal dominant manner. Abdominal pain is the most common symptom. Acute attacks may be manifested by anxiety, insomnia, depression, hallucinations, and paranoia.

   Intrinsic factor deficiency (**choice D**) is one of the causes of vitamin B_{12} deficiency. However, it occurs in postgastrectomy patients or in patients with pernicious anemia. The history of ileal resection points to malabsorption of the vitamin B_{12}-intrinsic factor complex from the terminal small bowel as the cause of vitamin B_{12} deficiency.

   Iron deficiency anemia (**choice E**) could result from Crohn disease secondary to the chronic bloody diarrhea. However, this would result in a microcytic anemia.

38. **The correct answer is D.** This history is typical for metatarsal stress fracture. This common sports injury usually involves the second, third, or fourth metatarsals, which have thin diaphyses. Diagnosis is usually by history; radiography may not demonstrate the fracture until the second or third week after injury, when a callus forms. Palpating the swollen area of the foot causes pain. Risk factors include a cavus (high arched) foot, osteoporosis, and shoes with inadequate shock-absorption. This type of fracture rarely requires a cast, and healing typically takes 3-12 weeks.

Achilles tendinitis (**choice A**), epiphysitis of the calcaneus (**choice B**), and posterior Achilles tendon bursitis (**choice E**) cause heel pain.

Fracture of the posterolateral talar tubercle (**choice C**) causes pain behind the ankle.

39. **The correct answer is A.** The patient has disseminated intravascular coagulation (DIC), which can be caused by trauma, shock, malignancy, or obstetric complications. It involves massive activation of coagulation, overwhelming of inhibitors, and depletion of factors. This results in platelet consumption, elevation of PT and PTT, and appearance of schistocytes on peripheral blood smears.

    Choice B may be seen in a patient with coagulation factor deficiency and an acute infection. Platelets are an acute phase reactant that may rise in any condition in which the body is stressed.

    Choice C may be seen in a patient on warfarin, which inhibits the function of the extrinsic coagulation pathway.

    Choice D may be noted in a patient with thrombocytopenia who is on an anticoagulant, such as heparin. Factor deficiency in the intrinsic pathway may cause a similar increase in PTT.

    Choice E may be seen in isolated thrombocytopenia, rather than DIC.

40. **The correct answer is D.** This is the classic presentation of ischemic colitis. Patients are typically in the sixth to eighth decade of life, and can be of any race. In this condition, there is an inflammation of the colon resulting from ischemic damage to the colon wall. Classic x-ray findings are mucosal edema with associated hematoma formation. This is often referred to as thumbprinting. Gas in the wall of the colon (pneumatosis coli) is highly suggestive of ischemic colitis. There are many possible causes of ischemic damage, including occlusion of a major artery or vein, small vessel disease, severe hypotension, and intestinal obstruction. Severe ischemic colitis usually requires surgical resection of the involved bowel segment.

    Appendicitis (**choice A**) involves the right lower quadrant of the abdomen.

    Colon cancer (**choice B**) would produce an ulcer or a mass visible on barium enema.

    Newly diagnosed Crohn disease (**choice C**) or ulcerative colitis (**choice E**) would be unusual in a 75-year-old, and would produce larger areas of mucosal ulceration and irregularity on barium enema.

41. **The correct answer is E.** Wegener granulomatosis develops over a period of months, usually presenting with upper or lower respiratory symptoms, such as sinusitis, otitis, and hemoptysis. Renal manifestations are due to the same pathologic process, namely a necrotizing granulomatous vasculitis. IgG and complement deposits are found in renal biopsies, but the most specific laboratory finding is the presence of circulating c-ANCA. This form of glomerulonephritis is classified among the *pauci-immune glomerulonephritides*, which also include Churg-Strauss syndrome (**choice A**) and polyarteritis nodosa (**choice C**). The latter two, however, are usually associated with circulating p-ANCA. Asthma and blood eosinophilia are characteristic of Churg-Strauss syndrome, whereas palpable purpura is associated with polyarteritis nodosa. The cytoplasmic pattern of ANCA (c-ANCA) is due to antibodies directed to the neutrophil *proteinase-3*, and the perinuclear pattern of ANCA (p-ANCA) is due to antibodies against *myeloperoxidase*.

    Goodpasture syndrome (**choice B**) is not associated with circulating ANCA. It manifests with hemoptysis and severe glomerulonephritis, often evolving to acute renal failure. Its pathogenesis is related to antibodies against the globular domain of type IV collagen, depositing in a linear pattern along the glomerular and pulmonary basement membranes. Antiglomerular basement membrane antibodies are also detected in the serum.

    Tuberculosis (**choice D**) may affect the kidneys, but it does not produce a picture of necrotizing vasculitis and it is not associated with ANCA.

42. **The correct answer is D.** Pancreatic cancer typically has a subtle presentation. This case has many of the classic signs of pancreatic cancer, such as dull, persistent abdominal pain. This pain differs from the burning, episodic pain associated with ulcer disease. Weight loss is often a sign of malignancy, and glucose intolerance is suggestive of destruction of the beta islet cells, which produce insulin. Pancreatic cancer often causes a hypercoagulable state, which can lead to deep venous thrombosis, evidenced in this patient by Homans sign (increased resistance or pain on dorsiflexion of the foot). All this together strongly suggests pancreatic cancer.

    Chronic pancreatitis (**choice A**) presents with atypical abdominal pain radiating to the back, which is usually persistent and not relieved by antacids. Weight loss and signs of malabsorption, such as abnormal stool, are common. Alcoholism is the most common cause in adults, whereas cystic fibrosis is the most common cause in children.

    Patients with gastric cancer (**choice B**) usually present with chronic, noncolicky epigastric pain that ranges from postprandial fullness to severe, steady pain. There is associated anorexia, weight loss, and anemia from blood loss. Late signs include an enlarged liver, Virchow node (supraclavicular), and Sister Mary Joseph (periumbilical) nodule. Glucose intolerance is not a feature of gastric cancer.

Hepatic cancer (**choice C**) presents with right upper quadrant pain. A mass can often be palpated in the liver. Increased alpha-fetoprotein and alkaline phosphatase are common laboratory features. Patients usually have a history of chronic liver disease.

Type 2 diabetes mellitus (**choice E**) typically presents with polyphagia, polydipsia, and polyuria. Each of these symptoms is caused by elevated serum glucose. Type 1 diabetes is characterized by an acute onset over several days and may be associated with weight loss or may even present as diabetic ketoacidosis. Type 2 diabetes usually has a more gradual onset, classically occurring in obese patients who are often asymptomatic.

43. **The correct answer is B.** The combination of hypertension and bilaterally enlarged kidneys is highly suggestive of autosomal dominant (adult) polycystic kidney disease, which is often associated with microhematuria as well. A positive family history may be present. Ultrasonography is the diagnostic procedure of choice, since it is extremely sensitive for detecting cystic formations within the kidneys. The disease frequently manifests in young adult or middle-age life. Hypertension is frequently the presenting sign.

Cytologic examination of urine (**choice A**) would show no changes (besides hematuria) in this case. It is usually negative in patients with renal neoplasms as well.

CT scan of the abdomen (**choice C**) is also a sensitive diagnostic tool in the study of renal masses, but should follow ultrasonography in this setting.

Intravenous pyelography (IVP; **choice D**) results in good visualization of the kidneys and urinary tract and is a functional test as well. However, it requires contrast administration and does not discriminate between solid and cystic masses.

Renal biopsy (**choice E**) is not indicated for the study of polycystic renal disease. Fine needle aspiration may be used to analyze the content of an isolated cystic mass if imaging studies have failed to determine whether it is of benign or malignant nature.

44. **The correct answer is B.** The clinical manifestations are characteristic of *intermittent claudication*, characterized by intermittent ischemic pain arising from inadequacy of blood flow secondary to arterial stenosis. The pain manifests when muscle oxygen demands increase (usually during walking) and subsides at rest. The most common cause of this picture is atherosclerosis of the arteries to the lower extremities, affecting the external iliac or the superficial femoral/popliteal segments. In this case, the presence of normal femoral pulses and the weakening of popliteal and pedal pulses on the affected site point to the site of stenosis. The distal segment of the superficial

femoral artery is often the first to be affected by atherosclerotic change, which then progresses to involve the popliteal artery. Several risk factors for atherosclerosis (smoking, hypertension) are present in this patient.

Atherosclerotic stenosis of the common iliac artery (**choice A**) would give rise to similar clinical manifestations, but the femoral pulse would be weakened or absent.

The pain caused by peripheral polyneuropathy (**choice C**) usually affects the distal extremities in a symmetric fashion, manifests at rest and often at night, and is frequently associated with paresthesia/hypoesthesia and decreased reflexes. Diabetes and alcohol abuse are probably the most common causes in Western countries.

Prolapse of an intervertebral disk in the lumbar spine (**choice D**) produces manifestations due to compression of one of the spinal roots, most commonly L5 or S1. The patient experiences lumbar pain, as well as pain and paresthesias in a radicular distribution. Decreased sensation and reduced reflexes may develop in long-standing cases.

Thromboangiitis obliterans (**choice E**) usually occurs in young males who are heavy smokers. The disease results from acute inflammation of the whole neurovascular bundles, including major arteries, veins, and nerves. Thus, the symptomatology is due to obstruction of arterial and venous blood flow, as well as nerve involvement. Intermittent claudication is common but is associated with signs of venous thrombosis and pain at rest. The disorder often leads to amputation of fingers and toes.

45. **The correct answer is D.** Meigs syndrome usually consists of a triad of benign fibroma or other ovarian tumors, ascites, and large effusions (usually on the right side). The symptoms, which are most commonly seen shortly after menopause, consist of a chronic illness, chest pain, and increased abdominal girth. Fluid moves from the abdomen to the thorax through small diaphragmatic defects or via lymphatics. When the condition is suspected, an abdominal CT scan and a pelvic examination should be performed. The removal of the ovarian tumor results in resolution of the effusion within two to three weeks.

Alcoholic cirrhosis (**choice A**) is unlikely, not only because the patient denies alcohol use, but because she has normal liver function tests.

The presence of hepatitis B surface antibody and the absence of hepatitis B surface antigen imply immunity to hepatitis B, so she cannot have this type of cirrhosis (**choice B**).

It is unlikely that the patient would have hepatitis C cirrhosis (**choice C**) because she tested negative for hepatitis C antibody. Unlike hepatitis B, the antibody to hepatitis

C does not confer immunity. It marks the presence of an infection in most cases. The hepatitis C antibody test is extremely sensitive. A negative antibody test in the presence of cirrhosis is usually seen only in immunocompromised hosts.

Although the patient has a history of a positive PPD test many years ago, she does not have peritoneal tuberculosis (**choice E**). Patients with peritoneal TB almost always have an elevated leukocyte count, usually with lymphocyte predominance.

46. **The correct answer is A.** This patient has diverticulitis. This disorder classically presents with fever, left lower quadrant pain, and an elevated white count with a left shift. Most diverticula are right-sided, but most ruptured diverticula are on the left. Diverticular disease is associated with constipation and is a significant cause of lower gastrointestinal bleeding. With this patient, the physical and laboratory findings are highly suggestive of diverticulitis, but an abdominal CT scan has the required sensitivity to detect diverticula, as well as any possible abscess formation.

Abdominal ultrasound (**choice B**) has no role in diagnosing diverticular disease. Ultrasound is useful for detection of masses, stones, and gross changes in organ size or anatomy. Its sensitivity in detecting small diverticula is less than 10%.

Flat and upright abdominal radiographs (**choice C**) are not useful tests to diagnose diverticular disease, but are very useful in the ruling out intra-abdominal free air from perforation and small or large bowel obstruction.

Barium enema (**choice D**) at one time was the preferred method for diagnosing diverticulitis, since the leakage of the barium from the ruptured diverticulum was easily visualized. However, a number of studies have suggested that such leakage is in fact harmful. Largely because of these observations, as well as the readily available nature of CT scanners at most institutions, CT scanning has become the imaging modality of choice for making the diagnosis of diverticulitis.

Exploratory laparotomy (**choice E**) is a major surgical procedure and is limited to cases in which there is such a high suspicion of massive abdominal pathology that even the highly sensitive CT scan (>95%) is not adequate. An example of such a case would be perforating abdominal trauma.

47. **The correct answer is A.** In the presence of this classic symptomatology, the clinical judgment alone is sufficiently accurate. Thus, no further laboratory or radiologic investigations are needed to support a diagnosis of primary osteoarthritis in a patient with characteristic signs and symptoms. If there are atypical manifestations,

further investigations may be indicated to rule out other conditions.

Complete blood count and erythrocyte sedimentation rate (**choice B**) are not needed in this case, but may be occasionally helpful in excluding inflammatory causes of joint diseases.

A blood test for rheumatoid factor (**choice C**) would be indicated in the presence of signs and symptoms suggesting rheumatoid arthritis. Symmetric involvement of small joints, associated with low-grade fever, fatigue, and prolonged stiffness, suggests the need for rheumatoid factor testing.

A blood test for antinuclear antibodies (**choice D**) is useful in ruling out collagen vascular diseases. Among these, systemic lupus erythematosus may present with polyarticular inflammation, but this is usually associated with multiorgan involvement as well as constitutional symptoms.

X-ray studies (**choice E**) are not necessary in the diagnostic assessment of typical osteoarthritis. Radiologic signs of degenerative osteoarthritis include narrowing of joint space, osteophytes, subchondral sclerosis, and intra-articular bone fragments ("joint mice").

Bone densitometry (**choice F**) is indicated in patients with osteoporosis, as a part of diagnostic evaluation or during treatment follow-up.

Diagnostic arthrocentesis (**choice G**) allows microscopic examination of synovial fluid. With this procedure, the nature of the fluid (transudate or exudate) can be determined, microorganisms identified by Gram staining and culture, and crystals evaluated by polarized microscopy. It is rarely necessary in degenerative osteoarthritis.

48. **The correct answer is A.** AFP is the blood marker for hepatocellular carcinoma, the tumor most likely to be present in this man. Although moderate elevations of the marker will occur just because of the cirrhosis, higher levels are virtually diagnostic for the tumor.

CEA (**choice B**) is the marker for metastatic colon cancer. Had the background been the discovery of a liver mass in a patient who previously had had colorectal cancer resected, this would have been the correct answer.

5-HIAA (**choice C**) is diagnostic for the carcinoid syndrome. Liver masses also would be a feature in that condition, as patients do not develop the syndrome unless they have liver metastasis. The clinical picture would have included episodes of flushing of the face, diarrhea, and bronchoconstriction. Long-term damage to the right side heart valves might also have been present.

This man will have elevated titers for hepatitis C (**choice D**), and the levels will not be diagnostic for the development of cancer.

Should a surgical resection be planned, arteriograms might be done. Studies of the portal vein (**choice E**) would be less likely to be undertaken, and if done they would add only information about location and spread, rather than about the nature of the tumor.

49. **The correct answer is I.** The clinical presentation is that of listeriosis caused by *Listeria monocytogenes*. Patients at risk include pregnant women, the elderly, newborns, and immunodeficient patients after eating contaminated foods. *Listeria* is found in unpasteurized milk, delicatessen meats, cheese, and raw vegetables. In pregnant women, it can cause miscarriages, premature labor, and stillbirths. Half of all newborns who are infected with *Listeria* die from the illness.

50. **The correct answer is B.** The clinical presentation is that of *anthrax*, which is caused by *Bacillus anthracis*. Anthrax is a disease of sheep, cattle (**choice B**), horses, goats, and pigs, but the agent can be transmitted to humans through broken skin or mucous membranes, or through inhalation. This infection is now rare in the U.S. and is seen only in persons exposed to infected animals or animal products. Thus, farmers, veterinarians, and workers in the wool industry are susceptible to anthrax. Penicillin G is the treatment of choice.

Coyote bite (**choice A**) and raccoon bite (**choice K**) may expose the victim to the risk of rabies. In fact, several wild animals may transmit rabies virus. In the U.S., potentially rabid animals include raccoons in the East and New England, skunks in the West and Midwest, coyotes in Texas, and foxes in the Southwest, New England, and Alaska. Contrary to popular belief, rodents are very unlikely to have rabies.

Exposure to ticks (**choice C**) may result in a number of infective illnesses, which depend on the regional distribution of the ticks and organisms involved. The following is a list of infections known to be transmitted to humans by ticks: arbovirus encephalitis, babesiosis, Colorado tick fever, ehrlichiosis, hemorrhagic fever, Lyme disease, relapsing fever, Rocky Mountain spotted fever, and tularemia.

History of contact with rabbits or other rodents (**choice D**) may be found in humans affected by *tularemia*, caused by *Francisella tularensis*. It affects wild rodents, especially rabbits and muskrats. The disease may be acquired by contact with infected tissue (such as skinning rabbits) or from tick bites.

History of recent travel to tropical countries (**choice E**) may be linked to a great variety of exotic infectious processes, from innocuous and self-limiting, such as traveler's diarrhea, to potentially life-threatening, such as malaria. Suffice it to say that travel history should always be elicited when investigating the etiology of infectious diseases.

Ingestion of home-canned food (**choice F**) is typically associated with botulism, caused by *Clostridium botulinum*. This is a ubiquitous, strictly anaerobic, spore-forming bacillus that finds excellent growth conditions in the anaerobic environment of home-canned or vacuum-packed foods.

Ingestion of inadequately cooked pork (**choice G**) may result in parasitic diseases, such as *cysticercosis* (due to *Taenia solium*), trichinosis (*Trichinella spiralis*), and *toxoplasmosis* (*Toxoplasma gondii*).

Ingestion of inadequately cooked salmon (**choice H**) may result in tapeworm infection due to *Diphyllobothrium latum*. Cases of fish tapeworm are observed on the Pacific coast of the U.S. and many other temperate and subarctic lake regions in the world.

Ingestion of unpasteurized milk products (**choice I**) has become a very rare mode of transmission of infections. It was once commonly responsible for gastrointestinal tuberculosis and brucellosis.

Recent admission to a hospital (**choice L**) is a common predisposing condition for severe *hospital-acquired infections*, the most common of which are urinary tract infection and pneumonia. Hospital-acquired infections have become a major health problem, especially because hospital-acquired organisms are often resistant to most antibiotics.

Recent exposure to a child with chickenpox (**choice M**) exposes nonimmune individuals to chickenpox, but also to shingles.

Transfusion of blood and blood products (**choice J**), sexual contact (**choice N**), accidental needlesticks among health professionals and in dialysis units (**choice P**), and intravenous drug use (**choice O**) are all related to viral hepatitis transmission.

Working in an aviary (**choice Q**) is a risk factor for psittacosis, an atypical pneumonia caused by *Chlamydia psittaci*. Transmission is via dust from dry bird secretions and feces. Patients present with fever, nonproductive cough, myalgias, and x-rays that appear more severe than clinical presentations.

Internal Medicine: **Test Two**

1. A 25-year-old man comes to the physician because of the rapid onset of pain and swelling of his left knee, which began 24 hours ago. His temperature is 38.5° C (101.3° F), blood pressure is 125/70 mm Hg, pulse is 95/min, and respirations are 20/min. His personal history is significant for IV drug abuse. He denies a history of sexually transmitted diseases. The left knee is tender, swollen, and warm to the touch. Chest auscultation is normal. Which of the following is the most appropriate next step in management?

   (A) Blood studies including complete blood count (CBC)

   (B) HIV testing prior to instituting any treatment

   (C) Plain x-ray films of the joint

   (D) Nonsteroidal anti-inflammatory and empiric antibiotic therapy

   (E) Diagnostic arthrocentesis

2. A 28-year-old man presents to the emergency department with complaints of fever, chills, and malaise for the past three days. He also complains of nausea, headaches, and anorexia. The patient denies any homosexual practices but admits to occasional IV drug use. Examination of his palms and soles reveals painless macules; on auscultation, a loud holosystolic murmur is noted. Which of the following is the most appropriate next step in diagnosis?

   (A) ECG

   (B) Echocardiogram

   (C) Chest CT scan with contrast

   (D) RPR for syphilis

   (E) Cardiac catheterization

3. A 71-year-old man is brought to the emergency department with acute onset of headache, vomiting, and confusion. The family reports that he has a long history of poorly controlled hypertension with hypertensive renal disease and eye disease that were diagnosed three years ago. They report that, a few hours ago, he rapidly developed a very severe headache, and over the next half hour, became more lethargic and confused, and had five episodes of vomiting. His blood pressure is 235/140 mm Hg in both arms, and he appears to have a lateral gaze paralysis on the right. There is no nuchal rigidity, and the pupils appear reactive bilaterally; however, papilledema is evident on funduscopic exam. Which of the following is the most likely diagnosis?

   (A) Cerebellar hemorrhage

   (B) Epidural hematoma

   (C) Putamenal hemorrhage

   (D) Subarachnoid hemorrhage

   (E) Subdural hematoma

4. A 55-year-old woman presents to the emergency department because of chest pain. The pain, which has lasted three hours, is substernal and dull in nature, with no relation to respiration or position. The pain does not radiate and is accompanied by weakness, lightheadedness, and nausea. She has received oxygen, aspirin, a continuous infusion of nitroglycerin, and a beta blocker. Her chest x-ray film is normal, and her ECG is remarkable for inverted T waves in leads II, III, and aVF. Which of the following is the most important next step in management?

   (A) Nifedipine

   (B) IV heparin

   (C) IV thrombolytic therapy

   (D) Cardiac catheterization

   (E) Percutaneous coronary angioplasty

5. A 40-year-old man consults a physician because of dizziness. The patient has noticed that every time he lays with the right side of his head down, he develops a whirling sensation within a few seconds. This symptom will last as long as the position is maintained, but resolves when a new head position is taken. He does not experience tinnitis or hearing changes during these episodes. Otoscopic examination is within normal limits. Which of the following is the most likely diagnosis?

(A) Benign paroxysmal positional vertigo

(B) Cholesteatoma

(C) Herpes zoster oticus

(D) Ménière disease

(E) Presbycusis

6. A 62-year-old woman with a history of depression and hypertension presents complaining of recurrent falls over the past six months. She had been having difficulty with complex tasks at work and was recently asked to leave. On examination, her mental status is unremarkable. Her cranial nerve examination is notable for limited downward gaze. She has prominent, symmetric bradykinesia with more axial than limb rigidity. There is no resting tremor. Her gait is stiff with "en bloc" turning. Reflexes are normal, with downgoing toes. An MRI of the brain is read as showing a small lacunar infarct in the left putamen. She has recently been started on L-dopa/carbidopa but has had little to no improvement in her symptoms. Which of the following is the most likely diagnosis?

(A) Basal ganglia stroke

(B) Carbon monoxide poisoning

(C) Cervical stenosis

(D) Parkinson disease

(E) Progressive supranuclear palsy

7. A 22-year-old man presents with burning on urination and a milky urethral discharge for three days. He had unprotected sex five days prior to the onset of these manifestations. A smear of the urethral discharge demonstrates gram-negative diplococci in neutrophilic granulocytes. The patient reports no allergies. Which of the following is the most appropriate treatment?

(A) Amoxicillin

(B) Azithromycin

(C) Ceftriaxone

(D) Doxycycline

(E) Penicillin G

8. A 50-year-old woman presents with a chief complaint of dizziness when she gets out of bed in the morning. During the episodes of dizziness, she feels very warm and flushed. She also has had frequent episodes of abdominal cramping and severe watery diarrhea during the past year, and she recently began having dry, itchy skin. On physical examination, she has a 2/6 systolic murmur best heard at the left lower sternal border. No wheezing, rhonchi, or crackles are apparent on lung examination. Laboratory results are unremarkable. Which of the following is the most appropriate next step in diagnosis?

(A) Barium examination of the bowel

(B) Measurement of serum lipase and amylase levels

(C) Ultrasound of the abdomen

(D) Urinalysis for 5-hydroxyindoleacetic acid (5-HIAA)

(E) Small bowel biopsy

9. A 40-year-old woman consults a physician about a "mole" on her neck. The lesion is 2 cm in diameter and slightly irregular, and has a variegated dark red to brown/black color. Wide excision of the lesion demonstrates a malignant neoplasm that extends to a depth of 3 mm. This tumor would be most likely to stain for which of the following tumor markers?

    (A) Alpha-fetoprotein

    (B) CA-125

    (C) Leukocyte common antigen (LCA)

    (D) Prostate-specific antigen (PSA)

    (E) S-100

10. A 19-year-old homosexual college freshman presents to the student health clinic complaining of diarrhea of two days' duration. He returned nine days ago from a spring break trip to Mexico. His diarrhea is accompanied by prominent bloating, flatulence, nausea, and general malaise. On physical examination, he appears to be well hydrated, with a temperature of 36.9° C (98.4° F), blood pressure of 130/86 mm Hg, pulse of 89/min, and respirations of 18/min. Examination of the abdomen reveals diffusely hyperactive bowel sounds without tenderness or masses. A stool sample is negative for red and white blood cells. Which of the following is the most appropriate next step in management?

    (A) Supportive care with IV fluids

    (B) Treatment with ciprofloxacin

    (C) Treatment with mebendazole

    (D) Treatment with metronidazole

    (E) Treatment with trimethoprim-sulfamethoxazole

11. A 26-year-old woman has a 10-year history of type 1 diabetes mellitus. She has maintained strict glycemic control and has had no significant diabetic complications so far. On her last routine examination, her blood pressure is 125/78 mm Hg. Blood chemistry studies are within normal limits. Funduscopic examination reveals no evidence of diabetic retinopathy. Which of the following is the most appropriate next step in management to prevent diabetic nephropathy?

    (A) Periodic measurement of serum creatinine levels

    (B) Screening for microalbuminuria with dipstick examination of urine

    (C) Screening for microalbuminuria with 24-hour urine collection

    (D) Administration of ACE inhibitors

    (E) Renal biopsy

12. A 45-year-old woman consults a physician because of chronic fatigue. A review of systems reveals long-standing stomach problems characterized by slow digestion and delayed emptying of her stomach. A complete blood count demonstrates a moderately severe megaloblastic anemia. Serum vitamin B_{12} level is 85 pg/mL; serum folate is 3 ng/mL; and serum iron is 105 mg/dL. Autoantibodies to intrinsic factor are detected in the serum. A biopsy of the stomach is most likely to show which of the following?

    (A) Acute erosive gastritis

    (B) Gastric atrophy

    (C) Linitis plastica

    (D) Ménétrier disease

    (E) Peptic ulcer

13. A 72-year-old man who was recently diagnosed with lymphoma has been undergoing chemotherapy for the past three weeks. He now develops acute renal failure. His laboratory studies reveal a creatinine of 4 mg/dL, urea nitrogen of 15 mg/dL, and uric acid level of 20 mg/dL. Which of the following would most likely have prevented this patient's acute renal failure?

    (A) Allopurinol

    (B) Diphenhydramine

    (C) Furosemide

    (D) *N*-acetylcysteine

    (E) Nifedipine

    (F) Urinary acidification

14. A 30-year-old man consults a physician because of weight loss and fatigue. A complete blood count demonstrates an erythrocyte count of 2.2 million/mm^3, a leukocyte count of 105,000/mm^3, and a platelet count of 100,000/mm^3. The peripheral smear shows many abnormal white cells containing multiple Auer rods. Remission is achieved with chemotherapy, and the decision is made to treat the patient with total body irradiation followed by allogeneic bone marrow transplantation. Depletion of which of the following cells in the transplanted marrow tends to decrease the incidence of subsequent graft-versus-host disease?

    (A) B cells

    (B) Megakaryocytes

    (C) Promyelocytes

    (D) Pronormoblasts

    (E) T cells

15. A 40-year-old woman presents to her physician's office with a rash on her legs for the past four days. She recalls a recent respiratory infection. On examination, there is a small amount of blood in her nostrils. There are several hemorrhagic bullae in her oral cavity. Her lungs are clear, cardiac examination is unremarkable, and her abdomen is soft with no palpable spleen or liver. Both lower extremities have multiple dark blue ecchymoses. Laboratory analysis reveals:

Leukocyte count:	9,000/mm^3
Hemoglobin:	10.1 g/dL
Platelets:	9,000/mm^3
Peripheral smear:	Reticulocytosis with normal erythrocytes and megathrombocytes

An ultrasound examination is negative for masses or fluid collections. Which of the following is the most appropriate next step in management?

    (A) Cryoprecipitate

    (B) Immunoglobulins

    (C) Prednisone

    (D) Plasmapheresis

    (E) Splenectomy

16. A 30-year-old man presents with a rapidly enlarging, single, stony hard, palpable 2.5-cm nodule in his thyroid gland. Thyroid isotope scanning demonstrates the nodule to be "cold." On resection of the thyroid gland with subsequent pathologic examination, the nodule is found to contain follicular structures, some of which have inwardly protruding fibrovascular branching cores covered by epithelial cells. Many of the epithelial cells have "orphan Annie" nuclei. Which of the following is the most likely diagnosis?

    (A) Follicular carcinoma of the thyroid

    (B) Graves disease

    (C) Hashimoto disease

    (D) Nontoxic goiter

    (E) Papillary carcinoma of the thyroid

17. A 38-year-old man is admitted to the hospital after having a pulmonary embolism. The patient has a past medical history significant for two idiopathic deep venous thromboses and takes only an aspirin daily. Three hours ago, he developed acute shortness of breath, pleuritic chest pain, and palpitations. He was taken by ambulance to the hospital. In the emergency department, he was diagnosed with a pulmonary embolus on the basis of clinical signs and symptoms and a ventilation-perfusion scan. He was started on IV unfractionated heparin at that time. Which of the following laboratory tests would be most appropriate to guide therapy with this drug?

(A) Bleeding time

(B) Factor Xa levels

(C) Platelet count

(D) Prothrombin time (PT)

(E) Partial thromboplastin time (PTT)

18. A 48-year-old man presents to the physician's office with progressive hearing loss in his right ear for the past several months. He describes a ringing and hissing sound in his right ear, and he feels unsteady on his feet, as if he is losing his sense of balance. His past medical history includes syphilis, which was treated at age 20, and bronchial asthma, which is controlled with medications. On physical examination, right-sided facial numbness is noted, and a Rinne test shows air conduction that is greater than bone conduction. Routine laboratory profile is normal, and rapid plasma reagin is negative. Which of the following is the most likely diagnosis?

(A) Acoustic neuroma

(B) Benign positional vertigo

(C) Lyme disease

(D) Ménière disease

(E) Tertiary syphilis

19. A 22-year-old woman comes to the physician for her first physical health examination in several years. She says that she has always been in good health except for irregular menses in the past year. She does not take any medication or smoke. Her blood pressure is 137/80 mm Hg. Her height is 160 cm (63 in), and her weight is 83 kg (185 lb). Physical examination reveals a slight increase in upper lip and chin hair. She reports that she has been gaining weight since the age of 15 despite all attempts to both limit calorie intake and exercise. Which of the following is the most appropriate next step in management?

(A) No intervention needed at this time

(B) Explanation of risks of obesity and benefits of weight loss

(C) Laboratory investigations to exclude secondary causes of obesity

(D) Referral to weight reduction program for very-low-calorie diet

(E) Pharmacologic treatment with the serotonin reuptake inhibitor sibutramine

20. A 55-year-old man presents to a physician because of a two-month history of difficulty swallowing. At first, the difficulty was only with large bites of solid food, and he was able to limit it by taking smaller bites and washing them down with drinks. However, he now has trouble with small bites and liquids. He has a long history of heavy use of both alcohol and cigarettes. Esophagoscopy demonstrates a large, irregular polypoid mass that is nearly occluding the upper third of the esophagus. A biopsy of the tumor is most likely to show which of the following?

(A) Anaplastic squamous epithelial cells with numerous mitotic figures

(B) Large, lymphocytic cells with large, prominent nucleoli

(C) Mucin-producing glandular tissue with signet ring cells

(D) Small, lymphocytic cells with irregular nuclei and condensed chromatin

(E) Small, polygonal cells with neurosecretory granules

21. A 19-year-old African American woman with sickle cell anemia has had palpitations and dizziness for three days. She works part-time in a daycare center. Her temperature is 38.1° C (100.5° F), pulse is 110/min, and respirations are 18/min. The cardiac examination is significant for a systolic murmur heard best at the apex. Her lungs are clear, and her abdominal examination is unremarkable. Laboratory studies reveal a hemoglobin of 6.0 g/dL. A blood smear stained with Wright's stain demonstrates Howell-Jolly bodies and the absence of reticulocytes. Which of the following is the most likely pathogen?

    (A) Influenza virus

    (B) Parainfluenza virus

    (C) Parvovirus

    (D) *Salmonella*

    (E) *Streptococcus pneumoniae*

22. A healthy 20-year-old man presents with a history of recurrent episodes of severe throbbing headache. The headaches are triggered or aggravated by noise and stress and last for several hours. The pain is frequently preceded by visual disturbances, such as luminous stars or zigzags of light, and accompanied by nausea and vomiting. His father experienced a similar form of headache. The patient has found no relief with aspirin and ibuprofen. Which of the following is the most appropriate drug treatment during the acute attacks?

    (A) Acetaminophen

    (B) Calcium channel antagonists

    (C) Carbamazepine

    (D) Ergotamine

    (E) Prednisone

23. A 55-year-old man consults a physician because of weight loss and severe abdominal pain of several months' duration. The pain radiates to the mid-back and is slightly relieved when he assumes a bent forward position. On physical examination, the man appears emaciated, with mild jaundice. The liver edge is palpable and smooth; the liver depth is not increased. The clinician suspects pancreatic cancer. Which of the following tests is the most appropriate next step in diagnosis?

    (A) CT scan

    (B) MRI scan

    (C) Ultrasound

    (D) Arteriography

    (E) Endoscopic retrograde pancreatography

24. A 70-year-old man presents to his physician with complaints of blurred vision in his right eye along with intermittent loss of vision, which has been occurring for the past three days. He describes it as a "curtain passing vertically" across the visual field. He does not have any pain, fever, headache, nausea, or vomiting. He has a history of hypertension and diabetes and is a smoker. Current medications include captopril and twice-daily insulin. On examination, the conjunctivae are pink, the sclerae are clear, and the pupils bilaterally are 3-4 mm and reactive. Cranial nerves II-XII are intact, and there are no focal neurologic deficits. Which of the following is most likely diagnosis?

    (A) Amaurosis fugax

    (B) Diabetic retinopathy

    (C) Retinal artery occlusion

    (D) Retinal detachment

    (E) Retinal vein occlusion

25. A study by McGinnis and Foege, published in the *Journal of the American Medical Association* in 1993, showed that up to 43% of deaths occurring annually in the U.S. are potentially preventable. Which of the following is an example of a program of *primary* (versus secondary or tertiary) prevention?

    (A) Annual mammography for women older than 45

    (B) Controlling blood lipid levels

    (C) Controlling hypertension

    (D) Increasing cigarette taxes

    (E) Pap smear screening

    (F) Prophylactic aspirin after myocardial infarction

26. A 58-year-old man with a 12-year history of type 2 diabetes mellitus comes to the physician because of an ulcer in his right foot. Physical examination reveals a 1-cm irregular ulceration over the right metatarsal head, surrounded by an area of black gangrenous skin. The patient is admitted to the hospital and undergoes amputation of the right forefoot. Which of the following measures would have been most effective in preventing this complication?

    (A) Appropriate instructions on self-care of the feet

    (B) Doppler examination of the lower extremities

    (C) Neurophysiologic and electromyographic studies

    (D) Local application of platelet-derived growth factor

    (E) Prophylactic treatment with cholesterol-lowering agents

27. A 35-year-old woman presents with erythematous, round, scaling papules for several years. The lesions are 5-10 mm in diameter and show follicular plugging. Although the lesions are generalized in distribution, the highest number are on the malar prominences, bridge of the nose, scalp, and external auditory canals. Biopsy of the lesions is consistent with either discoid lupus erythematosus or systemic lupus erythematosus. Which of the following additional findings would most strongly tend to exclude discoid lupus?

    (A) Alopecia of the scalp

    (B) Anti-ds DNA

    (C) Noncontracting scars

    (D) Positive antinuclear antibody test

    (E) Sun sensitivity

28. A 25-year-old man with acute myelogenous leukemia is undergoing chemotherapy. One week after his therapy, he presents with a headache, fever, and confusion. On physical examination, he has nuchal rigidity, Kernig sign, and photophobia. Laboratory results are notable for a white count of 1,000 mm^3, hematocrit of 25%, and a differential of 10% neutrophils and 5% lymphocytes. Lumbar puncture is consistent with meningitis. Which of the following is the most likely pathogen?

    (A) *Bacteroides fragilis*

    (B) *Haemophilus influenzae*

    (C) *Pseudomonas aeruginosa*

    (D) *Staphylococcus aureus*

    (E) *Toxoplasma gondii*

29. A healthy 25-year-old woman comes to the physician for a health maintenance examination. Her blood pressure is 126/82 mm Hg, pulse is 75/min and regular, and respirations are 14/min. She denies any significant health problems and exercises regularly. Cardiac auscultation reveals a low-pitch grade III/VI mid-diastolic murmur near the apex. It begins with a snap and ends before the first heart sound. The lungs are clear to auscultation. An ECG shows no abnormalities. Which of the following is the most appropriate next step in diagnosis?

    (A) Antistreptolysin O titers

    (B) Doppler ultrasound

    (C) Echocardiography

    (D) Radionuclide angiography

    (E) Cardiac catheterization

30. A 30-year-old man presents to the emergency department with severe headache, visual changes, and palpitations. His temperature is 37.2° C (100° F), blood pressure is 190/130 mm Hg, pulse is 130/min, and respirations are 17/min. The remainder of the physical examination is unremarkable except for clamminess of the hands and increased sweating on the face. The patient's hypertension is treated. A 24-hour urine specimen demonstrates elevated metanephrine, vanillylmandelic acid (VMA), and homovanillic acid (HVA). On questioning, the patient notes that endocrine problems have been very common in his family. This patient most likely has a significantly increased risk of developing which of the following thyroid diseases?

    (A) Graves disease

    (B) Hashimoto disease

    (C) Medullary carcinoma

    (D) Multinodular goiter

    (E) Papillary carcinoma

31. A 12-year-old boy presents with acute onset of morbilliform rash, fever, malaise, and oliguria. These manifestations began one week after starting treatment with ampicillin for streptococcal pharyngitis. His temperature is 38.8° C (102° F), blood pressure is 115/76 mm Hg, pulse is 95/min, and respirations are 16/min. Urinalysis shows microhematuria, leukocyturia with numerous eosinophils, and occasional white blood cell casts. Proteinuria is absent. Blood studies show elevated antistreptolysin titers and moderate eosinophilia. BUN is 42 mg/dL, and serum creatinine is 2.5 mg/dL. Which of the following is the most likely diagnosis?

    (A) Acute interstitial nephritis

    (B) Acute pyelonephritis

    (C) Acute tubular necrosis

    (D) Henoch-Schönlein purpura

    (E) Post-streptococcal glomerulonephritis

32. An 18-year-old man presents with pain in his left knee and right ankle. There is no history of trauma. The young man states that he has not felt well since recovering from a two-week diarrheal illness one month ago. On physical examination, his temperature is 38.1° C (100.6° F), blood pressure is 100/70 mm Hg, pulse is 76/min, and respirations are 16/min. He has bilateral conjunctivitis. His right ankle and left knee are swollen, erythematous, warm, and tender. There is a small effusion present in the knee. His right Achilles tendon is also erythematous and tender. Synovial fluid from his knee shows a white blood cell count of 10,000/mm³ with 80% neutrophils. No organisms are seen on Gram stain. Which of the following is the most likely diagnosis?

    (A) Crohn disease

    (B) Felty syndrome

    (C) Gout

    (D) Juvenile rheumatoid arthritis

    (E) Reiter syndrome

    (F) Septic arthritis

33. A 25-year-old schizophrenic patient presents with painful oral ulcers. He was started on chlorpromazine treatment three months ago. He is currently afebrile, and there is no evidence of significant somatic disease on physical examination. Blood analyses show:

Hematocrit	45%
Platelet count	320,000/mm³
Leukocyte count	400/mm³
Differential	
Lymphocytes	85%
Monocytes	10%
Neutrophils	5%

    Morphology of red and white blood cells is normal on peripheral blood smears. Which of the following is the most appropriate next step in management?

    (A) Discontinue current pharmacologic treatment

    (B) Treat stomatitis by topical corticosteroids

    (C) Treat with myeloid growth factors (G-CSF and GM-CSF)

    (D) Admit patient for broad spectrum antibiotic treatment

    (E) Perform bone marrow aspirate examination

34. A 60-year-old man presents with shortness of breath and dull left-sided chest pain. Examination reveals decreased breath sounds on the left. A chest x-ray film is consistent with a large left-sided pleural effusion, for which the patient undergoes thoracentesis. The fluid is slightly turbid with a pH of 7.2, a white count of 60,000/mm³, an RBC count of 15,000/mm³, an LDH of 400 IU/L, and a serum LDH of 500 IU/L (normal 50-150 IU/L). A repeat chest x-ray film reveals a pneumonia in the right middle lobe. A pleural fluid Gram stain shows multiple gram-positive diplococci. Which of the following is the most appropriate next step in management?

    (A) Ampicillin

    (B) Diuresis

    (C) Pleural biopsy

    (D) Pleurodesis

    (E) Chest tube insertion

35. A 46-year-old housewife from Connecticut presents with complaints of malaise, arthritis, and a rash on her left thigh. ELISA and Western blot confirm infection with *Borrelia burgdorferi*. A 30-day course of oral doxycycline with follow-up in one week is prescribed. The patient cancels the follow-up appointment and returns three months later complaining of facial droop, confusion, daily fevers, and tingling in her hands and feet. She states that she felt markedly better after two weeks on the antibiotics and therefore discontinued her medication. Which of the following is the most appropriate next step in management?

    (A) A 14-day course of chloramphenicol

    (B) A 14-day course of IV ceftriaxone

    (C) A 28-day course of IV vancomycin

    (D) Prescribe a repeat 3-day course of oral doxycycline

    (E) Prescribe a 30-day course of oral amoxicillin

36. A 65-year-old man comes to the physician because of an increasingly severe tremor that affects the right hand. The tremor is present at rest and disappears when the limb is in movement. The man's speech is soft but not monotonous. There is increased resistance when the arms or neck are passively flexed. Sensation and muscle strength appear intact. Short-term memory is preserved. The patient's blood pressure is 134/82 mm Hg, temperature is 37° C (98.6° F), pulse is 70/min, and respirations are 10/min. The patient has a history of a previous episode of narrow-angle glaucoma. Which of the following drugs should be avoided in the treatment of his neurologic condition?

    (A) Amantadine

    (B) Benztropine

    (C) Bromocriptine

    (D) Levodopa

    (E) Selegiline

37. A patient presents to a physician with severe jaundice. Physical examination reveals a nodular, enlarged liver. In addition to the generalized nodularity of the liver, the physician can feel one nodule that is much larger than the others. CT of the abdomen confirms multinodular cirrhosis and demonstrates a 7-cm mass near the lower border of the liver. CT-guided biopsy of this mass shows a malignant tumor derived from hepatic parenchymal cells. Which of the following risk factors is most strongly associated with the development of this tumor?

    (A) Aflatoxin exposure

    (B) Hemochromatosis

    (C) Hepatitis B virus infection

    (D) *Opisthorchis* infection

    (E) Thorotrast exposure

38. A 37-year-old florist comes to the employee health clinic for a routine evaluation. He is healthy and without complaints. Five units of tuberculin protein (PPD) is injected intradermally. He returns to the clinic 48-72 hours later. Which of the following would indicate a positive reaction in this patient?

    (A) 5 mm of erythema and 5 mm induration

    (B) 10 mm of erythema and 5 mm induration

    (C) 15 mm of erythema and 5 mm induration

    (D) 15 mm of erythema and 15 mm induration

    (E) 20 mm of erythema and 10 mm induration

39. A 18-year-old woman comes to medical attention because of fever and a red papule on her left forearm, which developed one week after being scratched by her cat. She has had temperatures to 38.5° C (101.3° F) and malaise for two days. Examination reveals enlarged and tender lymph nodes in the epitrochlear and axillary regions. Which of the following is the most likely pathogen?

    (A) *Bartonella henselae*

    (B) *Bartonella quintana*

    (C) *Calymmatobacterium granulomatis*

    (D) *Chlamydia psittaci*

    (E) *Pasteurella multocida*

40. A 56-year-old woman with a long history of painful osteoarthritis of the hip and lower back comes to medical attention because of polyuria for three months. She denies any previous urinary tract infection or renal disease. Her blood pressure is 135/80 mm Hg. Urine dipstick test shows hematuria and mild proteinuria. Blood studies reveal mild microcytic anemia, hyperkalemia, and normal uric acid levels. Ultrasonography shows kidneys of normal size. Intravenous pyelography (IVP) demonstrates the presence of characteristic "ring shadow" defects at the tips of renal papillae. Which of the following is the most likely cause of this condition?

    (A) Analgesic nephropathy

    (B) Lead exposure

    (C) Multiple myeloma

    (D) Obstructive uropathy

    (E) Polycystic kidney disease

    (F) Vesicoureteral reflux

41. An 82-year-old woman is accompanied to the physician by her daughter because of repeated falls without apparent cause. The patient reports that she fell to the ground because of a sudden loss of strength in her legs without losing consciousness or feeling dizzy. She lay on the floor for a few minutes until she recovered strength and became able to stand up and walk again. She is otherwise in good health and takes alendronate for osteoporosis. Examination reveals mild resting tremor of her hands, but there is no rigidity or slowing of movements. Her blood pressure is 125/80 mm Hg, pulse is 68/min and regular, and respirations are 13/min. On auscultation, a bruit is heard over the right carotid artery. Which of the following is the most likely cause of this patient's falls?

    (A) Adverse drug reaction

    (B) Lateral medullary infarction

    (C) Parkinson disease

    (D) Postural hypotension

    (E) Transient ischemia in the carotid territory

    (F) Transient vertebrobasilar ischemia

42. A 39-year-old man presents to the emergency department with acute onset of shortness of breath, hemoptysis, and left-sided pleuritic chest pain. His past medical history includes medication-controlled asthma, peptic ulcer disease, and a recent onset of idiopathic nephrotic syndrome. His blood pressure is 180/100 mm Hg, pulse is 110/min, and respirations are 28/min. Cardiac and lung examinations are normal. Laboratory data are remarkable for a serum lactate dehydrogenase of 300 U/L. An ECG shows sinus tachycardia, prominent S waves in lead 1, inversions of the T wave, and a prominent Q wave in lead III. Which of the following is the most likely cause of the chest pain?

    (A) Aortic dissection

    (B) Esophageal spasm

    (C) Myocardial infarction

    (D) Pneumonia

    (E) Pulmonary embolism

    (F) Variant angina

43. A 45-year-old woman with systemic lupus erythematosus (SLE) comes to the physician for a routine checkup. Her condition has been stable for several years, and she currently is not taking any medication. Blood chemistry studies and hematologic parameters are remarkable for a blood urea nitrogen (BUN) of 23 mg/dL, a creatinine of 1.6 mg/dL, and a mild normocytic anemia. The erythrocyte sedimentation rate is 18 mm/min. Urinalysis shows microhematuria and mild proteinuria. Which of the following is the most appropriate next step in management?

    (A) Repeat urinalysis at next routine examination

    (B) Sequential serum complement and ANA studies

    (C) Treatment with corticosteroids

    (D) Treatment with cyclophosphamide

    (E) Renal biopsy

44. A 62-year-old man presents with complaints of severe pain in his left wrist that he says is episodic and has increased in frequency over the past year. He says that he cannot move the wrist when this happens. His father had similar problems before he died of kidney problems due to diabetes. The patient is also diabetic and is taking insulin. His physical examination is normal, except for the limitation of motion of the left wrist. A CBC is normal, and serum chemistry findings are as follows:

Sodium	139 mEq/L
Potassium	3.9 mEq/L
Chloride	98 mEq/L
Calcium	9.2 mEq/L
Uric acid	4 mg/dL

    Synovial fluid analysis reveals a white blood cell count of 32,000/μL with 60% neutrophils. Rhomboid-shaped, positive, birefringent crystals are seen under polarized light. Which of the following is the most likely diagnosis in this patient?

    (A) Charcot arthropathy

    (B) Degenerative joint disease

    (C) Gout

    (D) Pseudogout

    (E) Rheumatoid arthritis

    (F) Septic arthritis

45. A 52-year-old woman from Southeast Asia comes to medical attention because of slowly growing nodular lesions on her nose and auricles. Examination also reveals bilateral hypoesthesia in the upper extremities along the ulnar nerve distribution. Biopsies of the skin lesions demonstrate a florid granulomatous reaction with numerous acid-fast bacilli (AFB) within multi-nucleated giant cells. Cultures on blood agar and special media, however, yield no growth. Which of the following is the most likely diagnosis?

    (A) Lepromatous leprosy

    (B) Lupus vulgaris

    (C) *Mycobacterium avium-intracellulare* (MAI)

    (D) Sarcoidosis

    (E) Tuberculoid leprosy

46. A 42-year-old man presents with a chief complaint of severe, sharp chest pain that started suddenly while lifting heavy objects. The pain began in a midsternal location, then radiated to both shoulders as well as to his back. It has been constant for 18 hours but started to get worse during the past 2 hours. On physical examination, the patient is in severe distress, with a temperature of 36.9° C (98.5° F), blood pressure of 160/90 mm Hg, pulse of 92/min, and respirations of 18/min. Heart sounds are normal without rubs or murmur. An ECG reveals a normal tracing. Which of the following is the most appropriate next step in diagnosis?

    (A) Chest x-ray film

    (B) CT scan of chest

    (C) MRI

    (D) Ventilation-perfusion (V/Q) scan

    (E) Angiogram

47. A 55-year-old homeless, alcoholic man who has recently been binge drinking complains of two weeks of fever, malaise, productive cough, and pain on deep inspiration. He has smoked two packs of cigarettes per day for the past 30 years. A chest x-ray film reveals an infiltrate of the superior portion of the right lower lobe, with a cavity containing an air fluid level. A biopsy is likely to show which of the following?

    (A) Acid-fast bacilli and caseating granulomas

    (B) Anaplastic squamous cells with numerous mitotic figures

    (C) Fibrosis and needle-like ferruginous bodies

    (D) Gram-positive, lancet-shaped diplococci in short chains

    (E) Mixture of anaerobic organisms

48. An 83-year-old woman presents with a 1-year history of increasing forgetfulness and inattentiveness. She has had episodes of confusion, usually occurring at night when she wanders around in her house, disoriented to time and place. According to a family member, she has recently developed paranoid ideation. On a Mini-Mental Status examination, she is unable to recall one of three words, but she is able to follow a three-stage command. There is no history of alcohol abuse, major physical illness, or current pharmacologic therapy. Physical examination is unrevealing, and blood and thyroid function tests are within normal limits. Which of the following is the most appropriate next step in diagnosis?

    (A) Electroencephalographic studies

    (B) MRI of the brain

    (C) Cerebral angiographic studies

    (D) Lumbar puncture for CSF examination

    (E) Brain biopsy

The response options for items 49-50 are the same. You will be required to select one answer for each item in the set.

(A) Acute respiratory distress syndrome

(B) Asthma

(C) Bronchiectasis

(D) Carcinoma of the lungs

(E) Chronic aspiration of gastric contents

(F) Chronic obstructive pulmonary disease (COPD)

(G) Cystic fibrosis

(H) Pleural effusion

(I) Pneumocystis carinii pneumonia

(J) Pulmonary hypertension

(K) Pulmonary thromboembolism

(L) Sarcoidosis

(M) Spontaneous pneumothorax

(N) Tuberculosis

For each patient with dyspnea, select the most likely diagnosis.

49. A 45-year-old man presents with respiratory difficulty and right chest pain. His temperature is 37.7° C (99.9° F) and respirations are 24/min and shallow. Chest examination reveals decreased tactile fremitus over the right hemithorax, with an extensive area of dullness to percussion and marked diminution of breath sounds on auscultation. Just above this area, egophony is appreciated.

50. A 38-year-old African American woman presents with the insidious onset of shortness of breath, chest pain, and fatigue. Physical examination reveals enlarged cervical lymph nodes and scattered brown-red papules on the skin. A chest x-ray film shows bilateral pulmonary infiltrates and enlarged hilar lymph nodes. Biopsies of skin lesions and lymph nodes show non-necrotizing granulomas. Special stains for fungi and mycobacteria are negative.

Internal Medicine Test Two:
Answers and Explanations

ANSWER KEY

1.	E	26.	A
2.	B	27.	B
3.	C	28.	C
4.	B	29.	C
5.	A	30.	C
6.	E	31.	A
7.	C	32.	E
8.	D	33.	A
9.	E	34.	E
10.	D	35.	B
11.	C	36.	B
12.	B	37.	C
13.	A	38.	D
14.	E	39.	A
15.	C	40.	A
16.	E	41.	F
17.	E	42.	E
18.	A	43.	E
19.	C	44.	D
20.	A	45.	A
21.	C	46.	A
22.	D	47.	E
23.	A	48.	B
24.	A	49.	H
25.	D	50.	L

1. **The correct answer is E.** This clinical picture is consistent with *septic arthritis*. IV drug abusers are prone to developing joint infections (as well as endocarditis) due to *Staphylococcus aureus*. Fever and local inflammatory changes restricted to a single joint (i.e., monoarthritis) are sufficient clues to the correct diagnosis. Swelling of the joint indicates that there is probably an effusion within the articular cavity. The next step is to confirm the diagnosis and isolate the offending agent by performing aspiration of the joint fluid. Microscopic examination will allow confirming the nature of the effusion (transudate versus exudate) and ruling out crystal-related joint disease (gout and pseudogout). Culture of the fluid will most likely yield *S. aureus* in this case.

   Blood studies, including complete blood count (CBC; **choice A**), are useful additional investigations. However, arthrocentesis is more important in management.

   HIV testing (**choice B**) is appropriate in this case, considering the high frequency of HIV infection among IV drug abusers. However, the results would not have any influence on the specific therapy for septic arthritis.

   Plain x-ray films of the joint (**choice C**) are not helpful in diagnosis or management of infectious arthritis.

   Nonsteroidal anti-inflammatory and empiric antibiotic therapy (**choice D**) prior to arthrocentesis would be a mistake in this context, since isolation of the pathogen is necessary to institute appropriate antibiotic therapy.

2. **The correct answer is B.** This patient is displaying signs and symptoms of acute bacterial endocarditis (ABE), with fever, chills, a heart murmur, Janeway lesions, and a positive history of drug use. A thoracic echocardiogram is the most appropriate first step for finding the vegetations of ABE on heart valves, which are diagnostic. Blood cultures are also diagnostic, but take two days for a result and confirm only the bacteremia itself, not its source. Since the mortality is great for ABE, empiric antibiotics should be initiated after three sets of blood cultures are drawn. The organism is most likely *Staphylococcus aureus*, and the right-sided valves are more commonly affected in IV drug users. The tricuspid regurgitation murmur (a holosystolic murmur along the sternal border that increases with inspiration) should always suggest the diagnosis of *S. aureus* endocarditis.

   ECG findings (**choice A**) are not sensitive for diagnosing endocarditis.

   There is no role for CT (**choice C**) or cardiac catheterization (**choice E**) in this case. The findings do not suggest syphilis; however, both an HIV test and an RPR (**choice D**) would provide useful information, although neither would aid in the diagnosis of ABE.

3. **The correct answer is C.** This patient is having a hypertensive hemorrhage. The caudate and the putamen are the most common sites for such bleeds (70%), which can lead to dangerous elevations in intracranial pressure (ICP), as in this patient. The signs and symptoms of increased ICP, when present, portend imminent herniation of the brain and certain death. These patients require urgent intervention to lower their blood pressure.

   The cerebellum (**choice A**) is an uncommon site (<5%) for hypertensive hemorrhage. When cerebellar hemorrhages occur, urgent intervention is required because they can cause brainstem compression and/or obstructive hydrocephalus.

   Epidural hematoma (**choice B**) is usually the result of trauma to the squamous portion of the temporal bone of the skull and is not associated with hypertension.

   Subarachnoid hemorrhage (SAH; **choice D**) is infrequently associated with severe hypertension and is usually accompanied by meningismus. Once the SAH is identified, neurosurgical intervention to stop the bleeding can be performed, and the patient thereafter has a normal life expectancy. The most common nontraumatic cause for SAH is a berry aneurysm in the anterior portion of the circle of Willis.

   Subdural hematoma (**choice E**) results from tearing of the bridging subdural veins, most often due to trauma or shearing forces. It is uncommon without trauma and, even when present, does not tend to produce headache and increased ICP unless very severe.

4. **The correct answer is B.** The patient has unstable angina. Unstable angina with ECG changes is associated with critical coronary artery stenosis in most cases. One goal of therapy is to prevent thrombus formation on complex atherosclerotic plaques; heparin is the most effective proven treatment to prevent progression of unstable angina to myocardial infarction. Heparin is also required to maintain vessel patency when using relatively fibrin-specific thrombolytics, such as tPA. Heparin may cause delayed thrombocytopenia in about 10% of cases.

   Nifedipine (**choice A**), a calcium channel blocker, has no proven benefit in the therapy of acute myocardial infarction. The drug decreases afterload and may cause a reflex tachycardia.

   The patient does not meet the criteria for thrombolytic therapy (**choice C**). The best candidate for thrombolytic therapy is one in whom the ECG has distinct regional ST segment elevation or new left bundle branch block. Thrombolytic therapy has not been shown to benefit patients with inverted T waves, ST segment depression, or nonspecific ST-T waves changes and chest pain.

   The patient may eventually require catheterization (**choice D**) to see the extent of the coronary artery disease, but it is not the appropriate next step in management.

Angioplasty (**choice E**) should be considered if chest pain refractory to medical management persists, but it is not the appropriate next step in management.

5. **The correct answer is A.** This patient has benign paroxysmal positional vertigo. The pathophysiology appears to involve granular masses (tiny rocks) that sit on the cupola in the inner ear, pushing the cilia (hairs) on the sensory cells down. Certain positions compress the cells more, producing vertigo. Patients should be instructed to avoid the position that sets off the vertigo. A canalith repositioning maneuver is effective in most cases, but chronic cases may require surgical treatment. Some cases resolve spontaneously within a year.

    Cholesteatoma (**choice B**) is a tumor-like, benign lesion that can destroy the middle ear and occurs in the setting of chronic otitis media.

    Herpes zoster oticus (**choice C**), or herpes infection of the ganglion of CN VIII, causes severe ear pain, vertigo, hearing loss, and sometimes facial nerve paralysis.

    Ménière disease (**choice D**) causes the triad of vertigo, tinnitus, and fluctuating hearing loss, but is usually not triggered by positional changes.

    Presbycusis (**choice E**) is a progressive loss of sensitivity to high frequency sounds with age.

6. **The correct answer is E.** Progressive supranuclear palsy is a degenerative disorder that predominantly affects the midbrain and basal ganglia. The clinical hallmarks are symmetric parkinsonism with vertical gaze limitation and axial rigidity. These patients tend to have falls as their earliest symptoms. There is an associated mild-to-moderate dementia that usually involves frontal lobe functions more than hippocampal/memory systems. These patients tend to show a very modest response, if any, to L-dopa/carbidopa. Imaging is typically unremarkable.

    The basal ganglia (**choice A**) is a common site of small lacunar strokes in patients with hypertension and/or diabetes. Most of these tend to be asymptomatic, and vascular parkinsonism requires a heavier burden of disease in the basal ganglia. In addition, a unilateral left putamenal lacunar infarct would result in right-sided, rather than symmetric, symptoms.

    Carbon monoxide poisoning (**choice B**) results in bilateral pallidal (globus pallidus) necrosis. These patients develop symmetric parkinsonian symptoms but would not be expected to have vertical gaze problems. In addition, an MRI would demonstrate bilateral lesions in the putamen.

Cervical stenosis (**choice C**) with impingement on the spinal cord can present with falls and a spastic gait but should not affect eye movements or cognition. These patients should have hyperreflexia and upgoing toes.

Idiopathic Parkinson disease (**choice D**) typically begins asymmetrically, with resting tremor and rigidity worse on one side of the body. Vertical eye movements are not usually affected. Falls occur but normally a few years into the course of the disease. Patients with idiopathic Parkinson disease will usually experience a pronounced improvement in symptoms when started on carbidopa-levodopa.

7. **The correct answer is C.** This is the typical presentation of gonorrhea in men. The infection may regress spontaneously, progress to involve the epididymis and prostate, or become chronic, resulting in urethral strictures. In women, the infection is more often clinically silent, but when symptomatic, the manifestations frequently begin during menses, with frequency, dysuria, and urethral discharge. Chronic cervicitis is an important reservoir of gonococci. If gonococci cannot be demonstrated in smears of the discharge, cultures become necessary. For uncomplicated urethritis or cervicitis, a single intramuscular injection of ceftriaxone, 125 mg, is the treatment of choice and guarantees compliance.

    Amoxicillin (**choice A**) and penicillin G (**choice E**) are no longer recommended because of the increasing prevalence of penicillin-resistant strains of gonococcus.

    Chlamydial infection develops frequently in association with gonorrhea. Thus, therapy with ceftriaxone should be combined with a drug effective against chlamydia. Erythromycin, 500 mg four times daily for one week, or alternatively azithromycin (**choice B**) in a single oral dose of 1 g, may be used.

    Doxycycline (**choice D**) is also effective against chlamydia and should be administered at a dosage of 100 mg twice daily for one week.

8. **The correct answer is D.** This woman has carcinoid syndrome. The classic triad of this disorder is flushing (present in 85%), watery diarrhea, and valvular heart disease. The first test for screening carcinoid syndrome is the determination of 5-HIAA (metabolite of serotonin, 5-HT) in a 24-hour urine sample (carcinoid patients may excrete more than 25 mg/day). Carcinoid syndrome is also associated with hypotension, bronchospasm, telangiectasia, and abdominal cramps due to the release of serotonin and vasoactive peptides, especially in bronchial carcinoid. There may also be a secondary niacin deficiency, causing dermatitis, depression, and diarrhea. Symptomatic treatment of carcinoid syndrome consists of giving the synthetic peptide octreotide.

KAPLAN) MEDICAL

Barium examination of the bowel (**choice A**) will often not demonstrate the primary carcinoid tumor, most commonly located in the distal ileum.

Measurement of serum lipase and amylase levels (**choice B**) is indicated in the diagnosis of pancreatitis.

Ultrasound examination (**choice C**) would be indicated if she had symptoms pointing to an abdominal mass or gallbladder disease.

Small bowel biopsy (**choice E**) is invasive and would not aid in the diagnosis.

9.   **The correct answer is E.** The tumor is a malignant melanoma, which is a neoplastic proliferation of melanocytes. The cells in these tumors are related to neuroendocrine cells and often stain immunohistochemically for S-100. The prognosis in malignant melanoma is closely related to the depth of the lesion, therefore shallow lesions are much less likely to metastasize than lesions of 1 mm or more thickness, which have reached the rich lymphatic plexus of the superficial dermis. Shallow melanomas have a close to 100% cure rate with wide (typically 1 cm) excision, whereas deep melanomas have a dreadful prognosis since they typically have already metastasized by the time of surgical removal and usually fail to respond to chemotherapy.

Alpha-fetoprotein (**choice A**) is a marker for testicular and ovarian tumors with a yolk sac component, as well as hepatocellular carcinoma.

CA-125 (**choice B**) is a marker for some ovarian tumors.

LCA (**choice C**) is a marker for some lymphoid neoplasms.

PSA (**choice D**) is a marker for prostatic carcinoma.

10.   **The correct answer is D.** This patient probably has giardiasis, caused by *Giardia lamblia*. The diagnosis of giardiasis can often be made clinically on the basis of symptoms of flatulence and bloating appearing several days after a trip to Mexico. Metronidazole is the treatment of choice for giardiasis.

Supportive care with IV fluids (**choice A**) is used for patients with *Escherichia coli* "traveler's diarrhea" who are severely dehydrated. Patients generally have diarrhea the day after they return from their trip, rather than one week later.

Ciprofloxacin (**choice B**) is effective for *Shigella* and *Salmonella* infections. Patients usually have fever and blood or leukocytes in the stool, since these agents are invasive.

Mebendazole (**choice C**) is indicated for infection with helminths.

Trimethoprim-sulfamethoxazole (**choice E**) is not effective against *Giardia lamblia*.

11.   **The correct answer is C.** Diabetes mellitus is the most common cause of chronic renal failure in the U.S. (and probably in all industrialized countries). Diabetic nephropathy is one of the most severe complications and manifests on average 10-15 years after the onset of diabetes. The earliest expression of diabetic nephropathy is microalbuminuria, while the patient is otherwise asymptomatic. This is the rationale for screening diabetic patients for microalbuminuria, which should be performed by 24-hour urine collection or on an early morning urine sample. In the latter case, dipstick screening (**choice B**) may not be sufficiently sensitive. The *albumin:creatinine ratio* in an early morning urine sample is a convenient alternative to 24-hour collection. A ratio <3.5 is normal and >10 is abnormal between these two values; reevaluation is recommended. During the phase of microalbuminuria, aggressive treatment, including strict glycemic and blood pressure control, is in order.

Measurement of serum creatinine levels (**choice A**) would not be valuable in detecting preclinical renal damage.

Treatment with ACE inhibitors (**choice D**) has been shown to slow progression of renal nephropathy, possibly because of the reduction of intraglomerular pressure. This treatment is not widely used if microalbuminuria is absent and the patient is normotensive.

Renal biopsy (**choice E**) is not indicated in asymptomatic diabetic patients as a method for prevention of renal disease.

12.   **The correct answer is B.** The patient has pernicious anemia, in which gastric atrophy causes megaloblastic anemia due to vitamin B_{12} deficiency. The gastric atrophy characteristically involves the corpus, with sparing of the antrum. Most cases appear to have an autoimmune basis, with antibodies to parietal cells detected in 90% of patients; antibodies to intrinsic factor and the proton pump (H^+/K^+ ATPase) are also commonly present. The lack of parietal cells and the damage to the proton pump lead to markedly decreased acid secretion by the stomach. Lack of intrinsic factor leaves the small bowel unable to absorb vitamin B_{12}, leading to megaloblastic anemia.

Acute erosive gastritis (**choice A**) is seen most often in severely ill patients, who develop multiple small gastric ulcers.

Linitis plastica (**choice C**) is an aggressive form of adenocarcinoma of the stomach that produces a "leather bottle" stomach.

Ménétrier disease (**choice D**) is characterized by markedly thickened gastric folds with mucous gland hyperplasia. It presents with weight loss and severe protein wasting because of protein loss from the gastric mucosa.

Peptic ulcer disease (**choice E**) usually occurs in the setting of *Helicobacter pylori* infection or NSAID use and is very rare in pernicious anemia, since gastric acid secretion is markedly diminished.

13. **The correct answer is A.** Instituting chemotherapy in this patient has resulted in tumor lysis syndrome (TLS). TLS results from the acute lysis of lymphoma cells and acute renal failure from the precipitation of uric acid and hypoxanthine in the renal collecting tubules. Patients should receive allopurinol, a xanthine oxidase inhibitor that reduces the synthesis of uric acid, and should be aggressively hydrated prior to the initiation of chemotherapy to reduce the incidence of TLS.

Diphenhydramine (**choice B**) is an antihistamine that may be used in allergic conditions. Because TLS is not due to a drug allergy, diphenhydramine has no role in its prevention or management.

Furosemide diuretic (**choice C**) is reserved for well hydrated patients with insufficient diuresis. It increases the excretion of water but has not been proven to be beneficial as front-line therapy in TLS. It may contribute to uric acid or calcium phosphate precipitation in renal tubules in volume-contracted patients.

N-acetylcysteine (**choice D**) is used in the treatment of acetaminophen overdose and may be used to reduce hemorrhagic cystitis due to cyclophosphamide and ifosfam. However, it has no role in the prevention of TLS.

Nifedipine (**choice E**) is a calcium channel blocker used to treat hypertension and angina. It has no role in the prevention of TLS.

Urinary alkalinization, not urinary acidification (**choice F**), is a method of managing TLS. Intravenous sodium bicarbonate promotes alkaline diuresis and acts to solubilize (and thus minimize) intratubular precipitation of uric acid.

14. **The correct answer is E.** The patient has acute myeloid leukemia (AML). Auer rods are pathognomonic for AML. Patients who have this disease and undergo bone marrow transplantation in the first remission have a 50% to 60% chance of long-term, disease-free survival. The major complications of allogeneic bone marrow transplantation are infection, failure of graft survival, recurrent leukemia, and graft-versus-host disease. The incidence of graft-versus-host disease can be reduced by removal of T cells from the donor marrow by using monoclonal antibodies, rosetting techniques, or mechanical separation.

B cells (**choice A**) are not as important as T cells in graft-versus-host disease.

Megakaryocytes (**choice B**), promyelocytes (**choice C**), which are granulocyte precursors, and pronormoblasts

(**choice D**), which are erythrocyte precursors, play no role in graft-versus-host disease.

15. **The correct answer is C.** This woman most likely has idiopathic thrombocytopenic purpura (ITP). ITP is most common in adults (women > men) aged 20-40 years. Spontaneous bleeding, epistaxis, oral bleeding, or menorrhagia can occur, and isolated thrombocytopenia (<10,000) is characteristic. Ten percent of patients will have coexistent autoimmune hemolytic anemia (note the reticulocytosis and anemia). The first-line therapy is prednisone if the patient is not actively bleeding. Patients who are bleeding may require IV immunoglobulin (**choice B**) to block phagocytic activity; in severe and refractory cases, splenectomy (**choice E**) may be required.

Cryoprecipitate (**choice A**) is an effective treatment for von Willebrand disease.

Plasmapheresis (**choice D**) is the treatment of choice for hemolytic uremic syndrome (HUS) in a coagulation disorder setting. The most striking features of HUS are fever, fragmented RBC, and renal failure without neurologic signs. HUS is often seen after a diarrheal illness, particularly after infection with *Escherichia coli* 0157:H7.

16. **The correct answer is E.** Papillary structures within follicles that have epithelial cells with nuclei with cleared centers ("orphan Annie eyes") indicate the presence of papillary carcinoma of the thyroid. It does not matter whether the papillary structures are present in only a percentage of the follicles; the condition is still considered to be papillary carcinoma. Of all thyroid cancers, 60% to 70% are papillary carcinomas. The condition is more frequent in younger patients but tends to be more aggressive in the elderly. There is usually a single dominant nodule that is "cold" (does not take up radioactive iodine) on thyroid scan. Among the different types of thyroid cancers, papillary carcinoma tends to be the one with the best overall prognosis, and smaller lesions can be treated with thyroid lobectomy alone. Large or more diffusely spreading lesions require complete thyroidectomy, sometimes with ablation of any residual thyroid tissue with large doses of ^{131}I.

Follicular carcinoma of the thyroid (**choice A**) would not exhibit the papillary structures or orphan Annie nuclei seen in this case. Well-differentiated follicular carcinoma can be very difficult to distinguish from normal thyroid tissue.

Graves disease (**choice B**) would be characterized by prominent hyperthyroid symptoms and would show smaller than normal amounts of colloid on biopsy. This disease is not characterized by a single hard nodule; a symmetric, diffusely enlarged goiter may be found.

Hashimoto disease (**choice C**) would produce a diffuse goiter and would show an intense lymphocytic infiltrate with destruction of follicles on biopsy. Symptoms of hypothyroidism are often apparent.

Nontoxic goiter (**choice D**) produces a goiter that may be either smooth or multinodular, but does not usually have a single dominant nodule. On biopsy, the follicles are typically of a wide range of sizes, and the patient is usually clinically euthyroid.

17. **The correct answer is E.** The dose of traditional unfractionated heparin required for anticoagulation can be determined by following the partial thromboplastin time (PTT). Heparin prolongs the PTT. This test is performed by adding particulate matter to a patient's blood sample to activate the intrinsic coagulation cascade; the PTT therefore reflects activity of the intrinsic coagulation pathways.

Bleeding time (**choice A**) reflects the interaction of platelets with the vascular endothelium leading to the formation of an initial clot. An abnormal bleeding time usually reflects abnormal or diminished platelets.

Factor Xa levels (**choice B**) can be used to follow the dosing of the newer, low-molecular-weight heparins.

Platelet count (**choice C**) should be followed while giving IV heparin, since a minority of patients will develop heparin-induced thrombocytopenia. The platelet count, however, is not the test used to monitor efficacy of heparin therapy and any dosing changes.

Prothrombin time (PT; **choice D**) is a measure of the extrinsic coagulation system. This value, and the corresponding international normalized ratio (INR) of patient and normal PTs, is particularly sensitive to deficiencies in factor VII. It is usually used to help guide warfarin therapy.

18. **The correct answer is A.** Acoustic neuroma, also known as neurilemoma or schwannoma, is a benign tumor that typically arises from the neurilemmal sheath of the vestibular portion of the acoustic nerve in the auditory canal. Symptoms are produced by compression or displacement of the cranial nerves, brainstem, and cerebellum and by obstruction of CSF flow. The trigeminal (CN V) and facial (CN VII) nerves are often affected because of their anatomic location and relationship to the acoustic nerve. Clinical findings include insidious onset of sensorineural hearing loss, tinnitus, and a sensation of fullness in the ear. Facial numbness, facial weakness, headache, and gait ataxia may also be present; vertigo ultimately develops in 20% to 30% of patients. The most useful diagnostic test is MRI of the cerebellopontine angle. Treatment is surgical excision of the lesion.

Patients with benign positional vertigo (**choice B**) experience vertiginous symptoms only when their head is in a specific position. Symptoms are usually most severe when the patient is in the lateral decubitus position with the affected ear down. Hearing loss is not a feature of this condition.

There is no specific reason to suspect Lyme disease (**choice C**), although it should be included in the differential.

Ménière disease (**choice D**) is characterized by repeated episodes of vertigo lasting minutes to days, tinnitus, and progressive sensorineural hearing loss.

Tertiary syphilis (**choice E**) or neurosyphilis presents 3 to 10 years after untreated syphilis, with personality changes, ataxia, blurred vision, headache, dizziness, and hearing loss. Pupillary response to light is lost (Argyll Robertson pupils), and there is loss of proprioception and vibration sense. Although this patient has a history of syphilis at age 20, he was treated and his present rapid plasma reagin test is negative. Therefore, neurosyphilis is unlikely.

19. **The correct answer is C.** Obesity can be defined by using the nomograms based on the statistical studies of the National Center for Health Statistics on large population samples in the U.S. These data allow estimating the body mass index (BMI) from height (in inches) and weight (in pounds) [To calculate this index more rigorously, BMI = weight/(height)^2, where weight is in kilograms and height is in meters]. Most authors agree that obesity is present when the BMI is higher than 30 kg/m^2. This patient has a BMI of 33 kg/m^2. Once obesity is identified, the most appropriate next step is to determine whether obesity is secondary to underlying pathologic conditions. Physical examination and history should focus on detecting signs and symptoms of the three most common causes of secondary obesity, namely hypothyroidism, Cushing syndrome, and genetic conditions. In this case, menstrual irregularities and slight hirsutism are features that suggest the need to undertake additional investigations to rule out endocrinologic or genetic causes. Stein-Leventhal syndrome (in addition to those mentioned) should be considered in this case.

No intervention at this time (**choice A**) would not be appropriate. Active diagnostic and therapeutic interventions are needed for all patients whose BMI is >30 kg/m^2, and patients with BMI >27 kg/m^2 should be encouraged to lose weight. In fact, it is well established that obesity is associated with increased risk of developing hypertension, diabetes, cardiovascular disease, cholelithiasis, pulmonary dysfunction, osteoarthritis, and some forms of cancer.

The physician should explain the risks of obesity and benefits of weight loss (**choice B**) to all overweight patients, even if they are already painfully aware of the disadvantages inherent to obesity, with regard to both health risks and social stigma.

Treatment options for obese patients include decreasing calorie intake and/or increasing energy expenditure, variably combined with techniques of behavioral modification. A weight reduction program for a very-low-calorie diet (**choice D**) is an aggressive approach that replaces the whole daily food intake with a diet or a beverage containing no more than 800 kcal/day, 1 g protein/kg of body weight, plus all of the necessary vitamins and minerals. This diet is used as part of a comprehensive weight-loss program, in which the patient is closely monitored by a medical specialist to prevent possible serious adverse effects.

Pharmacologic treatment with the serotonin reuptake inhibitor sibutramine (**choice E**) has been approved by the FDA for treatment of obesity. However, the long-term effects of this therapy are still under investigation. Hypertension has been observed in some patients. In any case, this type of treatment should be used only after secondary obesity has been excluded.

20. **The correct answer is A.** Cancers involving the upper third of the esophagus are usually squamous cell in origin; histologically, they are described as anaplastic squamous cells with numerous mitotic figures. Lower esophageal cancers may be either squamous cell carcinomas or adenocarcinomas (usually arising in Barrett esophagus). Esophageal cancer has a very poor prognosis (most patients die within two years) because the cancer usually has advanced through the esophageal wall by the time the patient presents with dysphagia. Because the esophageal wall is thin, it is easy for the cancer to penetrate to the level of the lymphatics (less than 1 mm), where metastasis can occur, or penetrate completely through the esophagus (2 to 4 mm) to directly involve nonresectable mediastinal structures, such as the aorta, heart, or vicinity of the carina of the bronchial tree. Predisposing factors for squamous cell carcinoma of the esophagus include alcohol and tobacco use, human papillomavirus, esophageal scarring (lye ingestion, irradiation), sclerotherapy, and chronic achalasia.

Large, lymphocytic cells with large, prominent nucleoli (**choice B**) describe large cell lymphoma, whereas small, lymphocytic cells with irregular nuclei and condensed chromatin (**choice D**) describe small cell lymphoma. Both of these cancers are unlikely to be found in this patient.

Mucin-producing glandular tissue with signet ring cells (**choice C**) is the classic description of adenocarcinoma, which is unlikely to be found in the upper third of the

esophagus. It usually arises in patients who have had long-standing metaplastic changes of Barrett esophagus.

Small, polygonal cells with neurosecretory granules (**choice E**) describe small cell carcinoma of the lung, which is also called oat cell carcinoma. This cancer is strongly associated with cigarette smoking and usually presents as a central or hiker lung tumor.

21. **The correct answer is C.** This patient is experiencing an aplastic crisis due to parvovirus infection. Parvovirus exposure is common in daycare centers. Individuals with sickle cell disease, like those with other chronic hemolytic diseases, are susceptible to infection with parvovirus. Patients usually present with weakness, lethargy, and severe anemia often preceded by a few days of nonspecific symptoms. These patients have intense reticulocytopenia and the bone marrow contains no erythroid precursor cells, despite a normal myeloid series. A transient aplastic crisis due to parvovirus infection may produce life-threatening anemia and may require urgent transfusion. Note that Howell-Jolly bodies are consistent with asplenism.

Influenza virus (**choice A**) and parainfluenza virus (**choice B**) present with fever and systemic symptoms, including myalgia, headache, and malaise. Sudden development of severe anemia with reticulocytopenia is not seen in these infections.

Salmonella infection (**choice D**) is more common in sickle cell patients because of splenic hypofunction, but it presents either as typhoidal illness or diarrhea. Selective red cell aplasia is not a feature of *Salmonella* infection. Note that osteomyelitis due to *Salmonella* is more common in sickle cell patients.

Infection due to *Streptococcus pneumoniae* (**choice E**), although common in sickle cell disease patients because of splenic hypofunction, more frequently manifests as pneumonia or, less commonly, as meningitis.

22. **The correct answer is D.** The clinical picture is virtually pathognomonic of migraine, especially considering the premonitory visual symptoms (the aura), the throbbing quality of the pain, and the positive family history. However, migraine does not always present classically. A common form of migraine may be more frequent, with diffuse (not unilateral) throbbing pain of moderate intensity, which is not preceded by visual disturbances or associated with nausea. Acute treatment is based on the administration of antimigraine drugs at the onset of symptoms. Effective drugs include ergotamine tartrate or similar compounds, and sumatriptan. Prophylactic treatment is aimed at decreasing the frequency of attacks. Calcium channel blockers (**choice B**), for example, have been used for prophylaxis.

Acetaminophen (**choice A**) is very unlikely to provide relief in classic migraine, especially if aspirin and ibuprofen have already failed to do so.

Carbamazepine (**choice C**) has been found particularly helpful in the treatment of trigeminal neuralgia (*tic douloureux*), but not in migraine.

Prednisone (**choice E**) should be used to treat patients manifesting signs and symptoms strongly suggestive of giant cell arteritis (temporal arteritis), which may lead to blindness in the absence of effective anti-inflammatory therapy. However, temporal arteritis is much more common in the elderly and would not be in the differential diagnosis in this 20-year-old.

23. **The correct answer is A.** Ductal carcinoma of the pancreas is often devastating because, in roughly 90% of cases, it presents late in the clinical course, when it is no longer resectable. Therefore, the first step when this disease is suspected on clinical grounds is a CT scan, which is now recommended as the most cost-effective method of both diagnosing and staging the tumor (i.e., determining whether it is potentially resectable). If unresectable disease is detected, then definitive tissue diagnosis (for choice of chemotherapy) can be made on the basis of CT-guided percutaneous needle aspiration or biopsy. If a potentially resectable lesion is identified, endoscopic ultrasound (not yet widely available) can be used to search for small metastatic lesions not visible with CT.

MRI (**choice B**) is no more accurate than CT in detecting and staging pancreatic cancer, and is more expensive.

Ultrasound (**choice C**) is still frequently used, but usually is followed by CT scan. Therefore, the current thinking is to eliminate this test and go directly to CT, since the ultrasound is less sensitive.

Arteriography (**choice D**) is rarely used and is primarily for determining vascular invasion and tumor resectability.

Endoscopic retrograde pancreatography (**choice E**) is still commonly used in working up pancreatic cancer. However, this is an invasive procedure and would not be the first step in diagnosis.

24. **The correct answer is A.** A sensation of a curtain passing across the visual field can be characteristic of either amaurosis fugax or retinal detachment (**choice D**). In this case, the phenomenon is transient, so amaurosis fugax is more likely than retinal detachment. Fleeting blindness is characteristically caused by retinal emboli from ipsilateral carotid disease. The visual loss is described as a curtain passing vertically across the visual field, with complete monocular visual loss lasting a few minutes. Amaurosis fugax may be due to cholesterol plaque release and is a precursor of retinal artery occlusion.

Diabetic retinopathy (**choice B**) is the most common cause of blindness in the U.S. in adults aged 20-65 years, but the clinical description favors a diagnosis of amaurosis fugax.

Retinal artery occlusion (**choice C**) is characterized by sudden profound visual loss. Pupils are unreactive to direct light, and there is a cherry-red spot on the fovea.

Retinal detachment (**choice D**) causes progressive, unilateral, and painless blurred/loss of vision in one eye. There is often a sensation of a curtain passing down over the eyes.

Retinal vein occlusion (**choice E**) produces a sudden decrease or loss of vision; the pupils react sluggishly to light. Younger patients may present with near normal vision, whereas older patients may have significant obscuration.

25. **The correct answer is D.** Preventive programs are aimed at reducing the likelihood that a disease develops or worsens. Preventive programs can be divided into three types. *Primary prevention* attempts to prevent disease before it develops. Examples of primary prevention include all those programs aimed at reducing the risk of specific diseases: avoidance of cigarette smoking to prevent lung cancer and cardiovascular disease, immunizations to reduce the risk of infectious illnesses, and so on. Often, public health programs for primary prevention are more effective than an individual-based approach. For example, increasing taxes on cigarettes has been shown to reduce cigarette smoking more effectively than has advice to quit smoking given by physicians. Nevertheless, the beneficial role of physicians in individual-based prevention is undeniable.

Secondary prevention is based on early detection of an existing pathologic state before it causes damage to the organism. Examples of secondary prevention include the following: annual mammography for women older than 45 (**choice A**) to detect breast cancer in early stages, controlling hypertension (**choice C**) and blood lipid levels (**choice B**) to reduce the risk of atherosclerotic complications, and Pap smear screening (**choice E**) to detect early stages of cervical cancer or its histologic precursors.

Tertiary prevention is based on rehabilitative interventions or other methods to improve the clinical evolution of a disease that has already developed. Prophylactic aspirin after myocardial infarction (**choice F**) is a classic example of tertiary prevention.

26. **The correct answer is A.** Diabetic patients are particularly prone to gangrene of the feet. Sensory loss due to peripheral neuropathy, small vessel disease leading to ischemia, and secondary infections are the pathogenetic factors underlying this pathology. Diabetes is the leading cause of nontraumatic amputations. In addition to strict

glycemic control to prevent vascular and neurologic complications, the most effective method of prevention is self-care. The patient should receive instructions on daily foot self-examination (to look for abrasions and blisters), wearing appropriate shoes, cutting toenails straight across, and avoiding barefoot walking.

Doppler examination of the lower extremities (**choice B**) assesses vascular insufficiency. However, since the arteries may become rigid because of calcific atherosclerosis, falsely elevated blood pressure readings may be obtained with this test.

Periodic neurophysiologic and electromyographic studies (**choice C**) are not useful to prevent foot complications. Neurophysiologic and electromyographic studies may be performed when there are symptoms of peripheral neuropathy.

Local application of platelet-derived growth factor (**choice D**) has some efficacy in treating nonhealing ulcers refractory to debridement and antibiotic therapy.

Prophylactic treatment with cholesterol-lowering agents (**choice E**) should be considered for diabetic patients with high cholesterol levels to prevent or slow atherosclerotic change.

27. **The correct answer is B.** The skin manifestations of discoid lupus and systemic lupus erythematosus can be indistinguishable. Although the two conditions probably represent extremes of a spectrum, it is convenient to separate them into discoid lupus, which can have absent to minimal systemic effects, and systemic lupus, which often has significant effects on other organ systems. A real clinical question arises in newly diagnosed patients who may have either just skin manifestations or skin manifestations that are the earliest feature of what will become systemic disease. The identification of antibodies to double-stranded DNA, which are more specific than antinuclear antibodies, can exclude discoid lupus, since they are not encountered in this variant. Unfortunately, not all patients with systemic lupus develop these antibodies, so a negative result is not helpful. In these cases, the progression over time will permit disease classification.

Alopecia, or hair loss, of the scalp (**choice A**) can be seen in both conditions.

Noncontracting scars (**choice C**), usually at the centers of old lesions, can be seen in both conditions.

A positive antinuclear antibody test (**choice D**) is almost always seen in systemic lupus, but can also be seen in up to 10% of discoid patients.

Sun sensitivity (**choice E**) is seen in both conditions.

28. **The correct answer is C.** The patient is neutropenic with an absolute neutrophil count (ANC) of 100 (1,000 × 10%). He has symptoms of meningitis. By definition, a patient with an ANC less than 500 is neutropenic. Such patients are susceptible to gram-negative bacteria, such as *Pseudomonas*, and would be treated with IV ceftazidime.

Bacteroides (**choice A**) is an anaerobic agent and, along with *Clostridium*, is a typical pathogen in abscesses and gangrene. Infection with *Bacteroides* would require treatment with IV metronidazole.

Haemophilus (**choice B**) is the most common cause of meningitis in children. It is a gram-negative organism and would require treatment with an IV antibiotic, such as a third-generation cephalosporin.

Staphylococcus (**choice D**) could cause meningitis after a penetrating wound and would require treatment by a IV penicillinase-resistant antibiotic, such as nafcillin or vancomycin.

Toxoplasma (**choice E**) is a serious CNS infection in patients with HIV. Patients with *Toxoplasma* encephalitis will have focal or multifocal abnormalities demonstrable on CT or MRI. Common neurologic symptoms include seizures, meningoencephalitis, and headaches.

29. **The correct answer is C.** The clinical presentation is consistent with mitral stenosis, with its typical opening snap followed by a diastolic "rumbling" murmur. Echocardiography is the technique of choice to evaluate mitral valve abnormalities; it can confirm an auscultatory diagnosis of mitral stenosis.

Rheumatic fever continues to be one of the most frequent causes of mitral valve stenosis. Rheumatic fever is usually a sequela of a pharyngitis due to group A beta-hemolytic streptococci. Elevated antistreptolysin O titers (**choice A**) are used to confirm recent streptococcal infection but would have no value in the assessment of long-term complications of rheumatic heart disease.

Doppler ultrasound (**choice B**) can give quantitative estimates of transvalvular gradients and mitral valve area, but this is usually performed after echocardiography.

Radionuclide angiography (**choice D**) is mainly used to assess left and right ventricular ejection fraction. This technique also allows the study of segmental wall motion, and can be used to estimate valvular regurgitation and measure pulmonary-to-systemic flow ratio in left-to-right shunts. It is not commonly used in the diagnosis of mitral valve disease.

Most of the information needed in cases of mitral stenosis can be obtained by clinical and usually echocardiographic studies. Thus, cardiac catheterization (**choice E**) is not necessary, unless surgery is being considered and additional information is necessary.

KAPLAN MEDICAL

30. **The correct answer is C.** The patient has a pheochromocytoma, which has produced the severe hypertension with excess urinary metabolic products of epinephrine and norepinephrine demonstrated in the 24-hour urine collection. The family history of "endocrine problems" suggests the possibility of multiple endocrine neoplasia (MEN), of which medullary carcinoma of the thyroid may be a part, particularly in type IIa (Sipple syndrome) and type IIB (mucosal neuroma syndrome).

    Graves disease (**choice A**) and Hashimoto disease (**choice B**) can be associated with other autoimmune diseases, but are not associated with the MEN syndromes.

    Multinodular goiter (**choice D**) can be associated with iodine deficiency.

    Papillary carcinoma of the thyroid (**choice E**) can be associated with history of neck irradiation.

31. **The correct answer is A.** Acute interstitial nephritis is probably the second most common cause of intrinsic renal failure (after acute tubular necrosis). The most frequent causative factors are drugs, including penicillins (especially methicillin), cephalosporins, sulfonamides, NSAIDs, rifampin, and phenytoin. Coexistence of skin rash, eosinophils in the urine, and blood eosinophilia is an important diagnostic clue.

    Acute pyelonephritis (**choice B**) often develops in the setting of some underlying urologic diseases. In children, the most common underlying factor is vesicoureteral reflux. High fever, flank pain, and abundant pyuria are the main clinical manifestations.

    Acute tubular necrosis (**choice C**) develops as a result of severe hypoxia, prolonged prerenal azotemia, exogenous nephrotoxic agents (e.g., aminoglycosides), or endogenous substances (e.g., myoglobinuria, hemoglobinuria, or severe hyperuricemia). Granular casts, but not eosinophils, are found in the urine.

    Henoch-Schönlein purpura (**choice D**) is due to a small-vessel vasculitis secondary to IgA deposition. It manifests with some combination of purpura (due to dermal vessel involvement), nephritic syndrome, abdominal pain, melena, and arthralgia.

    Poststreptococcal glomerulonephritis (**choice E**) is associated with a classic nephritic syndrome, which manifests with pedal and periorbital edema, hypertension, hematuria, and mild proteinuria. Red blood cell casts are seen in the urine.

32. **The correct answer is E.** This young man has developed asymmetric, noninfectious polyarthritis, conjunctivitis, and Achilles tendinitis following a self-limited diarrheal episode. This is called Reiter syndrome, or reactive arthritis. The other features of this syndrome are urethritis, circinate balanitis, keratoderma blennorrhagica, anterior uveitis, and an association with HLA-B27.

    Abdominal pain and chronic diarrhea are the main features of Crohn disease (**choice A**). Intestinal malabsorption and significant weight loss may be present. Arthritis is seen in some patients with Crohn disease and affects lumbosacral and sacroiliac joints, as well as peripheral joints. However, Crohn disease is usually not characterized by an acute, self-limited diarrheal episode.

    Felty syndrome (**choice B**) consists of chronic rheumatoid arthritis, splenomegaly, neutropenia, and, on occasion, anemia and thrombocytopenia. It is most common in individuals with long-standing disease. These patients frequently have high titers of rheumatoid factor, subcutaneous nodules, and other manifestations of systemic rheumatoid disease.

    In gout (**choice C**), the initial attack typically affects only one joint, most commonly the first metatarsal joint. Monosodium urate crystals in the joint fluid, which appear long, needle-shaped, and negatively birefringent, are diagnostic. The synovial fluid leukocyte count tends to be higher, in the 25,000 to 50,000/mm^3 range.

    Juvenile rheumatoid arthritis (**choice D**) is a particular arthritis involving mainly the knees and hips. Achilles tendinitis is not a feature of this disease.

    Septic arthritis (**choice F**) should always be considered with sudden-onset inflammatory arthritis in one or more joints. It can lead to rapid destruction if it is untreated. Septic arthritis is classified as gonococcal or nongonococcal, and it is presumptively diagnosed when synovial fluid has a white blood cell count over 50,000/mm^3 and over 90% neutrophils. Organisms are often found on Gram stain of synovial fluid.

33. **The correct answer is A.** This patient presents with clinical manifestations consistent with drug-induced neutropenia. Neutropenia is defined as a blood cell count lower than 1,500/mm^3. Neutropenic patients are susceptible to bacterial and fungal infections. Drugs that may cause neutropenia include chlorpromazine, sulfonamides, procainamide, methimazole, propylthiouracil, penicillins, cephalosporins, and multiple chemotherapeutic agents. Clinical severity may vary considerably in relation to the degree of neutropenia. Sore throat and oral ulcers (stomatitis) are the mildest signs, but life-threatening infections may be the presenting manifestation. If signs of infection are absent, the patient may be followed on an outpatient basis, and, of course, suspected drugs should be immediately discontinued.

    Topical corticosteroid therapy for stomatitis (**choice B**) is not useful in this case. It is occasionally beneficial in aphthous ulcers (i.e., small but painful erosions of the buccal mucosa). Oral ulcers associated with neutropenia will resolve as soon as leukocyte counts return to normal levels.

Treatment with myeloid growth factors (G-CSF and GM-CSF; **choice C**) may be used to hasten recovery of bone marrow in patients with neutropenia secondary to chemotherapy.

Admitting the patient for broad-spectrum antibiotic treatment (**choice D**) is not recommended unless there is fever or other signs of infection. Hospitalization may indeed be more risky than useful to neutropenic patients, since it exposes them to nosocomial infections.

Examination of bone marrow aspirate (**choice E**) is not useful in this case, since both the condition and its under-lying cause (i.e., neutropenia due to chlorpromazine toxicity) are relatively obvious, and are reversible with discontinuation of the drug.

34.   **The correct answer is E.** Pleural effusions may be tran-sudative or exudative. This effusion is exudative since the pleural fluid/serum LDH ratio is greater than 0.6. Causes of exudates include parapneumonic effusion, tuberculo-sis, pulmonary infarct, malignancy, and bacterial infec-tion. Organisms in the fluid, a pleural fluid leukocyte count of 50,000, and a low pH constitute a complicated parapneumonic effusion. Such collections tend to locu-late and form adhesions if not immediately drained with a chest tube.

This infection may prove too tenacious to eradicate with antibiotic coverage alone (**choice A**). The risk of mortality increases with age and extent of hemodynamic compromise. This patient probably has a streptococcal infection and would need coverage with a penicillin in association with chest tube placement.

Diuresis (**choice B**) would be an option if this patient had heart failure that was compromising his respiratory status, but such effusions are simple transudates.

Biopsy (**choice C**) will not be helpful in the diagnosis in this patient with an obvious parapneumonic effusion; thoracentesis must be performed, and the fluid exam-ined. A common complication of a biopsy is pneumo-thorax.

Pleurodesis (**choice D**) might be an option if this were a malignancy and the patient had recurring effusions, compromising his pulmonary function. This is often achieved by injecting talc or bleomycin in the pleural space, thereby causing adhesions between the two layers of pleura and preventing future fluid collections.

35.   **The correct answer is B.** This patient now has neuro-logic manifestations of Lyme disease. Approximately 15% of patients at some point develop frank neurologic abnormalities, including meningitis, encephalitis, chorea,

cranial neuritis (including bilateral facial palsy), motor and sensory radiculoneuritis, or mononeuritis multiplex. The usual pattern is fluctuating meningoencephalitis with superimposed cranial nerve (particularly facial) palsy and peripheral radiculoneuropathy, but Bell's palsy may occur alone. The best treatment is admission to the hospital for IV ceftriaxone (2 g daily for 10-21 days). An alternative is IV penicillin G (20 million units a day for 10-20 days).

Chloramphenicol (**choice A**) and vancomycin (**choice C**) are not appropriate drugs for the treatment of Lyme disease.

Oral antibiotic therapy (**choices D and E**) is not appro-priate for treating advanced neurologic Lyme disease.

36.   **The correct answer is B.** The clinical picture is consistent with Parkinson disease at a relatively early stage. Resting tremor may be unilateral at first. Anticholinergic drugs, such as benztropine, are frequently used initially and are effective in alleviating tremor and rigidity. The key to the correct answer is the fact that the patient's history includes narrow-angle glaucoma. Use of anticholiner-gic drugs may lead to an acute increase of intraocular pressure in predisposed individuals and precipitation of narrow-angle glaucoma. Other contraindications to the use of anticholinergics include prostatic hyperplasia (or symptoms of urinary retention) and gastrointestinal obstruction (or severe constipation).

Amantadine (**choice A**) is also used for mild parkin-sonism, although its mechanism of action is unclear. Depression, postural hypotension, and cardiac arrhyth-mias are the most serious adverse effects.

Bromocriptine (**choice C**) is one of the dopamine agonists used for Parkinson disease. This drug was used before the introduction of levodopa; currently, it is sometimes used in association with low doses of levodopa-carbidopa. Bromocriptine is contraindicated in patients with neuropsychiatric disturbances, recent myocardial infarction, or peptic ulcer.

Levodopa (**choice D**) is the drug of choice for treatment of Parkinson disease. Nausea, vomiting, and hypotension are the most common side effects.

Selegiline (**choice E**) is an inhibitor of monoamine oxi-dase B. It is used as an adjunctive treatment along with levodopa. Available evidence suggests that selegiline might be effective in retarding progression of the disease.

37.   **The correct answer is C.** The tumor is a hepatocellu-lar carcinoma, which usually develops in the setting of cirrhosis because of a variety of damaging agents. By far the most commonly implicated etiologic factor, both worldwide and in the U.S., is infection with hepatitis B

or C. Other important risk factors include alcohol abuse, hemochromatosis, and aflatoxin exposure.

Aflatoxin (**choice A**) is a fungal toxin found in contaminated bean products, including soy beans and soy products (e.g., soy sauce).

Hemochromatosis (**choice B**) is a disease of disordered iron metabolism, which particularly damages the liver, pancreas, heart, and skin.

Opisthorchis (**choice D**) is a liver fluke that infects the biliary tract and predisposes to cholangiocarcinoma, not hepatocellular carcinoma.

Thorotrast (**choice E**) is a radiologic contrast medium that is no longer used because it caused predisposition to cholangiocarcinoma, not hepatocellular carcinoma.

38. **The correct answer is D.** The tuberculin skin test is usually applied to the forearm. Reaction should be read measuring the transverse diameter of induration as detected by gentle palpation at 48-72 hours. Reaction of >15 mm is considered a positive test in patients from a low-risk population. The degree of erythema is unimportant.

An induration of 5 mm (**choices A, B, and C**) is considered positive in patients at high risk to be infected (i.e., immunocompromised patients) and household contacts of tuberculosis patients.

An area of induration measuring 10 mm (**choice E**) is considered positive only in patients from population groups at elevated risk of tuberculosis (i.e., health care workers).

39. **The correct answer is A.** *Cat-scratch disease* is an acute infection due to *Bartonella henselae* that is transmitted to humans by a cat scratch or bite. A papule or an ulcer develops at the site of the scratch/bite, followed one to two weeks later by fever, malaise, and regional lymphadenopathy. The disease is self-limiting and does not require any treatment. Rarely, biopsies of lymph nodes are necessary to establish a diagnosis. Affected lymph nodes will exhibit a necrotizing granulomatous reaction with characteristic stellate-shape areas of necrosis. *B. henselae* also causes bacillary angiomatosis in immunocompromised patients.

Bartonella quintana (**choice B**) is the etiologic agent of *trench fever*, which is transmitted by the human body louse.

Calymmatobacterium granulomatis (**choice C**) causes a sexually transmitted disease known as *granuloma inguinale*. A slowly enlarging, painless ulcer develops at the inoculation site, followed by granulomatous inflammation in the inguinal lymph nodes and, subsequently, scarring and adhesions.

Chlamydia psittaci (**choice D**) is the etiologic agent of *psittacosis*, transmitted by infected birds (parrots, parakeets, pigeons, and others). The disease manifests one to two weeks after exposure. It consists of atypical pneumonia indistinguishable from that caused by either viruses or bacteria.

Pasteurella multocida (**choice E**) is part of the normal mouth flora of cats and dogs. It is the most common pathogen causing early infection secondary to cat and dog bites. This manifests within 24 hours after the bite with local swelling and pain, regional lymphadenopathy, and fever.

40. **The correct answer is A.** The long history of osteoarthritis should suggest chronic analgesic abuse as the underlying etiology of this renal condition, which is chronic tubulointerstitial nephritis. Analgesic nephropathy affects patients who consume significant amounts of aspirin, NSAIDs, phenacetin, or acetaminophen for at least three years. Clinical surveys have shown that patients often underestimate the amount of analgesics that they ingest daily. Note the main diagnostic clues of chronic tubulointerstitial nephritis: progressive polyuria because of inability of the renal tubules to concentrate urine, hyperkalemia, presence of radiologic signs of papillary necrosis (often associated with this condition), concomitant microhematuria, and mild proteinuria. Microcytic anemia may develop because of gastrointestinal blood loss secondary to the same drugs.

Lead exposure (**choice B**) is now a rare cause of chronic tubulointerstitial nephritis in the U.S. Lead intoxication also results in impaired tubular secretion of uric acid and hyperuricemia (note normal uric acid levels in this case); consequently, "saturnine" gout may ensue. Peripheral neuropathy may also manifest, leading to wrist drop. Suspect lead intoxication in alcoholics who drink "moonshine" alcohol prepared in old automobile radiators.

Multiple myeloma (**choice C**) is associated with bone involvement that manifests with pain and pathologic fractures. The resulting monoclonal gammopathy may cause renal damage. These patients are generally the elderly and may also present with a normochromic, normocytic anemia and hypercalcemia.

Obstructive uropathy (**choice D**) is another frequent cause of tubulointerstitial nephritis and papillary necrosis. It is commonly accompanied by an underlying disease, such as urolithiasis or prostatic hyperplasia. This patient does not have a history of renal disease.

Polycystic kidney disease (**choice E**) is an inherited renal disorder, presenting as multiple bilateral cysts that increase renal size and reduce functioning renal tissue. Patients may develop renal failure in the fourth to sixth decade of life. Abdominal pain, hypertension, hematuria, and impaired concentrating ability of the kidneys are common findings. Multiple bilateral cysts in the renal parenchyma and enlarged kidneys are seen on ultrasound and intravenous pyelography.

Vesicoureteral reflux (**choice F**) manifests in children and young adults with recurrent urinary tract infections. It is associated with hydronephrosis (dilatation of renal pelvis) and would not present for the first time in a 56-year-old.

41. **The correct answer is F.** The clinical symptomatology is strongly suggestive of "drop attacks" resulting from transient ischemia in the vertebrobasilar territory. Ischemia of the pyramidal tract in the brainstem is the most probable pathogenetic mechanism. Transient ischemic attacks (TIAs), by definition, last less than 24 hours (usually less than 1 hour). TIA is often a harbinger of stroke, especially when involving the carotid circulation.

Adverse drug reaction (**choice A**) must be considered as a potential etiology of frequent falls in an elderly patient, especially when hypotension is the suspected mechanism and there is a history of antihypertensive medication. The most common adverse effect of alendronate is esophagitis.

Lateral medullary infarction (**choice B**) follows occlusion of the vertebral or posterior inferior cerebellar artery. Manifestations include ataxia, vertigo, nystagmus, impaired pain and temperature sensation on the ipsilateral face and contralateral body, dysphagia, and hoarseness.

Parkinson disease (**choice C**) leads to resting tremor, rigidity, and bradykinesia. Falls due to Parkinson disease result from loss of postural reflexes, which can be assessed by the *pull-test*.

Postural hypotension (**choice D**) is a frequent cause of falls in the elderly and is often the result of medication. Typically, the patient reports a light-headed sensation on standing or getting up from bed, and the fall may be accompanied by a transiently obtunded consciousness.

The carotid bruit in this case is probably secondary to atherosclerotic stenosis of the carotid artery but not to the patient's symptoms. Transient ischemia in the carotid territory (**choice E**) manifests with motor deficits, sensory symptoms, or alterations in language expression or comprehension (aphasia).

42. **The correct answer is E.** Clinical features suggestive of pulmonary embolism in this patient are pleuritic chest pain, hemoptysis, tachycardia, tachypnea, and elevated serum lactate dehydrogenase (suggestive of lung infarction). Individuals with nephrotic syndrome are at increased risk of pulmonary embolism because of an underlying hypercoagulable state. Possible mechanisms responsible for the underlying hypercoagulability include loss of anticoagulant proteins in the urine and intravascular volume depletion. The ECG findings are indicative of acute cor pulmonale, which may mimic inferior myocardial infarction (MI); however, an inferior

wall MI is characterized by prominent Q waves and ST segment elevations in leads II, III, and AVF.

Aortic dissection (**choice A**) typically causes severe, tearing chest pain radiating to the back. Loss or decrease of a peripheral pulse, new-onset aortic insufficiency, and pericardial tamponade are possible physical findings of aortic dissection.

Esophageal spasm (**choice B**) can cause retrosternal chest pain and is usually associated with a history of dysphagia. The pain is typically substernal and usually not pleuritic in nature. It accounts for about 10% of noncardiac causes of chest pain.

Myocardial infarction (**choice C**) classically presents with retrosternal chest pain that may radiate to the left arm, neck, or jaw. The pain is described as a dull ache, heaviness, or pressure in the chest and may be associated with dyspnea, diaphoresis, light-headedness, nausea, and vomiting.

Pneumonia (**choice D**) may cause unilateral pleuritic chest pain if there is pleuritis or pleural effusion complicating the pneumonia. However, the patient would have fever and cough, indicating the presence of infection.

Variant angina (**choice F**) presents with chest pain or pressure at rest and classic transient elevation of the S-T segment on ECG. Reduced coronary blood flow results from transient coronary spasm. Variant angina is not associated with elevated serum LDH or Q and T wave inversions on ECG.

43. **The correct answer is E.** Renal involvement is one of the most common manifestations of systemic lupus erythematosus (SLE) and a major cause of morbidity and mortality. When renal abnormalities are detected in patients with SLE, a renal biopsy must be performed. SLE may, in fact, lead to various types of morphologic changes, which can be evaluated only by tissue examination and have fundamental implications for choosing the most appropriate therapy. Such changes have been divided into five types. Type I and II lesions (normal and mesangial proliferative, respectively) require no treatment. Type III and IV lesions (focal segmental proliferative and diffuse proliferative, respectively) require aggressive immunosuppressive treatment. Type V lesions (membranous glomerulopathy) require immunosuppression if superimposed proliferative lesions are found.

A repeat urinalysis at the next routine examination (**choice A**), while adequate in patients with type I and II lesions, is not appropriate in SLE patients in whom the underlying glomerular changes are still unknown.

Sequential serum complement and ANA studies (**choice B**) are useful to monitor response to treatment, or to follow patients with type I and II lesions. A return to normal values of markers such as C3, C4 and dsDNA antibodies indicates remission, whereas rising levels in patients with type I and II lesions suggest the need of repeat biopsy studies.

Treatment with corticosteroids (**choice C**) represents the mainstay of therapy for SLE patients with proliferative glomerular lesions (types III and IV). If these patients do not respond to corticosteroids, cyclophosphamide is used (**choice D**).

44. **The correct answer is D.** The presence of rhomboidal, positively birefringent crystals in the joint aspirate is diagnostic of pseudogout. This type of crystal arthropathy usually occurs in persons older than 60 years. The crystals consist of calcium pyrophosphate and tend to deposit on the joint cartilage. Pseudogout is associated with a variety of metabolic disorders, such as diabetes, hypothyroidism, hyperparathyroidism, and hemochromatosis. Management consists of NSAID administration for acute episodes. Colchicine can be used for prophylaxis.

Charcot arthropathy (**choice A**), which is also called neuropathic arthropathy, is a rapidly destructive arthropathy due to impaired pain perception and position sense. Repetitive injury is unnoticed and causes relatively painless destruction of the joint. Charcot arthropathy is most commonly associated with diabetic neuropathy and tabes dorsalis. The presence of crystals and an inflammatory pattern are not seen on synovial fluid examination of Charcot joints.

Degenerative joint disease (**choice B**) does not produce crystals in the joint fluid.

Gout (**choice C**) typically presents with pain in the first metatarsophalangeal joint or in the knee joint. The joint aspirate would show negatively birefringent needle-shaped crystals.

Rheumatoid arthritis (**choice E**) usually presents with pain in small joints (e.g., hands and wrists), is symmetric, and is accompanied by morning stiffness greater than one hour in duration. It is associated with rheumatoid factor.

Septic arthritis (**choice F**) is associated with evidence of microorganisms in the joint aspirate or elsewhere in the body, and large numbers of neutrophils in the joint fluid.

45. **The correct answer is A.** Leprosy is endemic in many parts of Africa, Asia, and South America. The patients seen in the U.S. are usually immigrants from endemic regions. *Mycobacterium leprae*, the etiologic agent, cannot be cultured in artificial media. A characteristic feature of this mycobacterium is that it tends to affect cooler parts of the body, such as the nose, ears, and scrotum, and has a special tropism for peripheral nerves. In lepromatous leprosy, granulomas contain numerous acid-fast bacilli (AFB), which are easily identifiable on

tissue sections. This form results from defective cellular immunity and is the most contagious. Nodular lesions in the skin and areas of anesthesia are the most characteristic manifestations. Bilateral ulnar neuropathy is highly suggestive of lepromatous leprosy. It should be treated with a triple-agent combination therapy, including dapsone, clofazimine, and rifampin, for at least two years.

Lupus vulgaris (**choice B**) results from reactivation tuberculosis and is most commonly associated with nonnecrotizing granulomas, in which acid-fast bacilli are difficult to demonstrate by special stains.

Mycobacterium avium-intracellulare (MAI) (**choice C**) is an opportunistic infection that may cause fevers, lymphadenopathy, pneumonia, and hepatos plenomegaly. It does not typically produce the skin lesions described in this patient.

Sarcoidosis (**choice D**) of the skin may mimic leprosy, lupus vulgaris (i.e., skin tuberculosis), lupus erythematosus, and other conditions. It is characterized by nonnecrotizing granulomas, in which no infectious agent can be demonstrated by special stains, polymerase chain reaction (PCR) techniques, or culture. In most cases, the lungs and lymph nodes are involved. Sarcoidosis is a diagnosis "of exclusion," to be considered only after infectious and noninfectious etiologies have been ruled out.

Lepromatous leprosy differs significantly from tuberculoid leprosy (**choice E**), which is a milder form due to hypersensitivity to infecting bacilli. In tuberculoid leprosy, acid-fast bacilli are rarely found in the dermal histiocytic collections. It is treated with dapsone and rifampin for 6-12 months.

46. **The correct answer is A.** Of all the possible diagnoses, the one that will kill the patient the fastest, but is surgically treatable if caught early, is aortic dissection. Aortic dissection must be ruled out before heparin can be administered. A chest x-ray film can provide important information about a possible dissection. In 90% of patients with aortic dissection, widening of the aorta will be seen on chest x-ray. A left pleural effusion is also common. The diagnosis can also be made by transesophageal echocardiography (TEE), MRI, dynamic CT scan, or catheterization. These three methods have comparable accuracy, but TEE is preferred if available because it is the fastest and does not require the patient to lay still for a long period of time. Chest x-ray is available in more centers and will give the quickest results.

47. **The correct answer is E.** This patient's signs and symptoms indicate aspiration pneumonia with a resultant lung abscess. Lung abscesses in an unconscious or obtunded patient result from aspiration of infected

material from the upper airway. The causative organisms are usually mixed anaerobes from oral flora. This patient's infiltrate is in the superior portion of the right lower lobe, a common site of aspiration pneumonia. Sputum is copious in lung abscesses and often malodorous. Patients have risk factors for aspiration (drugs, CNS disease, general anesthesia, coma, or excessive sedation), and many patients have periodontal infection.

Acid-fast bacilli and caseating granulomas (**choice A**) refer to pulmonary tuberculosis. Although it may be seen in homeless alcoholics, tuberculosis more often presents with a protracted, rather than an acute, illness. Additionally, cavity formation classically occurs in the upper lung lobes.

Considering this patient's long history of tobacco use, a possible diagnosis is squamous cell carcinoma (**choice B**), which may lead to a mass with an air-fluid level that resembles a lung abscess radiographically. Additionally, some lung cancers can present with a postobstructive pneumonia with resultant lung abscess. However, lung cancer usually presents with symptoms over longer periods of time.

Fibrosis and needle-like ferruginous bodies (**choice C**) are the classic histology for asbestosis. Asbestosis results from long-term exposure to asbestos fibers and presents with progressive exertional dyspnea and fibrosis. Symptoms are not as acute as those found in this patient, and a history of asbestos or occupational exposure is needed for the diagnosis.

Pneumococcal pneumonia (**choice D**) is the most common community-acquired pneumonia. It is a lobar pneumonia that does not cavitate or cause lung abscesses. Additionally, presentation of fever, chest pain, dyspnea, and cough occurs more acutely than the two-week presentation seen in this patient.

48. **The correct answer is B.** Even when the clinical history and neurologic evaluation are consistent with Alzheimer disease, as in this case, MRI studies of the brain may rule out other conditions that may mimic this disorder. Marked ventricular dilatation without significant cortical atrophy, for example, would suggest normal pressure hydrocephalus, which may respond to CSF shunting. A subdural hematoma may manifest with dementia. An entirely normal-appearing brain may suggest nonorganic causes of dementia.

Electroencephalographic studies (**choice A**) are of limited value in the evaluation of dementing illnesses, except in the case of Creutzfeldt-Jacob disease.

Cerebral angiographic studies (**choice C**) are useful in evaluating the morphology of the cerebral vasculature to detect the location and degree of atherosclerotic ste-

nosis, as well as the presence of aneurysms or vascular malformations.

Lumbar puncture for CSF examination (**choice D**) is uninformative in most cases of dementia. Despite extensive research, a diagnostically useful CSF marker of Alzheimer disease has yet to be found.

Brain biopsy (**choice E**) is reserved for those rare cases in which clinical and radiologic investigations have failed to disclose any apparent cause of dementia, and there is evidence of a mass lesion in imaging studies.

49. **The correct answer is H.** The physical findings of pleural effusion on chest examination depend on the amount of fluid accumulating within the pleural space. If the amount is small, a pleural friction rub may be the only sign, sometimes associated with decreased tactile fremitus and breath sounds. If the pleural effusion is large, there is an extensive area of dullness to percussion, usually demarcated by a peripheral zone where compression of the lung parenchyma creates the acoustic conditions for transmission of bronchial breathing and egophony.

50. **The correct answer is L.** Sarcoidosis frequently involves the lungs and hilar lymph nodes. Other commonly affected sites include skin, lymph nodes (in regions other than the lung hila), eyes, peripheral nerves, liver, kidneys, and heart. Fever, weight loss, and malaise may be present. Respiratory symptoms are due to interstitial lung disease secondary to diffuse granulomatous inflammation and scarring. A picture of restrictive pulmonary disease, with reduced total lung capacity, develops. Nonnecrotizing granulomas are found on biopsy, but other conditions (such as mycobacterial and fungal infections) must be ruled out by special stains. Sarcoidosis, in other words, is a diagnosis "of exclusion."

Acute respiratory distress syndrome (**choice A**) manifests with rapid onset of shortness of breath and signs of acute respiratory failure poorly responsive to oxygen therapy. Acute predisposing conditions are usually present, the most common of which include sepsis, trauma, gastric aspiration, and shock.

Asthma (**choice B**) is characterized by recurrent paroxysmal episodes of respiratory difficulty due to bronchospasm. Severe asthma exacerbations are associated with loud respiratory wheezes. The patient may have no symptoms between asthma attacks.

Bronchiectasis (**choice C**) is due to progressive and irreversible bronchial dilatation, usually secondary to inflammatory destruction of bronchial walls. Cystic fibrosis is currently the most frequent cause of bronchiectasis in young adults, whereas COPD is more common in older patients, particularly smokers. Chronic cough productive of copious sputum is characteristic of bronchiectasis.

Carcinoma of the lungs (**choice D**) would be evident on a chest x-ray film as a mass, not as diffuse pulmonary infiltrates. It usually manifests in smokers with productive cough, recurrent bronchopneumonia, and weight loss.

Chronic aspiration of gastric contents (**choice E**) may lead to asthma attacks, bronchiectasis, or pulmonary fibrosis. It develops in patients with esophageal diseases (e.g., achalasia, progressive sclerosis, and, most commonly, gastroesophageal reflux) and is facilitated by smoking and alcohol.

COPD (**choice F**) is a clinical designation that applies to a picture in which airway obstruction is the predominant pathophysiologic element. It results from varying combinations of emphysema, chronic bronchitis, and bronchiectasis.

Cystic fibrosis (**choice G**) involves the lungs in virtually every affected patient, causing recurrent pneumonia (especially with *Pseudomonas*) and bronchiectasis. Respiratory involvement accounts for most deaths in cystic fibrosis.

Pneumocystis carinii pneumonia (**choice I**) manifests with fever, abrupt onset of shortness of breath, and rapid evolution to acute respiratory failure. It is a disease of immunocompromised patients, especially those with AIDS.

Pulmonary hypertension (**choice J**) typically develops as a complication secondary to other conditions, leading to increased pulmonary arterial resistance (most commonly COPD) or, rarely, as a primary disorder. Patients present with progressive dyspnea, fatigue, and chest pain. Chest x-ray films demonstrate right ventricular hypertrophy and enlarged pulmonary arteries.

Pulmonary thromboembolism (**choice K**) develops in the presence of predisposing conditions that result in venous thrombosis, usually affecting the deep veins in the legs. Abrupt onset of dyspnea, tachypnea, tachycardia, and chest pain are the most characteristic manifestations. Because chest x-ray films may be normal, the diagnosis relies on more specific imaging studies, namely ventilation-perfusion scans and pulmonary angiography.

Spontaneous pneumothorax (**choice M**) occurs in young adults and manifests with sudden onset of dyspnea. Hyperresonance and absent breath sounds on the affected side are present. Chest x-ray will demonstrate air within the pleural space.

Tuberculosis (**choice N**) of the lungs may be asymptomatic (usually the case in primary tuberculosis) or may manifest with productive cough, low-grade fever, malaise, and weight loss. Chest x-ray shows pulmonary infiltrates and cavitary lesions in the upper lobes.

Internal Medicine: **Test Three**

1. A 60-year-old man comes to his physician with complaints of easy fatigability and palpitations for the past six months. Physical examination is remarkable for pallor of skin and mucous membranes. No evidence of cardiac or respiratory disease is found. Hematologic studies show:

Hemoglobin	8.4 g/dL
Mean corpuscular volume (MCV)	75 fl
Leukocyte count	9,000/mm^3
Platelet count	380,000/mm^3

Serum chemistry studies show a ferritin of 25 ng/L and serum bilirubin within normal values. Peripheral blood smear shows small erythrocytes with marked variability in size. Which of the following is the most appropriate next step in management?

(A) Bone marrow biopsy

(B) Coombs test for anti-red blood cell antibodies

(C) Hemoglobin electrophoresis

(D) Test for occult blood in the stool

(E) Therapeutic trial with oral ferrous sulfate

(F) Treatment with vitamin B$_{12}$ and folic acid

2. A 28-year-old woman presents with painful swelling of her right hand and fingers of two days' duration. She has a low-grade fever and is currently menstruating. She denies a past history of sexually transmitted diseases. On examination, her temperature is 38.6° C (101.4° F), blood pressure is 130/70 mm Hg, pulse is 110/min, and respirations are 20/min. The digits on her right hand are swollen and held in mild flexion, with papules and vesicles in the web spaces. Her left knee and ankle are swollen and tender to touch. Laboratory evaluation shows:

Leukocytes	12,000 with 86% neutrophils
Hemoglobin	14.0 g/dL
Platelets	220,000/mm^3
Erythrocyte sedimentation rate	43 mm/h

X-ray films of the hand, knee, and ankle show no evidence of fracture. Which of the following tests is most likely to confirm the likely diagnosis?

(A) Cultures of cervix, rectum, throat, and blood

(B) Blood cultures

(C) Arthrocentesis for bacterial cultures

(D) Synovial fluid analysis for cell count

(E) Synovial fluid Gram stain

KAPLAN MEDICAL

3. A 39-year-old California rancher consults a physician because of chronic abdominal pain. The man has been a sheepherder for 23 years. Physical examination is notable for a palpable liver mass but is otherwise unremarkable. Ultrasound demonstrates a 15-cm cyst bearing multiple daughter cysts in the liver. CT confirms the presence of the cysts and demonstrates the presence of a finely calcified rim around the cysts. Which of the following is the most likely diagnosis?

    (A) Ascariasis

    (B) Echinococcosis

    (C) Fascioliasis

    (D) Schistosomiasis

    (E) Toxocariasis

4. A solitary nodule is detected on a chest x-ray film in an otherwise healthy 25-year-old man. The patient has been smoking 10 cigarettes daily for 3 years. The nodule is located in the right middle lobe and measures approximately 1.5 cm. Previous chest x-ray films are not available for comparison. CT scan reveals a solitary lung nodule with a smooth contour and diffuse calcifications. No other pulmonary lesions are found. Physical examination and routine laboratory tests are normal. Which of the following is the most likely diagnosis?

    (A) Aspergilloma

    (B) Bronchogenic carcinoma

    (C) Hamartoma

    (D) Pulmonary abscess

    (E) Sarcoidosis

    (F) Secondary (reactivated) tuberculosis

5. A 65-year-old woman is admitted with a three-week history of headache over the right temporal region, malaise, fever, morning stiffness, and weight loss. On physical examination, scalp tenderness is appreciated. Her temperature is 38.5° C (101.3° F), blood pressure is 142/84 mm Hg, pulse is 85/min, and respirations are 14/min. There is no loss of visual acuity, and funduscopic examination is unremarkable. Laboratory studies show the following:

Hematocrit	40.3%
Hemoglobin	11.9 g/dL
Leukocytes	7,800/mL (neutrophils 68%)
Erythrocyte sedimentation rate (ESR)	80 mm/h

    After reviewing the results, the physician initiates high-dose prednisone therapy. Which of the following is most likely to confirm the diagnosis?

    (A) CT scan of the head

    (B) Lumbar puncture

    (C) Muscle biopsy

    (D) Temporal artery biopsy

    (E) Visual evoked potentials

6. A 35-year-old man goes to the emergency department because he has developed a severe case of hives. He has never had hives before. Physical examination demonstrates multiple wheals and erythematous patches over his body, which respond to subcutaneous epinephrine. The patient's sclera are slightly yellow-tinged. Results of the chest and abdomen examination are within normal limits. Screening biochemistry tests demonstrate an AST (SGOT) of 350 U/L and an ALT (SGPT) of 300 U/L. Which of the following is the most likely diagnosis?

    (A) Alcoholic cirrhosis

    (B) Alpha$_1$-antitrypsin deficiency

    (C) Hemochromatosis

    (D) Hepatitis A

    (E) Hepatitis B

7. A 47-year-old Brazilian immigrant presents with fatigue and dyspnea. He has been healthy for the past 10 years. The patient denies fever, cough, chills, or weight loss. On physical examination there are no murmurs, the pulse and the rhythm are regular, S_1 is normal, and S_2 is split. This split increases with inspiration and persists with expiration. Which of the following ECG findings is most consistent with the auscultatory findings in this patient?

   (A) Acute ST segment elevation in the anterior leads

   (B) Decreased PR interval

   (C) Early repolarization

   (D) Marked T wave inversion

   (E) Right bundle branch block

8. An otherwise healthy 60-year-old man undergoes a health maintenance examination. Physical examination and medical history are unremarkable. A blood chemistry panel is normal except for a serum calcium level of 11 mg/dL when corrected for serum albumin. The measurement is repeated two times, giving values of 10.5 mg/dL and 11.2 mg/dL, respectively. Serum phosphorus is 2.5 mg/dL, and alkaline phosphatase is 50 U/L. Immunoradiometric assay (IRMA) reveals higher than normal serum levels of parathyroid hormone. Urine calcium excretion is within normal limits. The patient denies previous renal colic or urinary tract infections. Which of the following is the most appropriate next step in management?

   (A) Bone x-ray films

   (B) Extensive cancer screening

   (C) Generous fluid intake

   (D) Treatment with bisphosphonates (e.g., alendronate)

   (E) Surgical exploration of the neck

9. A 27-year-old African American man visits his primary care physician because of recent onset of "yellowness in the white of his eyes." His recent history is significant for a "chest cold" for which he is taking trimethoprim-sulfamethoxazole; he is also taking fluoxetine for depression. On examination, the sclera are icteric and the mucosa beneath the tongue appears yellow. No hepatosplenomegaly is present. Laboratory studies are as follows:

Hemoglobin	11.1 g/dL
Hematocrit	34%
Total bilirubin	6.2 mg/dL
Conjugated (direct) bilirubin	0.8 mg/dL
Alkaline phosphatase	77
AST (SGOT)	24
ALT (SGPT)	22

Which of the following is the most likely explanation for this patient's jaundice?

   (A) Acute infectious hepatitis

   (B) Cholestatic liver disease

   (C) Drug reaction from fluoxetine

   (D) Drug reaction from trimethoprim-sulfamethoxazole

10. A 26-year-old woman complains of painful and frequent urination for two days. She has no significant medical history and has had a monogamous sexual relationship with another woman for the past year. Her temperature is 37.2° C (99° F), blood pressure is 120/70 mm Hg, pulse is 68/min, and respirations are 12/min. There is no costovertebral angle tenderness, the abdomen is soft, and there is mild suprapubic tenderness. The pelvic examination is within normal limits except for tenderness at the urethral meatus. Urinalysis reveals 23 white blood cells per high-power field. Which of the following is the most likely pathogen?

   (A) *Chlamydia trachomatis*

   (B) *Escherichia coli*

   (C) *Klebsiella pneumoniae*

   (D) *Proteus* sp.

   (E) *Staphylococcus saprophyticus*

11. A 72-year-old man complains of malaise and easy fatigability for the past three weeks. His past medical history is significant for gout and pneumonia. He lives alone and usually drinks two six-packs of beer daily. His temperature is 36.9° C (98.4° F), blood pressure is 160/90 mm Hg, pulse is 88/min, and respirations are 19/min. Thyroid palpation is normal, and heart, lung, and abdomen examination results are within normal limits. There is a diffuse ecchymotic rash spreading out from hair follicles on the limbs and trunk. The patient most likely has a deficiency of which of the following vitamins?

(A) Niacin

(B) Thiamin

(C) Vitamin B_{12}

(D) Vitamin C

(E) Vitamin D

12. A 40-year-old man with a history of type V hyperlipoproteinemia is brought to the emergency department three hours after the abrupt onset of severe deep epigastric pain, nausea, and vomiting. The pain is steady and radiates to the back. The patient is agitated and has cool, clammy skin. His temperature is 38.5° C (101° F), blood pressure is 100/70 mm Hg, pulse is 110/min, and respirations are 22/min. Abdominal examination reveals tenderness in the upper abdomen, without guarding. A plain x-ray film shows an air-filled intestinal loop in the left upper quadrant. Laboratory investigations show:

Glucose	150 mg/dL
LDH	150 U/L
ALT	90 U/L
AST	80 U/L
Amylase	120 U/L
Lipase	30 U/L
Calcium	7 mg/dL
C-reactive protein	1.2 mg/dL

Which of the following is the most likely diagnosis?

(A) Acute cholecystitis

(B) Acute hepatitis

(C) Acute pancreatitis

(D) Bowel perforation

(E) Mesenteric ischemia

(F) Ureteral lithiasis

13. An 18-year-old man has had rhinorrhea and a sore throat for two days. He has no significant past medical history. His temperature is 39.3° C (102.6° F), pulse is 110/min, and respirations are 20/min. He has tender anterior and posterior cervical lymphadenopathy and an erythematous pharynx with white exudates on the tonsils. The remainder of his examination is normal. Which of the following is the most likely causal organism?

(A) *Candida albicans*

(B) *Haemophilus influenzae*

(C) *Staphylococcus aureus*

(D) *Streptococcus pneumoniae*

(E) *Streptococcus pyogenes*

14. Due to a recent and sudden death of a rival college football player, a local university wishes to implement changes in its health care policies. The school is particularly concerned about the risk for sudden cardiac death in players with previously undiagnosed heart conditions. A preparticipation evaluation is to be performed on all of the school's athletes. Which of the following is considered the most cost-effective method of screening young athletes at risk for sudden cardiac death?

(A) Careful medical history and examination

(B) Chest x-ray

(C) Echocardiography

(D) Exercise electrocardiography

(E) Resting electrocardiography

15. A 20-year-old male college student is participating in the New York City Marathon and collapses one-third of the way through the race. He is a well developed, athletic man who frequently plays basketball and tennis. He has no past medical history, except for a tonsillectomy at nine years of age. He had no symptoms before he collapsed to the ground and lost consciousness. The patient is immediately rushed to the nearest emergency room but is pronounced dead on arrival. Which of the following is the most likely underlying cause of his sudden death?

(A) Aortic stenosis

(B) Arrhythmogenic right ventricular dysplasia

(C) Coronary anomalies

(D) Hypertrophic cardiomyopathy

(E) Isolated left ventricular hypertrophy

(F) Myocarditis

(G) Ruptured aorta

16. A seriously ill AIDS patient is admitted to a hospital. He has multiple infections, including *Pneumocystis carinii* pneumonia, pulmonary cytomegalovirus infection, and candidiasis of the esophagus and possibly other sites. Screening chemistry studies are drawn, including electrolytes. Which of the following abnormalities would be most likely seen in this setting?

    (A) Hyperkalemia

    (B) Hypermagnesemia

    (C) Hypocalcemia

    (D) Hyponatremia

    (E) Hypophosphatemia

17. A 31-year-old man is admitted to the hospital for suspicion of gastrointestinal bleeding. He has no significant past medical history but takes daily nonsteroidal anti-inflammatory agents for pain in his knee. He presented to the hospital six hours ago after he noticed melanotic stools while at home. He is observed to have copious bright red blood per rectum. On physical examination, he is tachycardic, and his peripheral pulses are faint but present. His mental status appears normal. His extremities are cool to the touch. An intravenous line is placed. Which of the following is the most appropriate next step in management?

    (A) Order an urgent type and cross match for blood

    (B) Order an urgent hematocrit level

    (C) Begin parenteral administration of large volumes of normal saline solution

    (D) Begin parenteral administration of large volumes of colloid solution

    (E) Place two additional large bore peripheral intravenous catheters

18. A 40-year-old man presents to the physician for recent onset of exertional dyspnea. The patient appears comfortable at rest but says that he becomes short of breath with minimal effort. His temperature is 37° C (98.6° F), blood pressure is 162/65 mm Hg, pulse is 92/min with a rapid rise and fall, and respirations are 15/min. Chest examination reveals a prominent and laterally displaced apical impulse. A soft diastolic decrescendo murmur is heard along the left sternal border. Bilateral crackles are present at the lung base. The liver is not palpable, and there is no sign of peripheral edema. Which of the following is the most likely diagnosis?

    (A) Aortic insufficiency

    (B) Aortic stenosis

    (C) Hypertrophic obstructive cardiomyopathy

    (D) Infective endocarditis

    (E) Mitral stenosis

    (F) Ventricular septal defect

19. A 42-year-old man with AIDS presents with a chief complaint of persistent watery, nonbloody diarrhea. He is not on any medications and denies recent travel or fever. On physical examination, his abdomen is slightly bloated, with mild tenderness to palpation. There is no occult blood in his stool. Stool samples for leukocytes, culture, ova, and parasites are all negative × 3. Which of the following is the most appropriate next step in diagnosis?

    (A) Abdominal CT

    (B) Cytomegalovirus (CMV) antigenemia

    (C) Modified acid-fast stain of the stool

    (D) PPD test

    (E) Small bowel biopsy

20. A previously healthy 23-year-old man comes to the physician because of a febrile illness that developed over a two-day period. He has had temperatures to 39.4° C (102.9° F), with rigors, cough productive of mucopurulent sputum, and right chest pain. At this time, his temperature is 38.7° C (101.7° F), blood pressure is 132/80 mm Hg, pulse is 110/min, and respirations are 22/min. There is no cyanosis. Diminished tactile fremitus, dullness on percussion, and bronchial breathing are present in the right lower lung. A chest x-ray film shows consolidation of the right lower lobe. Microscopic examination of the sputum reveals gram-positive diplococci. The patient denies previous allergic drug reactions. Which of the following is the most appropriate pharmacotherapy?

    (A) Cefazolin

    (B) Erythromycin

    (C) Penicillin

    (D) Tetracyclines

    (E) Trimethoprim-sulfamethoxazole

    (F) Vancomycin

21. An otherwise healthy 22-year-old woman presents to her physician because of daily headaches over the past two weeks. The headaches have a vise-like character, seem to be more intense in the back of the head, and are often precipitated by emotional stress. Physical examination fails to disclose focal neurologic or visual deficits. Which of the following is the most appropriate initial step in patient care?

    (A) Antidepressant drugs

    (B) Calcium channel antagonists

    (C) Ergotamine-containing preparations

    (D) Nonsteroidal anti-inflammatory drugs (NSAIDs)

    (E) Sumatriptan

22. A 42-year-old woman presents to her physician because of recent urinary tract infections (UTIs). She has been on an unknown oral antibiotic chronically. She has a temperature of 37.2° C (99° F), and costovertebral angle tenderness is noted on the left side. A plain film of the abdomen reveals a radiopaque density filling the left renal pelvis and calyces. Which of the following is the most likely pathogen?

    (A) *Bacteroides fragilis*

    (B) *Clostridium difficile*

    (C) *Escherichia coli*

    (D) *Proteus mirabilis*

    (E) *Streptococcus bovis*

23. A 35-year-old woman has developed marked thickening of the skin of her hands, particularly her fingers. This thickening is accompanied by hyperpigmentation and is marked enough to limit the range of motion of her fingers. If this patient goes on to develop gastrointestinal problems, which of the following is most likely?

    (A) Carcinoid tumor

    (B) Duodenal peptic ulcer

    (C) Esophageal dysfunction

    (D) Pneumatosis cystoides intestinalis

    (E) Sacculations of the colon

    (F) Small bowel adhesions

24. A 23-year-old man presents with a three-month history of cough with blood-tinged sputum, shortness of breath, and gross hematuria. His temperature is 37.5° C (99.5° F), blood pressure is 158/94 mm Hg, pulse is 87/min, and respirations are 22/min. Examination reveals bilateral crackles at the lung base and mild edema of the palpebrae and feet. A chest x-ray film shows scattered pulmonary infiltrates in a distribution different from that present on a film taken two months ago. Examination of the sputum shows hemosiderin-laden macrophages but no microorganisms. Laboratory investigations show modest iron-deficiency anemia and no evidence of ANCA-type antibodies. Urinalysis shows gross hematuria and modest proteinuria. A renal biopsy demonstrates the presence of glomerulonephritis with linear deposition of IgG and complement components along the glomerular basement membrane. Which of the following is the most likely diagnosis?

    (A) Churg-Strauss syndrome

    (B) Goodpasture syndrome

    (C) Idiopathic pulmonary hemosiderosis

    (D) Postinfectious glomerulonephritis

    (E) Wegener granulomatosis

25. A 67-year-old man comes to the physician because of insomnia, irritability, and palpitations for three months. He is currently taking amiodarone for cardiac arrhythmias, fluoxetine for depression, and enalapril for hypertension. His blood pressure is 130/70 mm Hg, and his pulse is 90/min and regular. Which of the following is the most appropriate next step?

    (A) Measurements of thyroxine and TSH

    (B) Administration of propranolol

    (C) Referral for psychiatric consultation

    (D) Substitution of antidepressant drug

    (E) Substitution of antihypertensive drug

26. An unconscious 35-year-old man is brought to the emergency department by his wife. She explains that the patient takes phenytoin for chronic epilepsy. An hour ago, the patient had a seizure but did not regain consciousness. Physical examination reveals that his temperature is 38.5° C (101.3° F), blood pressure is 92/40 mm Hg, pulse is 110/min, and respirations are 20/min. During the examination, the physician observes the sudden onset of tonic-clonic convulsions. Which of the following is the most common precipitating cause of this emergency?

    (A) Alcohol withdrawal

    (B) Drug noncompliance

    (C) Head trauma

    (D) Hypoxia

    (E) Intracranial infection

    (F) Intracranial tumor

    (G) Metabolic alterations

27. A 26-year-old librarian presents with chronic daytime somnolence, which has frequently caused him to fall asleep at work. He does not smoke but drinks one to two glasses of wine daily. He says he frequently awakens at night but denies any visual or auditory hallucinations. His height is 186 cm (73 in), and his weight is 60% greater than expected. Chest examination reveals no specific findings other than distant breath sounds. Arterial blood gas analysis during normal ventilation shows:

Pa_{O_2}	82 mm Hg
Pa_{CO_2}	55 mm Hg

    After the patient voluntarily hyperventilates for one minute, blood gas analysis returns within normal limits. Which of the following will have the greatest benefit on this patient's symptoms?

    (A) Benzodiazepines at bedtime

    (B) Daily acetazolamide

    (C) Morning administration of dextroamphetamine

    (D) Supplemental oxygen at night

    (E) Weight loss

28. A 35-year-old man with a history of chronic heroin abuse comes to the physician because of progressive swelling of his hands and feet. His blood pressure is 155/90 mm Hg. Laboratory studies show:

Blood, serum

Creatinine	1.6 mg/dL
BUN	20 mg/dL

Urinalysis

Protein	4+
Erythrocytes	10/hpf

The amount of protein measured in a 24-hour urine collection is 4.5 g. Which of the following is the most likely diagnosis?

(A) Acute proliferative glomerulonephritis

(B) Crescentic glomerulonephritis

(C) Focal segmental glomerulosclerosis

(D) Minimal change disease

(E) Nodular glomerulosclerosis (Kimmelstiel-Wilson disease)

29. A 61-year-old man presents for an elective surgical incision and drainage procedure. The patient has an eight-year history of hepatitis C infection with well-documented cirrhosis and portal hypertension. He has a large hematoma on his thigh that is suspected to have necrotic tissue underlying it and therefore requires debridement. On preoperative screening, his prothrombin time is noted to be 17.4 seconds. Transfusion of which of the following is the most appropriate next step in management of this patient prior to his procedure?

(A) Cryoprecipitate

(B) Fresh frozen plasma

(C) Packed red blood cells

(D) Platelets

(E) Whole blood

30. A 55-year-old woman with long-standing diabetes mellitus and a two-year history of progressive renal failure comes to medical attention because of chest pain for 12 hours. The pain is substernal and continuous, with radiation to the neck. She is on a strict dietary regimen with protein, fluid, and salt restriction. Her temperature is 37.2° C (99° F), blood pressure is 150/85 mm Hg, pulse is 82/min and regular, and respirations are 16/min. There is no jugular vein distention or pitting edema. Auscultation reveals a rubbing sound in the precordial region and slightly distant but normal heart sounds. Lungs are clear to auscultation. The patient is admitted, and laboratory studies show:

Hematocrit	33%
Hemoglobin	11.2 g/dL
Leukocyte count	12,500/mm^3
Serum	
Urea nitrogen	102 mg/dL
Glucose	128 mg/dL
Na	142 mEq/L
K	5.3 mEq/L
Cl	103 mEq/L
Arterial blood	
pH	7.38
PO_2	92 mm Hg
PCO_2	39 mm Hg

A chest x-ray film shows a normal cardiac outline, and an ECG shows nonspecific ST changes. Echocardiogram reveals mild fluid collection within the pericardial sac. Which of the following is the most appropriate next step in management?

(A) Water and salt intake reduction

(B) Antibiotic treatment

(C) Antihypertensive treatment

(D) Anti-inflammatory treatment

(E) Erythropoietin administration

(F) Hemodialysis

(G) Pericardiocentesis

(H) Pericardial biopsy

(I) Partial pericardiectomy

31. A 28-year-old man comes to the emergency department complaining of abdominal pain. He has no significant past medical history, has had no recent illnesses, and denies any alcohol or drug abuse. He reports that three days ago, he developed acute pain in his right upper quadrant. The pain was nonradiating and was associated with nausea and two episodes of nonbloody, nonbilious emesis. He also reports that two days ago, he began to turn "yellow." On examination, he is afebrile and has scleral icterus with mild jaundice of his skin. His right upper quadrant is tender, with no palpable gallbladder and no Murphy's sign. Determination of which of the following is the most appropriate next step in diagnosis?

    (A) Serum hepatitis A IgG titer

    (B) Serum hepatitis A IgM titer

    (C) Serum hepatitis B surface antibody titer

    (D) Serum hepatitis C antibody

    (E) Serum hepatitis C RNA level

32. A 40-year-old woman comes to the physician because of a six-month history of increasing respiratory difficulty that occurs during mild exercise, such as walking uphill. She is 165 cm (65 in) tall and weighs 58 kg (129 lb), but says that she has lost 4 kg (9 lb) over the past three months. Her blood pressure is 120/75 mm Hg, pulse is 85/min, and respirations are is 16/min. Chest examination reveals crackles at both lung bases and a diastolic murmur near the cardiac apex. The characteristics of the murmur change with the patient's position. Echocardiography reveals a solid mass that partially fills the left atrium and results in obstruction of the mitral flow. Which of the following is the most likely diagnosis?

    (A) Fibroelastoma

    (B) Metastasis

    (C) Mural thrombus

    (D) Myxoma

    (E) Sarcoma

33. A 45-year-old woman with rheumatoid arthritis develops pain, erythema, and swelling of the cartilaginous portion of both of her external ears. This is accompanied by pain localized to the costochondral joints. Which of the following is the most likely diagnosis?

    (A) Ankylosing spondylitis

    (B) Behcet syndrome

    (C) Gout

    (D) Reiter syndrome

    (E) Relapsing polychondritis

34. An otherwise healthy 40-year-old woman comes to the physician because she discovered a painless nodule in her neck. On physical examination, palpation reveals a firm 1-cm nodule in the left cervical region, which moves upward as the patient swallows. Thyroid function tests are normal. Fine needle aspiration is positive for papillary carcinoma. Which of the following is a recognized risk factor for this form of cancer?

    (A) Amiodarone treatment

    (B) Dietary iodine supplementation

    (C) Family history of multiple endocrine neoplasia (MEN)

    (D) Graves disease

    (E) Hashimoto thyroiditis

    (F) Radiation to the neck

    (G) Subacute thyroiditis

    (H) Thyroglossal duct anomalies

35. A 40-year-old man is admitted for chemotherapy for treatment of acute myelogenous leukemia. A central line through his subclavian vein is inserted to facilitate infusion of chemotherapeutic agents. Ten days after this procedure, he develops a temperature of 39.4° C (103.0° F). Physical examination is remarkable for tachycardia and tenderness around the central line insertion site. Blood cultures and a chest x-ray film are negative. Which of the following is the most appropriate next step in management?

    (A) Repeat blood cultures and wait for culture results to guide therapy

    (B) Administer amphotericin

    (C) Administer vancomycin

    (D) Remove the central line

    (E) Remove the central line and insert a new one over a guide wire

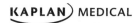

36. A recently widowed 35-year-old woman with an anxiety disorder, for which she has been taking alprazolam and imipramine, is brought to the emergency department for a multiple drug overdose. Her daughter states that she may have taken 30-40 tablets of 50-mg imipramine and 35-40 tablets of 1-mg alprazolam. On route to the hospital, she became apneic and was intubated. Her blood pressure is 130/84 mm Hg, and her pulse is 120/min. The patient is unresponsive to painful stimuli, and her pupils react very sluggishly, but there are no other neurologic findings. The ECG shows a normal sinus rhythm with a widened QRS complex. Which of the following is the most appropriate intervention?

    (A) DC cardioversion

    (B) Flumazenil

    (C) Ipecac

    (D) Lidocaine bolus

    (E) Maintenance of serum pH at 7.5

37. A 38-year-old woman visits the clinic because of oral tenderness and soreness in her jaw for the past two months. She admits that swallowing food has become more painful. She notices that her mouth is chronically dry and that drinking lots of fluids seems to reduce the pain. She has a normal appetite but reports that she has lost 2 kg (5 lb) and is eating less because of the pain associated with swallowing most foods. Physical examination reveals parched lips, dry oral mucous membranes, and bilaterally enlarged parotid glands with a firm, smooth texture. Needle biopsy of the salivary gland tissue reveals a dense, lymphocytic infiltrate with loss of many glands. Residual glands have prominent intraductal cellular proliferation. Which of the following is the most likely diagnosis in this patient?

    (A) Mucoepidermoid carcinoma

    (B) Pleomorphic adenoma

    (C) Sarcoidosis

    (D) Sjögren syndrome

    (E) Squamous cell carcinoma

    (F) Warthin tumor

38. A 52-year-old man with a 30-pack-year history of cigarette smoking presents to a physician after moving to a new city. He was told that he had "high cholesterol" about two years ago, and he has a history of mild hypertension for which he has never been treated. He had a myocardial infarction (MI) six months ago. His post-MI course has been uncomplicated, his exercise stress test was satisfactory, and he has experienced no subsequent chest pain. His medications include one aspirin tablet every other day. Physical examination is normal except for a fourth heart sound. Which of the following is the most appropriate next step in management to prevent significant morbidity and mortality?

    (A) Add a beta blocker

    (B) Add enalapril

    (C) Add nifedipine

    (D) Increase the aspirin to one tablet three times daily

    (E) Prescribe nitroglycerin for angina

39. A 17-year-old boy of Jewish descent is taken to the emergency department by his mother because of bloody diarrhea. Over the past two weeks, the boy has reported frequent urges to defecate that are accompanied by abdominal cramping. Over the past several days, the stools have become looser, and mucus was present around the feces. One hour ago, he saw fresh blood on his stool. On questioning, the boy notes that similar symptoms have occurred over the past two years, except for the blood in his stool. His temperature is 37.5° C (99.5° F), blood pressure is 120/70 mm Hg, pulse is 65/min, and respirations are 16/min. His abdomen is soft, without guarding, and there is localized tenderness in the right lower quadrant. Which of the following is the most likely diagnosis?

    (A) Appendicitis

    (B) Colon cancer

    (C) Diverticulitis

    (D) Mesenteric lymphadenitis

    (E) Pseudomembranous colitis

    (F) Ulcerative colitis

40. A 32-year-old man with AIDS has a CD4+ T cell count of 40/mm^3. He complains of a gradual onset of decreased vision in his right eye over the past few days. He is afebrile and has temporal wasting. There is a thick, cheesy, white exudate on his tongue and oropharynx, and there are deficits in the acuity and the visual fields of his right eye. The remainder of the cranial nerve examination is normal. Infection with which of the following pathogens is the most likely cause of his decreased vision?

    (A) *Candida albicans*

    (B) Cytomegalovirus (CMV)

    (C) Herpes simplex virus 1 (HSV-1)

    (D) *Mycobacterium avium-intracellulare* (MAI)

    (E) *Pneumocystis carinii*

    (F) Toxoplasmosis

41. A 5-year-old boy is brought to the emergency department four hours after sudden onset of fever and chills. He was bitten in his right hand by the family's dog 24 hours ago. Examination reveals superficial lacerations of the ulnar aspect of the right hand consistent with a history of dog bite. The wound is surrounded by extensive skin erythema and soft tissue swelling. Palpable lymph nodes are found in the right axilla. His temperature is 38.9° C (102° F). Which of the following is the most likely pathogen or pathogens?

    (A) *Capnocytophaga canimorsus*

    (B) *Eikenella corrodens*

    (C) Mixed aerobic and anaerobic bacteria

    (D) *Pasteurella multocida*

    (E) Staphylococci

    (F) Streptococci

42. A 65-year-old woman consults a physician with complaints of severe pain and stiffness of the neck, shoulders, and hips. These symptoms are worst in the morning and after inactivity. The woman has also been experiencing a variety of systemic symptoms, including malaise, low-grade fever, depression, and some weight loss. On physical examination, there is no evidence of erosive or destructive joint disease, no point tenderness when pressure is applied to small joints, no selective muscle weakness or muscle atrophy, and no rheumatoid nodules. Blood studies demonstrate a mild normochromic normocytic anemia, dramatically elevated erythrocyte sedimentation rate, and elevated c-reactive protein. Thyroid-stimulating hormone (TSH) is 0.75 mIU/mL. Rheumatoid factor is negative. Electromyography and muscle biopsy fail to demonstrate conclusive evidence of muscle disease. This patient's most likely condition has the strongest association with which of the following?

    (A) Crohn disease

    (B) Dermatomyositis

    (C) Discoid lupus erythematosus

    (D) Sjögren syndrome

    (E) Temporal arteritis

43. A 71-year-old man with a long history of poorly controlled hypertension presents to the emergency department with headache and visual changes. His blood pressure is 220/130 mm Hg. Current medications include atenolol, nifedipine, thiazide, and clonidine. An IV sodium nitroprusside drip is started. The patient is then transferred to the intensive care unit, where his blood pressure is 135/75 mm Hg; however, he becomes hypoxemic with room air saturations falling to 80%. Which of the following is the most likely reason for this patient's hypoxemia?

    (A) Elevation of carboxyhemoglobin levels

    (B) Elevation of methemoglobin level

    (C) Hypoventilation

    (D) Loss of hypoxic pulmonary vasoconstriction

    (E) Pulmonary embolism

44. A 45-year-old man with alcoholism is admitted with a diagnosis of acute pancreatitis. He requires large volumes of fluid to maintain blood pressure and urine output, but 24 hours after admission, he appears in stable condition. On the fourth hospital day, the patient develops rapidly progressive respiratory distress, with labored breathing and tachypnea. His temperature is 37.0° C (98.6° F), pulse is 100/min, blood pressure is 128/75 mm Hg, and respirations are 24/min. Intercostal retraction and crackles are appreciated on chest examination. Blood tests show:

Hematocrit	42%
Leukocytes	9,800/mm^3
Glucose	110 mg/dL
BUN	20 mg/dL
AST	98 U/L
ALT	60 U/L
Amylase	280 U/L
Arterial blood gas (room air)	
pH	7.32
Pa$_{O_2}$	52 mm Hg
Pa$_{CO_2}$	51 mm Hg

A chest x-ray film reveals diffuse bilateral infiltrates and air bronchograms, a normal cardiac silhouette, and minimal pleural effusions. Which of the following is the most likely diagnosis?

(A) Acute bilateral bronchopneumonia

(B) Adult respiratory distress syndrome (ARDS)

(C) Cardiogenic pulmonary edema

(D) Exacerbation of acute pancreatitis

(E) Pulmonary embolism

45. A 47-year-old woman comes to the physician because she has had several episodes of severe chest pain that awoke her in the early morning. She has no significant past medical history, denies smoking or drug abuse and drinks alcohol only occasionally. Her temperature is 37.0° C (98.6° F), blood pressure is 126/78 mm Hg, pulse is 78/min and regular, and respirations are 12/min. An ECG reveals no abnormalities. No further studies are undertaken, and the physician tells the patient that her pain is probably of psychological origin. After a few days, the patient comes to the emergency department at 5 A.M. complaining of chest pain. An ECG reveals sinus rhythm with ST segment elevation. The patient is admitted, and coronary arteriography is performed, revealing no stenotic lesions. Intravenous administration of ergonovine during arteriography triggers chest pain accompanied by ST elevation on ECG. Which of the following is the most likely diagnosis?

(A) Myocardial infarction

(B) Prinzmetal angina

(C) Psychological chest pain

(D) Stable angina

(E) Unstable angina

46. A 34-year-old female flight attendant presents with a recurring, sharp pain radiating from her left ear to her mouth. She describes the pain as intense but intermittent, precipitated by cold, light touch, and chewing. Neurologic examination is normal. A tentative diagnosis of trigeminal neuralgia is made, and carbamazepine is prescribed. She returns six weeks later complaining of the same pain on both sides of her face and a new onset of urinary incontinence. Which of the following is the most likely diagnosis?

(A) Acoustic neuroma

(B) Amyotrophic lateral sclerosis

(C) Bell's palsy

(D) Multiple sclerosis

(E) Myasthenia gravis

47. A 32-year-old woman is brought to the emergency department following the rapid onset of profound malaise and fever. On arrival, the patient's temperature is 39.7° C (103.5° F), blood pressure is 110/75 mm Hg, pulse is 110/min and regular, and respirations are 17/min. On examination, needle tracks and scars are noted on the forearms and thighs. Chest examination reveals a systolic murmur along the left lower sternal border. Blood tests show 16,000 leukocytes/mm^3 and an erythrocyte sedimentation rate of 90/min. Which of the following is the most appropriate next step in management?

(A) Broad spectrum antibiotic therapy

(B) Echocardiographic studies

(C) Three sets of blood cultures

(D) Toxicologic studies on blood and urine

(E) Ventilation-perfusion lung scans

48. An 18-year-old man comes to clinic for evaluation of weakness and fatigue lasting six weeks. Before these past six weeks, he reports being fairly healthy. He did, however, have a recent case of "the flu." On reviewing his medical records, it seems that approximately two months ago the patient had a mild hepatitis of unclear etiology (serologies for hepatitis A, B, and C were negative) that has since resolved. Before this illness, he has been healthy, takes no medications, and knows of no diseases that run in his family. He does not use illicit substances, does not smoke, rarely drinks alcohol, has never received a blood transfusion, has never had sex, and does not have any tattoos. Physical examination reveals marked pallor and a 2/6 nonradiating systolic murmur heard best at the right upper sternal border. Abdominal examination reveals a few scattered petechiae but no hepatosplenomegaly. Laboratory studies show:

Hematologic

Hematocrit	15%
Hemoglobin	5.0 g/dL
Leukocytes	4,000/mm^3 (normal differential)
Platelets	15,500/mm^3
Reticulocytes	0.5%

The rest of the patient's laboratory studies, including a set of chemistries and liver function tests, are unremarkable. The patient is admitted to the hospital and receives a transfusion with leukocyte-reduced blood products. A bone marrow biopsy is performed the next morning that shows cellularity of less than 5% with normal cellular morphology and no organisms on Gram stain. Which of the following is the most appropriate treatment?

(A) Antithymocyte globulin

(B) Bone marrow transplant

(C) Broad-spectrum antibiotics

(D) Colony-stimulating factor

(E) Intravenous corticosteroids

The response options for items 49-50 are the same. You will be required to select one answer for each item in the set.

(A)   Allergen skin testing

(B)   Bacterial cultures of skin scrapings

(C)   Blood glucose measurement

(D)   Gluten-free diet trial

(E)   HIV testing

(F)   Microscopic examination of KOH-treated skin scrapings

(G)   Serum IgE assays (RAST or ELISA)

(H)   Stroking on skin lesions with a blunt object

For each patient with recent onset of skin lesions, select the most appropriate initial diagnostic test.

49.   A 70-year-old woman has been in good health until three months ago, when she noted the appearance of plaques in her axillae and groin. She has also experienced anorexia and easy fatigability for the past few months. The patient has no history of major disease, and her family history is unremarkable. She is 165 cm tall (65 in) and weighs 53 kg (117 lb). Examination reveals several slightly raised, brown plaques with a velvety surface in the flexural regions of neck, axilla, and groin. A biopsy is consistent with acanthosis nigricans.

50.   A 40-year-old man presents with numerous brown spots on the skin. He reports a history of chronic diarrhea and generalized itching, the latter manifesting frequently after he takes aspirin or drinks alcoholic beverages. He has noticed that slight rubbing on affected skin results in redness and itching. He has had recurrent asthmatic episodes in the past few years. His recent medical history is also significant for 8-kg (18-lb) weight loss in the past six months. On examination, there are dozens of small, red-brown macules on the trunk and upper limbs. The spleen is palpable 4 cm below the left costal arch. A biopsy of these macules reveals a dense dermal infiltrate of cells that stain positively for toluidine blue.

Internal Medicine Test Three:
Answers and Explanations

ANSWER KEY

1.	D	26.	B
2.	A	27.	E
3.	B	28.	C
4.	C	29.	B
5.	D	30.	F
6.	E	31.	B
7.	E	32.	D
8.	C	33.	E
9.	D	34.	F
10.	B	35.	D
11.	D	36.	E
12.	C	37.	D
13.	E	38.	A
14.	A	39.	F
15.	D	40.	B
16.	D	41.	D
17.	C	42.	E
18.	A	43.	D
19.	C	44.	B
20.	C	45.	B
21.	D	46.	D
22.	D	47.	C
23.	C	48.	B
24.	B	49.	C
25.	A	50.	H

KAPLAN MEDICAL

1. **The correct answer is D.** Microcytic anemia with low ferritin levels is characteristically due to iron deficiency. Low serum ferritin indicates depletion of body iron stores, as does transferrin saturation below 15%. Severe iron deficiency will result not only in reduced mean corpuscular volume (MCV) of red blood cells, but also in variability in their size (anisocytosis) and shape (poikilocytosis). Iron-deficiency anemia is often accompanied by a high platelet count. In industrialized countries, iron-deficiency anemia should be assumed to result from chronic blood loss. The most important step in management is to identify the source of bleeding. In men, gastrointestinal hemorrhage is the most common underlying cause of iron-deficiency anemia. Thus, a test for occult blood in the stool is the initial screening study in this situation. Proper investigations must then be carried out to disclose the source of bleeding, which may be due to conditions such as peptic ulcer, gastritis, or colon cancer.

Bone marrow biopsy (**choice A**) is not necessary in classic cases of microcytic anemia secondary to iron deficiency. It is sometimes helpful to rule out anemia of chronic disease, which is associated with normal or elevated serum ferritin and increased iron stores in the marrow.

Coombs test for anti-red blood cell antibodies (**choice B**) is one of the initial diagnostic studies performed when there are hematologic signs of hemolytic anemia (e.g., normocytic red blood cells, reticulocytosis, and high unconjugated bilirubin). A positive Coombs test indicates the presence of circulating anti-red blood cell antibodies responsible for hemolysis.

Hemoglobin electrophoresis (**choice C**) is mainly used for the diagnosis of qualitative or quantitative disorders of hemoglobin, namely sickle cell anemia and thalassemias. Sickle cell anemia is associated with the typical sickle-shaped red blood cells on peripheral smear. Thalassemias manifest with microcytosis (MCV <75 fl), but ferritin levels are normal/elevated. In addition, morphologic abnormalities of erythrocytes are more pronounced in thalassemia compared with iron-deficiency anemia. Alpha-thalassemia trait and beta-thalassemia minor are often accompanied by normal or increased numbers of red blood cells.

Oral ferrous sulfate (**choice E**) is the most appropriate treatment for iron-deficiency anemia. However, this form of anemia is usually a *manifestation* of an underlying condition that should be identified and treated. Anemia itself is usually not life-threatening, but the underlying cause may be.

Treatment with vitamin B_{12} and folic acid (**choice F**) is effective for megaloblastic anemia secondary to vitamin B_{12} or folic acid deficiency. In contrast to iron-deficiency anemia, megaloblastic anemia is characterized by *macro-cytes* (i.e., red blood cells with high MCV [usually >110 fl]) and often associated with mild hyperbilirubinemia.

2. **The correct answer is A.** The acute onset of tenosynovitis is often the initial manifestation of gonococcal arthritis. Risk factors specific to this patient include female sex, menses, and pregnancy. Signs and symptoms include fever and involvement of the knee and ankles. Obtaining cultures from the cervix, rectum, pharynx, and blood will give a higher probability of a positive result than cultures from the joint fluid alone. Gonococcal arthritis is confirmed by prompt response to antibiotics.

Blood cultures (**choice B**) are positive in only 40% of patients.

The immunologic reaction to nonviable fragments of the organism's cell wall will interfere with culture of the organism from skin or joints (**choice C**). These cultures will be positive in less then 50% of cases.

A synovial fluid cell count (**choice D**) is helpful in making the diagnosis of septic arthritis, but not in identifying the pathogen causing the infection.

Synovial fluid Gram stain (**choice E**) is typically positive in only 25% of cases.

3. **The correct answer is B.** This is hydatid disease, due to infection with *E. granulosus* (rarely *Echinococcus multilocularis*). The life cycle of this parasitic worm usually alternates between sheep and canine carnivores (including sheep herding dogs). Man is an accidental host. Endemic areas correspond to the major sheepherding areas of the world: the Mediterranean, the Middle East, Australia, New Zealand, South Africa, and South America. Smaller foci of the disease are found in California, Canada, and Alaska. The ingested egg hatches in the intestine, and the larva migrates to the human liver, lungs, or, less commonly, other body sites. Over years, the larva forms the hydatid cyst, which is a large, fluid-filled bladder that develops multiple brood capsules in its periphery, each of which contains numerous small infective scolices. So long as the cyst does not rupture, the patient may be asymptomatic. However, rupture (including accidental surgical rupture) can cause an anaphylactic reaction (the cyst fluid is highly antigenic) or a "metastatic" infection, because millions of infectious scolices can be released. Treatment can be either with very careful surgical resection or with percutaneous aspiration under CT guidance followed by instillation of a scolecoidal agent and then reaspiration. If the case is inoperable, or if an intraoperative spillage occurs, albendazole can be used to suppress growth or kill the cysts.

Ascariasis (**choice A**) can cause biliary obstruction by the adult worms and granulomas in the liver by the larvae.

Fascioliasis (**choice C**) can acutely cause tender hepatomegaly with fever and eosinophilia, and can chronically cause cholangitis and biliary fibrosis.

Schistosomiasis (**choice D**) can cause a severe granulomatous reaction to the ova, producing hepatosplenomegaly, pipestem fibrosis, and portal hypertension.

Toxocariasis (**choice E**) can cause visceral larva migrans and hepatomegaly with granulomas.

4. **The correct answer is C.** This case raises the problem of the clinical approach to a solitary pulmonary nodule radiographically detected in an otherwise healthy subject. In large surveys, 60% of solitary pulmonary nodules are benign, and granulomas represent the most common benign lesion. However, there is no infallible clinical or radiologic set of criteria that can discriminate between benign and malignant lesions. Factors favoring a benign lesion include young age (<45 years), small size (<2 cm), smooth margins of the lesion, absence of symptoms, and slow growth on successive films. Generally, calcification is not a malignant feature, and presence of "popcorn-like" calcifications definitely favors hamartoma. A hamartoma is a malformative lesion resulting from a random admixture of tissues normally present in the lung, including cartilage, bronchial mucosa, and smooth muscle. It is usually discovered incidentally.

    An aspergilloma (**choice A**) is a fungus ball (mycetoma) that develops in a preexisting lung cavity. It may be seen as an asymptomatic radiographic abnormality (a crescent of air outlining a solid mass that moves with position changes) that is usually in the upper lobe. An aspergilloma can cause hemoptysis, and there are often other systemic signs. Hemoptysis is frequently present, and signs and symptoms of the underlying disease should be found.

    Bronchogenic carcinoma (**choice B**) may present as a solitary nodule, but patients are typically older and have a much longer exposure to cigarette smoking. Calcifications usually are not seen in malignant pulmonary tumors.

    Pulmonary abscess (**choice D**) manifests as a pulmonary infiltrate with cavitation and, frequently, an air-fluid level. Accompanying symptomatology, such as fever and cough, is usually present.

    Sarcoidosis (**choice E**) frequently affects the lungs. A diffuse multinodular infiltrate is seen on chest x-ray, most commonly associated with hilar lymphadenopathy. The patient may have signs and symptoms of restrictive pulmonary disease.

    Secondary (reactivated) tuberculosis (**choice F**) manifests with multiple nodular and cavitary infiltrates in the upper lobes; the patient has low-grade fever, malaise, weight loss, and cough. However, primary tuberculosis may result in a calcified nodule within the lung parenchyma, which is the remnant of an old Ghon complex.

5. **The correct answer is D.** The patient has signs, symptoms, and laboratory findings consistent with giant cell arteritis, which is a systemic disease overlapping with polymyalgia rheumatica. It affects the superficial temporal artery most commonly but may involve any medium-sized or large caliber artery in the body. The most characteristic elements in the diagnosis include scalp tenderness (sometimes associated with palpation of a nodular and tender temporal artery), elevated ESR, a frequently normal leukocyte count, and age older than 55 years. The major risk of this condition is blindness deriving from extension of the inflammatory process to the ophthalmic artery. Prednisone therapy must be immediately started, and a biopsy of the temporal artery should be obtained to confirm the diagnosis.

    CT scan of the head (**choice A**) would be useful to obtain information in case of suspected intracranial lesions, especially bleeding, infarct, or a space-occupying mass.

    Lumbar puncture (**choice B**) for CSF examination would have no diagnostic value in this patient. Meningitis would develop more rapidly, usually with nuchal headache and rigidity. Subarachnoid hemorrhage results in thunderclap headache followed by changes in mental status.

    Muscle biopsy (**choice C**) is useful in investigating muscular disorders. Myalgia, arthralgia, and stiffness in the pelvic and shoulder girdles are often present in this condition, which may mimic a myopathy.

    Visual evoked potentials (**choice E**) are especially useful in evaluation of optic nerve involvement in demyelinating diseases.

6. **The correct answer is E.** Urticaria, or hives, is a common condition that can be quite difficult to manage because there are such a wide variety of triggers. The underlying basis of the condition is mediator- (histamine, serotonin, leukotrienes) driven vasodilation with accompanying dermal edema. The triggers for mediator release from mast cells or basophils may be either allergic (IgE bound to antigen) or nonimmunologic direct pharmacologic effects. Although there is a wide range of possible triggers for urticaria, it is important to note that up to 25% of cases of acute hepatitis B present with urticaria. It is therefore well worth checking the sclera (the most visible site in tanned or dark-skinned individuals) for jaundice in patients with newly diagnosed hives. Other triggers include contact chemicals, drugs, food allergens, pressure, sunlight, insect stings, and hereditary predispositions.

All the other choices can produce acute or chronic hepatitis but do not have a significant association with urticaria.

7. **The correct answer is E.** A persistently wide split S_2 is typically seen in patients with right bundle branch block, pulmonic stenosis, pulmonary embolus, and ectopic or pacemaker beats originating in the left ventricle. All these conditions produce delayed function of the right ventricle. In a Brazilian patient, Chagas disease (caused by *Trypanosoma cruzi*) should be considered as a possible cause of heart block. This trypanosomal infection is endemic in Central and South American countries, and is a cause of rhythm disturbances, cardiomyopathy, and thromboembolism.

ST segment elevation (**choice A**) is seen in acute anterior myocardial infarction.

A short PR interval (**choice B**) is associated with a loud S_1 (when the mitral valve slams shut).

Early repolarization (**choice C**) will produce ECG changes only, with no specific findings on auscultation.

Although modest T wave changes can sometimes be associated with right bundle branch block, marked T wave inversions (**choice D**) are more typical of right or left ventricular hypertrophy and myocardial ischemia or infarction.

8. **The correct answer is C.** *Hyperparathyroidism* is one of the most frequent endocrinologic conditions, found in 1 in 1,000 adults. In most cases, hyperparathyroidism is asymptomatic, manifesting only with hypercalcemia often discovered incidentally in the course of routine laboratory investigations conducted for other reasons. The most common cause is a parathyroid adenoma. Calcium levels should be corrected for albuminemia, since most of the calcium is bound to serum albumin. If hypercalcemia is the only clinical sign, without associated complications such as renal stones, bone disease, or cataracts, abundant fluid intake is the only measure recommended to prevent formation of calcium stones in the urinary system.

Bone x-ray films (**choice A**) are not necessary for the diagnostic work-up of hypercalcemia and hyperparathyroidism, unless bone pain or pathologic fractures are present. X-ray films may reveal bone rarefaction, which is often more pronounced in the phalanges and in subperiosteal locations.

Extensive cancer screening (**choice B**) would be appropriate if hypercalcemia were suspected to be secondary to neoplasms (e.g., lung, breast, renal cell carcinoma, multiple myeloma). Hypercalcemia of malignancy can be due to secretion of PTH-like substances or bone destruction by metastases. In either case, plasma levels of PTH

detected by IRMA would be low. In fact, the PTH-like peptides produced by some tumors (lung cancer) are not identified by IRMA. Alkaline phosphatase would be high in the presence of osteolysis.

Treatment with bisphosphonates (e.g., alendronate; **choice D**) may serve as an alternative treatment to prevent excessive bone resorption.

Surgical exploration of the neck (**choice E**) is aimed at finding the source of increased PTH production, which is usually a parathyroid adenoma. Removal of the adenoma is recommended when patients have symptomatic hyperparathyroidism, with recurrent renal stones or bone disease. Indications for surgical treatment in asymptomatic patients include very high calcium levels, high urinary excretion of calcium, extreme bone loss, or difficulty in medical follow-up.

9. **The correct answer is D.** This man has glucose-6-phosphate dehydrogenase (G6PD) deficiency (as do 10% of African American males). G6PD serves to protect the RBCs from oxidative damage by maintaining high intracellular levels of NADPH. People of Mediterranean descent can also have G6PD deficiency, but to a much greater degree. Therefore, hemolytic episodes in this population are more severe (and can be fatal), as compared with those in the African American population, which are usually mild and self-limited. Common oxidative stressors that initiate hemolysis are drug reactions (especially sulfa drugs), febrile illnesses, and fava bean ingestion.

Acute infectious hepatitis (**choice A**) would more likely present with fatigue, fever, abdominal pain, hepatomegaly, and high elevations of AST and ALT (often into the thousands).

Cholestatic liver disease (**choice B**) more often presents with elevation of alkaline phosphatase, along with mild elevations of AST and ALT. This patient has elevated unconjugated bilirubin levels, as in hemolytic disorders. Both hepatocellular (hepatitis) and cholestatic liver disease cause more conjugated (as opposed to unconjugated) hyperbilirubinemia.

The most common side effects of fluoxetine (a selective serotonin reuptake inhibitor; **choice C**) are anxiety, agitation, and insomnia.

10. **The correct answer is B.** *Escherichia coli*, a coliform bacteria, is the most common cause of urinary tract infection (UTI) and is therefore seen much more often than *Klebsiella* (**choice C**) and *Proteus* (**choice D**). *E. coli* causes about 80% of UTIs in patients without urologic abnormalities. Coliform bacteria colonize the urethra, and ascending infection may lead to cystitis or pyelonephritis.

Chlamydia trachomatis (**choice A**) is part of the differential diagnosis for UTI in a sexually active patient with dysuria. However, the patient often has a vaginal discharge.

Urine culture usually shows <100 organisms. On physical examination, the patient with *Chlamydia* may have cervical motion tenderness if cervicitis is present.

Staphylococcus saprophyticus (**choice E**) is another common cause of UTIs in young women, often after heterosexual intercourse.

11. **The correct answer is D.** This question examines the different aspects of vitamin deficiencies. Scurvy is a deficiency of vitamin C that may occur in older men who cook for themselves and alcoholics. The features are perifollicular hemorrhage and purpura, splinter hemorrhages, and gum involvement. Normochromic, normocytic anemia is common.

Niacin deficiency (**choice A**), known as pellagra, is a chronic wasting disease associated with dermatitis, dementia, and diarrhea. The skin lesions are characterized by hyperkeratosis, hyperpigmentation, and desquamation. The course is progressive over several years. Niacin is found in cereals.

Vitamin B_1 (thiamine) deficiency (**choice B**), known as beriberi, occurs in alcoholics and food faddists. Two manifestations of deficiency include cardiovascular disease (high output failure) and neurologic disorders (e.g., Wernicke-Korsakoff syndrome, characterized by peripheral neuropathy, a global confusional state, retrograde amnesia, and confabulation).

Vitamin B_{12} deficiency (**choice C**) causes a macrocytic anemia. Patients may complain of a sore tongue or weight loss. Neurologic manifestations, including weakness and ataxia from demyelination, are the most worrisome. Causes include pernicious anemia, gastrectomy, and ileal abnormalities.

Vitamin D deficiency (**choice E**) causes disorders of bone mineralization, namely rickets in children and osteomalacia in adults.

12. **The correct answer is C.** Although the whole clinical presentation is characteristic of acute pancreatitis, normal or slightly elevated serum levels of pancreatic enzymes seem to contrast with such a diagnosis. Types I and V hyperlipoproteinemia are rare conditions predisposing to acute pancreatitis (the two most frequent are cholelithiasis and alcoholism). However, hypertriglyceridemia itself may often falsely depress amylase and lipase levels in the presence of otherwise typical clinical features of pancreatitis. Note, however, other classic laboratory and radiologic signs of acute pancreatitis present in this case: neutrophilic leukocytosis, hyperglycemia, hypocalcemia, elevated C-reactive protein, and the "sentinel loop" (air-filled loop of small bowel in the left upper quadrant). The latter parameter is often used as a radiologic marker of pancreatic damage.

Acute cholecystitis (**choice A**) is associated with gallstones in the great majority of cases. Often, it develops when a stone occludes the cystic duct. Severe pain in the right upper quadrant or epigastrium and leukocytosis are present, but none of the other signs characteristic of acute pancreatitis are seen.

Acute hepatitis (**choice B**) is associated with increased levels of serum aminotransferases. Pain is relatively mild compared with the extreme pain of acute pancreatitis. Jaundice is often present, although pancreatitis may also cause mild elevation of direct bilirubin because the pancreas becomes swollen and the common bile duct is blocked.

Bowel perforation (**choice D**) also presents with a dramatic clinical picture of pain of sudden onset, shock, and rigid abdomen. Pancreatic enzymes may be elevated. A plain x-ray film taken in upright position reveals air underneath the diaphragm.

Mesenteric ischemia (**choice E**) due to cardioembolism or artherosclerosis of mesenteric vessels presents with acute abdominal pain that is typically out of proportion to physical examination findings. The typical patient is over 50 years old and presents with acute left-sided abdominal pain that begins in the left iliac fossa, with nausea, vomiting, diarrhea, and abdominal guarding. The patient may have had similar previous episodes, or there may be associated symptoms of cardiovascular disease. Plain films show thickened bowel walls, indicating a paucity of gas in the intestines. Specific radiologic signs are pneumatosis intestinalis (i.e., submucosal gas), bowel wall thumbprinting, and portal vein gas. Although patients with hypertriglyceridemia are at risk for cardiovascular diseases, the most likely cause of this patient's symptoms is acute pancreatitis.

Ureteral lithiasis (**choice F**) is in the differential diagnosis of conditions mimicking acute pancreatitis. However, the pain is often referred to the flank region and radiates toward the ipsilateral perineum. Gross or microscopic hematuria is usually present. Pancreatic enzymes are not elevated, and neutrophilic leukocytosis is absent.

13. **The correct answer is E.** This patient has the classic triad of fever, exudative pharyngitis, and cervical lymphadenopathy, strongly suggestive of streptococcal infection (group A beta hemolytic *Streptococcus*).

Candida albicans (**choice A**) rarely causes the above clinical scenario. It is seen commonly in immunosuppressed patients, diabetics, and those recently on antibiotics. It causes characteristic white patches of exudate on mucosa.

Haemophilus influenza (**choice B**), *Staphylococcus aureus* (**choice C**), and *Streptococcus pneumoniae* (**choice D**) rarely cause exudative pharyngitis.

14. **The correct answer is A.** Sudden cardiac death (SCD), defined as any unexpected death of proven cardiac origin, is a rare event in young, competitive athletes. However, it raises the question of which preparticipation screening methods should be used for prevention. A consensus document published by the American Heart Association in 1996 (*Circulation* 1996;94:850) indicates that the most feasible and cost-effective approach is to perform a careful medical history (including personal and family history) and cardiac examination to identify subjects at risk. Pertinent histories, cardiac auscultation, and assessment of exercise-induced symptoms are all essential to primary prevention of SCD in the athletic population.

Chest x-ray (**choice B**) would not be an adequate screening test to detect cardiac abnormalities that may result in sudden death.

Echocardiography (**choice C**) is certainly an effective test to demonstrate cardiac abnormalities, such as left ventricular hypertrophy or valvular disease, but its cost as a preparticipation screening in all competitive athletes would be exorbitant.

Both exercise cardiography (**choice D**) and resting cardiography (**choice E**) would also result in excessive costs.

15. **The correct answer is D.** A fatal arrhythmia is the immediate cause of demise in sudden cardiac death (SCD), but the underlying conditions are extremely variable. Nonatherosclerotic causes are prevalent in the young population, but coronary artery disease becomes more frequent in athletes older than 40. Hypertrophic cardiomyopathy has been found in approximately one-third of cases of SCD in young athletes. This condition is frequently hereditary (hence the need for a careful family history) and may manifest with arrhythmias, chest pain, and signs of subaortic stenosis. Coronary anomalies (**choice C**), including atherosclerotic changes, represent the second most frequent cause of SCD in competitive athletes.

Aortic stenosis (**choice A**), arrhythmogenic right ventricular dysplasia (**choice B**), isolated (and otherwise unexplained) left ventricular hypertrophy (**choice E**), myocarditis (**choice F**), and ruptured aorta (**choice G**) are rare causes of SCD. Some studies have shown that an increased myocardial mass, per se, is a risk factor for SCD, even without coexisting pathologic changes.

16. **The correct answer is D.** You should be aware that roughly half of all hospitalized AIDS patients have hyponatremia. There are many reasons for abnormal sodium metabolism in seriously ill AIDS patients, who may have multiple organ system involvement. Some of the drugs these patients receive impair renal water excretion, hypotonic fluids may be administered during the course of therapy, and they may also have impaired renal function. Cytomegalovirus or mycobacteria may cause destructive adrenalitis, or ketoconazole may impair adrenal glucocorticoid and mineralocorticoid synthesis. Pulmonary and CNS infections may induce the syndrome of inappropriate ADH secretion (SIADH). All of these causes, often more than one in an individual case, contribute to the high incidence of hyponatremia in AIDS patients. If a specific cause can be identified and corrected, that will often improve the hyponatremia. Otherwise, fluid restriction is used for mild abnormalities; administration of hypertonic saline can be used to (slowly) correct more severe hyponatremia.

Disorders of potassium (**choice A**), magnesium (**choice B**), calcium (**choice C**), and phosphate (**choice E**) can occur but are much less common than disorders of sodium in AIDS patients.

17. **The correct answer is C.** The management of acute hemorrhage is the same for almost all patients, regardless of the etiology. In this case, a patient who is actively bleeding with apparent marginal vital signs requires immediate restoration of blood pressure via fluid resuscitation with at least 3 L of crystalloid solution (normal saline or lactated Ringer's) for every liter of blood lost. Tachycardia and hypotension are signs of a moderate to severe loss of blood volume, and no delay in initiating fluid therapy is warranted.

Ordering an urgent type and cross match for blood (**choice A**), although appropriate for the overall short-term management of this patient, is not an acceptable therapeutic option in the face of active bleeding with no fluid resuscitation in progress.

Ordering an urgent hematocrit level (**choice B**) is not useful in this case because hematocrit levels do not change for at least four hours after an acute bleed. In addition, it offers no therapeutic benefit and will not change the short-term management of this patient.

Beginning parenteral administration of large volumes of colloid solution (**choice D**) is not indicated in this case. In fact, colloid (albumin, Hetastarch, Hetaspan) is rarely indicated for fluid resuscitation since it may actually precipitate pulmonary edema. The only clear indication for colloid is in the therapy of early burns, as these patients have capillary leaks and are losing protein and albumin.

Placing two additional large bore peripheral IV catheters (**choice E**) is indicated only AFTER fluid resuscitation has been started through whatever peripheral or central access is available. The concept here is that large bore IV catheters or central catheters are required for aggressive fluid resuscitation, but not at the expense of delaying therapy through an already available route.

18. **The correct answer is A.** The patient manifests early left ventricular failure secondary to aortic regurgitation. The diastolic murmur in decrescendo along the left sternal border and the wide differential between systolic pressure and diastolic pressure are highly characteristic. The rapid rise and fall of peripheral pulses is known as Corrigan pulse. Similar hemodynamic changes (hyperdynamic circulation) may be observed in hyperthyroidism, large arteriovenous fistulas, beriberi, and patent ductus arteriosus.

Aortic stenosis **(choice B)** produces a "diamond-shaped" (crescendo-decrescendo) systolic murmur often radiating to the neck. In contrast to aortic regurgitation, aortic stenosis is associated with a narrow differential between systolic and diastolic pressures.

Hypertrophic obstructive cardiomyopathy (HOCM; **choice C)** may simulate aortic stenosis or coronary artery disease in symptoms. HOCM often presents with symptoms of exertional angina, dyspnea, and/or syncope. It is also widely known to be a cause of sudden cardiac death in young athletes. Diagnosis is usually made by recognizing the signs associated with outflow obstruction and the symptoms that are predominantly characterized by diastolic dysfunction. Characteristic findings on physical examination include a bifid carotid pulse, an S_4 heart sound, and a harsh systolic crescendo-decrescendo located at the apex and left sternal border. The murmur increases with the Valsalva maneuver upon standing and with amyl nitrite, and it decreases with sudden squatting, leg raising, and handgrip exercises.

Infective endocarditis **(choice D)** may be accompanied by murmurs, usually secondary to valvular insufficiency, but systemic signs and symptoms of infection would be present.

Mitral stenosis **(choice E)** leads to a diastolic rumbling murmur audible at the apex or central precordium. An opening snap soon after S_2 often precedes the murmur and is related to the forced opening imposed by the atrial contraction on rigid mitral valve leaflets.

Ventricular septal defect (VSD; **choice F)**, the most frequent congenital cardiac anomaly, is associated with a pansystolic murmur at the left sternal border, often accompanied by a thrill.

19. **The correct answer is C.** In cases of HIV and persistent diarrhea, the differential diagnosis includes *Cryptosporidium* and *Isospora*. A fresh stool specimen should be examined for parasites using a modified acid-fast stain for both pathogens. These protozoal infections are the most common enteric protozoal infections in AIDS patients throughout the world.

Abdominal CT scan **(choice A)** may show changes in the colon wall consistent with inflammation and edema. However, the scan will probably not be helpful in the principal diagnosis of this patient's condition.

CMV antigenemia **(choice B)** is an index of infection with CMV, which is common in an immunocompromised host such as a patient with HIV or one undergoing chemotherapy. GI symptoms are the result of ulcers in the esophagus, stomach, small intestine, or colon, which may cause rectal bleeding, bloody diarrhea, or perforation. Ganciclovir is used in the alleviation of symptoms.

The PPD test **(choice D)** is used to determine whether a patient has had prior exposure to *Mycobacterium tuberculosis*. Biopsy may show caseating granulomas. In a condition such as this, the patient would also complain of bloody diarrhea and weight loss.

If diagnostic studies are negative and diarrhea persists, patients should undergo endoscopy. Biopsy **(choice E)** of the duodenum or small bowel may show histologic evidence of cryptosporidial, microsporidial, mycobacterial, or cytomegalovirus (CMV) infection.

20. **The correct answer is C.** The symptomatology, x-ray evidence of lobar consolidation, and the finding of gram-positive diplococci in the sputum all support a diagnosis of acute pneumonia due to pneumococcus. Microscopic examination of gram-stained sputum is more sensitive than culture in identifying pneumococcus. Penicillin is the agent of choice, administered orally (penicillin V) on an outpatient basis in uncomplicated pneumonia, or parenterally (IV penicillin G) for seriously ill patients.

Patients with a history of mild allergic reactions to penicillin, but without anaphylaxis or other serious reactions, should be treated with cefazolin **(choice A)**.

Erythromycin **(choice B)** is a safe alternative to penicillin for pneumococcal pneumonia and covers the other common bacterial pathogens of community-acquired pneumonia, including (besides pneumococcus) *Mycoplasma pneumoniae*, *Chlamydia pneumoniae*, and *Legionella*.

Tetracyclines **(choice D)**, such as doxycycline, are the preferred drugs against *Chlamydia pneumoniae* and a good alternative to erythromycin for infections due to *Mycoplasma pneumoniae* and *Moraxella catarrhalis*.

The combination of trimethoprim and sulfamethoxazole **(choice E)** can be used as a second-line treatment in penicillin-allergic patients. It can also be used in case of pneumonia caused by highly penicillin-resistant strains of pneumococcus.

Vancomycin **(choice F)** is used against strains of pneumococcus highly resistant to penicillin or in case of severe allergic reaction to previous penicillin administration.

21. **The correct answer is D.** The clinical features of these headaches, with their characteristic vise-like quality, immediately suggest *tension headaches*, which are often associated with tightness of the neck muscles. Anxiety, fatigue, and noise may act as precipitating triggers. Exploration of underlying causes of anxiety is often useful, but a trial with aspirin or other NSAIDs may be sufficient in most cases. Tension headaches may show overlapping features with migraine.

Antidepressant drugs (**choice A**) are used to treat depression and its manifestations, including depression headaches. A full neuropsychiatric evaluation is necessary to begin such treatment.

Calcium channel antagonists (**choice B**) are effective in decreasing the frequency of attacks of migraine, although they do not influence the intensity and duration of pain.

Ergotamine-containing preparations (**choice C**) and sumatriptan (**choice E**) represent the treatments of choice for acute migraine.

22. **The correct answer is D.** The patient is experiencing recurrent UTIs associated with the presence of kidney stones (the radiopaque density in the renal pelvis and calyces). Urease-producing organisms, such as *Proteus mirabilis*, create a high urinary pH, contributing to the development of struvite kidney stones. The stone may cause obstruction and urinary stress, leading to infection. These stones are relatively soft and are usually amenable to percutaneous nephrostomy. Acetohydroxamic acid is an effective urease inhibitor. *Pseudomonas* and *Providencia* are less common urease-producing organisms that may cause struvite calculi.

Bacteroides fragilis (**choice A**) is associated with peritonitis in patients with an intra-abdominal abscess.

Clostridium difficile (**choice B**) is associated with pseudomembranous colitis.

Escherichia coli (**choice C**) is the most common cause of UTI.

Streptococcus bovis (**choice E**) is a nonenterococcal type of group D *Streptococcus*.

23. **The correct answer is C.** The changes seen are those of scleroderma; if other organs become involved, the term systemic sclerosis is appropriate. This disease is characterized by diffuse fibrosis, degenerative changes, and vascular abnormalities. The most common significant internal involvement in these patients is esophageal dysfunction (which predisposes to disease with risk of Barrett esophagus and cancer of the esophagus), which occurs as a result of replacement of the muscle of the esophagus by densely fibrotic, scar-like tissue. Other gastrointestinal complications include pneumatosis cystoides intestinalis (see below), sacculations of the colon and ileum (see below), biliary cirrhosis, and malabsorption secondary to bacterial overgrowth in the poorly functional small bowel.

Carcinoid tumor (**choice A**) does not have an increased incidence in systemic sclerosis.

Duodenal peptic ulcer (**choice B**) does not have an increased incidence in systemic sclerosis, although esophageal peptic ulcer, secondary to reflux problems, does.

Pneumatosis cystoides intestinalis (**choice D**) is an uncommon intestinal complication of systemic sclerosis in which degeneration of the muscularis mucosa allows the entry of air into the intestinal wall.

Sacculations of the colon (**choice E**) and ileum are broad outpouchings (very fat diverticula) that can sometimes complicate systemic sclerosis as a result of smooth muscle atrophy.

Small bowel adhesions (**choice F**) are not a feature of systemic sclerosis. They are commonly seen following abdominal surgery (e.g., for appendicitis) and in inflammatory conditions, such as Crohn disease. Small bowel adhesions typically present with symptoms of small bowel obstruction.

24. **The correct answer is B.** Goodpasture syndrome is an autoimmune disease mediated by autoantibodies against a domain of type IV collagen in the basement membranes of both glomerular and alveolar capillaries. Consequently, the lungs develop hemorrhagic interstitial pneumonia manifesting with hemoptysis, whereas the kidneys develop necrotizing glomerulonephritis leading to *nephritic syndrome* (responsible for hematuria, pitting edema, and hypertension in this case). Linear deposition of IgG and complement along the basement membrane of the alveolar and glomerular capillaries is the pathognomonic feature. The latter alone is sufficient to support a diagnosis of Goodpasture syndrome. Corticosteroids and immunosuppressants are necessary to treat this serious condition.

Churg-Strauss syndrome (**choice A**) must be considered in the differential diagnosis. This condition is associated with blood and tissue eosinophilia and, frequently, with circulating ANCA (i.e., *antineutrophil cytoplasmic antibodies* [specifically p-ANCA]).

Idiopathic pulmonary hemosiderosis (**choice C**) may appear similar to Goodpasture syndrome in its pulmonary manifestations—hemoptysis and pulmonary infiltrates—but this condition does not involve the kidneys nor is it associated with linear IgG deposition along basement membranes.

Postinfectious glomerulonephritis (**choice D**) most commonly follows a streptococcal infection and manifests with nephritic syndrome. Pulmonary manifestations are not present. Immunofluorescence of kidney biopsies reveals *granular* deposition of IgG and complement in the mesangium and glomerular basement membrane.

Wegener granulomatosis (**choice E**) enters the differential diagnosis of any condition manifesting with concomitant involvement of lungs and kidneys. It is characterized by a necrotizing granulomatous vasculitis and frequent presence of circulating c-ANCA.

25. **The correct answer is A.** Insomnia, irritability, and palpitations are nonspecific symptoms that may be caused by a variety of diseases and drugs, but they are frequent manifestations of hyperthyroidism. Furthermore, the fact that the patient takes amiodarone should prompt investigations for hyperthyroidism. Amiodarone causes symptomatic hyperthyroidism in a small percentage of patients (2% to 3%) and asymptomatic elevation of T_3 and T_4 with much greater frequency. Thus, thyroid hormone measurements should be combined with measurement of TSH, which is suppressed in the presence of significant thyroid hyperfunction.

Administration of propranolol (**choice B**) is effective in relieving symptoms of hyperthyroidism due to abnormal sympathetic activation, namely tachycardia, excessive sweating, anxiety, and tremor. It should be used for temporary relief until hyperthyroidism has resolved, but is not adequate treatment in this case.

Referral for psychiatric consultation (**choice C**) implies that the symptoms are due to an underlying psychiatric etiology, which is a plausible explanation in a patient with history of depression. However, hyperthyroidism should be ruled out first.

Substitution of a different antidepressant drug (**choice D**) would be justified if the symptoms were due to fluoxetine administration. Treatment with fluoxetine, as well as other serotonin-selective reuptake inhibitors (SSRI), may cause insomnia and nervousness. Again, amiodarone-related hyperthyroidism should be ruled out before attributing the symptoms to the SSRI side effects.

Substitution of a different antihypertensive drug (**choice E**) would not be justified in this case. Enalapril, as any other angiotensin-converting enzyme (ACE) inhibitors, is a remarkably safe drug with few and rare adverse effects. Hypotension is one of these, but the patient in this example has a blood pressure within a fairly normal range.

26. **The correct answer is B.** *Status epilepticus* is a life-threatening emergency that should be treated promptly. It is diagnosed when a generalized convulsive seizure lasts longer than ten minutes or when a seizure episode is followed by another episode without recovery of consciousness. There are two types of status epilepticus:

convulsive and nonconvulsive. The convulsive type is the most dangerous. It can lead to metabolic and cardiovascular disturbances, including hypoxemia, hypoglycemia, hypotension, and hyperthermia, that may cause death or permanent brain damage. About 50% of patients presenting with status epilepticus do not have history of epilepsy. The most frequent precipitating factor in adults with a diagnosis of epilepsy is drug noncompliance.

Alcohol withdrawal (**choice A**), head trauma (**choice C**), hypoxia (**choice D**), intracranial infection (**choice E**), intracranial tumor (**choice F**), and metabolic alterations (**choice G**) are other precipitating factors for status epilepticus. Of these, infection is the most common in childhood.

27. **The correct answer is E.** The clinical picture and results of blood gas analysis before and after hyperventilation are characteristic of *obesity-hypoventilation syndrome* (also known as *pickwickian syndrome*, after a character in Charles Dickens' *The Pickwick Papers*). Hypoventilation results from a combination of reduced drive on respiratory centers and physical impediment on respiration imposed by obesity. Improvement of hypoxemia and hypercapnia following voluntary hyperventilation differentiates this condition from chronic obstructive pulmonary disease. Most patients with pickwickian syndrome also have obstructive sleep apnea and consequent daytime sleepiness. Weight loss is the single most effective therapeutic intervention.

Benzodiazepines at bedtime (**choice A**) are contraindicated, as are any other hypnotic agents. Alcohol should also be avoided.

Treatment with daily acetazolamide (**choice B**) has been tried in obstructive sleep apnea but with disappointing results.

Morning administration of dextroamphetamine (**choice C**) is used for the treatment of *narcolepsy*. This disease is hereditary and manifests with sudden sleep attacks, cataplexy (abrupt loss of muscle tone), and hypnagogic hallucinations. None of these symptoms are present in this case.

Supplemental oxygen at night (**choice D**) has been found to have some benefit in reducing the severity of nocturnal episodes of hypoxemia in obstructive sleep apnea, but it may also increase the duration of apneic episodes.

28. **The correct answer is C.** The clinical presentation is consistent with nephrotic syndrome, since proteinuria is within the nephrotic range (i.e., >3 g/day). The history of heroin abuse makes focal segmental glomerulosclerosis (FSG) the most likely diagnosis. FSG may occur in an idiopathic form or in association with three conditions: morbid obesity, HIV infection, and heroin abuse. A renal

biopsy will reveal sclerosis occurring in some, but not all, glomeruli (focal), with each glomerulus showing partial involvement (segmental). Electron microscopy shows detachment of epithelial podocytes from the glomerular basement membrane, an alteration also seen in minimal change disease. Note in this clinical case, the coexistence of nephrotic features (marked proteinuria and edema) with nephritic signs (hypertension and microhematuria), which is often present in FSG.

Acute proliferative glomerulonephritis (**choice A**) is characterized by proliferation of endothelial and mesangial cells with influx of leukocytes. The glomeruli are hypercellular, and immune deposits are epimembranous in location. This pattern is associated with nephritic syndrome: proteinuria <3 g/day, hematuria, hypertension, and pedal and periorbital edema. The prototype of this glomerular disease is postinfectious glomerulonephritis.

Crescentic glomerulonephritis (**choice B**) owes its designation to the crescent-shaped masses of cells (epithelial and inflammatory) that accumulate within the urinary space of Bowman capsule, obliterating the glomerular tuft. This results in rapidly progressive renal failure, requiring aggressive immunosuppressive therapy.

Minimal change disease (**choice D**) is mostly a disease of childhood. It manifests with full-blown nephrotic syndrome. On light microscopy, the glomeruli appear normal, only to reveal alterations in epithelial podocytes on electron microscopy.

Nodular glomerulosclerosis (Kimmelstiel-Wilson disease; **choice E**) is pathognomonic for diabetic nephropathy. Round PAS-positive (i.e., glycoprotein-rich) globules are seen within the glomeruli. This feature, along with diffuse mesangial sclerosis due to accumulation of altered glycoproteins of plasma origin, constitutes the pathologic substrate of diabetes-related renal dysfunction.

29. **The correct answer is B.** A basic understanding of blood product and blood component replacement is crucial. The use of such products is extremely common, and there is misuse. Patients with liver disease have a deficiency of one or more clotting factors produced by the liver. A blood product that specifically raises such factors is indicated for treatment. Fresh frozen plasma (FFP) generally increases plasma anticoagulation factors by 30%. Like all blood products, it is type specific. There is a correlation for prothrombin times greater than 15 and the risk of bleeding with invasive procedures such as paracentesis. For this reason, FFP is usually indicated in such patients prior to undergoing their procedure.

Cryoprecipitate (**choice A**) is prepared from FFP and contains concentrated factor VIII, factor XIII, fibrinogen, and von Willebrand factor. Indications for use are hypofibrinogenemia (DIC), von Willebrand disease, and hemophilia A.

Packed red blood cells (**choice C**) are prepared from all the red cell mass in a pint of donated blood. It has no plasma or buffy coat and therefore no proteins (coagulation factors) or platelets. It is used to restore red cell mass.

Platelets (**choice D**) are a blood component therapy used to restore platelet count. One unit of platelets increases the platelet count by 5,000-10,000 cells/mm^3, assuming no ongoing destruction or sequestration. Platelets are usually transfused as a "six-pack." Each unit is the product of one unit of donated whole blood; thus, a "six-pack" represents pooled platelets from multiple donors.

Transfusion of whole blood (**choice E**) is not a current practice. Whole blood is the content of 1 pint of donated blood. It is unfiltered and contains plasma, platelets, white cells, and red cells. This product is usually processed so that each of these components is removed (except white cells) and used for transfusions in specific clinical situations.

30. **The correct answer is F.** A friction rub on auscultation indicates that the patient's chest pain is due to acute fibrinous pericarditis. ECG changes in this condition are often nonspecific, but echocardiography is a sensitive diagnostic tool. Renal failure is one of the most common causes of acute pericarditis (*uremic pericarditis*), which usually occurs when BUN exceeds 100 mg/dL (often earlier in diabetic patients). Fever is usually absent in uremic pericarditis. Institution of hemodialysis (or more aggressive hemodialysis) promptly leads to resolution of pericarditis. The onset of acute pericarditis is an absolute indication to start hemodialysis treatment.

Further reduction of water and salt intake (**choice A**) would not be sufficient to treat uremic pericarditis and might be counterproductive in this specific case.

Antibiotic treatment (**choice B**) is useful in cases of infective (purulent) pericarditis, but uremic pericarditis is the result of circulating toxins, not infection.

Antihypertensive treatment (**choice C**) is often necessary in renal failure but has no effect on uremic pericarditis. In this case, the blood pressure is within "borderline" values.

Anti-inflammatory treatment (**choice D**) is helpful in reducing symptoms but does not affect the natural course of the process. Indomethacin or corticosteroids may be used.

Erythropoietin administration (**choice E**) is used to treat anemia of renal failure. It is usually started when hematocrit falls below 30% to 35%.

Pericardiocentesis (**choice G**) and partial pericardiectomy ("pericardial window"; **choice I**) are used to treat pericardial tamponade, which is an accumulation of large amounts of pericardial fluid (inflammatory or hemorrhagic) that impairs diastolic filling and causes acute heart failure. In this case, the amount of exudate within the pericardium and the hemodynamic conditions do not warrant such therapy.

Pericardial biopsy (**choice H**) is advisable when the etiology is not clear, which is not the case in the presence of an obvious clinical picture of renal failure.

31. **The correct answer is B.** This patient likely has acute hepatitis A infection. The prodrome of this infection is very similar to this patient's presentation, and within 10-14 days after infection, many patients will manifest varying degrees of abdominal pain as well as jaundice. The disease is self-limiting, usually transmitted by contaminated shellfish or oral-anal contact with an infected person or their feces, and does not predispose patients to the same long-term risks as infection with the other hepatitis viruses. In the acute setting, serum IgM antibody may be positive.

A positive serum hepatitis A IgG titer (**choice A**) would be seen months after the acute infection has passed and is a marker for previous infection.

A positive serum hepatitis B surface antibody titer (**choice C**) is a marker for previous hepatitis B exposure.

A positive serum hepatitis C antibody (**choice D**) is a marker for hepatitis C infection. Although both B and C varieties can cause acute viral illnesses similar to the one in this patient, the epidemiology of their transmission is quite different from this patient's risk factors. Both agents are transmitted via blood-to-blood contact, and current epidemiology indicates this is primarily by IV drug abuse and exposure to infected blood (e.g., health care workers and needle sticks). Unlike hepatitis A, which has no long-term sequelae and is self-limited, both hepatitis B and C infections are associated with significant long-term morbidity and mortality. Hepatitis C is the most common cause of nonalcoholic cirrhosis and liver failure.

A positive serum hepatitis C RNA level (**choice E**) is a test ordered after initial exposure to hepatitis C and is used to follow the activity of disease over time. Unless hepatitis C infection was suspected in this patient, this test is not appropriate.

32. **The correct answer is D.** Myxoma is the most common primary cardiac tumor. It affects women more frequently than men and grows in the left atrium in 80% of cases. It may present with a systemic illness mimicking infective endocarditis, give rise to systemic embolism, or present with signs and symptoms of mitral valve obstruction (as in this case). The change in murmur when the patient changes position is suggestive of an atrial myxoma. The tumor sometimes produces a diastolic sound due to the tumor motion (*tumor plop*). Echocardiography is diagnostic.

Fibroelastoma (**choice A**) results from organization of a mural thrombus and is usually clinically silent. It represents an incidental postmortem finding.

Metastasis to the heart (**choice B**) is a relatively rare event that affects the pericardial sac or ventricular wall. Melanoma is the most common malignancy metastasizing to the heart. In addition, malignant neoplasms from the lungs, breast, pleura, and mediastinal organs may involve the heart.

A mural thrombus (**choice C**) is a frequent complication of abnormalities in wall motion resulting, for example, from myocardial infarction or atrial fibrillation. Mural thrombosis, however, does not appear as a mass filling the left atrium and does not produce mitral valve obstruction. Its most significant risk is embolization.

Sarcoma of the heart (**choice E**) is an exceptionally rare event that would not manifest with an intra-atrial mass.

33. **The correct answer is E.** The patient has relapsing polychondritis, which is an autoimmune condition that occurs as an isolated process or together with other autoimmune diseases, including rheumatoid arthritis, systemic vasculitis, and systemic lupus erythematosus. Presentations can include bilateral swelling of the external ears, nasal involvement, arthralgias to symmetric arthritis (with a predilection for the costochondral joints), and involvement of the larynx, trachea, and bronchi. The condition can also involve the cardiovascular system, kidney, and skin. In severe cases, the cartilage destruction may be disfiguring (floppy ears, saddle nose).

Ankylosing spondylitis (**choice A**) causes arthritis of the lower back.

Behcet syndrome (**choice B**) is characterized by oral ulcers, genital ulcers, and arthritis.

Gout (**choice C**) can cause both arthritis and ear involvement with tophi, but has no particular predilection for the costochondral joints.

Reiter syndrome (**choice D**) produces uveitis, urethritis, and arthritis, often triggered by an infection.

34. **The correct answer is F.** Papillary carcinoma is the most common variant of thyroid carcinomas, and the one associated with the best prognosis. Previous radiation to the neck, whether iatrogenic (for Hodgkin lymphoma, acne, tonsillitis, etc.) or resulting from accidental exposure, is a risk factor for both papillary carcinoma and follicular carcinoma (the latter being the second most

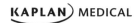

common type). The frequency of thyroid cancer is also increased in areas of high goiter incidence.

Amiodarone treatment (**choice A**) is associated with a 2% to 3% incidence of hyperthyroidism in patients treated with this drug, but not with thyroid cancer.

Dietary iodine supplementation (**choice B**) in salt and water has become standard practice in areas of low iodine concentration as a public health measure to prevent goiter. This has virtually eliminated goiter due to environmental iodine deficiency.

A family history of multiple endocrine neoplasia (MEN) (**choice C**) is not a risk factor. None of the three types of MEN is associated with papillary or follicular carcinoma of the thyroid. MEN types IIa and IIb predispose to medullary carcinoma of the thyroid, which originates from C cells.

Clinical evidence linking either Graves disease (**choice D**) or Hashimoto thyroiditis (**choice E**) to thyroid cancer is still controversial, but it is safe to assume that if there is any increased risk for patients with either disorder, it is very small.

Subacute thyroiditis (**choice G**), also known as *de Quervain thyroiditis,* manifests as painful enlargement of the thyroid, accompanied by dysphagia. It does not confer any increased risk for thyroid cancer.

Thyroglossal duct anomalies (**choice H**) include thyroglossal cysts and fistulas. These embryologically related conditions do not increase the risk of thyroid cancer. Exceptionally, squamous cell carcinoma has been reported arising in one of these anomalies.

35. **The correct answer is D.** Unfortunately, nosocomial infections are very common in hospitals. Given this patient's physical examination and history, it is most likely that the central line is the site of the current infection. Anything short of removal of the line will not remove the source of the infection, and it will be almost impossible to treat the infection.

Waiting until the blood cultures grow the offending organism (**choice A**) would be risky since the patient's infection would remain untreated and get out of control. If the infecting pathogen is not known, broad coverage is preferred; therapy can be narrowed once the pathogen, and its sensitivity to antibiotics, is known.

Administering an antifungal agent, such as amphotericin (**choice B**), would be an option if this patient were septic from an infection such as *Candida* or *Aspergillus.* This is likely in this patient with leukemia; his immunity is probably suppressed, and he is prone to fungal infections. However, treatment with amphotericin would not address the underlying problem related to the indwelling central line.

Administering vancomycin (**choice C**) would be helpful if this patient were infected with *Staphylococcus*, which is likely in the setting of a line infection. In fact, vancomycin is preferred in this setting; however, it will not be successful until the contaminated line is removed.

Replacement over the guide wire (**choice E**) will simply reintroduce the line infection.

36. **The correct answer is E.** Any unknown overdose with QT prolongation on ECG should raise the suspicion of tricyclic antidepressant (TCA) overdose. We know that the patient ingested both TCAs and benzodiazepines in overdose amounts. The ECG changes (QRS widening) are signs of TCA intoxication. The treatment is to maintain an alkalemic state, by hyperventilation if the patient is intubated or with IV bicarbonate. Gastric aspiration and lavage should be performed to eliminate unabsorbed drug if more than 750 mg of TCA has been taken. Seizures may occur in TCA overdose, but this patient also took an overdose of a benzodiazepine, which is likely suppressing the seizures.

DC cardioversion (**choice A**) would not be indicated, since this patient is in sinus rhythm.

Flumazenil (**choice B**) would reverse the effects of the benzodiazepine and might precipitate life-threatening seizures.

Ipecac (**choice C**) would be contraindicated in a comatose patient. Gastric aspiration and lavage would be more suitable.

Lidocaine (**choice D**) is indicated for ventricular dysrhythmias, but this patient was in sinus rhythm.

37. **The correct answer is D.** This is Sjögren syndrome, which is an autoimmune condition that can damage the salivary glands and/or the tear glands. The presence of dry eyes or dry mouth is common, but be aware that about one-third of patients have significant parotid gland enlargement (one or both sides) and may present with parotid masses and dry mouth with pain upon swallowing. In cases where a parotid mass is not present, biopsy of the lip may show characteristic changes in minor salivary glands, without the risk of damage to the facial nerve. Patients with Sjögren syndrome may have other autoimmune diseases as well, notably rheumatoid arthritis, scleroderma, and systemic lupus erythematosus.

Mucoepidermoid carcinoma (**choice A**) is characterized by nests of tumor cells without a dense lymphocytic infiltration.

Pleomorphic adenoma (**choice B**) is characterized by a variety of histologic patterns with nests, cords, or sheets of benign tumor cells.

Sarcoidosis (**choice C**) can destroy salivary glands but is characterized by prominent granulomas.

Squamous cell carcinoma (**choice E**) typically presents as an asymptomatic, white oral patch in a person who smokes, chews tobacco, or drinks alcohol. There is no associated parotid gland enlargement or salivary gland damage.

Warthin tumor (**choice F**) is a tumor composed of lymphoid tissue resembling tonsils that is covered by a distinctive, two-cell deep epithelium.

38. **The correct answer is A.** Beta blockers have been shown to decrease the incidence of nonfatal reinfarction and recurrent ischemic events. They decrease both infarct size and mortality.

Enalapril (**choice B**) is recommended for the first six weeks in patients with a large anterior wall infarction to decrease mortality by preventing infarct remodeling and expansion, although angiotensin converting enzyme (ACE) inhibitors may be harmful if hypotension is present.

Calcium channel blockers, especially diltiazem and verapamil, may be beneficial if the ejection fraction is adequate. Nifedipine (**choice C**) has been shown to increase mortality in patients following an MI.

The patient is already taking one aspirin every other day. Increasing the dose to three tablets daily (**choice D**) will not help and, in fact, may hurt him.

Adding nitroglycerin (**choice E**) would be appropriate symptomatic treatment if the patient developed angina, but at present he has none.

39. **The correct answer is F.** Ulcerative colitis has a bimodal distribution of age of onset, with a large peak between ages 15 and 30 and a smaller peak between ages 50 and 70. It occurs in both sexes and all races, although there is a somewhat increased rate in the Jewish population. The underlying etiology of the condition is still poorly defined. The presentation illustrated is typical, and many patients have had developing disease for several years before the diagnosis is made. The process usually starts in the rectum, and the stool may be hard unless the involved segment of bowel is extensive. Stool mixed with mucus and fresh blood is typical of an exacerbation. With severe disease, accompanying findings can include malaise, fever, anemia, anorexia, weight loss, and leukocytosis. The diagnosis should be confirmed by sigmoidoscopy.

Appendicitis (**choice A**) can occur in teenagers but usually causes left lower quadrant pain and would not produce stool with blood and mucus.

Colon cancer (**choice B**) can produce similar symptoms but is extremely rare among teenagers.

Diverticulitis (**choice C**) can produce similar symptoms, but it is a disease of middle-aged to elderly individuals and is not associated with rectal bleeding.

Mesenteric lymphadenitis (**choice D**) refers to inflammation of the mesenteric lymph nodes. It often presents acutely in children and is clinically difficult to differentiate from acute appendicitis and enterocolitis. Clinical features of an associated enterocolitis or ileitis in a *Yersinia* infection, such as right lower quadrant pain, fever, diarrhea, nausea, and vomiting, may be present. However, bloody stools are not a feature of mesenteric lymphadenitis.

Pseudomembranous colitis (**choice E**) is due to a clostridial infection that is usually seen as a complication of broad-spectrum antibiotic use.

40. **The correct answer is B.** This patient has a very low CD4+ count, predisposing him to a variety of opportunistic infections. This patient's visual symptoms are most likely due to cytomegalovirus (CMV) retinitis, the most common cause of HIV-associated retinitis. Other manifestations of CMV infection include constitutional symptoms, gastrointestinal disturbances, bone marrow suppression, adrenalitis, and lower respiratory tract infections. CMV is treated with ganciclovir or foscarnet.

Although the thick, cheesy white exudate on the tongue and oropharynx is likely due to *Candida albicans* (**choice A**), which is also common in AIDS patients, this pathogen does not cause visual deficits.

Herpes simplex virus 1 (HSV-1; **choice C**) causes herpes labialis and keratitis. Herpes keratitis occurs initially as conjunctivitis with vesicular blepharitis. Recurrences are termed "dendritic keratitis" and are characterized by branched corneal lesions that look like the veins of a leaf. A foreign body sensation, along with lacrimation, photophobia, and conjunctival hyperemia, may occur at the onset of the condition.

AIDS patients with CD4+ counts $<100/mm^3$ are particularly susceptible to infection with *M. avium-intracellulare* (MAI; **choice D**). For this reason, such patients are routinely administered MAI prophylaxis with azithromycin, clarithromycin, or rifabutin. The most common manifestations of MAI infection are fever of unknown origin, weight loss, and gastrointestinal disease.

Pneumocystis carinii (**choice E**) is a common cause of pneumonia in HIV+ patients and is often the first presenting sign of AIDS. Patients with CD4+ counts $<200/mm^3$ should receive prophylaxis against *P. carinii* pneumonia (PCP) with double-strength trimethoprim-sulfamethoxazole (TMP-SMX). In sulfa-allergic patients, dapsone or pentamidine may be used.

Toxoplasmosis (**choice F**) is a rare cause of chorio-retinitis in AIDS patients, but the most likely cause of this patient's ocular changes is still CMV. When *Toxoplasma* does affect the eyes, it causes decreased vision, eye pain, and necrotizing lesions seen on fundoscopy. Most commonly, *Toxoplasma* affects the brain, with or without focal lesions. Clinical findings in the CNS include an altered mental state, seizures, weakness, cranial nerve disturbances, sensory abnormalities, cerebellar signs, meningismus, movement disorders, and neuropsychiatric manifestations.

41. **The correct answer is D.** Dog bites are the least likely to become infected compared with cat and human bites. The infection rate for dog bites is only 5%, for cat bites 30% to 50%, and an intermediate figure for human bites. The pathogens accounting for infection are different depending on the biting animal and the time of onset of infection. *Early* infections (in the first day) due to dog or cat bites are usually secondary to *Pasteurella multocida*. This agent is sensitive to penicillin or tetracyclines; however, the response is slow, and treatment should be continued for at least two weeks. Early infections following human bites are usually due to mixed aerobic and anaerobic bacteria (**choice C**), which are normal components of the oral flora.

Capnocytophaga canimorsus (**choice A**), *Eikenella corrodens* (**choice B**), and especially staphylococci (**choice E**) and streptococci (**choice F**) are responsible for *late* infections, occurring more than 24 hours after a bite. *Capnocytophaga canimorsus* is a gram-negative organism of the canine mouth flora, whereas *Eikenella corrodens* is a saprophyte of the human mouth. The pathogens involved in human bite infections are so variable that therapy should be adjusted once antibiotic sensitivity has been determined on the pathogen(s) isolated from cultured wounds.

42. **The correct answer is E.** This patient has polymyalgia rheumatica, which affects older individuals with a 2 to 1 female to male predominance. The disease is characterized by both severe muscle pain with stiffness and usually prominent systemic symptoms, such as malaise, fever, and weight loss. The muscle pain and stiffness tend to involve areas near the trunk and are not accompanied by muscle wasting or evidence of muscle damage on electromyography or biopsy. This condition is associated with temporal arteritis (which can cause blindness). Patients should be warned to inform their physician promptly if they develop severe headaches, visual changes, or significant jaw pain on repeated chewing.

Crohn disease (**choice A**) is associated with ankylosing spondylitis and a peripheral arthritis.

Dermatomyositis (**choice B**) is associated with polymyositis, skin rash, and polyarthralgias, sometimes with joint swelling and effusions.

Discoid lupus erythematosus (**choice C**) is occasionally accompanied by relatively mild arthralgias.

Sjögren syndrome (**choice D**) may be accompanied by rheumatoid arthritis-like or lupus-like symptoms.

43. **The correct answer is D.** Nitroprusside is a nonselective veno- and arteriodilator that works via release of nitric oxide. The intrinsic ability of the lungs to match ventilation with perfusion via vasoconstriction in relatively underventilated lung areas is abolished with this therapy. Therefore, large areas of V/Q mismatch are created that can result in profound hypoxia.

Elevation of carboxyhemoglobin levels (**choice A**) is incorrect. Carboxyhemoglobin is the result of binding of carbon monoxide to hemoglobin. This moiety cannot bind oxygen and results in a drastically reduced oxygen-carrying capacity. This patient has not been exposed to carbon monoxide. The byproduct of nitroprusside administration is cyanide.

Methemoglobin (**choice B**) is an oxidized form of hemoglobin in which the iron is in the Fe^{3+} configuration. This often results from blood being exposed to strong oxidizers such as nitrites. Methemoglobinemia is suspected in a cyanotic patient with normal oxygen tension. This form of hemoglobin cannot carry oxygen.

Hypoventilation (**choice C**), which is one of the four mechanisms underlying hypoxemia, is usually quite apparent on clinical inspection.

Pulmonary embolism (**choice E**) would certainly produce hypoxia, but in the absence of any clinical or historical evidence for this diagnosis, it is very unlikely at this time.

44. **The correct answer is B.** The clinical picture is consistent with ARDS, a disorder that may be triggered by a number of different conditions, including acute pancreatitis. Typically, ARDS develops 12 to 48 hours following the initiating event (3 to 4 days after acute pancreatitis) and is characterized by acute respiratory failure unresponsive to supplemental oxygen. Therapy includes treatment of the underlying condition and mechanical ventilation with positive end expiratory pressure (PEEP). The overall mortality rate is 50%.

Acute bilateral bronchopneumonia (**choice A**) may result in shortness of breath; however, it usually does not cause such severe respiratory failure and is commonly accompanied by productive cough and fever. Furthermore, chest x-ray findings, especially diffuse infiltrates and air bronchograms, are consistent with ARDS and not with bronchopneumonia.

Cardiogenic pulmonary edema (**choice C**) must be ruled out because specific treatment is available. A normal cardiac silhouette and the pulmonary changes on chest x-ray do not support a diagnosis of cardiogenic pulmonary edema. In uncertain cases, it may be necessary to measure the pulmonary capillary wedge pressure by Swan-Ganz catheter.

Exacerbation of acute pancreatitis (**choice D**), per se, is excluded by the clinical symptomatology and laboratory findings. There is no hyperglycemia, and leukocytes are only mildly elevated. However, the symptoms of acute pancreatitis can appear to improve while the extrapancreatic complications (i.e., ARDS) worsen.

Pulmonary embolism (**choice E**) usually arises from venous thrombosis in the pelvis or in the legs in patients with prolonged immobility or hypercoagulable states. It manifests as acute breathlessness, pleuritic chest pain, tachypnea, and tachycardia. Chest x-ray is often normal or may show oligemia of the affected lung segment, and an arterial blood gas (ABG) study will show hypoxemia and hypocapnia. This patient developed progressive respiratory distress and signs and symptoms of diffuse alveolar lung damage, both of which are inconsistent with acute pulmonary embolism.

45. **The correct answer is B.** The clinical presentation is characteristic of Prinzmetal angina, a form of recurrent myocardial ischemia due to transient coronary vasospasm. ST elevation on ECG during ischemic episodes is highly characteristic. This condition is most often seen in women younger than 50. Coronary angiography frequently fails to disclose any stenotic segments, but the ergonovine test (to be performed with great caution) triggers vasospasm and anginal pain.

Myocardial infarction (**choice A**) usually manifests with intense precordial pain that persists for more than 30 minutes associated with characteristic ECG changes.

Psychological chest pain (**choice C**) may manifest with variable clinical patterns and is usually associated with other symptoms, such as depression, anxiety, or panic attacks. ECG changes, such as ST elevation, are absent.

Precordial pain due to stable angina (**choice D**), by definition, manifests with a predictable pattern, usually following constant amounts of physical exertion, emotional stress, or exposure to cold temperatures.

Unstable angina (**choice E**) usually follows a period of stable angina. The attacks of precordial pain become more frequent and less predictable, and tend to occur at rest. Increasing degrees of coronary artery stenosis and/or platelet thrombi are thought to be the underlying pathologic substrate.

46. **The correct answer is D.** The most likely diagnosis in this young woman is multiple sclerosis. Trigeminal neuralgia typically occurs in patients older than 50; however, onset at a young age, bilaterality, and presence of objective signs of sensory loss on the affected side raises the suspicion of multiple sclerosis (MS). MS should be suspected in a patient with multiple neurologic findings that are "separated by time and location."

Acoustic neuroma (**choice A**) is a tumor at the cerebellopontine angle. It is associated with sensory hearing loss, facial nerve palsy, cerebellar dysfunction on the affected side, and headache. It is common in patients with neurofibromatosis, type 2.

Amyotrophic lateral sclerosis (**choice B**) is a form of progressive motor neuron disease characterized by both upper and lower motor neuron involvement; fasciculations, muscle wasting, and weakness are observed. Even in the late stages of illness, sensory, bowel, bladder, and cognitive functions are preserved. Dementia is unusual. The illness is relentlessly progressive, leading ultimately to death.

Bell's palsy (**choice C**) is characterized by loss of facial nerve function. Facial paralysis, loss of taste sensation, and hyperacusis may all be produced.

Myasthenia gravis (**choice E**) is an autoimmune neuromuscular disorder involving skeletal muscles. The fundamental defect is a decrease in the number of available acetylcholine receptors at the postsynaptic muscle membrane. Sensory changes, bladder and bowel involvement, and loss of tendon reflexes are not usually seen.

47. **The correct answer is C.** The rapid progression of a febrile illness, the systolic murmur, and the objective evidence indicating intravenous drug abuse point to infective endocarditis as the underlying etiology. The current recommendation is to obtain three different blood samples for culture over a 24-hour period before initiating antibiotic therapy, unless the patient's condition is critical. This allows identification of the infectious agent and aids in the choice of the most appropriate antibiotic regimen. Intravenous drug abusers are particularly prone to right-sided infective endocarditis, especially *Staphylococcus aureus* infections on the tricuspid valve. Note that murmurs are infrequent in right-sided infections.

Broad spectrum antibiotic therapy (**choice A**) should be started immediately after obtaining the necessary blood cultures. Until culture results are available, the combination of antibiotics should cover the three most frequent organisms responsible for infective endocarditis affecting native valves: viridans streptococci, *Staphylococcus aureus*, and *Enterococcus*.

Echocardiographic studies (**choice B**) may document the presence of vegetations. Transthoracic echocardiography has a sensitivity of approximately 60%, whereas transesophageal is 90% sensitive in identifying vegetations.

Toxicologic studies on blood and urine (**choice D**), although generally useful to document use of illicit drugs, would not be helpful as a diagnostic tool in this case.

Ventilation-perfusion lung scans (**choice E**) are used for the diagnosis of pulmonary infarction, which may occur as a result of embolism from right-sided vegetations.

48. **The correct answer is B.** Patients with severe aplastic anemia need a bone marrow transplant. If the patient needs blood products, they should be leukocyte-reduced to reduce allosensitization in likely transplant candidates (even in bone marrow transplant patients). The cause of this patient's aplastic anemia is not clear. Up to 50% of cases are idiopathic, though many of these may be from an undiagnosed viral infection that induces a host immune response or is directly marrow toxic. A small subset of cases follows an undiagnosed hepatitis, though there is no link with known viral hepatitis subtypes.

Immune-modulating drugs, such as antithymocyte globulin (**choice A**), azathioprine, methotrexate, and corticosteroids (**choice E**) are used in different bone marrow transplant protocols. In older patients or patients without good graft matches, they may be used as definitive therapy. The primary treatment of severe aplastic anemia, however, is bone marrow transplantation.

Broad-spectrum antibiotics (**choice C**) are not indicated, as there is no evidence of a bacterial infection causing this patient's symptoms.

Colony-stimulating factors (**choice D**) do not treat aplastic anemia, which is primary marrow failure. Transplantation is necessary.

49. **The correct answer is C.** *Acanthosis nigricans* is a benign skin condition histologically characterized by papillomatous hypertrophy of the epidermis with hyperpigmentation. The lesions involve flexural regions of the body, particularly the posterior neck, axilla, and groin. Although the lesions are benign, the sudden appearance of acanthosis nigricans in an elderly woman should raise the suspicion of an underlying malignancy, most commonly gastric cancer. Thus, extensive clinical and radiologic screening must be undertaken to rule out this possibility. Acanthosis nigricans is also associated with endocrinopathies, such as acromegaly, Cushing syndrome, hyperthyroidism, and glucose intolerance. Laboratory tests to screen for such diseases, including fasting glycemia (**choice C**), are thus appropriate. Glucose intolerance in elderly patients with acanthosis nigricans is due to insulin resistance resulting from autoantibodies to insulin receptors.

50. **The correct answer is H.** The clinical history alone is highly characteristic of *systemic mastocytosis* (*urticaria pigmentosa*), which is a proliferative disorder of mast cells. The infantile type is usually confined to the skin, whereas the adult type affects visceral organs as well. The most telling signs include the brown macules that urticate on stroking or rubbing (**choice H**), itching triggered by aspirin or alcohol ingestion, asthma, and splenomegaly. Development of a wheal on gentle stroking with a blunt object (e.g., the handle of the reflex hammer) is a useful diagnostic test. Loss of weight and splenomegaly suggest systemic involvement. The bone marrow is the most commonly involved organ (besides the skin), and x-ray investigations will reveal osteolytic foci. Skin biopsies show accumulation of mast cells in the dermis. Metachromatic staining with toluidine blue is used for visualization of mast cells in tissue sections.

Allergen skin testing (**choice A**) and serum IgE assays (RAST or ELISA; **choice G**) are used in the diagnosis of allergic disorders and may allow identification of the inciting agents. Neither test is indicated in the diagnosis of urticaria pigmentosa (systemic mastocytosis).

Bacterial cultures of skin scrapings (**choice B**) are useful in identifying bacterial pathogens in skin lesions suspected to be of infectious nature. Neither of the above conditions is due to bacterial organisms.

Gluten-free diet trial (**choice D**) is a diagnostic and therapeutic approach to cases of suspected *dermatitis herpetiformis/celiac disease*. Dermatitis herpetiformis manifests with pruritic vesicles on the trunk, which shows characteristic IgA deposition in the tips of dermal papillae, whereas celiac disease is associated with chronic diarrhea and malabsorption. Often, these disorders occur in the same patient and probably result from an abnormal immunologic reaction to gliadin, a protein in the gluten.

HIV testing (**choice E**) would not be diagnostic in either case. HIV infection is associated with a number of skin conditions, including opportunistic infections (e.g., candidiasis, herpes simplex, herpes zoster, *Staphylococcus*, and bacillary angiomatosis) and neoplastic conditions (e.g., Kaposi sarcoma and lymphoma). Neither acanthosis nigricans nor mastocytosis has been reported in AIDS.

Microscopic examination of KOH-treated skin scrapings (**choice F**) allows identification of fungal organisms in skin lesions.

Internal Medicine: **Test Four**

1. A 21-year-old man is brought to the emergency department by his roommate because of abrupt onset of shortness of breath, mild chest pain, and a sensation of rapid heart beating. The patient says that in the past he had similar episodes, which resolved with the Valsalva maneuver or breath holding. This time, these measures were unsuccessful. He does not take any medication and is otherwise in good health. An ECG documents supraventricular tachycardia with a pulse of 200/min. Under ECG monitoring, gentle massage over the right carotid sinus is attempted, but the attack does not cease. Which of the following is the most appropriate next step in treatment?

   (A) Further carotid sinus massage

   (B) IV lidocaine

   (C) IV procainamide

   (D) IV verapamil

   (E) Oral verapamil

2. A 45-year-old African American man is taken to the emergency department because he is vomiting fresh blood. His temperature is 37° C (98.6° F), blood pressure is 65/30 mm Hg, pulse is 120/min, and respirations are 24/min. The patient is stabilized, then taken for emergency endoscopy. The source of bleeding is a tortuous vein near the gastroesophageal junction. The bleeding is successfully stopped by banding of the vessel. Which of the following is the most likely underlying condition predisposing this patient for this complication?

   (A) Alcoholism

   (B) Alpha$_1$-antitrypsin deficiency

   (C) Hemochromatosis

   (D) Hepatitis A infection

   (E) Hepatitis B infection

3. A 32-year-old man with AIDS develops right-sided weakness over the course of one week. He is on a combined drug regimen of zidovudine (AZT) and a protease inhibitor, and his CD4 cell count is 190 cells/mL. MRI of the brain reveals a single 2-cm mass in the left cerebral white matter that appears as an area of low signal surrounded by a rim of contrast enhancement ("ring-enhancing lesion"). A trial of sulfadiazine and pyrimethamine is started. Three weeks after beginning this treatment, the patient's neurologic status is unchanged, and imaging studies show that the lesion has not regressed. Which of the following is the most likely diagnosis?

   (A) Cryptococcal meningoencephalitis

   (B) Glioblastoma multiforme (GBM)

   (C) Metastatic tumor

   (D) Primary brain lymphoma

   (E) *Toxoplasma* abscess

4. A 68-year-old woman complains of two days of cough associated with purulent sputum and right-sided chest pain exacerbated by breathing. She has had mid-back pain unassociated with trauma for the past two months. One month ago, she was hospitalized briefly for pneumonia. On physical examination, her temperature is 39.0° C (102.2° F), blood pressure is 110/80 mm Hg, pulse is 98/min, and respirations are 28/min. There are crackles and egophony over the right lower lung field. There is no occult blood in the stool. Blood tests show a white blood cell count of 16,000/mm³, a hematocrit of 18%, and a platelet count of 189,000/mm³. The mean corpuscular volume is 82 μm³. A chest x-ray film shows consolidation of the right middle and lower lobes, diffuse osteopenia, and multiple lytic lesions of the ribs and thoracic spine. Which of the following is the most likely laboratory finding?

(A) Decreased serum ferritin

(B) Elevated serum protein

(C) Hyperphosphatemia

(D) Hypertriglyceridemia

(E) Hypocalcemia

5. A 38-year-old woman is complaining of shortness of breath that started suddenly on the morning of presentation. She is an otherwise healthy woman. She takes oral contraceptive pills, and she has a ten-year history of smoking a pack of cigarettes daily. She appears anxious and is rapidly breathing at 30 breaths/min. Her pulse is 110/min, and her blood pressure is 120/80 mm Hg and stable. The rest of her physical examination is unremarkable. Which of the following is the most appropriate initial step in management?

(A) Aspirin

(B) Warfarin

(C) Heparin

(D) IV fluid

(E) Streptokinase

6. A 35-year-old man is brought to the emergency department after he faints and cannot be revived. Stat chemistries are notable for a plasma glucose of 23 mg/dL. The patient is promptly given IV glucose and recovers consciousness. Careful questioning reveals that he has a family history of endocrine abnormalities. Follow-up studies performed on the remainder of the blood drawn for the screening studies demonstrate insulin levels of 120 mU/mL (reference range 5-25 mU/mL). A CT scan of the abdomen demonstrates a 2-cm mass in the tail of the pancreas. Which additional finding will most likely be seen this patient?

(A) Marfanoid habitus

(B) Medullary carcinoma of the thyroid

(C) Mucosal neuromas

(D) Parathyroid adenoma

(E) Pheochromocytoma

7. A 45-year-old man presents to a physician because of repeated episodes of fainting. The radial pulse is erratic, with multiple skipped beats at a rate of 45 beats/min. An ECG shows a normal sinus rhythm at a rate of 60/min. An echocardiogram reveals a 2-cm mass that is acting like a "ball valve" to produce intermittent obstruction of flow. Which of the following is the most likely location of this patient's lesion?

(A) Aorta

(B) Left atrium

(C) Left ventricle

(D) Right atrium

(E) Right ventricle

8. A diabetic patient is undergoing a routine physical examination. During the review of systems, the patient comments that he has been having pain on swallowing. He localizes the pain to below his sternum. Barium swallow shows slightly raised plaques throughout the esophagus. Endoscopy demonstrates plaques covered with white, curdy, cheese-like material. A biopsy of one of the lesions will most likely demonstrate which of the following?

   (A) Acute-angled, branching, septated filaments

   (B) Anaplastic squamous cells with numerous mitotic figures

   (C) Intranuclear and cytoplasmic inclusion bodies with "owl's-eye" appearance

   (D) Loss of ganglion cells in the myenteric plexus

   (E) Multinucleated epithelial giant cells on Giemsa stain

   (F) Pseudohyphal mycelia and budding yeast cells

9. A 45-year-old woman comes to the physician because of persistent blurred vision for the past month. She also reports three episodes of *Candida* vaginitis during the past year. She is 167 cm (66 in) tall, and weighs 84 kg (185 lb). Her blood pressure is 130/84 mm Hg. Funduscopic examination reveals dot retinal hemorrhages and increased tortuosity of retinal veins. Her family history is significant for obesity, coronary artery disease, and type 2 diabetes mellitus in several relatives. Examination reveals no significant abnormalities. Dipstick urinalysis is normal. Which of the following is the most appropriate next step in diagnosis?

   (A) Blood test for C-peptide

   (B) Fasting blood glucose level

   (C) Glucose tolerance test

   (D) Glycosylated hemoglobin

   (E) Urine glucose levels

   (F) Urine protein

10. A 61-year-old woman presents with complaints of two months of low-grade fevers and malaise. She states that she has been having frequent right-sided headaches without any other associated neurologic symptoms. On physical examination, she has a temperature of 37.9° C (100.2° F), and her neurologic examination is unremarkable. Laboratory results reveal a white blood cell count of 11,200/mm^3 and a hematocrit of 36%. Serum electrolytes are normal, and her erythrocyte sedimentation rate (ESR) is 86/min. Which of the following is the most appropriate next step in management?

    (A) Carotid artery Doppler flow studies

    (B) Ergotamine

    (C) High-dose IV penicillin

    (D) High-dose steroids

    (E) Oral nonsteroidal anti-inflammatory drugs (NSAIDs)

11. A 55-year-old man comes to medical attention because of a long history of recurrent bouts of deep epigastric pain, associated with elevation of amylase and lipase. He also reports bulky, foul-smelling stools for the past two months. A plain x-ray film of the abdomen reveals multiple calcifications in the pancreatic region. At this time, serum levels of amylase and lipase are within normal limits. Which of the following is the most common etiologic factor associated with this condition in the U.S.?

    (A) Alcoholism

    (B) Biliary stone disease

    (C) Cystic fibrosis

    (D) Familial predisposition

    (E) Hyperlipidemia

    (F) Hyperparathyroidism

    (G) Malnutrition

    (H) Pancreatic neoplasms

12. A 60-year-old woman presents with complaints of chronic fatigue and mild pruritus. She has a history of rheumatoid arthritis and autoimmune thyroiditis. On examination, her liver is modestly enlarged, firm, and nontender; skin xanthomas are noted. Routine serum chemistry studies show:

Sodium	141 mEq/L
Potassium	5.1 mEq/L
Chloride	102 mEq/L
Bicarbonate	25 mEq/L
Albumin	4.1 g/dL
Urea nitrogen	25 mg/dL
Bilirubin, total	1.3 mg/dL
Creatinine	0.8 mg/dL
AST	55 U/L
ALT	48 U/L
Alkaline phosphatase	240 U/L

Follow-up laboratory studies demonstrate a serum gamma-glutamyl transpeptidase level of 150 U/L, and a serum cholesterol of 240 mg/dL. Immunoglobulin studies reveal a marked elevation of serum IgM. Ultrasound demonstrates diffuse enlargement of the liver without marked echogenicity. Endoscopic retrograde cholangiography demonstrates an intact extrahepatic biliary tree accompanied by stricture and loss of ducts within the liver itself. Liver biopsy shows a florid bile duct lesion with patchy inflammation and destruction of septal and interlobular bile ducts. Antibodies directed against which of the following antigens are present in up to 95% of patients with this disease?

(A) Double-stranded DNA

(B) Hepatitis A virus

(C) Hepatitis B core antigen

(D) Hepatitis C virus

(E) Mitochondria

13. A 62-year-old man comes to the physician because of episodic chest pain that manifests as a sensation of precordial tightness, occurs after physical exertion, and is relieved promptly by rest. The patient has noted that the amount of activity sufficient to trigger the pain is relatively constant, such as climbing three flights of stairs or walking uphill for a few minutes. An ECG recorded at rest fails to show any abnormalities. Which of the following is the most appropriate next step in diagnosis?

(A) Ambulatory ECG monitoring

(B) Echocardiography

(C) Exercise ECG

(D) Myocardial perfusion scintigraphy

(E) Coronary arteriography

14. A 49-year-old man with acute pancreatitis develops severe shortness of breath 15 minutes after undergoing placement of a catheter in his subclavian vein. His blood pressure is 100/60 mm Hg, pulse is 124/min, and respirations are 50/min. He is cyanotic and in obvious distress. His neck veins are distended, and his trachea deviates to the left. Breath sounds are diminished on the right side of his chest. Which of the following is the most appropriate next step in management?

(A) Chest x-ray

(B) Removal of the catheter

(C) Endotracheal intubation

(D) Needle thoracostomy in the second right intercostal space

(E) Tube thoracostomy in the left fifth intercostal space

15. A 31-year-old Asian American man presents to the clinic for an annual physical. He has a 19-year history of type 1 diabetes, requiring 10 units NPH insulin each morning and 8 units NPH in the evening, with frequent blood glucose checks and regular insulin dosing throughout the day. He does not keep a log of his blood glucose values. A urine dipstick test shows 2+ albumin. His hemoglobin A_{1c} (HbA_{1c}) is 7.9%. Which of the following is the most appropriate next step in management to prevent morbidity?

(A) Add a standing regular insulin dose at lunchtime

(B) Begin ACE inhibitor therapy

(C) Discuss options for using an insulin pump

(D) Increase his morning NPH insulin dose

(E) Send a 24-hour urine collection specimen for total protein

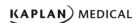

16. A 55-year-old patient presents with chronic cough. In addition to the cough, the patient has gained weight recently with development of a "buffalo hump" and Cushingoid features. A chest x-ray film demonstrates a mass involving the central area of the chest. Bronchoscopy is performed, and they are able to biopsy the tumor during the procedure. Which of the following is the most likely diagnosis?

    (A) Adenocarcinoma

    (B) Bronchioloalveolar carcinoma

    (C) Large cell carcinoma

    (D) Small cell carcinoma

    (E) Squamous cell carcinoma

17. A 61-year-old man is hospitalized after receiving an implantable cardiac defibrillator (ICD). The patient has a long history of coronary disease and sustained an anterior wall myocardial infarction three years ago. Two weeks ago, he had an episode of pulseless ventricular tachycardia and was successfully resuscitated. This episode led to the ICD placement. In addition to the ICD, the cardiologist also plans to initiate antiarrhythmic therapy with amiodarone. Which of the following is the most important side effect of this therapy?

    (A) Hypotension

    (B) Pulmonary fibrosis

    (C) Prolongation of the QT interval

    (D) Recurrent ventricular arrhythmia

    (E) Skin discoloration

18. A 32-year-old woman is referred to a neurologist for evaluation of unsteady gait and numbness in the right foot. Examination reveals weakness of the right lower extremity with muscle spasticity and decreased vibratory sensation. MRI studies show cerebral and spinal cord changes suspicious for demyelinating lesions. A lumbar puncture is performed for examination of CSF. Which of the following CSF findings would be most consistent with a diagnosis of demyelinating disorder?

    (A) Elevated protein with marked lymphocytosis

    (B) Elevated protein with normal cell count

    (C) Marked neutrophilic leukocytosis with reduced glucose

    (D) Mildly increased protein with oligoclonal IgG bands

    (E) Normal protein with mild lymphocytosis

19. A 70-year-old man is brought to the emergency department by his family because of the rapid onset of right-sided weakness and confusion. On arrival, the patient is drowsy, but examination confirms a right hemiparesis associated with left sided deviation of the eyes. The patient is admitted with a preliminary diagnosis of cerebral infarction. A CT scan of the head performed 12 hours following symptom onset reveals changes consistent with ischemic necrosis in the territory of the middle cerebral artery. The patient's neurologic status deteriorates rapidly on the third hospital day, and he lapses into coma. He dies the next day. An autopsy confirms a large infarct in the territory of the middle cerebral artery, associated with massive swelling of the left hemisphere, transtentorial herniation, and pontine Duret hemorrhages. Which of the following treatments might have prevented such an outcome?

    (A) Anticoagulants

    (B) Barbiturates

    (C) Calcium channel blockers

    (D) Corticosteroids

    (E) NMDA receptor antagonists

20. A 60-year-old woman is hospitalized with a severe case of pneumonia that is treated with cephalosporins. Her condition improves over the course of therapy, and after six days, she develops loose stools that progresses to frequent bouts of foul-smelling, watery diarrhea with small amounts of blood over the course of ten hours. There is associated abdominal pain, nausea and vomiting, fever, leukocytosis, and hypotension. Physical examination reveals diffuse pain on palpation, and an abdominal x-ray shows marked dilatation of the transverse colon and mucosal edema. Sigmoidoscopy is performed and reveals diffuse pseudomembranes over the colon that reveal an erythematous, inflamed muscosa when removed. Which of the following is this patient at greatest risk for?

    (A) Colon cancer

    (B) Colonic perforation

    (C) Fistula formation

    (D) Gangrenous necrosis

    (E) Hemorrhage

    (F) Malabsorption

    (G) Vitamin deficiency

21. A 35-year-old man with a history of chronic hepatitis B presents to the emergency department with severe abdominal pain. The patient states that he has had intermittent fevers and a 15-lb weight loss over the past six months. His temperature is 38° C (100.4° F), blood pressure is 160/120 mm Hg, pulse is 60/min, and respirations are 15/min. Abdominal examination demonstrates guarding and diffuse pain. Examination of his legs is remarkable for purpura and several distinctive pea-sized nodules along the course of superficial arteries. The erythrocyte sedimentation rate is 30 mm/hr. Urinalysis reveals proteinuria, hematuria, and proteinaceous casts. Biopsy of one of the pea-shaped lesions of the leg would likely show which of the following in vessels walls?

(A) Atherosclerotic plaques

(B) Fungal hyphae

(C) Giant cells

(D) Granulomas

(E) Neutrophils

22. A 22-year-old woman presents with a one-week history of an itchy rash, which manifested a few weeks after coming back from a trip with her friends. One of the friends has developed a similar rash. The patient reports that the itching keeps her awake at night. Physical examination reveals a linear papulovesicular eruption along the waistline, axillary folds, and finger webs. Linear burrows are evident on close inspection. Which of the following is the most appropriate next step in diagnosis?

(A) Microscopic examination of skin scrapings obtained after placing oil on lesions

(B) Microscopic examination of skin scrapings treated with potassium hydroxide

(C) Measurement of serum IgE levels

(D) Allergen challenge tests

(E) Skin biopsy

23. A 35-year-old man being treated with phenytoin for epilepsy comes to the physician for a routine check-up examination. He has been seizure-free for the past year. Physical examination reveals pallor of skin and mucosae, slightly jaundiced discoloration of sclerae, and a red and shiny tongue. He denies paresthesias, and sensation is normal on neurologic examination. Significant results of blood and serum studies include:

Hematocrit	28%
Hemoglobin	8.5 g/dL
Mean corpuscular volume	130 fL
Reticulocytes	0.2%
Platelets	140,000/mm^3
Leukocytes	4,800/mm^3
Bilirubin	
Total	2.0 mg/dL
Direct	0.3 mg/dL
Lactate dehydrogenase	600 U/L

A peripheral blood smear reveals macrocytes, ovalocytes, and hypersegmented neutrophils. Which of the following is the most likely cause of this patient's anemia?

(A) Autoimmune hemolysis

(B) Bone marrow aplasia

(C) Folate deficiency

(D) Iron deficiency

(E) Vitamin B$_{12}$ deficiency

24. A 35-year-old man comes to the emergency department because he is experiencing palpitations and is afraid he is having a heart attack. On questioning, the patient has had a number of these episodes in the past few months, although the present one is the worst. His temperature is 37° C (98.6° F), blood pressure is 170/135 mm Hg, pulse is 140/min, and respirations are 17/min. Physical examination is remarkable only for diaphoresis. Within the hour, before definitive therapy is begun, the patient's blood pressure drops spontaneously to 140/85 mm Hg, and his symptoms improve. Measurement of which of the following in a 24-hour urine collection is most likely to confirm the probable diagnosis?

(A) 17-Hydroxycorticosteroids

(B) Porphobilinogen

(C) Pregnanediol

(D) Tetrahydrocortisol

(E) Vanillylmandelic acid

25. A 55-year-old white man presents to the emergency department with severe abdominal pain that has been radiating to his back for the past two days. The man appears acutely ill and is sitting in a markedly bent-over position, holding his arms over his abdomen. The patient states that this posture makes him feel slightly better, and comments that sudden movements and deep breathing make the pain worse. He has also been throwing up, even when there is nothing in his stomach. He describes the pain as "terrible" and begs for narcotics. On questioning, he admits to heavy drinking for the past five or ten years. He denies use of street drugs. His temperature is 38.1° C (100.6° F), blood pressure is 85/60 mm Hg when lying down and 60/45 mm Hg when sitting, pulse is 120/min and regular, and respirations are 22/min and shallow. His lungs are clear to auscultation. Pressure on the upper portion of the abdomen intensifies the pain. Examination of the extremities reveals multiple bruises but no needle marks. The liver edge can be felt and has a nodular character. A complete blood count shows an erythrocyte count of 3.5 million/mm^3, white blood cell count of 18,000/mm^3 with predominately neutrophils and increased band forms, and a platelet count of 200,000/mm^3. Which of the following is the most appropriate next step in diagnosis?

    (A) Blood urea nitrogen

    (B) Chest x-ray

    (C) Serum amylase level

    (D) Serum transaminase levels

    (E) Esophagogastroduodenoscopy

26. A 40-year-old woman presents to the physician because of increased nervousness for the past three months. She reports insomnia, frequent palpitations without an identifiable cause, and weakness. She has no significant past medical history and takes no medications. Vital signs are remarkable for a blood pressure of 150/60 mm Hg and a pulse of 135/min. She appears anxious, and despite being in the middle of winter, is dressed in a t-shirt and shorts. Physical examination reveals proptosis and eyelid retraction, moist skin, mild hand tremor, and a palpable diffuse goiter. Which of the following is the most likely diagnosis?

    (A) Euthyroid sick syndrome

    (B) Follicular carcinoma of the thyroid

    (C) Graves disease

    (D) Hashimoto thyroiditis

    (E) Subacute thyroiditis

27. A malnourished and dehydrated 54-year-old man with a history of alcoholism is brought to the emergency department. His temperature is 36.9° C (98.4° F), blood pressure is 105/65 mm Hg, pulse is 98/min, and respirations are 14/min. Neurologic assessment reveals decreased reflexes and sensation in the legs, and an ataxic gait. On admission, laboratory tests show:

Albumin	2.9 g/dL
Sodium	105 mEq/L
Potassium	3.9 mEq/L
Chloride	101 mEq/L
Plasma osmolality	256 mOsm/kg
Na fractional excretion	<0.5%

    He is treated with parenteral administration of 100 mg of thiamin and IV infusion of isotonic saline and glucose. Twelve hours after treatment is started, the patient becomes quadriplegic and mute, although he appears to be able to communicate by slow eye blinking. A blood sample at this time shows the following values:

Sodium	126 mEq/L
Potassium	4.0 mEq/L
Chloride	105 mEq/L

    Despite adequate therapeutic interventions, the patient dies on the third hospital day. Which of the following postmortem findings will most likely be obtained at autopsy?

    (A) Alzheimer type 2 glia, consistent with hepatic encephalopathy

    (B) Central pontine myelinolysis

    (C) Cerebellar vermis atrophy

    (D) Subacute combined degeneration of the spinal cord

    (E) Wernicke encephalopathy

28. A 64-year-old man is brought to the emergency department because of sudden onset of tearing chest pain that originates in the anterior chest and radiates to the back in the interscapular region. A few weeks ago, he had a dental abscess, which resolved with extraction followed by a full course of ampicillin. On examination, he is oriented to person, place, and time; however, he appears in acute distress, is diaphoretic, and is breathing with difficulty. His temperature is 37.1° C (98.8° F), blood pressure is 174/68 mm Hg, pulse is 206/min, and respirations are 25/min. There is no jugular vein distention or hepatomegaly. Auscultation reveals a diastolic murmur along the left sternal border. The lungs are clear to auscultation. The ECG shows no signs of myocardial ischemia. A chest x-ray film demonstrates widening of the mediastinum. Which of the following is the most likely diagnosis?

    (A) Aortic dissection

    (B) Acute mediastinitis

    (C) Acute pericarditis

    (D) Cardiac tamponade

    (E) Myocardial infarction

29. A 25-year-old man is admitted to a burn unit after an automobile accident in which he lost consciousness and then was burned over 65% of his body. Two days after his accident, the nurse notices that small amounts of blood are returned through his nasogastric tube when she checks it prior to administering fluids. Endoscopy shows multiple, tiny to small (2-20 mm in diameter) ulcers in the corpus of the stomach. Which of the following is the most likely diagnosis?

    (A) Acute erosive gastritis

    (B) Chronic erosive gastritis

    (C) Gastric atrophy

    (D) Nonerosive gastritis

    (E) Superficial gastritis

30. A 56-year-old woman with a long history of untreated hypertension is brought to the emergency department because of severe headache and confusion. The patient is oriented to person, but not to time or place. Her blood pressure is 230/140 mm Hg, pulse is 86/min, and respirations are 18/min. Funduscopic examination reveals optic disc edema, and a dipstick test shows protein in the urine. Which of the following is the most appropriate pharmacotherapy?

    (A) Clonidine

    (B) Enalaprilat

    (C) Esmolol

    (D) Furosemide

    (E) Hydralazine

    (F) Nifedipine

    (G) Nitroglycerin

    (H) Sodium nitroprusside

31. A 29-year-old man consults a physician because he has developed chronic weakness and fatigue. He also feels dizzy when he first stands up in the morning. On further questioning, he reports cold intolerance and frequent urination. Physical examination is notable for facial puffiness; coarse, sparse, hair; and a hoarse voice. Laboratory studies show:

Sodium	125 mEq/L
Potassium	5.5 mEq/L
Bicarbonate	25 mEq/L
Urea nitrogen (BUN)	22 mg/dL
Serum glucose	380 mg/dL
Thyroid-stimulating hormone (TSH)	9.5 IU/mL

    Which of the following is the most likely diagnosis?

    (A) Multiple endocrine neoplasia (MEN), type I

    (B) MEN, type IIA

    (C) MEN, type IIB

    (D) Polyglandular deficiency syndrome, type I

    (E) Polyglandular deficiency syndrome, type II

32. A 55-year-old white man is taken to the emergency department because he is vomiting fresh blood. For the past several hours, he had been vomiting, then dry heaving; 30 minutes ago, he suddenly started vomiting fresh blood. The patient's temperature is 35.6° C (96° F), blood pressure is 110/55 mm Hg, pulse is 75/min, respirations are 16/min. Endoscopy demonstrates several lacerations in the mucosa near the gastroesophageal junction. Which of the following underlying conditions is likely present in this patient?

    (A) AIDS

    (B) Alcoholism

    (C) Chagas disease

    (D) Diabetes mellitus

    (E) Scleroderma

33. A 34-year-old woman undergoes clinical investigations because of chronic dyspeptic symptoms, such as mild nausea, bloating after meals, and mild right upper abdominal pain. She is otherwise healthy and takes oral contraceptives only. Physical examination and laboratory studies are normal. Liver ultrasonography reveals a 5-cm, well-circumscribed mass in the right hepatic lobe. A percutaneous needle biopsy shows a lesion consistent with hepatic adenoma. When symptomatic, which of the following is the most common clinical presentation of this tumor?

    (A) Abdominal pain

    (B) Jaundice

    (C) Metastatic disease

    (D) Portal hypertension

    (E) Rupture into peritoneal cavity

34. A 40-year-old man presents with the acute onset of severe pain in his left great toe for the past 24 hours. He denies trauma, fever, chills, or changes in appetite. He is a chronic smoker but does not abuse alcohol. He is currently on day four of a course of erythromycin for bronchitis. Examination shows his blood pressure is 120/80 mm Hg, pulse is 80/min, and respirations are 18/min. The left great toe is red, swollen, and tender to touch, with no fluctuation. Laboratory evaluation shows the following:

Sodium	139 mEq/L
Potassium	4.5 mEq/L
Hemoglobin	13.5 g/dL
Leukocytes	$9,000/mm^3$
Platelets	$350,000/mm^3$
Uric acid	14 mg/dL

Which of the following is the most appropriate initial step in management?

    (A) Allopurinol

    (B) Colchicine

    (C) Indomethacin

    (D) Intra-articular corticosteroids

    (E) Probenecid

35. A 38-year-old engineer presents with complaints of epistaxis, severe sinus pain, and purulent sinus drainage over the past six months. One year ago, he had frequent episodes of cough, and a chest x-ray film obtained at that time showed pulmonary infiltrates. He recalls that his cough was poorly responsive to antibiotics. The man also admits to general weakness and diffuse muscle aches. Over the past eight months he has lost more than 5 kg (10 lb). The patient has no other medical problems, denies smoking, is not taking any medications, and reports no other symptoms. On physical examination, his lungs are clear without wheezing or rhonchi. Small ulcerative lesions are apparent on his nasal septum, and many tender subcutaneous nodules are present on his back and arms. Laboratory values are as follows:

Erythrocyte sedimentation rate	66 mm/h
Leukocytes	12,000/mm^3 (70% segmented neutrophils, 20% lymphocytes, 10% monocytes)
Hemoglobin	13 g/dL
Hematocrit	41%

A chest x-ray film is obtained that shows multiple 1- to 2-cm nodules in both upper lung fields. Which of the following is most likely to confirm the diagnosis?

(A) Antiribonucleoprotein

(B) Elevated serum IgE

(C) Positive antiglomerular basement membrane antibody

(D) Positive c-ANCA

(E) Positive p-ANCA

(F) Positive rheumatoid factor

36. An 87-year-old woman with advanced Alzheimer disease is transferred from a nursing home to a hospital unit after a deterioration in her condition. Physical examination demonstrates a nearly immobile, emaciated woman with poor skin turgor and a dry mouth. Her temperature is 35.6° C (96° F), blood pressure is 90/60 mm Hg, pulse is 90/min, and respirations are 15/min. Blood chemistry studies demonstrate a sodium of 151 mEq/L, a potassium of 5.3 mEq/L, and a chloride of 112 mEq/L. Which of the following is the most appropriate next step in management?

(A) Oral water administration

(B) IV 0.9% saline

(C) IV 5% D/W

(D) IV colloid and 0.9% saline

(E) IV distilled water

37. A 28-year-old man presents to a physician because of sores on his penis and scrotum. He also has lesions in his oral cavity, which began a few days before the sores on his genitalia. He has had several similar episodes in the past, but they resolved before he consulted a physician. During these periods, his eyes often hurt when he goes into bright light. He has also had recent intermittent pain in his knees. Physical examination demonstrates oral lesions resembling aphthous ulcers, as well as small ulcers on the genitalia. Tzanck smear of the genital and oral ulcers is negative for multinucleated giant cells. Blood studies demonstrate an elevated erythrocyte sedimentation rate (ESR), elevated alpha-2 and gamma globulins, and mild leukocytosis. Which of the following is the most likely diagnosis?

(A) Behcet syndrome

(B) Herpes simplex infection

(C) *Neisseria gonorrhoeae* infection

(D) Psoriasis

(E) *Treponema pallidum* infection

38. A 65-year-old man reports feeling increasingly tired and short of breath. He had been well until a year ago, when he started losing weight despite any dietary change. He also complains of pencil thin stools. His wife has commented that he seems very pale. He is on no medications. Physical examination shows a pale-appearing man with an elevated heart rate. Rectal examination is positive for occult blood. Laboratory studies are remarkable for a hematocrit of 25%. Which of the following is the most appropriate next step in diagnosis?

    (A) KUB (x-ray film showing the kidney, ureters and bladder)
    (B) Colonoscopy
    (C) Esophagoduodenoscopy
    (D) Sigmoidoscopy
    (E) Open laparotomy

39. A 42-year-old woman with a history of rheumatoid arthritis develops tingling, pain, and focal numbness of one hand. These sensations involve the palmar aspect of the thumb and fingers, with the exception of the ulnar edge of the little finger. The woman works as a secretary and has noticed that her symptoms are worst at night, particularly after she has done a considerable amount of typing during the preceding workday. Tapping on the volar surface of the wrist with a reflex hammer reproduces the symptoms. Which of the following is the most likely diagnosis?

    (A) Carpal tunnel syndrome
    (B) Cubital tunnel syndrome
    (C) Radial tunnel syndrome
    (D) Reflex sympathetic dystrophy
    (E) Scapholunate ligament rupture

40. An 18-year-old student comes to the physician five hours after sustaining an injury to his right ankle while playing football. He says that he "rolled his ankle over," but denies feeling any snap or crack at the time of injury. He walks with a slight limp. Examination shows swelling of the right ankle, especially on the lateral side. Pulses and sensation are normal. Pain is most pronounced in the area of the calcaneofibular ligament. The "drawer" test is normal, but the "talar tilt" test reveals increased excursion on the right compared with the uninjured side. There is no tenderness on palpation of the lateral malleolus. Which of the following is the most appropriate next step in management?

    (A) Referral to orthopedic specialist
    (B) Treatment with nonsteroidal anti-inflammatory drugs without ankle immobilization
    (C) Treatment for acute ankle sprain with rehabilitation within 72 hours
    (D) Treatment for acute ankle sprain with rehabilitation after ten days of ankle rest
    (E) X-ray examination

41. One week following an uncomplicated delivery, a 27-year-old woman comes to the physician because of polyuria and excessive thirst. Her pregnancy was normal, but she reports that she began to feel an unusual craving for ice water in the last month of gestation. She is forced to get up at night several times to void and drinks large amounts of water. Her blood pressure is 120/80 mm Hg. Serum electrolytes are within normal limits. A 24-hour urine collection during ad libitum water intake yields the following results:

Total volume	10 L
Specific gravity	<1.006
Glucose	Absent
Protein	<150 mg

Which of the following is the most appropriate next step in management?

    (A) Advise the patient to reduce water intake
    (B) Perform vasopressin challenge test
    (C) Order MRI studies of the pituitary-hypothalamic region
    (D) Refer for psychiatric evaluation of compulsive water drinking
    (E) Refer to nephrologist for evaluation of nephrogenic diabetes insipidus

42. A 74-year-old man is hospitalized for treatment of enterococcal pneumonia. He has a history of gout and hyperuricemia, for which he takes allopurinol. In the hospital, the patient receives treatment with ampicillin and gentamicin for seven days. Despite antibiotic therapy, he remains persistently febrile. On the eighth hospital day, he manifests signs of rapidly progressive renal insufficiency. His temperature is 38.2° C (100.8° F), blood pressure is 100/60 mm Hg, pulse is 100/min, and respirations are 20/min. Laboratory investigations show:

Blood, serum:

Sodium	145 mEq/L
Potassium	6.5 mEq/L
Chloride	110 mEq/L
Bicarbonate	20 mEq/L
Urea nitrogen	40 mg/dL
Creatinine	3.5 mg/dL
Uric acid	8.5 mg/dL

Urine:

Sodium	23 mEq/L
Creatinine	35 mg/dL
Pigmented granular casts	Present
Protein	Negative
Erythrocytes	Negative

Which of the following is the most likely cause of this patient's renal failure?

(A) Allopurinol toxicity

(B) Ampicillin toxicity

(C) Gentamicin toxicity

(D) Hyperuricemia

(E) Hypotension

(F) Sepsis

43. A 72-year-old woman is driven to the emergency department because ten minutes earlier she had developed painless, sudden, unilateral blindness. When light is shined on the affected eye, the pupil fails to constrict. When the light is shined on the opposite eye, the affected eye's pupil constricts briskly. Tonometry of both eyes is within normal limits. Ophthalmoscopy demonstrates a pale, opaque fundus with a red fovea. The arteries are markedly attenuated. Which of the following is the most likely diagnosis?

(A) Age-related macular degeneration

(B) Central retinal artery occlusion

(C) Central retinal vein occlusion

(D) Hypertensive retinopathy

(E) Retinitis pigmentosa

44. A 45-year-old woman presents to a physician with marked swelling of her hands. Five years previously, she had developed multiple arthralgias, and early rheumatoid arthritis was suspected; however, no confirmatory immunologic studies had been performed at that time. Since then, she has experienced difficulty swallowing and mild dyspnea on exertion. On physical examination, the hands are strikingly swollen, producing a sausage-like appearance to the fingers. Other findings include erythematous patches over the knuckles, a mild malar rash, and slight violaceous discoloration to the eyelids. No joint deformity is noted, although many joints are tender. A chest x-ray film demonstrates diffuse interstitial infiltrates. In antibody studies, high titers of antibodies directed against which of the following antigens will most likely be present?

(A) c-ANCA

(B) dsDNA

(C) p-ANCA

(D) Scl-70

(E) RNP

45. A 41-year-old high school teacher comes to the physician for a health maintenance examination. He has been in good health except for occasional episodes of acute upper respiratory infections. His blood pressure is 137/83 mm Hg. His height is 175 cm (69 in), and his weight is 81 kg (180 lb). He has no family history of early coronary artery disease, hypertension, or hyperlipidemia. He drinks alcohol on social occasions and has been smoking 30 cigarettes daily since the age of 20. He smokes his first cigarette soon after getting up in the morning, finds it extremely difficult to refrain from smoking while teaching in school, and does not quit even when he is sick in bed. With respect to smoking cessation, which of the following is the most appropriate next step in management?

(A) Ask patient if he intends to quit smoking in the near future

(B) Try to elicit a quitting date even if patient appears unwilling

(C) Prescribe nicotine patch and gum

(D) Recommend group behavior treatment

(E) Refer to a psychiatrist for alcohol and nicotine dependence

46. A 21-year-old woman presents to the emergency department with several days of fever and fatigue. Her temperature is 39.0° C (102.2° F), her pulse is 90/min, and her blood pressure is 96/64 mm Hg. Her chest is clear to auscultation, and her abdomen is soft and nontender. A grade III/IV holosystolic murmur that increases on inspiration is best heard along the left sternal border. A CBC shows normochromic normocytic anemia. Chest x-ray films reveal several well-circumscribed, round infiltrates in multiple lobes. Echocardiography and blood cultures suggest a diagnosis of acute bacterial endocarditis limited to the tricuspid valve. Which of the following is the most likely explanation for these findings?

(A) Congenital heart disease

(B) Illicit drug use

(C) Rheumatic fever

(D) Rheumatoid arthritis

(E) Systemic lupus erythematosus

47. A 22-year-old man is brought to the emergency department several hours after sustaining a severe head trauma during a soccer game. He became unconscious for a short time soon after the accident, regained consciousness for three hours, and subsequently relapsed into coma. On arrival, the patient appears unresponsive to verbal or painful stimuli. A scalp lesion consistent with prior contusion is found in the right parietal region. The right pupil is dilated and poorly reactive to light, and funduscopic examination reveals early papilledema. X-ray films of the head show a linear fracture in the right calvarial wall. Which of the following is the most likely diagnosis?

(A) Epidural hemorrhage

(B) Fracture without associated brain injury

(C) Intracerebral hypertensive hemorrhage

(D) Subarachnoid hemorrhage

(E) Subdural hemorrhage

48. A 72-year-old man suffers severe pleuritic chest pain on the seventh postoperative day after surgical pinning of an intertrochanteric hip fracture. He was not on anticoagulants at the time. He is hemodynamically stable, but is short of breath and has distended neck veins. Spiral CT scan shows the presence of a pulmonary embolus on the left side, and echocardiogram does not show signs of right ventricular strain. Which of the following is the most appropriate management at this time?

(A) Anticoagulation with heparin

(B) Infusion of thrombolytic agents into the left pulmonary artery

(C) Insertion of vena cava filter

(D) Surgical embolectomy

(E) Systemic infusion of thrombolytic agents

The response options for items 49-50 are the same. You will be required to select one answer for each item in the set.

(A) Alzheimer disease

(B) Chronic subdural hematoma

(C) Creutzfeldt-Jakob disease

(D) Dementia pugilistica

(E) Depression

(F) Diffuse Lewy body disease

(G) Glioblastoma multiforme

(H) HIV encephalopathy

(I) Meningioma

(J) Normal pressure hydrocephalus

(K) Parkinson disease

(L) Pellagra

(M) Pick dementia

(N) Vascular dementia

(O) Wernicke encephalopathy/Korsakoff syndrome

For each patient with dementia, select the most likely diagnosis.

49. A 60-year-old man presents to the physician with his daughter, who is concerned about her father's insidious onset of inattention and slowing of thought processes. The man reports difficulty walking and a recent onset of urine incontinence. On physical examination, his gait is noted to be unsteady, slow, and wide-based with a shuffling quality. His past medical history and family history are noncontributory. MRI of the brain is performed and reveals dilated ventricular spaces with a relatively preserved cortical mantle. A shunting procedure is performed, which leads to an improvement of his clinical condition.

50. A 60-year-old woman is referred to a neurologist because of progressive loss of memory, disturbance of language, and social withdrawal. On examination, she is noted to have poor personal hygiene, and she acts in a disinhibited manner. Mental status examination reveals difficulty in naming objects, echolalia, and poor insight and judgment. There is a mild disturbance of memory, but visual-spatial functions are preserved. An MRI of the brain is performed and reveals marked cortical atrophy of the frontal lobes and anterior temporal lobes, with relative sparing of the remaining cortex.

Internal Medicine Test Four:
Answers and Explanations

ANSWER KEY

1.	D	26.	C
2.	A	27.	B
3.	D	28.	A
4.	B	29.	A
5.	C	30.	H
6.	D	31.	E
7.	B	32.	B
8.	F	33.	E
9.	B	34.	C
10.	D	35.	D
11.	A	36.	C
12.	E	37.	A
13.	C	38.	B
14.	D	39.	A
15.	B	40.	C
16.	D	41.	B
17.	B	42.	C
18.	D	43.	B
19.	D	44.	E
20.	B	45.	A
21.	E	46.	B
22.	A	47.	A
23.	C	48.	A
24.	E	49.	J
25.	C	50.	M

1. **The correct answer is D.** Paroxysmal supraventricular tachycardia is the most common paroxysmal arrhythmia with a rapid heart rate. It is often associated with a perfectly normal heart. Depending on heart rate, manifestations may vary from a subjective sensation of increased heart rate to mild chest pain, shortness of breath, or syncope. The pulse is usually between 160 and 220/min. Patients may be instructed to carry out maneuvers that stimulate the vagal nerve (e.g., Valsalva maneuver, breath holding, and arm and body stretching), which may interrupt the attacks. Carotid sinus massage should be performed for 10-20 seconds on the patient in a semi-recumbent position and only on one side. Presence of carotid bruits is an absolute contraindication to carotid sinus massage. IV verapamil (a calcium channel blocker) or IV *adenosine* is the treatment of choice if other non-pharmacologic measures have failed.

    Further carotid sinus massage (**choice A**) would most probably be unsuccessful.

    IV lidocaine (**choice B**) is reserved for treatment of ventricular tachyarrhythmias, especially in the setting of acute myocardial infarction.

    IV procainamide (**choice C**) is not a choice for treatment of supraventricular tachycardia. Oral procainamide may be used for prevention of attacks as an alternative to digoxin, verapamil, or beta blockers.

    Oral verapamil, 80-120 mg/4-6 hours (**choice E**), can be tried on patients with mild symptoms, but this is not the case in this patient.

2. **The correct answer is A.** The patient has a bleeding esophageal varix. These are dilated vessels that usually develop when cirrhosis blocks blood flow from the portal venous system through the liver, and back to the systemic circulation. Hypersplenism and arteriovenous malformations that markedly increase blood flow in the portal system can also cause esophageal varices, even in the absence of cirrhosis. Although any type of cirrhosis can potentially cause bleeding esophageal varices, you should be aware that the most common cause is alcoholism, possibly because it is both very common and may be accompanied by gastritis, which makes it easier for the varices to start to bleed. While individual incidents of bleeding varices can often be handled by either sclerotherapy or endoscopic banding of the bleeding vessel, the long-term prognosis remains poor for these patients, who often eventually either exsanguinate or die of other complications of advanced cirrhosis.

    Alpha$_1$-antitrypsin deficiency (**choice B**) is a rare cause of cirrhosis.

    Hemochromatosis (**choice C**) is much less common than alcoholism as a cause of cirrhosis.

Hepatitis A infection (**choice D**) may cause fulminant hepatic failure but does not cause cirrhosis.

Hepatitis B infection (**choice E**) is also a relatively common cause of cirrhosis, but it is not as strongly linked to bleeding varices as is alcoholism. In real life, coexistent alcoholism and hepatitis B infection are common.

3. **The correct answer is D.** The two most common causes of intracranial masses in AIDS patients are cerebral toxoplasmosis and primary brain lymphoma, both of which usually manifest as *ring-enhancing lesions* on CT or MRI. The central nonenhancing area of the lesion consists of necrosis, whereas the peripheral rim is due to viable tissue, inflammatory or neoplastic. A single ring-enhancing lesion in an AIDS patient is treated with a full course of anti-*Toxoplasma* agents (e.g., sulfadiazine and pyrimethamine). If there is no response following three weeks of therapy, an alternative diagnosis of primary brain lymphoma is investigated, and a brain biopsy is performed, if possible, to confirm the clinical diagnosis.

    Cryptococcal meningoencephalitis (**choice A**) is a frequent opportunistic infection associated with AIDS. It manifests with diffuse involvement of the leptomeninges, not with an intracerebral space-occupying lesion. The patient is severely ill and may become rapidly comatose, although localizing signs (meningismus) may be mild.

    Glioblastoma multiforme (GBM) (**choice B**) may also give rise to a nonenhancing lesion on MRI, but its incidence is not increased in AIDS patients compared with immune competent individuals. GBM would be unusual in a young adult.

    Metastatic tumor (**choice C**) is sometimes associated with the same MRI appearance as abscess or GBM. In an AIDS patient, however, metastases occur much less frequently than toxoplasmosis or lymphoma. Furthermore, metastases are usually multiple and located at the gray-white matter junction.

    A *Toxoplasma* abscess (**choice E**) responds to sulfadiazine and pyrimethamine treatment and shows signs of shrinkage on follow-up MRI.

4. **The correct answer is B.** This case describes the presentation of multiple myeloma, a plasma cell dyscrasia, characterized by multiple bone marrow tumor foci. Multiple myeloma is associated with osteomalacia, hypercalcemia, and normochromic, normocytic anemia. Susceptibility to infections occurs because of depression of functioning immunoglobulins. Pneumonia and pyelonephritis are the most common types of bacterial infection. Elevated serum protein is caused by clonal overproduction of immunoglobulin.

    Patients often are anemic because of bone marrow suppression of erythrocyte production. The iron level is not affected. In addition, this patient's mean corpuscular volume is greater than 80 μm^3, which is not consistent with iron deficiency. Therefore, decreased serum ferritin (**choice A**) would not be expected.

Hyperphosphatemia (**choice C**) is not associated with multiple myeloma but is seen with disorders of the parathyroid.

Hypertriglyceridemia (**choice D**) is not related to multiple myeloma but is a disorder of lipid metabolism.

Multiple myeloma is associated with hypercalcemia (due to lytic effects on bone), not hypocalcemia (**choice E**).

5. **The correct answer is C.** This patient probably has a pulmonary embolism (PE). Oral contraceptive pills and smoking place her at an increased risk for thromboembolic disease. The most common symptoms of PE include tachypnea and tachycardia. Shock may also ensue, and a massive PE can result in loss of blood pressure. This patient has a stable blood pressure at this time. Thus, placing her on heparin immediately would be appropriate to prevent the clot burden from further increasing.

Aspirin (**choice A**) would succeed in inhibiting platelet aggregation and would be appropriate if the patient had a coronary syndrome, such as myocardial infarction.

Warfarin (**choice B**) would be appropriate as a long-term choice for anticoagulation in this patient. However, it would take several days before the drug would be an effective anticoagulant and would not be of use in this acute setting. Ultimately, this patient would be switched to warfarin.

IV fluids (**choice D**) would be useful if this patient's blood pressure were falling in order to support her circulation. Since she is hemodynamically stable, she needs heparin before any other supportive therapy.

Streptokinase (**choice E**) could be used to immediately lyse the PE, but this would be indicated only if the patient were hemodynamically unstable with a low blood pressure or refractory hypoxemia. Because she is currently maintaining her blood pressure and is not exhibiting signs of right heart failure, streptokinase need not be given, avoiding the associated risk of bleeding and stroke.

6. **The correct answer is D.** This is a question about multiple endocrine neoplasia (MEN) type I, also known as Wermer syndrome. The patient has a probable pancreatic islet cell tumor that is secreting insulin. In MEN I, 30% to 75% of the patients develop pancreatic islet cell tumors, and about 40% of those develop insulin secreting tumors. The remainder of the islet cell tumors are derived from non-B cell elements and can secrete a variety of substances, most commonly gastrin (producing the multiple peptic ulcers of Zollinger-Ellison syndrome). Other features of MEN 1, which may occur

either sequentially or concurrently, include parathyroid adenomas (more than 90% of cases) and pituitary adenomas (50% to 65% of cases). Parathyroid adenomas are also found in 25% of MEN IIA cases and rarely in MEN IIB. Pancreatic islet cell tumors and pituitary adenomas are not a feature of MEN IIA or MEN IIB.

Marfanoid habitus (**choice A**) is a feature of MEN IIB.

Medullary carcinoma of the thyroid (**choice B**) is a feature of MEN IIA and MEN IIB.

Mucosal neuromas (**choice C**) are a feature of MEN IIB.

Pheochromocytoma (**choice E**) is a feature of MEN IIA and MEN IIB.

7. **The correct answer is B.** The most common primary cardiac tumor of adults is benign atrial myxoma. Ninety percent of these lesions involve the left atrium, where they can produce intermittent obstruction when they prolapse into the mitral orifice during diastole. Resection is curative.

Other tumors occur less commonly. Lipomas may involve the left ventricle (**choice C**), right atrium (**choice D**), or atrial septum. Rhabdomyomas are found in children and usually involve the left ventricle (**choice C**) or the right ventricle (**choice E**). The aorta (**choice A**) is not a common site of tumor formation.

8. **The correct answer is F.** White, curdy, cheese-like material specifically suggests thrush due to *Candida albicans*, whether it occurs in the mouth, vagina, or esophagus. This fungus occurs in both yeast and fungal forms, with both hyphae and pseudohyphae and budding yeast cells. *Candida* is usually a mouth and vagina commensal organism but can cause clinical disease, particularly among the immunosuppressed. Diabetics are particularly likely to develop clinical *Candida* infections because they are both immunosuppressed and have body secretions with a high sugar content on which the fungi like to feed.

Acute-angled, branching, septated filaments (**choice A**) describe *Aspergillus*, a much less common esophageal pathogen seen most often in AIDS patients. Although it can produce mucosal thickening, it does not cause the white, cheesy curd of *Candida*.

Anaplastic squamous cells with numerous mitotic figures (**choice B**) describe squamous cell carcinoma of the esophagus. Diabetics are at no greater risk for esophageal carcinoma. Risk factors include alcohol use and cigarette smoking. Esophageal carcinoma typically presents with weight loss and progressive difficulty in swallowing.

Intranuclear and cytoplasmic inclusion bodies with "owl's-eye" appearance (**choice C**) describe cytomegalovirus, a cause of esophageal ulcers, especially in AIDS patients.

Achalasia presents with pain upon swallowing, and a loss of ganglion cells in the myenteric plexus (**choice D**) is seen on biopsy. However, there are are no visible lesions seen on endoscopy, and there is no association with diabetes.

Multinucleated epithelial giant cells on Giemsa stain (**choice E**) describe herpes simplex virus, a cause of esophageal ulcers especially in AIDS patients.

9. **The correct answer is B.** This patient most likely has type 2 diabetes mellitus. This form represents 90% to 95% of all cases of diabetes mellitus in the U.S. The most common presentation of type 2 is that of an individual found to have hyperglycemia on routine laboratory investigations. Otherwise, patients present most frequently with symptoms due to diabetic complications, such as recurrent vulvovaginitis/balanitis, blurred vision, impotence, and peripheral neuropathy. Type 2 diabetes patients are often obese and older than 30 years. In this example, ophthalmoscopy reveals some of the findings associated with the *nonproliferative* stage of diabetic retinopathy, which accounts for decreased vision. Fasting blood glucose level is the recommended first-line test to screen for diabetes.

Blood test for C-peptide (**choice A**) documents function of pancreatic beta cells but is not useful in the diagnosis of diabetes. It may be useful in the diagnosis of insulinoma or factitious insulin injection.

Glucose tolerance test (**choice C**) is no longer used for screening or diagnostic purposes because of its low specificity. It is performed by measuring glucose levels after the patient is given a load of 75 g of glucose following overnight fasting. It is still useful in the diagnosis of gestational diabetes.

Glycosylated hemoglobin (**choice D**) reflects the mean blood glucose levels in the preceding three months. Normal values are below 7%. This test is generally not used for screening or diagnosis, but rather to check the adequacy of long-term glycemic control.

Urine glucose levels (**choice E**) do not detect hyperglycemia if the blood glucose is below 180 mg/dL (the renal threshold for glucose excretion). Furthermore, this test may be affected by many conditions that can cause false negative or false positive results.

Measurement of urinary protein (**choice F**) to detect microalbuminuria is the standard test for the diagnosis of early diabetic nephropathy, not diabetes.

10. **The correct answer is D.** This case describes a typical presentation of temporal arteritis, a systemic disease of inflammation of medium and large arteries. The disease affects older patients (>55 years) and has a female preponderance. Fever, anemia, elevated ESR, and headaches make up the classic complex of symptoms. Although definitive diagnosis is made by biopsy of the temporal artery, the condition is usually suspected on the basis of the clinical presentation. If steroids are not administered immediately (at the first suspicion of the disease), the patient has a high likelihood of developing blindness.

The presentation is not suggestive of narrowing of the carotid artery. If atherosclerosis of the carotid artery were present, the patient may have experienced transient ischemic attacks or stroke, or may have been found to have a bruit over the artery, indicating the need for a carotid artery Doppler flow study (**choice A**).

Ergotamine (**choice B**) is used to treat migraine headaches. The ESR would be normal, and the patient afebrile. Migraines typically last 4-72 hours and may have associated neurologic symptoms. In addition, the age at initial presentation is typically younger.

The presentation is not suggestive of a bacterial process. The fever is low grade, and the white cell count is within the normal range. Temporal arteritis would not respond to antibiotics (**choice C**).

NSAIDs (**choice E**) are for treatment of headache. The presentation of this case suggests a more systemic disease. Temporal arteritis would not respond to NSAIDs.

11. **The correct answer is A.** The condition described is *chronic pancreatitis* resulting in malabsorption. Steatorrhea (greasy, bulky, foul-smelling stools) is a common, although relatively late, manifestation. Chronic alcohol abuse is the most common etiologic factor (probably up to 60%) in chronic pancreatitis in the U.S. and other industrialized countries. Alcohol is thought to act by different pathogenetic mechanisms that result in direct injury to acinar cells and blockage of the ducts by inspissated secretion. Loss of parenchyma and fibrosis with calcification develop.

Biliary stone disease (**choice B**) is associated with a minority of cases. Small gallstones impacted in the distal end of the common bile duct may reverse the flow of pancreatic secretions or allow bile to enter the pancreatic duct.

Cystic fibrosis (**choice C**) is consistently associated with pancreatic damage, resulting in loss of pancreatic parenchyma and fibrosis but usually presents in childhood or early adulthood. Inflammation plays a minor role, but the ultimate result is similar to chronic pancreatitis (i.e., pancreatic insufficiency and malabsorption).

Familial predisposition (**choice D**) is seen in a very small percentage of cases associated with an autosomal dominant mutation manifesting with chronic pancreatitis in young age. The mutated gene encodes *trypsinogen*.

Hyperlipidemia (**choice E**), types I and V, is one of the rare predisposing conditions for both acute and chronic pancreatitis. The pathogenetic mechanism is uncertain. High serum triglycerides may falsely depress amylase and lipase levels, making the diagnosis of acute pancreatitis in such cases more problematic.

Hyperparathyroidism (**choice F**) may result in pancreatitis. Hypercalcemia probably triggers inappropriate activation of pancreatic enzymes.

Malnutrition (**choice G**) is the most common cause of acute and chronic pancreatitis in poor countries of southeast Asia and Africa. These cases are often referred to as *tropical pancreatitis*, but they are in fact simply related to protein-calorie malnutrition.

Pancreatic neoplasms (**choice H**) are often associated with some degree of chronic pancreatitis, and it is difficult to determine whether both conditions stem from the same underlying pathogenetic factors or one results from the other.

12. **The correct answer is E.** The disease is primary biliary cirrhosis. This autoimmune disease is characterized by progressive destruction of intrahepatic bile ducts. In early stages, intense inflammation of the bile ducts can be seen on biopsy, often accompanied by bile duct proliferation as the liver attempts to compensate. Later stages are characterized by initial portal fibrosis that eventually evolves to frank cirrhosis. Patients tend to be women, aged 35-70 years, who typically present with insidious disease and often have a history of other autoimmune disease. Chronic fatigue and pruritus are common initial complaints. Hepatomegaly, or hepatosplenomegaly, may be present, as may skin xanthomas or hyperpigmentation. In lab studies, elevations of alkaline phosphatase and gamma-glutamyl transpeptidase are usually out of proportion to those of serum bilirubin and aminotransferases. Endoscopic retrograde cholangiography can be helpful in distinguishing the condition from the related primary sclerosing cholangitis, which damages both the extrahepatic and the intrahepatic biliary system. Biopsies early in the disease may demonstrate florid bile duct destruction; later biopsies are more likely to show nonspecific hepatic fibrosis or cirrhosis. A very helpful test is to measure autoantibodies directed against mitochondrial antigens, since this test is positive in up to 95% of patients with primary biliary cirrhosis; a few patients with "autoimmune" chronic active hepatitis may also have these antibodies.

Anti-double-stranded DNA (**choice A**) is quite specific for systemic lupus erythematosus.

Hepatitis A (**choice B**) usually produces acute hepatitis with much more marked elevation of transaminases.

Determination of antibodies to hepatitis B core antigen (**choice C**) and hepatitis C virus (**choice D**) is usually used for evaluation of chronic viral hepatitis, which microscopically may show portal inflammation and fibrosis but does not show selective damage to bile ducts.

13. **The correct answer is C.** The patient's symptomatology is consistent with angina pectoris. During ischemic attacks, ECG usually shows a flat or down-sloping ST depression. The resting ECG may be normal in up to 25% of patients with typical angina between the attacks. In patients without ECG abnormalities at rest, exercise ECG is the most useful and cost-effective test to document myocardial ischemia.

Ambulatory ECG monitoring (**choice A**) is mainly used to document clinically silent (i.e., painless) episodes of myocardial ischemia, which may be more frequent than the clinically apparent ones in some patients.

Echocardiography (**choice B**) may reveal abnormalities in ventricular wall motion, which can be a result of current ischemia or prior myocardial infarction. It allows the study of left ventricular function, which is an important prognostic factor that influences treatment strategies as well.

Myocardial perfusion scintigraphy (**choice D**) is performed by injection of radiotracers (thallium-201 and technetium-99m are the most frequently used), which are taken up by viable myocardium. Scintigraphic defects indicate areas of ischemia. This is usually done after exercise ECG.

Coronary arteriography (**choice E**) is the gold standard for the diagnosis of coronary artery disease since it documents site and severity of stenotic lesions. Generally, it is indicated when coronary artery revascularization is being considered; it is not a first diagnostic procedure. It has a mortality of 1/1,000.

14. **The correct answer is D.** A significant risk associated with catheterization of the subclavian veins is a closed traumatic pneumothorax due to puncture of the apex of the lung. Hypotension, tachycardia, tachypnea, and cyanosis all favor this diagnosis. Classic clues in the patient's presentation are the distended neck veins, diminished breath sounds on the right side of the chest, and tracheal deviation to the opposite side. The most appropriate immediate treatment is needle thoracostomy at the second right intercostal space followed by chest tube insertion at the right fifth intercostal space.

Chest x-ray (**choice A**) is not necessary in this patient since the clinical examination was sufficient for making the diagnosis. Waiting for chest x-ray results before treating this unstable patient could prove fatal. Note, however, that chest x-rays are routinely performed after catheterizations to rule out subclinical pneumothoraces. On x-ray films, a pneumothorax appears as a region of air without peripheral lung markings limited by a distinct pleural boundary with medial lung markings.

Removal of the catheter (**choice B**) would not treat the punctured lung. Note that future attempts at central line placement should be attempted on the right side in this patient to avoid the possibility of creating bilateral pneumothoraces.

Endotracheal intubation (**choice C**) would not relieve the pneumothorax and would not be expected to improve respiratory status until the pneumothorax was successfully treated.

Tube thoracostomy in the left fifth intercostal space (**choice E**) would be on the wrong side in this patient with a right pneumothorax.

15. **The correct answer is B.** The concepts underlying this question are those of diabetes mellitus and the prevention of its complications. Many clinical trials have shown the beneficial effects of ACE inhibitors on preventing nephropathy and slowing the progression of established nephropathy in diabetics. This patient has microalbuminurial as shown by his urine dipstick, suggesting developing renal disease. It is the standard of care that all diabetics be given an ACE inhibitor if they are able to tolerate its blood pressure effects.

Adding a standing regular insulin dose at lunchtime (**choice A**) or increasing his morning NPH insulin dose (**choice D**) may be appropriate, although we do not know the details of his daily glucoses since he does not keep a glucose log. His nonoptimal HbA$_{1c}$ clearly indicates that his blood glucose control needs to be improved, but at this time we do not yet know the best way to accomplish this goal. The standard of care is for a goal HbA$_{1c}$ less than 7%.

Discussing options for using an insulin pump (**choice C**), similar to **choices A and D**, may be an option, depending on the details of this patients daily blood glucoses and his ability to comply with a stricter regimen.

Sending a 24-hour urine collection specimen for total protein (**choice E**) is not appropriate at this stage given the likelihood that this patient is developing diabetic nephropathy. Quantifying urine protein will not change this patient's management, namely, the addition of an ACE inhibitor.

16. **The correct answer is D.** The patient has bronchogenic lung cancer, which has produced Cushing syndrome as a paraneoplastic syndrome related to secretion of substances similar to ACTH. Small cell carcinoma of the lung is particularly notorious as a secretor of bioactive substances, including ADH, ACTH, parathormone, prostaglandins, calcitonin, gonadotropins, and serotonin. Small cell carcinoma of the lung has a strong association with smoking.

Adenocarcinoma of the lung (**choice A**), when used in questions, usually refers to adenocarcinoma without further differentiating features. This form of cancer can be seen in bronchi, as a coin lesion in the lung periphery, or involving scarred areas of lungs.

Remember bronchioloalveolar carcinoma (**choice B**) as the type that is not associated with smoking.

Large cell carcinoma (**choice C**) is an aggressive, undifferentiated form of lung cancer.

Associate squamous cell carcinoma of the lung (**choice E**) with the specific paraneoplastic syndrome of hypercalcemia.

17. **The correct answer is B.** Amiodarone is a class III antiarrhythmic agent with many electrophysiologic, as well as a number of potential, side effects. The most feared side effect, causing the greatest amount of long-term morbidity and mortality, is pulmonary fibrosis, occurring in up to 17% of patients in some series (average 10%). The incidence is clearly related to the total daily dosing, which is taken into account when the drug is prescribed in the U.S. Hyper- and hypothyroidism are also common side effects of amiodarone.

Hypotension (**choice A**) is common with the IV formulation of this drug but, once past the loading dose, is usually not an issue.

Prolongation of the QT interval (**choice C**) is very common with amiodarone therapy and could lead to a polymorphic ventricular arrhythmia termed "torsades de pointes." However, the incidence of torsades among patients on amiodarone with prolonged QTs is very low, less than 1%.

Recurrent ventricular arrhythmia (**choice D**) is a problem for any patient who has had a previous arrhythmia. In theory, amiodarone at therapeutic levels will decrease, but not eliminate, the possibility of recurrence.

Skin discoloration (**choice E**) is a common occurrence with this medication but, despite its cosmetic appearance, is not a significant issue for the patient.

18. **The correct answer is D.** Clinical symptomatology and MRI findings constitute the mainstay for the diagnosis of *multiple sclerosis*, but CSF examination may add confirmatory evidence. An abnormality frequently found in multiple sclerosis is the presence of oligoclonal bands of IgG detected by CSF electrophoresis. This appears to result from activation of lymphocytic subsets directed against specific white matter antigens, such as myelin basic protein. CSF cell count may be normal or slightly elevated.

Elevated protein with marked lymphocytosis (**choice A**) is usually associated with viral or mycobacterial meningitis/meningoencephalitis. CSF glucose is normal in viral infections but is reduced in mycobacterial infections.

Elevated protein with a normal cell count (**choice B**) is characteristic (but not pathognomonic) of Guillain-Barré syndrome.

Marked neutrophilic leukocytosis with reduced glucose (**choice C**) is highly characteristic of bacterial meningitis. Elevated CSF protein would also be present.

Normal protein with mild lymphocytosis (**choice E**) is nonspecific and may develop as a reaction (*neighborhood reaction*) to intracranial processes, such as abscess, mastoiditis, and tumor.

19. **The correct answer is D.** The edema (swelling) that develops around a cerebral infarct becomes particularly pronounced 48-72 hours following ischemic necrosis and may be of massive proportions if infarction is extensive. This leads to increased intracranial pressure, often resulting in cerebral herniations. Duret hemorrhages along the midline of the pons are secondary to transtentorial (uncal) herniation. Corticosteroids, such as prednisone (up to 100 mg/day) and dexamethasone (16 mg/day), are used to reduce cerebral edema following brain infarction and prevent herniation syndromes.

Anticoagulants (**choice A**) are not used in the acute management of stroke unless there is a proven source of thromboemboli, such as cardiac disease (e.g., atrial fibrillation and mitral valve prolapse). Heparin is the drug of choice. Anticoagulation can be started only if intracerebral hemorrhage has been ruled out by CT.

Several compounds that may minimize death of hypoxic neurons in the "penumbra" of the infarcted region have been used or are under investigation. These compounds include barbiturates (**choice B**), which diminish neuronal metabolism and energy requirements; calcium channel blockers (**choice C**), such as nimodipine, which have been shown to reduce neurologic deficits from stroke; and drugs that block receptors for glutamate, such as NMDA receptor antagonists (**choice E**), which seem to reduce infarct extent in experimental models.

20. **The correct answer is B.** This woman has antibiotic-associated pseudomembranous colitis, which has resulted in toxic megacolon, a known complication of severe pseudomembranous colitis. The causative organism of this colitis is *Clostridium difficile*, a gram-positive, spore-forming, anaerobic bacillus that overgrows in the setting of broad-spectrum antibiotic use, especially clindamycin, amoxicillin, ampicillin, or cephalosporins. Symptoms range from malodorous loose stools in the mildest cases to toxic megacolon (fever, nausea, vomiting, ileus) and colonic perforation (rigid abdomen, rebound tenderness) in the most severe cases. In most cases, the diagnosis can be made on clinical grounds without the need for colonoscopy. If colonoscopy is performed, it may show either a nonspecific colitis or, in severe cases, pathognomonic pseudomembranes. Many cases occur after antibiotic use (of up to six weeks). Mild cases resolve with the discontinuation of antibiotics, but severe cases

require treatment with oral metronidazole (first line of therapy) or oral vancomycin (in resistant and severe cases) to prevent toxic megacolon and resultant colonic perforation. Two-thirds of patients with toxic megacolon require surgical intervention.

Colon cancer (**choice A**) is not associated with pseudomembranous colitis. There is a significantly higher risk in patients who have had ulcerative colitis for more than 10 years, a family history of colon cancer, or a history of multiple colonic polyps.

The formation of fistulas (**choice C**) and colonic hemorrhages (**choice E**) are complications of diverticular disease. This patient's condition was not diverticulitis, and because this patient did not show evidence of diverticular disease on colonoscopy, it is unlikely that either of these complications will occur.

Gangrenous necrosis (**choice D**) is not a complication of pseudomembranous colitis. It may occur as a complication of mesenteric vessel occlusion. Typically, gangrenous necrosis is found in a patient with an underlying cause of embolism or atherosclerosis, and there is often a history of abdominal pain after eating (mesenteric angina). However, there is no association with antibiotic use, and the presence of pseudomembranes on endoscopy confirms a different diagnosis.

Malabsorption (**choice F**) and vitamin deficiency (**choice G**) are not complications of pseudomembranous colitis. Furthermore, they would unlikely be complications in conditions affecting the colon because vitamin and nutrient absorption is a function of the small, not large, intestine.

21. **The correct answer is E.** Polyarteritis nodosa (PAN) is a vasculitis of medium-sized arteries that can occur at any age and has a 2:1 male predominance. An important feature of the vasculitis is its spotty distribution, with individual lesions involving typically only 1 cm or shorter lengths of blood vessel. Some patients have hepatitis B antigenemia, and it is suspected that circulating immune complexes related to the chronic hepatitis may trigger the vasculitis. Diagnosis can be difficult because a variety of organ systems may be affected. Most patients have nonspecific constitutional findings, including hypertension, weight loss, fever, and elevated erythrocyte sedimentation rate (a marker for chronic disease with an immune component). Many patients seek medical attention because of an acute abdomen or gastrointestinal bleeding. Other presentations involving other systems, such as myocardial infarction, progressive renal failure, or infarction of individual abdominal organs, can occur. Urinalysis may be helpful in that the findings may suggest the possibility of multisystem disease. Particularly helpful, if present, are distinctive pea-shaped nodules along the superficial arteries

of the legs. The nodules may be accompanied by vasculitic purpura, urticaria, or even subcutaneous hemorrhage with gangrene. Microscopically, the acute lesions of PAN show fibrinoid necrosis and neutrophil infiltration into the vessel wall. With healing, the infiltrating cell population shifts to macrophages and plasma cells. In the healed lesion, residual damage in the form of vessel wall fibrosis and fragmentation of the internal elastic membrane can be seen.

Atherosclerotic plaques (**choice A**) severe enough to cause the patient's symptoms would be unusual in a 35-year-old man. Atherosclerotic plaques most often involve the aorta and the more proximal regions of its branches.

Associate fungal hyphae (**choice B**) with *Aspergillus*, or less frequently with *Candida*, both of which can destroy blood vessels, most often in patients with underlying immunosuppression.

Associate giant cells (**choice C**) with giant cell (temporal) arteritis, which most commonly involves the arteries of the head, notably the temporal and ophthalmic arteries.

Associate granulomas (**choice D**) of blood vessels with giant cell arteritis, Churg-Strauss syndrome, and Wegener granulomatosis.

22. **The correct answer is A.** The symptomatology and findings on physical examination are strongly suggestive of *scabies*, due to infestation by *Sarcoptes scabiei*. This mite is acquired by direct contact with an infected person and penetrates into the skin, producing burrows that are visible on close (or hand lens) examination. The areas of the body most frequently affected include the axillary and genital regions, waistline, and finger webs. Pruritus tends to be particularly intense at night. The most effective way to confirm a diagnosis of scabies is to place a drop of mineral oil on a suspected area (one of the burrow holes), then unroof the burrow hole with a curette ring and obtain scrapings that are examined under a microscope.

Microscopic examination of skin scrapings treated with potassium hydroxide (**choice B**) is the method of choice to demonstrate fungal organisms in skin lesions. To perform this test, skin scrapings are obtained by using a ring curette or a no. 15 blade. The scrapings are placed on a glass slide and treated with a drop of 10% to 20% KOH. After a few minutes, a cover slip can be applied on the glass slide, and the preparation examined under the microscope or a magnifying lens. Hyphae and spores can be identified. KOH treatment is necessary to dissolve the keratin.

Measurement of serum IgE levels (**choice C**) and allergen challenge tests (**choice D**) are appropriate investigations when an allergic disorder is suspected. Clinical history and physical examination clearly indicate that this is not the case.

Skin biopsy (**choice E**) is an invaluable investigative tool that should be resorted to when the clinical approach (i.e., history and objective findings) is insufficient to reach a diagnosis. Scabies can be easily diagnosed without resorting to biopsy.

23. **The correct answer is C.** This patient's anemia is clearly of the macrocytic/megaloblastic type, as evidenced by strikingly high mean corpuscular volume (MCV). Hypersegmented neutrophils also represent a characteristic accompanying feature. Glossitis (with red and shiny tongue) is another typical manifestation. The key to the correct answer is the history of treatment with phenytoin. This drug acts as an antimetabolite of folic acid and may induce folic acid-deficiency anemia even in the presence of adequate dietary intake. Besides drug-induced cases, the most frequent forms of folic acid deficiency result from inadequate diet with insufficient amounts of fresh fruits and vegetables. Alcoholics and anorexic patients are at increased risk.

Autoimmune hemolysis (**choice A**) is due to reduced survival of red blood cells resulting from antibodies to erythrocyte antigens. In this condition, reticulocytosis is prominent, since the bone marrow maintains the ability to compensate for the red blood cell loss. Unconjugated hyperbilirubinemia is a feature present in all hemolytic anemias and, to some extent, in megaloblastic anemia. However, the striking increase in MCV is characteristic of megaloblastic anemia, whereas hemolytic anemias are associated with normal MCV.

Bone marrow aplasia (**choice B**) will lead to severe anemia (aplastic anemia) accompanied by neutropenia and thrombocytopenia. The disorder results from injury to the marrow precursors of myeloid, erythroid, and megakaryocytic lines. It may be idiopathic or associated with immunologic conditions, radiation, toxins, and drugs (among the latter, phenytoin itself). Anemia due to bone marrow depression is normocytic and normochromic.

Iron deficiency (**choice D**) results in *microcytic anemia*, with MCV values often less than 80 fL. The most common cause of iron-deficiency anemia in the U.S. is chronic blood loss secondary to an underlying disorder (e.g., menstrual loss in women and gastrointestinal malignancies in both men and women).

Vitamin B_{12} deficiency (**choice E**) causes macrocytic anemia identical to that secondary to folic acid deficiency. However, vitamin B_{12} deficiency also results in neurologic deficits, such as paresthesias, ataxia, and decreased vibration and position sense. The most common cause of vitamin B_{12} deficiency in the U.S. is *pernicious anemia* due to autoimmune-related atrophic gastritis.

24. **The correct answer is E.** Pheochromocytomas are rare neoplasms of the adrenal medulla (or of extra-adrenal

sites) that produce epinephrine and/or norepinephrine, thereby causing episodic or continuous hypertension. Since the epinephrine and norepinephrine secretion tends to be episodic, plasma levels of these hormones may be normal. Therefore, it has become customary to look for metabolites of epinephrine and norepinephrine in 24-hour urine collections, thereby averaging out the periodicity. The specific compounds analyzed are the metanephrines, vanillylmandelic acid (VMA), and homovanillic acid (HVA).

17-Hydroxycorticosteroids (**choice A**) include cortisol, cortisone, and 11-deoxycortisol. These steroid hormones are unrelated to the amino acid-derived structure of epinephrine and norepinephrine.

Porphobilinogen (**choice B**) is a porphyrin precursor that is elevated in some of the porphyrias.

Pregnanediol (**choice C**) is a metabolite of the steroid hormone progesterone.

Tetrahydrocortisol (**choice D**) is a derivative of the steroid cortisol that is found in urine.

25. **The correct answer is C.** This case is a fairly classic presentation of acute pancreatitis. These patients often have a history of either alcohol abuse or gallstone disease. Alcohol intake greater the 100 g/day favors precipitation of protein of the pancreatic enzymes within the ducts, which eventually (over a period of years) cause enough blockage to trigger pancreatitis. The pain described is typical of acute pancreatitis, but some patients with more chronic disease may have surprisingly little pain. Very early in the disease, the patient's temperature may be subnormal, but fever usually develops within a few hours of onset. An elevated white count is usually present. The most helpful laboratory tests are serum amylase and serum lipase, elevation of which are considered strongly supportive of a diagnosis of pancreatitis.

Blood urea nitrogen (**choice A**) is a marker for renal dysfunction.

A chest x-ray film (**choice B**) might show pneumonia but would probably not be helpful in this patient with clear lungs.

Serum transaminase levels (**choice D**) may very well be elevated in this alcoholic patient, but his most significant acute problem is his pancreatitis, not his probably damaged liver.

Esophagogastroduodenoscopy (**choice E**) might show peptic ulcer disease, but severe pain would usually be seen only with perforation, and the patient would probably be vomiting blood in that setting.

26. **The correct answer is C.** This patient is exhibiting the classic presentation of hyperthyroidism. Other signs and symptoms that may be seen include atrial fibrillation,

nervousness, increased appetite, weight loss, frequent bowel movements, diplopia, conjunctival injection, and pretibial myxedema. The most common cause of hyperthyroidism is Graves disease (diffuse toxic goiter); in fact, infiltrative ophthalmopathy (as well as pretibial myxedema) is a specific autoimmune manifestation of Graves disease. The disease has an autoimmune basis, with antibodies directed against the TSH receptors, causing continuous thyroid gland stimulation and subsequent release of thyroid hormone.

Euthyroid sick syndrome (**choice A**) causes asymptomatic thyroid hormone alterations, usually in patients with serious systemic disease.

Follicular carcinoma of the thyroid (**choice B**) usually does not cause hyperthyroidism.

Hashimoto thyroiditis (**choice D**) can cause transient hyperthyroidism early in its course, but this is uncommon compared with Graves disease.

Subacute thyroiditis (**choice E**) usually causes striking thyroid gland tenderness in the setting of an acute illness and may cause transient hyperthyroidism.

27. **The correct answer is B.** The clinical picture is consistent with a "locked-in" state that can be caused by central pontine myelinolysis. This condition consists of acute demyelination of the basilar pons, resulting in interruption of the corticobulbar (excluding the fibers to cranial nerve nuclei I-IV) and corticospinal tracts with preservation of sensory input. The patient can close his eyes by inhibition of the levator palpebrae muscle, innervated by the oculomotor nerve. One of the most common causes of this disorder is excessively rapid correction of hyponatremia. To prevent this complication, it is recommended that the increase in serum sodium level should not exceed 1 mEq/L/hr or 25 mEq/L within the first day of therapy.

Alzheimer type 2 glia (**choice A**) refers to modified astrocytes that develop in patients with chronic liver failure. Hepatic encephalopathy is certainly a consideration in an alcoholic patient, but it would manifest with mental status changes and characteristic flapping tremor (asterixis) without paralysis.

Cerebellar vermis atrophy (**choice C**) may be due to chronic alcoholism and is responsible for the ataxic gait frequently seen in chronic alcoholics.

Subacute combined degeneration of the spinal cord (**choice D**) results in ataxia, numbness, and spastic paresis of the lower extremities. Wernicke encephalopathy (**choice E**) manifests with nystagmus, ophthalmoparesis, and confusion. Both disorders are related to thiamin deficiency.

28. **The correct answer is A.** A tearing, excruciating chest pain that radiates to the back should always generate

the clinical suspicion of aortic dissection involving the aortic arch. The patient presents with extreme signs of distress. Aortic insufficiency, with its associated diastolic murmur and widened pulse pressure, frequently develops. A discrepancy in blood pressure or pulse between the right and left arms is an additional supporting sign. Mediastinal widening is often seen on chest x-ray, but the diagnosis should be confirmed by CT or MRI scans. Hypertension is the most common predisposing factor, but Marfan syndrome is a classic condition associated with aortic dissection.

Acute mediastinitis (**choice B**) is a rare infectious complication due to extension of suppurative processes from adjacent cervical organs (e.g., peritonsillitis, thyroiditis) or perforation of the esophagus or trachea. The patient has chest pain but lacks fever and other systemic signs of infections. The history of a recent dental abscess should not deceive you.

Acute pericarditis (**choice C**) produces chest pain, which is gradual in onset and usually accompanied by a friction rub. If pericardial effusion is particularly abundant, cardiac tamponade (**choice D**) may ensue. The latter will result in acute signs and symptoms of cardiac failure, necessitating emergency pericardiocentesis to relieve the pressure on the heart.

Myocardial infarction (**choice E**) is probably the most important differential diagnosis to consider in case of aortic dissection, but the absence of ECG changes suggesting myocardial ischemia argues against it in this patient.

29. **The correct answer is A.** This is acute erosive gastritis, or "stress" gastritis, which is important to diagnose early because it can cause fatal gastrointestinal bleeding. Patients who develop this condition are usually already severely ill and very vulnerable to the problems of acute hemorrhage. Risk factors include severe burns, CNS trauma, sepsis, shock, and other organ system failure (respiratory, liver, renal, or multiorgan). Less severely ill patients may develop acute erosive gastritis as a complication of drug therapy (particularly NSAIDs) or alcohol use. The pathogenesis of acute erosive gastritis in severely ill patients is thought to involve decreased mucosal defense mechanisms and localized mucosal ischemia, possibly compounded by acid hypersecretion (particularly in burns, CNS trauma cases, and sepsis), which promotes mucosal damage. Because of the potential seriousness of the condition, most intensive care units use measures such as early enteral feeding, IV H2 blockers, or antacids to prevent it.

Chronic erosive gastritis (**choice B**) can be seen with drugs (aspirin and NSAIDs), Crohn disease, and viral infections. It is characterized by punctate lesions on the ridges of thickened rugal folds by endoscopy.

Gastric atrophy (**choice C**) is a nonerosive lesion of the stomach with mucosal atrophy that can complicate long-standing gastritis of various etiologies. It can also occur in connection with autoantibodies to parietal cells, producing pernicious anemia.

Nonerosive gastritis (**choice D**) is related to *Helicobacter pylori* infection characterized by inflammation through the entire mucosa.

Superficial gastritis (**choice E**) is a nonerosive, and often asymptomatic, mild form of gastritis related usually to *H. pylori* infection.

30. **The correct answer is H.** The patient is exhibiting the clinical picture of *hypertensive emergency*, in which striking elevation of blood pressure (diastolic values often >130 mm Hg) is associated with signs and symptoms of end-organ damage, such as cerebral damage (headache, confusion, and optic disc edema) and renal damage (proteinuria). Aggressive management is required to avoid serious complications or death and is aimed at gradually lowering blood pressure within 1 hour. IV infusion of sodium nitroprusside is the treatment of choice, but its administration should be carefully titrated to obtain the desired effect without excessively rapid reduction in blood pressure.

Clonidine (**choice A**) and nifedipine (**choice F**) are oral antihypertensive agents that should be reserved for less severe cases of hypertension (so-called *hypertensive urgencies*), in which signs of cerebral or renal damage are not detectable.

Enalaprilat (**choice B**) is the active form of enalapril. Its antihypertensive action is delayed; thus, it should be used only in conjunction with other, faster-acting agents.

Esmolol (**choice C**) is a beta blocker drug that has been useful in treating hypertensive emergencies in the presence of myocardial ischemia. However, it should be combined with some other antihypertensive agent.

Furosemide (**choice D**), as well as other IV loop diuretics, may be useful in the presence of signs of cardiac failure or fluid retention, but their action is slow to manifest.

Hydralazine (**choice E**) is mainly used in hypertensive crises affecting children and pregnant women. It may induce dangerous reflex tachycardia.

Nitroglycerin (**choice G**), administered by IV infusion, is less effective than nitroprusside but is useful in patients with manifestations of myocardial ischemia.

31. **The correct answer is E.** The polyglandular deficiency syndromes are autoimmune disorders that cause subnormal functioning of several endocrine glands concurrently. This patient has the type II variant, which has peak incidence at age 30 and always involves the adrenal cortex. Thyroid and pancreatic islet involvement, producing type

1 diabetes mellitus, are also common. In this patient, adrenocortical insufficiency is suggested by the cluster of serum sodium <130 mEq/L, serum potassium >5 mEq/L, plasma bicarbonate <28 mEq/L, and BUN >20 mg/dL. Diabetes mellitus is suggested by the polyuria and the blood glucose of 380 mg/dL. Hypothyroidism is suggested by the elevated TSH. Patients with polyglandular deficiency syndrome, type II, may also present with transient hyperthyroidism secondary to destruction of follicles in the thyroid gland. Other features of the condition include antibodies directed against the target glands, particularly against cytochrome P_{450} adrenal cortical enzymes, and reduced systemic T cell-mediated immunity.

MEN type I (**choice A**) is characterized by tumors of the parathyroid glands, pancreatic islet cells, and pituitary gland.

MEN type IIA (**choice B**) is characterized by medullary carcinoma of the thyroid, pheochromocytoma, and hyperparathyroidism.

MEN type IIB (**choice C**) is characterized by multiple mucosal neuromas, marfanoid habitus, medullary carcinoma of the thyroid, and pheochromocytoma.

Polyglandular deficiency syndrome type I (**choice D**) is characterized by onset in childhood or before age 35, hypoparathyroidism, adrenocortical failure, and gonadal failure; diabetes mellitus is not usually seen with this condition.

32. **The correct answer is B.** These tears, called Mallory-Weiss lacerations, account for about 5% of cases of upper GI hemorrhage. They occur when the proximal part of the stomach is telescoped into the distal esophagus (stretching and tearing it) by severe vomiting, severe retching, or severe hiccups. The lacerations are usually superficial and often stop bleeding spontaneously. If the bleeding fails to stop spontaneously, the lacerations may be controlled endoscopically. The condition was initially described in alcoholics, but you should be aware that it occasionally occurs in many other types of patients as well.

AIDS (**choice A**) can predispose for esophagitis due to viruses (CMV, herpes) or fungi (usually *Candida*).

Chagas disease (**choice C**) can cause megaesophagus.

Diabetes mellitus (**choice D**) can predispose for fungal (particularly *Candida*) esophagitis.

Scleroderma (**choice E**) can involve the esophagus with fibrosis, leading to dysphagia.

33. **The correct answer is E.** Liver adenoma is an infrequent benign tumor composed of hepatocytes arranged with the same lamellar pattern as the normal hepatic lobule. It is usually clinically silent and occurs most frequently in association with oral contraceptives or anabolic steroids.

When symptomatic, its most common clinical presentation is rupture into the peritoneal cavity with consequent hemoperitoneum and shock.

Abdominal pain (**choice A**) is a symptom of many hepatobiliary diseases, including hepatitis, carcinoma, and cholelithiasis. The pain of hepatic origin is presumed to result from stretching of the capsule as occurs in acute hepatitis. The pain of biliary origin derives from acute distention of the gallbladder, usually because of gallstones blocking the cystic or common bile duct.

Jaundice (**choice B**) is not a manifestation of liver adenoma. Hemolytic disorders, diffuse hepatocellular damage, and obstruction of the biliary pathways are the most common conditions resulting in jaundice.

Metastatic disease (**choice C**) is not a consequence of liver adenoma, which is a benign tumor. Liver adenoma, however, may be extremely similar histologically to well-differentiated hepatocellular carcinoma, so that one may be mistaken for the other.

Portal hypertension (**choice D**) may result from prehepatic causes (thrombosis of the portal vein), hepatic causes (cirrhosis or other diffuse infiltrative conditions), and posthepatic causes (obstruction of the hepatic veins or right-sided cardiac failure). Well-demarcated tumors, such as liver adenoma, do not lead to portal hypertension.

34. **The correct answer is C.** The classic presentation, along with the hyperuricemia, makes gouty arthritis the most likely diagnosis. Nonsteroidal anti-inflammatory drugs (NSAIDs) are the treatment of choice of acute gouty arthritis. They are somewhat less specific than colchicine for gout but are better tolerated and work quickly.

Allopurinol (**choice A**) is used in the intercritical period between attacks, not in acute attacks.

Colchicine (**choice B**) is effective for acute gouty arthritis but is poorly tolerated at the high, frequent doses required for an acute attack.

Steroids (**choice D**) can be used in an acute episode, but not before a trial with NSAIDs and/or colchicine is attempted.

Probenecid (**choice E**) is a uricosuric agent used in the intercritical period, not during acute attacks, in patients who are under excreters of uric acid.

35. **The correct answer is D.** Wegener granulomatosis is a vasculitis that affects the upper respiratory tract and paranasal sinuses, the kidneys, and the lungs. It is associated with dermatologic symptoms (subcutaneous nodules and purple papules). Antineutrophil cytoplasmic antibodies yielding a cytoplasmic immunofluorescence pattern (c-ANCA) are found in more than 90% of patients with Wegener granulomatosis.

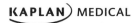

Antiribonucleoprotein (**choice A**) is found in high titer levels in mixed connective tissue disease (MCTD). MCTD is a distinct rheumatic syndrome characterized by overlapping clinical features of systemic lupus erythematosus, scleroderma, polymyositis or dermatomyositis, and rheumatoid arthritis.

Elevated levels of serum IgE (**choice B**) might be seen in bronchopulmonary aspergillosis.

Goodpasture syndrome is associated with anti-glomerular basement membrane antibody (**choice C**). This disorder affects the kidney and lungs, rather than the lungs or paranasal sinuses.

A positive p-ANCA (**choice E**) is seen in polyarteritis nodosa, a nongranulomatous vasculitis. Purple nodules can be seen in both polyarteritis nodosa and Wegener granulomatosis.

Rheumatoid factor is positive (**choice F**) in many patients with rheumatoid arthritis, but this marker is nonspecific and may be positive in several other disorders.

36. **The correct answer is C.** This is a dehydrated and malnourished patient with hypernatremia. The most probable cause is that she is no longer able to express thirst or hunger and cannot cooperate efficiently with caregivers when taking water or food. The most immediate goal of therapy is to replace water. The usual choice in this setting is 5% dextrose in water, which should be given relatively slowly to prevent glucosuria, followed by normal saline. This strategy would increase the salt-free water excretion and hypertonicity.

Oral water administration (**choice A**) will work with physically and mentally competent people who have been water deprived (e.g., stranded in the desert). However, this strategy has obviously already failed in this patient (the nursing home was probably not deliberately trying to dehydrate her) and is not the best choice.

IV 0.9% saline (**choice B**) by itself would not be used in this clinical setting.

IV colloid and 0.9% saline (**choice D**) is used as the initial hydrating fluid in patients who are in shock secondary to dehydration, but is not needed in this patient with adequate blood pressure and symptomatic hypernatremia.

IV distilled water (**choice E**) should never be given to patients—it will cause red cell lysis.

37. **The correct answer is A.** This is Behcet syndrome. The laboratory findings are usually nonspecific indications of an inflammatory process (such as those illustrated in the question stem), so the diagnosis is usually established by the history (and may take months to years since not all features are typically present from the beginning). Characteristic features include painful oral ulcers, painful genital ulcers (in men, in women they

may be painless), ocular disease (most often a relapsing iridocyclitis that causes pain and photophobia), skin lesions (papules, pustules, vesicles, or folliculitis), and mild arthritis of large joints. Other features that may be seen include CNS involvement and migratory thrombophlebitis.

Herpes simplex infection (**choice B**) can cause oral and genital ulcers, but the Tzanck smear would probably be positive and arthritis would be unlikely.

Neisseria gonorrhoeae infection (**choice C**) can affect both genitalia and joints, but does not usually cause ulcers.

Psoriasis (**choice D**) can cause both skin lesions and arthritis, but the skin lesions are characteristically scale-covered plaques.

Treponema pallidum infection (**choice E**) can cause ulcers (the chancre) but does not usually cause arthritis.

38. **The correct answer is B.** This patient may have colon cancer. The weight loss, pallor, and anemia are indicative of a chronic bleed, supported by the stool positivity for occult blood. Risk factors for colon cancer include a positive history of colon cancer or adenomatous polyps in a first-degree relative and a personal history of adenomatous polyps. Since our suspicion of colorectal cancer is high, it would be helpful to detect the lesion and remove it if possible. Colonoscopy provides the most efficient modality with which to achieve this goal.

A KUB (**choice A**) is usually a good modality for evaluating obstruction, which is a potential complication of colon cancer. This patient is not complaining of obstruction, and a KUB would not detect a soft tissue mass.

Esophagoduodenoscopy (**choice C**) would be done to evaluate the patient for a source of upper gastrointestinal bleeding, such as ulcers, varices, or gastric cancer.

Sigmoidoscopy (**choice D**) would be an effective screening test, but only 25% to 30% of colorectal cancers are detected by rigid sigmoidoscopy; the rate increases to 40% to 65% when flexible sigmoidoscopy is used. This patient has a high pre-test probability of having colorectal cancer, and since visualization of the entire colon will guide further action, sigmoidoscopy would be inadequate.

Open laparotomy (**choice E**) might ultimately be needed if the patient undergoes colonic resection; however, it would be premature to immediately proceed to this option.

39. **The correct answer is A.** The patient probably has carpal tunnel syndrome, which is caused by compression of the median nerve as it passes through the carpal tunnel in the wrist. The symptoms illustrated in the question stem are typical, as is the history of exacerbation of symptoms at night following heavy wrist use during the day. The test described is the Tinel test, which can be used to assess

other superficial nerves as well. Milder cases of carpal tunnel syndrome may respond to rest and nonsteroidal anti-inflammatory drugs; more severe cases may require surgical decompression.

Cubital tunnel syndrome (**choice B**) compresses the ulnar nerve at the elbow, producing numbness and paresthesias of the ring and little fingers.

Radial tunnel syndrome (**choice C**) involves compression of branches of the radial nerve in the arm or forearm. It causes pain of the back of the forearm and hand, sometimes with wrist drop.

Reflex sympathetic dystrophy (**choice D**) is pain and limited motion of the shoulder accompanied by ipsilateral involvement of the hand.

Scapholunate ligament rupture (**choice E**) usually occurs during a fall onto an outstretched hand and causes pain in the mid-wrist.

40. **The correct answer is C.** This patient presents with a lateral *ankle sprain*. Clinical assessment is usually sufficient to diagnose this condition, unless there are signs suggesting the presence of fracture. The drawer and talar tilt tests are used to assess ligament instability and confirm a diagnosis. A positive *talar tilt* test indicates injury to the calcaneofibular ligament, and a positive *drawer test* indicates injury to the anterior talofibular ligament. The history is also very important in clarifying the mode of traumatic injury. Currently recommended treatment for uncomplicated ankle sprains of mild-to-moderate degree includes *p*rotection of the injured joint by splinting or immobilizing boot; *r*est of the injured joint; *i*ce application several times daily; *c*ompression by elastic wrap, and *e*levation of the limb to reduce edema (which gives the *PRICE* mnemonic). Adjuvant anti-inflammatory or analgesic treatment may be used. Patients with lateral ankle sprains should start rehabilitation early, usually after 24-72 hours of ankle rest. Treatment for acute ankle sprain with rehabilitation after 10 days of ankle rest (**choice D**) has been found to be unnecessary compared with shorter periods of immobilization.

Referral to orthopedic specialist (**choice A**) is rarely necessary, unless there are complicating factors, such as associated injuries to other joints or fractures.

Treatment with nonsteroidal anti-inflammatory drugs without ankle immobilization (**choice B**) is definitely inappropriate in any case of ankle sprain, however mild.

X-ray examination (**choice E**) is indicated when there are signs suggestive of fractures, such as history of a snapping or popping sound at the time of injury, pain in the malleolar region, and tenderness on pressure on the lateral malleolus. It is recommended that patients older than 55 years should undergo routine x-ray control even in the absence of clinical signs of fractures because of the increased incidence of occult fractures in more advanced age.

41. **The correct answer is B.** The clinical picture is highly suggestive of *central diabetes insipidus*, a disorder due to deficiency of antidiuretic hormone (ADH) secretion from the posterior pituitary gland. Polydipsia is a consequence of polyuria (not an effect) because of abundant diuresis secondary to ADH deficiency. The vasopressin challenge test is given by administering *desmopressin* (a synthetic form) by the nasal route, and monitoring the urine output 12 hours before and 12 hours after administration. If the symptomatology is due to *central* diabetes insipidus, the patient will experience an immediate reduction in thirst and urine output. Diabetes insipidus may manifest in the third trimester of pregnancy or during the puerperium because of a circulating enzyme (*vasopressinase*) that degrades vasopressin. The enzyme is not effective against desmopressin. The disorder resolves spontaneously.

Besides the high likelihood of noncompliance, advising the patient to reduce water intake (**choice A**) would expose her to severe dehydration and hypernatremia due to loss of water and resultant hemoconcentration.

MRI studies of the pituitary-hypothalamic region (**choice C**) are performed to search for mass lesions that may be the underlying cause of central diabetes insipidus. These investigations should be performed after the diagnosis has received confirmation by a vasopressin challenge test.

Compulsive water drinking may require psychiatric evaluation (**choice D**), and may mimic diabetes insipidus, but this possibility should be undertaken once diabetes insipidus has been ruled out. In this particular case, the close temporal association with pregnancy and delivery makes the diagnosis of diabetes insipidus more likely.

Evaluation of nephrogenic diabetes insipidus (**choice E**) is the next appropriate step if the patient does not respond to vasopressin challenge test. Nephrogenic diabetes insipidus, in fact, is due to resistance of renal tubules to the action of vasopressin. A hereditary X-linked form is known, usually associated with hyperuricemia. Acquired forms are associated with a variety of conditions (e.g., pyelonephritis, multiple myeloma, chronic hypercalcemia, and lithium use).

42. **The correct answer is C.** Acute renal failure (ARF) is a common occurrence in hospitalized patients. It is crucial to determine whether ARF is secondary to *prerenal* or *renal* causes. In the former case, the underlying cause is reduction of blood flow to normal kidneys, resulting in a decreased glomerular filtration rate. In the latter, intrinsic renal damage is the underlying etiology. Of the *intrinsic* causes of ARF, *acute tubular necrosis* is the most common. How can one distinguish between prerenal

KAPLAN) MEDICAL

and renal forms of ARF? Sodium reabsorption is not impaired in prerenal azotemia, whereas creatinine reabsorption is deficient in both prerenal and intrinsic renal azotemia. Fractional excretion of sodium (FE_{Na}) is therefore a most useful parameter to distinguish between these two conditions. It can be calculated by the following formula: $Na_{URINE} \times Cr_{PLASMA}/Cr_{URINE} \times Na_{PLASMA}, \times 100$. In prerenal azotemia, $FE_{Na} <1\%$ because the undamaged renal tubules will avidly absorb sodium. In acute tubular necrosis, as well as other intrinsic renal causes of azotemia, damaged tubules will allow sodium to leak into urine, and FE_{Na} will be $>1\%$. In this particular case, the calculation yields $FE_{Na} = 1.6\%$. Gentamicin is the most nephrotoxic of the aminoglycoside antibiotics. Its toxicity usually manifests after 5-7 days of treatment.

The most frequent manifestation of allopurinol toxicity (**choice A**) is a pruritic rash due to hypersensitivity. Vasculitis and hepatitis are other, albeit rare, adverse effects.

Ampicillin toxicity (**choice B**) may manifest with renal damage, but usually in the form of acute interstitial nephritis, not acute tubular necrosis. Acute interstitial nephritis is associated with fever, rash, blood eosinophilia, and leukocyturia with eosinophils.

Hyperuricemia (**choice D**) may cause acute tubular necrosis, but only when serum uric acid levels rise rapidly as a result of rapid cell turnover. This may develop with hematologic malignancies or germ cell neoplasms treated with chemotherapy. Uric acid levels are often very high (>20 mg/dL).

Hypotension (**choice E**) is the underlying pathogenetic factor of most conditions leading to prerenal azotemia, such as hypovolemic, cardiogenic, or anaphylactic shock. Renal tubular function is preserved, but the fall in glomerular filtration rate results in oliguria/anuria and ARF. FE_{Na} is very low ($<1\%$). Clinical history is obviously an important aid in the differential diagnosis between prerenal and renal azotemia.

Sepsis (**choice F**) is a frequent cause of prerenal azotemia when associated with shock. In this case, the laboratory data rule out this possibility.

43. **The correct answer is B.** The presentation is classic for central retinal artery occlusion, which is a blockage of the central retinal artery by embolism or thrombosis that causes painless, sudden, unilateral blindness. Patients may have underlying atherosclerosis, endocarditis, or temporal arteritis. The retinal changes illustrated in the question stem are typical and are the result of a failure of blood to flow into the retina. Immediate treatment is imperative. Intermittent digital massage over the closed eyelids may dislodge the embolus and allow it to flow into a smaller blood vessel, where it will cause a small area of retinal

ischemia. If this fails, anterior chamber paracentesis will also sometimes dislodge the embolus.

Age-related macular degeneration (**choice A**) can also present with sudden, painless, unilateral blindness, but the fundus will show pigmentary changes with or without new vessel formation behind the retina.

Central retinal vein occlusion (**choice C**) can also cause painless, unilateral blindness. However, it tends to develop a little more slowly than central artery occlusion, and the retinal vessels appear congested.

Hypertensive retinopathy (**choice D**) does not usually cause sudden blindness.

Retinitis pigmentosa (**choice E**) develops over a period of years, with loss of peripheral vision.

44. **The correct answer is E.** This patient has mixed connective tissue disease. Clinically, it appears to be an overlap syndrome with features similar to rheumatoid arthritis, systemic lupus erythematosus, scleroderma, Sjögren syndrome, and polymyositis or dermatomyositis. It is now considered a separate disease because of a distinct autoantibody pattern, with very high levels of antibody directed against ribonucleoprotein. Rheumatoid agglutinins may also be present in high titers. Other antibodies characteristic of the individual diseases that mixed connective tissue disease mimics are usually absent or present only in low titers. The clinical presentation may be wildly diverse, depending on which disease pattern manifests first. With time, however, there should be clinical features suggestive of a variety of different autoimmune diseases. Mild disease may be controlled with measures similar to mild rheumatoid arthritis (salicylates, other NSAIDs, antimalarials, very-low-dose corticosteroids); more severe disease (which may be fatal with complications due to vascular lesions, renal failure, myocardial infarction, disseminated infection, or cerebral hemorrhage) usually requires large-dose steroids.

Associate c-ANCA (**choice A**) with Wegener granulomatosis.

Associate dsDNA (**choice B**) with systemic lupus erythematosus.

Associate p-ANCA (**choice C**) with microscopic polyarteritis.

Associate Scl-70 (**choice D**) with systemic sclerosis.

45. **The correct answer is A.** Cigarette smoking is considered the principal preventable cause of disease in the U.S., and approximately 20% of adults in this country smoke. The guidelines of the U.S. Agency for Health Care Policy and Research (AHCPR) and the National Cancer Institute recommend that all primary care physicians identify smokers and advise them to quit smoking. Several studies have found that 10% of all smokers will quit smoking if

they receive even three minutes of advice to quit from a clinician. However, the very first step in the physician's approach to a smoker is to establish his/her willingness to quit. With respect to smoking cessation, three stages have been identified: *precontemplation*, if there is no intention of quitting; *contemplation*, if there are some ideas but no clear plans of quitting soon; and *action*, if there is a definite intention of setting a quitting date. The next steps depend on the patient's response.

Trying to elicit a quitting date even if the patient appears unwilling (**choice B**) would be inappropriate. The physician should elicit a quitting date if the patient is already willing to do so (i.e., he/she is in the contemplation or action stage). The physician should discuss the reasons or obstacles that make a patient unwilling to stop if he/she is in the precontemplation stage. Information about risks of smoking should be provided.

Prescribing nicotine patch and gum (**choice C**) is most useful in smokers who are nicotine dependent. Several questionnaires have been developed to establish nicotine dependence (the *Fagerstrom* questionnaire is probably the most widely used). Nicotine dependence is present if a patient smokes the first cigarette within 30 minutes after awakening, smokes more than 20 cigarettes daily, finds it difficult to refrain from smoking in places where smoking is prohibited, and continues to smoke even during illness. Determining nicotine dependence allows a physician to individualize treatment strategies by prescribing nicotine replacement therapy.

Group behavior treatment (**choice D**) is mostly indicated for smokers who have already tried and failed to quit in the past. Recent studies have shown that combinations of intensive group counseling with nicotine replacement have the highest success rate (up to 40%) in obtaining long-term abstinence.

Maximal specialized care with intervention of a psychiatry specialist (**choice E**) may be indicated for patients with a high degree of nicotine dependence associated with other forms of drug abuse (alcohol being the most frequent).

46.   **The correct answer is B.** The most probable etiology of bacterial endocarditis involving the tricuspid valve is illicit IV drug use, which can introduce skin organisms into the venous system that then proceed to attack the tricuspid valve. *Staphylococcus aureus* accounts for between 60% and 90% of cases of endocarditis in IV drug users.

The endocarditis associated with congenital heart disease (**choice A**) typically involves either damaged valves or atrial or ventricular septal defects. The tricuspid valve is not particularly vulnerable.

Rheumatic fever (**choice C**) most commonly damages the mitral and aortic valves, and tricuspid damage is usu-

ally less severe and seen only when the mitral and aortic valves are heavily involved. Consequently, secondary bacterial endocarditis involving only the tricuspid valve in a patient with a history of rheumatic fever would be unusual.

Rheumatoid arthritis (**choice D**) is not associated with bacterial endocarditis.

Systemic lupus erythematosus (**choice E**) can produce small, aseptic vegetations on valves (Libman-Sacks endocarditis) but is not associated with bacterial endocarditis.

47.   **The correct answer is A.** The clinical presentation is highly characteristic of epidural bleeding, which usually is of traumatic origin and most often results from rupture of the middle meningeal artery. The initial concussion leads to a brief loss of consciousness, which is followed by a lucid interval lasting several hours. As the epidural hematoma progressively enlarges and pushes the underlying brain, the patient becomes comatose again and may display signs of uncal herniation. The herniating uncus pushes on the third cranial nerve, producing ipsilateral fixed pupillary dilatation. Papilledema is usually a late sign and indicates cerebral edema.

A calvarial fracture (**choice B**) would not cause such a severe neurologic state and evidence of uncal herniation unless associated with an intracranial hematoma.

Intracerebral hypertensive hemorrhage (**choice C**) usually occurs spontaneously and develops within the brain parenchyma (most commonly in the basal ganglia). Loss of consciousness develops in approximately 50% of patients. Headache, vomiting, and variable neurologic deficits are present.

Subarachnoid hemorrhage (**choice D**) characteristically manifests with sudden onset (thunderclap) of headache associated with vomiting and progressive impairment of consciousness. The most frequent cause is rupture of berry aneurysms.

The clinical manifestations of a subdural hemorrhage (**choice E**) may vary depending on the severity and location. Cerebral atrophy is a predisposing condition, as it leads to "stretching" of bridging veins that connect the veins on the cerebral convexities with the superior sagittal sinus. Minimal trauma may then result in tearing of such veins. Impaired consciousness and/or focal neurologic deficits follow the traumatic event after an interval of days or weeks.

48.   **The correct answer is A.** Anticoagulation with heparin is the standard therapeutic first step for pulmonary embolus.

Thrombolytic agents (**choices B and E**) still have a very limited role in the treatment of pulmonary embolus. They may be considered when overwhelming right-sided heart failure is life threatening, but bleeding remains a formidable potential complication; therefore, they are contraindicated after major surgery. When they are used, systemic administration (**choice E**) is as effective as direct delivery into the pulmonary artery (**choice B**).

Vena cava filters (**choice C**) are indicated only when pulmonary emboli recur while under anticoagulation, or if anticoagulation cannot be instituted (i.e., with pregnancy).

Surgical embolectomy (**choice D**) has the same restricted indications noted for the thrombolytic agents, and as a rule it is a major undertaking rarely feasible in a very sick patient.

49. **The correct answer is J.** The triad of dementia, gait disturbances, and incontinence ("wacky, wobbly, and wet") should immediately suggest normal pressure hydrocephalus as the underlying etiology (although such a complete clinical picture is often not present). MRI usually reveals an obvious discrepancy between the marked degree of ventricular dilatation (hydrocephalus) and the comparatively lesser extent of cortical atrophy. This cause of dementia is important because it is potentially treatable with a shunting procedure. However, long-standing cases lead to cortical atrophy and consequently become less responsive to shunting.

50. **The correct answer is M.** The clinical picture of Pick dementia may be confused with other forms of dementia, especially Alzheimer disease, although in its classic presentation, flat emotional affect and language disturbances are predominant. However, MRI evidence of marked atrophy limited to the frontal and anterior temporal cortex supports a diagnosis of Pick disease. If a cortical biopsy is performed, it will show neuron loss with other characteristic neuronal changes, namely intracytoplasmic argyrophilic inclusions.

Alzheimer disease (**choice A**) is the most frequent form of dementia and certainly should be suspected in all cases of gradually progressive memory loss accompanied by MRI evidence of diffuse cerebral atrophy. Dilatation of ventricles is secondary to loss of cerebral substance and is referred to as hydrocephalus ex vacuo.

Chronic subdural hematoma (**choice B**) refers to a subdural collection of blood resulting from tearing of bridging veins. This may slowly enlarge and compress the underlying brain, occasionally resulting in dementia. The diagnosis is easily made by CT/MRI studies.

Creutzfeldt-Jakob disease (**choice C**) causes a rapidly progressive form of dementia, accompanied by abnormal myoclonic movements and characteristic EEG changes. MRI does not reveal significant cerebral atrophy.

Dementia pugilistica (**choice D**) is associated with a history of boxing. Cerebral atrophy is evident on MRI.

Depression (**choice E**) is a major cause of pseudodementia, when intellectual impairment is not due to neurodegenerative changes. Other manifestations of depression are usually evident.

Diffuse Lewy body disease (**choice F**) is now ranked among the most common causes of dementia. Neuron loss and Lewy bodies (the same as in Parkinson disease) are found in the substantia nigra and in several neocortical fields, leading to parkinsonism, dementia, and other neurologic manifestations such as visual hallucinations.

Dementia is a very unusual presentation of intracranial tumors such as glioblastoma multiforme (**choice G**) and meningioma (**choice I**). Glioblastoma multiforme is the most frequent primary malignant tumor, and meningioma is the most frequent benign tumor of the brain. Both can be detected by MRI.

HIV encephalopathy (**choice H**) is referred to as AIDS-dementia complex or HIV-associated cognitive/motor complex. It manifests in AIDS patients with progressive deterioration of cognitive function and slowing of motor tasks (e.g., handwriting). MRI and CSF studies are necessary to exclude opportunistic infections or lymphoma.

One-quarter of Parkinson disease patients (**choice K**) present with dementia. Three cardinal signs of Parkinson disease are resting tremor, rigidity, and bradykinesia, two of which are required for clinical diagnosis. Postural instability is the fourth cardinal sign and emerges late, usually after eight years. Dementia also occurs late in the disease and affects short-term memory and visual spatial function.

Pellagra (**choice L**) is due to nicotinic acid deficiency, which in its advanced stages manifests with the classic triad of dermatitis, diarrhea, and dementia.

Vascular dementia (**choice N**) refers to dementia resulting from vascular causes, the most frequent of which are atherosclerosis of major cerebral arteries and hypertensive arteriolosclerosis. MRI would reveal multiple old infarcts in the cerebral cortex or lacunar infarcts in the basal ganglia, combined with variable white matter rarefaction.

Wernicke encephalopathy and Korsakoff syndrome (**choice O**) are both seen in chronic alcoholics and are due to thiamine deficiency. The former consists of nystagmus, ataxia, and confusion; the latter consists of impaired memory with confabulation.

Internal Medicine: **Test Five**

1. A 26-year-old man comes to the physician because of sore throat, fever, and malaise for one week, and a diffuse skin rash for one day. The skin rash developed after the patient took ampicillin. Examination reveals pharyngitis and tonsillitis, cervical lymphadenopathy, and splenomegaly. Laboratory studies show:

Hematocrit	40%
Leukocyte count	4,800/mm³
Segmented neutrophils	45%
Lymphocytes	40%
Platelet count	76,000/mm³
Alanine aminotransferase	80 U/L
Aspartate aminotransferase	70 U/L
Bilirubin, total	1.2 mg/dL

A peripheral blood smear show numerous atypical large lymphocytes with vacuolated cytoplasm. A heterophil antibody test is positive. Which of the following is the most likely diagnosis?

(A) Acute cytomegalovirus (CMV) disease

(B) Acute lymphocytic leukemia

(C) Drug-induced thrombocytopenia

(D) Infectious mononucleosis

(E) Streptococcal pharyngitis with leukemoid reaction

2. A 65-year-old man presents with a productive cough, fever, chills, and shortness of breath for three days. On physical examination, his temperature is 38.9° C (102° F), pulse is 96/min, and respirations are 28/min. There are decreased breath sounds and dullness to percussion over the left lower field. Laboratory findings are remarkable for a white cell count of 21,000/mm³ with 20% bands. A chest x-ray film demonstrates the presence of a large left pleural effusion. A thoracentesis is performed. Which of the following is the proper position for insertion of a thoracentesis needle within the sixth intercostal space?

(A) Inferior edge of the sixth rib at the midclavicular line

(B) Inferior edge of the sixth rib between the tip of the scapula and the posterior axillary line

(C) Superior edge of the seventh rib at the midclavicular line

(D) Superior edge of the seventh rib between the tip of the scapula and the posterior axillary line

3. A 66-year-old man comes to the physician for his annual health maintenance examination. He feels fine, and his vital signs are normal. Examination is remarkable only for enlarged lymph nodes in the cervical and supraclavicular regions. Liver and spleen are not palpable. Blood studies reveal:

Hematocrit	45%
Hemoglobin	13.5 g/dL
Platelet count	230,000/mm^3
Leukocyte count	28,000/mm^3
Lymphocytes	80%
Neutrophils	15%
Monocytes	5%

Peripheral blood smear shows a large number of mature lymphocytes. Bone marrow biopsy demonstrates diffuse infiltration by mature-looking lymphocytes. Which of the following is the most appropriate treatment at this time?

(A) No treatment

(B) Chlorambucil

(C) Fludarabine

(D) Prednisone

(E) Bone marrow transplantation

4. An 18-year-old Caucasian woman presents to her physician with complaints of excessive thirst over the past several months. Dipstick urinalysis demonstrates 4+ glucose in the urine. Blood chemistries demonstrate glucose of 420 mg/dL. In Caucasian patients, the condition affecting this woman is most strongly associated with which of the following HLA types?

(A) DR1 and DR2

(B) DR1 and DR3

(C) DR2 and DR3

(D) DR2 and DR4

(E) DR3 and DR4

5. A 45 year-old man undergoes a routine physical examination with screening blood studies. Physical examination is notable for an increased liver diameter; the liver edge is palpable and without irregularities. Blood studies show elevated liver enzymes. The clinician suspects alcoholic hepatitis. Which of the following findings would tend to support this diagnosis?

(A) Alanine aminotransferase = 2,000 U/L

(B) Aspartate aminotransferase (AST)/alanine aminotransferase (ALT) ratio = 2.5

(C) Gamma-glutamyl transferase (GGT) = 20 U/L (norm ≤65 U/L)

(D) Mean corpuscular volume (MCV) = 65 μm^3

(E) Platelet count = 600,000/mm^3

6. A 38-year-old man comes to his physician because of irregular jerky movements of his upper extremities for the past three months. The man's wife says that, over the past year, he has been acting irritable, moody, and restless. He stopped playing chess because he was unable to concentrate and sit quietly for long periods of time. He has no siblings. His father died at the age of 60 years after developing a dementing disorder in his forties. His grandmother died in a mental institution. During the examination, the patient displays erratic movements of his arms and fingers, which he tries to suppress or disguise. Mental status examination reveals difficulty in concentration and a mildly depressed mood, but intact short-term memory. No focal neurologic deficits are present. Which of the following is the most likely diagnosis?

(A) Creutzfeldt-Jacob disease

(B) Gilles de la Tourette syndrome

(C) Huntington disease

(D) Sydenham chorea

(E) Tardive dyskinesia

7. A 24-year-old woman presents with a chief complaint of "not feeling well" for the past several days. She describes generalized weakness and is at times confused and fatigued, but she denies fever, nausea, vomiting, or abdominal pain. She has been drinking a lot of fluids and urinates every one to two hours during the day. She also gets up once or twice at night to urinate. She has a history of major depression, for which she is regularly seeing a psychiatrist. Examination shows she is well hydrated. Her temperature is 37.1° C (98.8° F), blood pressure is 120/80 mm Hg, pulse is 70/min, and respirations are 18/min. Her heart is regular, with a grade 2/6 systolic murmur best heard along the left sternal boarder. Which of the following sets of laboratory findings is most compatible with the diagnosis?

(A) Hypernatremia and high urine sodium

(B) Hyponatremia and high urine sodium

(C) Hypernatremia and low urine sodium

(D) Hyponatremia and low urine sodium

(E) Hypernatremia and normal urine sodium

8. An elderly Asian man comes to the emergency department because of the rapid onset of severe pain and blurred vision in his right eye. He also reports seeing halos around lights. On examination, the eye is red with a fixed and dilated pupil. He is taking imipramine for treatment of depression. Which of the following diagnostic procedures should be performed at this time?

(A) Direct ophthalmoscopy

(B) MRI of the head

(C) Slit-lamp examination

(D) Tonometry

(E) Visual field assessment

9. A 19-year old HIV-positive female prostitute presents to the emergency department with complaints of high fever and shaking chills for the past 48 hours. She complains of difficulty breathing and a cough productive of sputum. On chest auscultation, coarse crackles can be heard, more prominently over the right lung fields. A chest x-ray film shows patchy consolidation of right middle and adjacent upper lobe areas. Her CD4 count was 150 two months ago. Which of the following is the most likely pathogen?

(A) *Isospora belli*

(B) *Mycobacterium avium-intracellulare*

(C) *Mycobacterium tuberculosis*

(D) *Pneumocystis carinii*

(E) *Streptococcus pneumoniae*

10. A 40-year-old woman presents with diffuse generalized edema and ascites. Laboratory studies show marked hypoalbuminemia, elevated serum creatinine, and severe proteinuria (10 g/day) without hematuria. A renal biopsy shows changes consistent with membranous glomerulopathy. Which of the following laboratory findings is most likely to be associated with this clinical condition?

(A) CD4 cell count less than 200 cells/mL

(B) Circulating C3 nephritic factor

(C) Elevated antistreptolysin levels

(D) Elevated serum IgA antibodies

(E) Positive antineutrophil cytoplasmic antibodies (ANCA)

(F) Positive antinuclear antibody test

(G) Positive serology for hepatitis B virus

11. A 45-year-old man comes to the physician because his "face and voice have changed." The patient came to this realization after meeting a nephew, who had not seen him for two years and could hardly recognize him. He also reports that he has had persistent joint pains in the past six months. His blood pressure is 140/90 mm Hg, but he says he has never had values over 120/80 mm Hg on previous health maintenance examinations. Physical examination reveals coarse facial features, a large tongue, and thick fingers. His handshake is moist and doughy, and his voice deep. Which of the following is the most appropriate next step in diagnosis?

(A) CT scans of the head

(B) MRI of the head

(C) Measurement of baseline growth hormone levels

(D) Measurement of growth hormone levels following glucose suppression test

(E) Measurement of TSH levels

12. A 30-year-old woman goes to her physician complaining of a whitish discharge from her nipples for the past three months. She denies headaches or visual problems. She notes that she often feels tired but attributes it to the fact that she has to take care of her 18-month-old daughter. She has not had a menstrual period since her delivery and has not nursed her baby for the past five months. She is not taking any medications. Her physical examination is unremarkable. She does not have any visual field defects. Laboratory results show a prolactin level of 200. Which of the following is the most appropriate next step in diagnosis?

(A) Chest x-ray film

(B) CT scan of the brain

(C) Measurement of thyroid hormone levels

(D) No additional investigation is warranted

(E) Pregnancy test

13. A 60-year-old man comes to his physician because of right flank pain. He has been smoking two packs of cigarettes daily for 30 years but has never had any renal diseases. His temperature is 37° C (98.6° F), blood pressure is 136/85 mm Hg, pulse is 70/min, and respirations are 14/min. Examination reveals tenderness on percussion of the right costovertebral angle and a deep abdominal mass in the right upper quadrant. Urine dipstick test shows microscopic hematuria. Which of the following is the most likely diagnosis?

(A) Adult polycystic kidney disease

(B) Angiomyolipoma

(C) Hydronephrosis

(D) Renal cell carcinoma

(E) Simple renal cyst

14. A 40-year-old woman comes to the physician because of fever and chills, jaundice, and right upper abdominal pain radiating to the shoulder for 24 hours. At present, the patient's temperature is 39° C (102° F), blood pressure is 100/60 mm Hg, pulse is 110/min, and respirations are 20/min. She is admitted for further diagnostic evaluation. Serum chemistry studies show:

ALT	100 U/L
AST	80 U/L
Alkaline phosphatase	800 U/L
Bilirubin	
Total	4.5 mg/dL
Direct	3.5 mg/dL
Prothrombin time	12 sec
Amylase	200 U/L

White blood cell count is 12,000/mm^3, with 70% neutrophils. Which of the following is the most likely diagnosis?

(A) Acute cholecystitis

(B) Acute hepatitis

(C) Acute pancreatitis

(D) Choledocholithiasis with cholangitis

(E) Cystic duct syndrome

15. A 30-year-old, dark-skinned man of racially mixed descent consults a physician because "his eyes turned yellow." Physical examination is remarkable for jaundice that is most visible in the sclera, palms, and nail beds. Serum chemistry studies show:

Sodium	141 mEq/L
Potassium	4.0 mEq/L
Chloride	102 mEq/L
Bicarbonate	26 mEq/L
Urea nitrogen	14 mg/dL
Creatinine	0.8 mg/dL
Uric acid	5.1 mg/dL
Total bilirubin	2.2 mg/dL
Direct bilirubin	0.3 mg/dL
Indirect bilirubin	1.9 mg/dL
Albumin	4.1 g/dL
Amylase	105 U/L
AST	20 U/L
ALT	25 U/L
Alkaline phosphatase	77 U/L

Which of the following is the most likely diagnosis?

(A) Carcinoma of the ampulla of Vater

(B) Cholesterol gallstone disease

(C) Dubin-Johnson syndrome

(D) Hepatic cirrhosis

(E) Sickle cell disease

16. A 45-year-old woman presents to clinic for a health maintenance visit. She has no complaints but has a history of diabetes and a family history of hypertension. On physical examination, the patient's blood pressure is 150/100 mm Hg. Laboratory results are normal. Which of the following agents would be most appropriate for the management of her hypertension?

(A) Atenolol

(B) Captopril

(C) Furosemide

(D) Hydrochlorothiazide

(E) Isordil

17. A 30-year-old man is brought to the emergency department because of acute chest pain for one hour. He is admitted with a diagnosis of myocardial infarction, which is confirmed by imaging and serum marker studies. The patient's family history is significant for early myocardial infarctions in several of his relatives. Nodular lesions are noted in his eyelids and several tendons, which are diagnosed as xanthomas by biopsy examination. Serum cholesterol level is 350 mg/dL, and triglycerides are within the normal range. An abnormality in which of the following proteins most likely accounts for this patient's condition?

(A) Apolipoprotein CII

(B) Apolipoprotein E

(C) 3-Hydroxy-3-methylglutaryl coenzyme A reductase

(D) LDL receptor

(E) Lipoprotein lipase

18. A 45-year-old woman comes to the physician because of muscle tenderness, pain on swallowing, hoarseness, and temperatures to 38° C (100° F). Several weeks ago, the patient returned from a trip to Greece, where she ate boar meat. Examination shows muscle swelling and tenderness involving the upper arms, neck, and masseters. Injected conjunctivae and periorbital edema are also noted. Laboratory investigations show:

Hematocrit	41%
Leukocyte count	9,000/mm³
Eosinophils	8%
Erythrocyte sedimentation rate	12/min
Creatine kinase	2,300 U/L
Albumin	4.0 g/dL
Globulins	4.3 g/dL

Which of the following is the most likely diagnosis?

(A) Cysticercosis

(B) Dermatomyositis

(C) Polyarteritis nodosa

(D) Systemic lupus erythematosus

(E) Toxoplasmosis

(F) Trichinosis

(G) Trypanosomiasis

19. A 26-year-old woman with a history of type 1 diabetes presents with nausea and vomiting for one day. She has had flu-like symptoms for the past three days, with mild abdominal pain but no fever or chills. She has cut her insulin dosage in half because she is not eating well. Examination shows her temperature is 37.7° C (99.8° F), blood pressure is 120/80 mm Hg, pulse is 110/min, respirations are 20/min. Examination of the lungs reveals crackles at the right base. Laboratory studies show the following:

Leukocyte count	13,000/mm^3
Hemoglobin	16.0 g/dL
Platelets	220,000/mm^3
Sodium	145 mEq/L
Potassium	4.5 mEq/L
Chloride	110 mEq/L
Glucose	322 mg/dL
Urine	Positive for ketones

Determination of arterial blood gases is likely to show which of the following sets of values?

(A) pH 7.33, PCO$_2$ 32, HCO$_3^-$ 14

(B) pH 7.33, PCO$_2$ 40, HCO$_3^-$ 15

(C) pH 7.43, PCO$_2$ 30, HCO$_3^-$ 24

(D) pH 7.45, PCO$_2$ 38, HCO$_3^-$ 34

(E) pH 7.23, PCO$_2$ 47, HCO$_3^-$ 18

20. A 45-year-old man is seen by a clinician because of chronic gastritis, which he has been self-treating with antacids. Screening blood chemistries demonstrate a plasma phosphate of 2.0 mg/dL. The physician suspects that the antacids may have caused the hypophosphatemia, but the man does not remember which brand of antacid he has been taking. Which of the following common antacid ingredients is most likely responsible for this man's hypophosphatemia?

(A) Aluminum hydroxide

(B) Calcium carbonate

(C) Magnesium hydroxide

(D) Simethicone

(E) Sodium alginate

21. A 43-year-old man with alcohol abuse has enrolled in a specialized program for alcohol-related disorders. Which of the following blood tests is useful in monitoring the patient's compliance with treatment?

(A) Carbohydrate-deficient transferrin

(B) γ-glutamyl transferase

(C) Mean corpuscular red blood cell volume

(D) Serum triglycerides

(E) Uric acid

22. A 38-year-old woman with rheumatoid arthritis presents to her physician because of increased joint pain. On physical examination, both passive and active range of motion of the hips are decreased. Her physician increases her dose of nonsteroidal anti-inflammatory drugs (NSAIDs). Which of the following should be prescribed as well to prevent peptic ulcer disease?

(A) Cimetidine

(B) Clarithromycin

(C) Misoprostol

(D) Omeprazole

(E) Sucralfate

23. A 22-year-old college student has had a nonproductive cough, low-grade fever, and severe headache for six days, as well as left ear pain for one day. His temperature is 38.3° C (101° F), pulse is 78/min, and respirations are 18/min. The left tympanic membrane is erythematous, and there are two small blebs present. Crackles are heard over the right lower lung field. The left lung fields are clear to auscultation. Laboratory studies reveal a white blood cell count of 6,000 with a normal differential. A chest x-ray film reveals a right lower lobe infiltrate with an area of platelike atelectasis. When an anticoagulated tube of blood is cooled with ice, a precipitate forms, clearing with rewarming. Which of the following is the most appropriate treatment?

(A) Amoxicillin

(B) Erythromycin

(C) Gentamycin

(D) Imipenem

(E) Vancomycin

24. A 40-year-old man presents to a physician because he has been experiencing episodes of severe vertigo accompanied by nausea and vomiting. The first time this happened, he thought he had picked up a gastrointestinal "bug," but he has now had five of these episodes over the past six months. The episodes frequently begin with a sense of fullness in his right ear, which is often accompanied by tinnitus and a sense of hearing loss in the affected ear. Each episode lasts hours to days and then resolves. Otoscopic examination of the affected ear is within normal limits. Which of the following is the most likely diagnosis?

    (A) Benign paroxysmal positional vertigo

    (B) Herpes zoster oticus

    (C) Ménière disease

    (D) Purulent labyrinthitis

    (E) Vestibular neuronitis

25. A 37-year-old woman complains of pain during intercourse. Several months ago, she noted the gradual onset of increasing vaginal discomfort, and she is now unable to have intercourse without significant pain. She uses oral contraceptives and does not use condoms or lubricants. During the interview, the patient stops several times to drink from a bottle of water that she carries with her. She reports that she has always had a dry mouth and dry eyes. On physical examination, her temperature is 37.2° C (98.9° F), blood pressure is 110/82 mm Hg, pulse is 74/min, and respirations are 14/min. There is bilateral parotid gland swelling. There are multiple dental caries and fillings. Cardiac examination is significant for a midsystolic click. Which of the following is the most likely diagnosis?

    (A) CREST syndrome

    (B) Dermatomyositis

    (C) Raynaud phenomenon

    (D) Scleroderma

    (E) Sjögren syndrome

26. A 35-year-old man consults a gastroenterologist because of chronic heartburn for several years. The heartburn tends to be worse at night, and he frequently tastes refluxed gastric contents when he goes to bed. He found that his symptoms were a little better when he avoided his customary late evening alcoholic drink; however, this modest improvement has subsequently deteriorated. The gastroenterologist performs esophageal manometry with pH monitoring, which demonstrates decreased pressure of the lower esophageal sphincter and the presence of acid in the esophagus. Esophagogastroduodenoscopy demonstrates a very irregular gastroesophageal junction with long "fingers" of reddened mucosa extending up to 7 cm above the lower esophageal sphincter. Biopsy of the proximal end of one of these fingers shows surface epithelium with regular columnar cells with small, ovoid nuclei admixed with goblet cells. Which of the following is the most likely diagnosis?

    (A) Achalasia

    (B) Barrett esophagus

    (C) Corrosive esophagitis

    (D) Esophageal adenocarcinoma

    (E) Zenker diverticulum

27. A previously healthy 22-year-old man comes to medical attention because of progressive exertional dyspnea punctuated by episodes of precordial pain. The patient's father and one of his elder siblings died of chronic heart disease in middle age. The most significant findings on physical examination include presence of a loud S_4 and a harsh systolic murmur. The latter increases with the Valsalva maneuver and decreases with squatting. Bibasilar rales are heard on lung auscultation. Blood pressure, pulse, and respiratory rate are within normal limits. A chest x-ray film shows no appreciable alterations in cardiac silhouette, but the ECG shows left axis deviation. Echocardiography reveals marked thickening of the interventricular septum, associated with delayed relaxation and filling of the left ventricle during diastole. Which of the following is the most appropriate initial step in management?

    (A) Beta blockers

    (B) Digitalis

    (C) Long-acting nitrates

    (D) Aortic valve replacement

    (E) Partial excision of myocardial septum

28. A 47-year-old alcoholic man is picked up by the police and taken to the emergency department. The police, who have had previous encounters with this man, are concerned that he seems particularly lethargic and confused. Stat blood chemistries demonstrate a plasma sodium of 115 mEq/L. The emergency department physician orders the administration of hypertonic saline; within four hours, the plasma sodium rises to 135 mEq/L. Over the next few days, the patient develops quadriparesis and weakness of the lower face and tongue. These symptoms never resolve. Damage to which of the following neural structures probably accounts for these findings?

    (A) Cerebellum

    (B) Cerebral cortex

    (C) Peripheral nerves

    (D) Pons

    (E) Spinal cord

29. A 61-year-old woman presents to her physician's office for a routine physical. She has a history of diabetes and hypertension and has a 30-pack-year history of cigarette smoking. Laboratory studies show:

Sodium	136 mEq/L
Potassium	4.5 mEq/L
Chloride	108 mEq/L
BUN	24 mg/dL
Creatinine	0.9 mg/dL
Calcium	11.5 mg/dL
Albumin	3.4 g/dL

    Which of the following is the most likely diagnosis?

    (A) Excess vitamin D intake

    (B) Occult malignancy

    (C) Paget disease

    (D) Parathyroid hormone (PTH) oversecretion

    (E) Sarcoidosis

30. A 35-year-old man with recurrent, active, genital herpes suddenly develops numerous erythematous macules, papules, wheals, and vesicles. The hands, feet, and face are most extensively involved. Careful examination demonstrates that many of the lesions have a "target" appearance. Some of the lesions involve the lips and buccal mucosa. Which of the following is the most likely diagnosis?

    (A) Erythema multiforme

    (B) Erythema nodosum

    (C) Granuloma annulare

    (D) Pemphigus

    (E) Toxic epidermal necrolysis

31. A 60-year-old woman comes to the physician because of jaundice, pruritus, and anorexia for two weeks. She has one or two alcoholic drinks on social occasions and has smoked one pack of cigarettes daily for 30 years. She is currently taking a thiazide diuretic for mild hypertension. Her temperature is 36.8° C (98° F), blood pressure is 130/80 mm Hg, pulse is 80/min, and respirations are 14/min. Physical examination confirms icteric discoloration of skin and mucosae. Abdominal examination is remarkable for slight tenderness in the right upper quadrant, and the liver is palpable 1 cm below the right costal arch. The spleen is not palpable. Serum chemistry tests show:

AST	60 U/L
ALT	40 U/L
Alkaline phosphatase	1,000 U/L
Total bilirubin	5.5 mg/dL
Direct bilirubin	4.0 mg/dL

    Which of the following is the most appropriate next step in diagnosis?

    (A) Abdominal ultrasound

    (B) Abdominal CT or MRI scan

    (C) Endoscopic retrograde cholangiopancreatography

    (D) Percutaneous liver biopsy

    (E) Percutaneous transhepatic cholangiography

32. A 45-year-old woman presents with recent onset of low back pain for the past three days. She has not sustained any significant trauma. She has a history of systemic lupus erythematosus and has been receiving chronic corticosteroid treatment. She is currently afebrile. Examination reveals tenderness on palpation of the lumbar spine. The pain does not radiate down the leg. Which of the following is the most likely diagnosis?

    (A) Ankylosing spondylitis

    (B) Cauda equina syndrome

    (C) Compression fracture

    (D) Herniated intervertebral disk

    (E) Infection

    (F) Neoplasm

    (G) Spinal stenosis

33. A 40-year-old man with a history of IV drug use presents with a two-week history of high-grade fevers. He has been seen in clinic before and is now found to have a new murmur on cardiac examination. He also has several dark painful spots on his feet. Which of the following is the most common cause of negative blood cultures in patients with this illness?

    (A) Fungal infection

    (B) Inadequate culture techniques

    (C) Prior administration of antibiotics

    (D) Prosthetic valve seeding

    (E) Right-sided endocarditis

34. A 45-year-old woman is taken to the emergency department with severe, colicky right upper quadrant pain for the past two days. She is on medications and denies alcohol use. Ultrasound studies show gallstones, and the patient is taken for cholecystectomy the next morning. Intraoperatively, it is noted that the liver has a yellowish color, and a liver wedge biopsy is submitted along with the gallbladder to pathology. The pathologist reports steatosis with a predominately macrovesicular pattern in the liver. Which of the following is the most likely explanation for these findings?

    (A) Breast cancer

    (B) Chronic pancreatitis

    (C) Diabetes mellitus

    (D) Peptic ulcer disease

    (E) Systemic lupus erythematosus

35. A 52-year-old woman consults a physician because of severe epigastric pain of several months' duration. Endoscopy demonstrates thickened gastric mucosa with several peptic ulcers in the stomach and duodenum. The basal acid secretion rate is 75% of that following a maximal stimulating dose of histamine. Serum gastrin levels are markedly elevated (1,200 pg/mL). Endoscopic ultrasound demonstrates a pancreatic mass, which is later resected. Following the resection, serum gastrin levels decrease to 50 pg/mL. In addition to the tumor that was resected, this patient would most likely develop which of the following during her lifetime?

    (A) Marfanoid habitus

    (B) Medullary carcinoma of the thyroid

    (C) Mucosal neuromas

    (D) Pheochromocytoma

    (E) Pituitary adenoma

36. A confused elderly man is taken to the emergency department. The patient was found wandering and complaining of severe abdominal pain, but is unable to give a coherent history. Urine dipstick demonstrates positive ketones but no glucosuria. Stat blood chemistries show a plasma glucose of 100 mg/dL. Which of the following is the most likely explanation for these findings?

    (A) Alcoholism

    (B) Congestive heart failure

    (C) Emphysema

    (D) Inflammatory bowel disease

    (E) Rheumatoid arthritis

37. A 70-year-old woman with metastatic lung cancer is brought to the hospital for increasing confusion and obtundation over the past several weeks. Her family denies recent head trauma. The woman is currently receiving chemotherapy for her malignancy, but no other medications. On physical examination, her vital signs are stable, her jugular venous pressure (JVP) is 7 cm H_2O, and her lungs are clear. Her heart rhythm is regular, and she has no edema in her legs. Laboratory analysis shows:

Sodium	124 mEq/L
Potassium	4.5 mEq/L
Chloride	109 mEq/L
Bicarbonate	25 mEq/L

A CT scan of her head indicates no brain metastases. What is the most appropriate next step in management?

(A) Administer diuretics and water

(B) Administer isotonic saline

(C) Administer water

(D) Restrict intake of salt

(E) Restrict intake of water

38. An 18-year-old female athlete undergoes successful arthroscopic repair of a torn right medial meniscus. She has been ambulating with the aid of crutches and now complains of profound weakness of her right arm. Physical examination is normal except for an inability to actively extend the right arm at the elbow or the right hand at the wrist. The muscle tone, reflexes, flexors, and intrinsic hand muscles are normal. There is a minor sensory deficit over the dorsolateral area of the right hand. Which of the following is the most likely diagnosis?

(A) Axillary nerve palsy

(B) Dorsal scapular nerve palsy

(C) Median nerve palsy

(D) Radial nerve palsy

(E) Ulnar nerve palsy

39. A 45-year-old woman presents with a yellowish discoloration of her body, first noted by her husband last week. Since then, she has been having severe itching at night, which disturbs her sleep, and complains of a tingling sensation of her hands and feet. On examination, xanthelasmas are seen around the eyes. The liver is firmly palpable 4 cm below the costal margin. Scratch marks are noted on her abdomen and limbs. Clubbing is observed in all the digits. Serum creatinine is 0.9 mg/dL, bilirubin is 2.3 mg/dL, albumin is 4.3 g/dL, alanine aminotransferase is 92 U/L, and alkaline phosphatase is 410 U/L. Which of the following is the most appropriate next step in diagnosis?

(A) Antimitochondrial antibody assay

(B) Antismooth muscle antibody assay

(C) Endoscopic retrograde cholangiopancreatography (ERCP)

(D) Serum protein electrophoresis

(E) Technetium (^{99m}Tc) liver-spleen scan

40. A 41-year-old man with alcoholic cirrhosis is admitted to the hospital for evaluation of increasing abdominal girth. The patient has a three-year history of cirrhosis due to 20 years of ethanol consumption. He has no known cardiac disease but has had two upper gastrointestinal bleeds secondary to portal hypertension from his cirrhosis. He underwent variceal banding on both occasions. He reports that since his last admission for ascites five months ago, he has continued to drink ethanol but has been taking his daily spironolactone and furosemide. On physical examination, his abdomen is distended with occasional spider angiomata and a fluid wave on palpation. A diagnostic paracentesis is planned. Monitoring which of the following laboratory values is most important in the continued care of this patient?

    (A) Bleeding time

    (B) Hematocrit

    (C) Partial thromboplastin time (PTT)

    (D) Platelet count

    (E) Prothrombin time (PT)

41. A 53-year-old man collapses while in the checkout line at the supermarket. A bystander administers CPR until an ambulance arrives after approximately ten minutes. During the ride to the hospital, the pulse is lost twice, and further resuscitation and electric defibrillation are required. At the emergency department, he has a steady sinus rhythm and normal, stable, vital signs, but he is in deep coma, with bilateral fixed, dilated pupils. His past medical and surgical history are unknown. Which of the following might ultimately improve his neurologic outcome?

    (A) Anticoagulation with heparin drip

    (B) High-dose systemic steroids (dexamethasone)

    (C) Hyperventilation to a P_{CO_2} of 25 mm Hg

    (D) Moderate hypothermia to 33.0° C (91.4° F) core temperature

    (E) Sedation with barbiturates

42. A 28-year-old man comes to medical attention because of sustained hypertension for the past year. During the same period, he also had paroxysmal episodes characterized by profuse sweating, headache, and a sensation of increased heart rate. At this time, his blood pressure is 160/95 mm Hg, with a pulse of 86/min on supine position. On standing, his blood pressure is 120/70 mm Hg and pulse is 110/min. A dipstick test reveals glucose in the urine. Which of the following is the most appropriate next step in diagnosis?

    (A) CT and/or MRI studies of the abdomen

    (B) Measurement of epinephrine and norepinephrine in the blood

    (C) Measurement of fasting glucose levels in plasma or serum

    (D) Pharmacologic provocative tests

    (E) Urinary assay for free catecholamines and vanillylmandelic acid

43. A 27-year-old man is brought to the hospital with a gunshot wound of the abdomen, and he is prepared quickly for emergency laparotomy. The endotracheal intubation is achieved with the help of succinylcholine, and he is then switched to nondepolarizing agents and inhaled halothane. Shortly thereafter, the anesthesiologist notices tachycardia, hypertension, and increased CO_2 production; subsequently the core body temperature rises to 40.6° C (105.0° F) and hyperkalemia develops. Which of the following is the intrinsic pathophysiology responsible for these abnormalities?

    (A) Bacteremia

    (B) Massive release of catecholamines

    (C) Massive release of thyroid hormone

    (D) Sustained muscular contracture

    (E) Unrecognized adrenal insufficiency

The response options for items 44-45 are the same. You will be required to select one answer for each item in the set.

(A) Aortic dissection

(B) Atherosclerotic disease

(C) Churg-Strauss syndrome

(D) Cryoglobulinemic vasculitis

(E) Giant cell arteritis

(F) Henoch-Schönlein purpura

(G) Kawasaki syndrome

(H) Microscopic polyangiitis

(I) Polyarteritis nodosa

(J) Syphilitic aortitis

(K) Takayasu arteritis

(L) Thromboangiitis obliterans

(M) Wegener granulomatosis

For each patient with signs and symptoms of peripheral vascular disease, select the most likely diagnosis.

44. A 25-year-old woman presents with a two-month history of recurrent transient episodes of visual blurring, dizziness, and focal neurologic deficits, such as limb weakness and paresthesias. She also reports numbness and coldness of her fingers. Physical examination discloses marked weakening of the pulses in the upper extremities. An aortic angiogram reveals proximal narrowing of the brachiocephalic, left common carotid, and left subclavian arteries. The aortic arch appears normal.

45. A 34-year-old woman presents with a six-month history of sinusitis and otitis media unresponsive to common antibiotic and anti-inflammatory treatments. She recently developed increasing malaise and a persistent cough productive of blood-tinged sputum. Her temperature is 38.2° C (100.8° F), blood pressure is 126/81 mm Hg, pulse is 80/min, and respirations are 16/min. Laboratory studies show mild anemia and leukocytosis, an erythrocyte sedimentation rate (ESR) of 87/min, and the presence of circulating antineutrophil cytoplasmic antibodies of c-ANCA type. Urinalysis shows more than five red blood cells/high-power field and red cell casts.

The response options for items 46-48 are the same. You will be required to select one answer for each item in the set.

(A) Allergic contact dermatitis

(B) Atopic dermatitis

(C) Hypothyroidism

(D) Immunodeficiency state

(E) Irritant contact dermatitis

(F) Langerhans cell histiocytosis

(G) Lupus erythematosus

(H) Nummular eczema

(I) Psoriasis

(J) Scabies

(K) Seborrheic dermatitis

(L) Tinea corporis

(M) Vitamin deficiency

For each patient with a rash, select the most likely diagnosis.

46. A 2-year-old boy is brought by his parents to the physician because of an itchy rash that has been a persistent problem since six months of age. The rash is dry, erythematous, and scaly, and chiefly involves the face and dorsal surfaces of hands and feet. The lesions undergo alternating periods of remission and exacerbations. Local steroid treatment has provided temporary relief. Examination also reveals dry skin and pronounced skin markings on plantar and palmar surfaces. Family history is significant for allergic rhinitis and asthma in several relatives. The child's development is otherwise normal.

47. A 50-year-old man comes to his physician because of a two-week history of pruritic rash on the extensor surfaces of legs and arms. The patient reports no family or personal history of allergic disorders. The rash is characterized by erythematous, crusted, coin-shaped plaques. Skin scrapings treated with KOH do not reveal any spores or hyphae on microscopic examination. Physical examination is otherwise unremarkable.

48. A 35-year-old man with AIDS develops a scaling, oily erythema involving the scalp, eyebrows, nasolabial folds, back, chest, and umbilicus.

The response options for items 49-50 are the same. You will be required to select one answer for each in the set.

(A) Chest x-ray film

(B) Dexamethasone suppression test

(C) Growth hormone glucose suppression test

(D) Measurement of urinary catecholamines

(E) Plasma lipids

(F) Plasma renin level

(G) Thyroid function tests

(H) Two-dimensional echocardiogram

For each patient with hypertension, select an appropriate initial diagnostic test.

49. A 50-year-old man comes to the physician for a health maintenance examination. On this occasion, and on two subsequent visits, his blood pressure is found to be elevated. On the last visit, his blood pressure is 145/98 mm Hg. He denies any significant medical problems, but his family history is significant for high blood pressure, premature coronary artery disease, and diabetes mellitus. Physical examination reveals no abnormalities.

50. A 30-year-old woman comes to the physician for a health maintenance examination. Her blood pressure is 145/65 mm Hg. Her pulse is irregular, with an average rate of 100/min. She admits having increasing anxiety, sleeplessness, and palpitations in the past three months. She also had a 4-kg (8.8 lb) weight loss over the same period. Examination reveals fine tremors of the hands, moist skin, and hyperreflexia.

Internal Medicine Test Five:
Answers and Explanations

ANSWER KEY

1.	D	26.	B
2.	D	27.	A
3.	A	28.	D
4.	E	29.	D
5.	B	30.	A
6.	C	31.	A
7.	D	32.	C
8.	D	33.	C
9.	E	34.	C
10.	G	35.	E
11.	D	36.	A
12.	E	37.	E
13.	D	38.	D
14.	D	39.	A
15.	E	40.	E
16.	B	41.	D
17.	D	42.	E
18.	F	43.	D
19.	A	44.	K
20.	A	45.	M
21.	A	46.	B
22.	C	47.	H
23.	B	48.	K
24.	C	49.	E
25.	E	50.	G

1. **The correct answer is D.** Characteristics of infectious mononucleosis include signs and symptoms similar to influenza, with lymphadenopathy (especially in the cervical chain) and splenomegaly. Skin rash is infrequent, but ampicillin administration is followed by a diffuse maculopapular rash in 90% of cases. Atypical lymphocytes are easily identified on blood smears. Granulocytopenia is present initially, and thrombocytopenia develops frequently. IgM antibodies to *Epstein-Barr virus* appear during the acute phase. The Monospot test is based on heterophil (sheep cell agglutination) antibody tests and becomes positive before the fourth week after the onset of the disease.

Acute cytomegalovirus (CMV) disease (**choice A**) may be indistinguishable in its clinical and laboratory manifestations from infectious mononucleosis, but the heterophil antibody test is negative in CMV infection. Most CMV infections, however, remain asymptomatic in immunocompetent hosts, producing severe disseminated infections in immunocompromised patients.

Acute lymphocytic leukemia (**choice B**) is a disease of children (peak between three and seven years) and is characterized by pancytopenia and the presence of circulating blasts.

Drug-induced thrombocytopenia (**choice C**) is not associated with other hematologic abnormalities or systemic illness. Currently, most cases are due to heparin. Other common drugs that may cause thrombocytopenia include sulfonamides, thiazides, and cimetidine.

Streptococcal pharyngitis with a leukemoid reaction (**choice E**) would be associated with marked neutrophilic leukocytosis with the presence of numerous circulating granulocytic precursors. Leukemoid reactions may give rise to leukocyte counts up to $50,000/mm^3$, but are not associated with the presence of blasts or thrombocytopenia.

2. **The correct answer is D.** The proper placement of the needle is at the superior edge of the seventh rib between the tip of the scapula and the posterior axillary line (rather than the midclavicular line, **choice C**). The superior border of the rib is used to avoid the neurovascular bundle, which runs along the inferior edge of each rib. Before the tap is done, a lateral decubitus film should be performed to confirm that the effusion is free flowing. The lungs should be percussed, and the needle should be placed below the point where fluid is detected. This usually occurs at the seventh rib. At least 200 mL of fluid should be present to be successfully tapped (otherwise it should be done with ultrasound guidance).

Insertion at the inferior edge (**choices A and B**) can result in damage to the neurovascular bundle.

3. **The correct answer is A.** The diagnosis is *chronic lymphocytic leukemia* (CLL). CLL is a neoplastic disorder of B lymphocytes, characterized by marked peripheral lymphocytosis. Circulating lymphocytes are extremely similar to normal lymphocytes and tend to accumu-

late progressively in the marrow and blood because of inactivation of the apoptosis-inhibiting *Bcl-2* gene. The manifestations are due to increasing immunosuppression, bone marrow replacement, and organ infiltration. Lymphocytosis due to CLL is often incidentally discovered in otherwise healthy older people. Lymphadenopathy, however, is frequently present. CLL follows an indolent course, and aggressive chemotherapy seems to have little impact on survival. In patients who present with only lymphocytosis and lymphadenopathy (stage I according to the *Rai system*), no treatment is necessary.

Chlorambucil (**choice B**) is the standard initial treatment for symptomatic CLL—that is, patients with progressive fatigue and organomegaly (stage II), severe anemia (stage III), and thrombocytopenia (stage IV). Chlorambucil is well tolerated.

Fludarabine (**choice C**) is usually used as a second-line treatment for patients who do not respond any longer to chlorambucil. It is associated with significant immunosuppression.

Prednisone (**choice D**) is useful for certain autoimmune-mediated manifestations of CLL, namely autoimmune hemolytic anemia or thrombocytopenia.

Bone marrow transplantation (**choice E**) is used only for the rare young patient who presents with an aggressive form of CLL. It is not a treatment option for most CLL patients. These are elderly persons who most often will die of causes unrelated to CLL.

4. **The correct answer is E.** This is a typical presentation of type 1 diabetes mellitus. Patients are typically diagnosed in childhood or adolescence, and this form of diabetes is the most prevalent type in patients younger than 30. Type 1 diabetics are particularly prone to develop diabetic ketoacidosis, as they produce little or no insulin. In Caucasian patients, there is a strong association between type 1 diabetes mellitus and the specific HLA phenotypes HLA-DR3, HLA-DR4, and the heterozygote form HLA-DR3/HLA-DR4. These patients often (but not always) have detectable serum islet cell cytoplasmic antibodies or antibodies to glutamic acid decarboxylase and to insulin. It is thought that their diabetes mellitus is the result of an immune-mediated selective destruction of the islet beta cells that usually secrete insulin. Pancreatic biopsies in these patients (usually done in research rather than clinical settings) show a dense lymphocytic infiltrate in pancreatic islets, with T and B lymphocytes, macrophages, and a loss of most beta cells.

HLA-DR1 and HLA-DR2 (**choices A to D**) are not associated with an increased incidence of type 1 diabetes and are actually relatively "protective" HLA types, since most type 1 diabetics instead have HLA-DR3 or HLA-DR4.

5. **The correct answer is B.** The diagnosis of alcoholic hepatitis has enough social implications that it is important

to be reasonably sure it is correct before suggesting it. A helpful rule of thumb in making the diagnosis is that the ratio of serum aspartate aminotransferase (AST) to serum alanine aminotransferase (ALT) is usually greater than 2 in alcoholic hepatitis. Other indices are affected by alcoholic hepatitis but are not as specific for the disease.

Very high ALT levels (**choice A**) are more characteristic of viral hepatitis, ischemic liver injury, or toxicity. In alcoholic hepatitis, elevation to around 250 U/L is more typical.

The gamma-glutamyl transferase (GGT) level (**choice C**) provides another helpful clue to alcoholic hepatitis, in that it is often markedly elevated in these patients. Normal levels for males are less than or equal to 65 U/L; for females, less than or equal to 45 U/L.

The erythrocyte mean corpuscular volume (MCV) (**choice D**) is frequently elevated and can be used as a marker of alcoholic hepatitis because it gradually returns to normal with drinking cessation.

Platelet count (**choice E**) is often decreased as either a direct toxic effect or secondary to hypersplenism.

6. **The correct answer is C.** The clinical manifestations and family history are consistent with Huntington disease, which is due to an autosomal dominant mutation of a gene on chromosome 4. The mutation consists of an unstable expansion of a CAG trinucleotide repeat in a gene encoding a novel protein named *huntingtin*. The age of clinical onset is commonly between 30 and 50 years, but may be as early as 5 years. Behavioral abnormalities often precede the characteristic choreiform movements. The patient may experience irritability, restlessness, and difficulty in concentration. Dementia subsequently develops.

Creutzfeldt-Jacob disease (**choice A**) manifests with a rapidly progressive dementia and mental status changes associated with myoclonic movements. A family history is usually absent.

Gilles de la Tourette syndrome (**choice B**) has an early clinical onset, commonly between 2 and 15 years of age. The manifestations include motor tics (sniffing, blinking, spitting, head and shoulder movements) or phonic tics (grunts, coughs, verbal sounds, coprolalia).

Sydenham chorea (**choice D**) accompanies rheumatic disease and is one of the *major Jones criteria* for the diagnosis of this condition.

Tardive dyskinesia (**choice E**) is a late complication of antipsychotic drugs that block dopamine D_2 receptors. It most commonly involves the lower face, manifesting with persistent chewing movements and intermittent protrusion of the tongue.

7. **The correct answer is D.** The combination of low serum sodium and low urine sodium indicates an increase in total body water due to primary polydipsia, leading to dilutional hyponatremia. This is caused by suppression of arginine vasopressin (AVP) secretion. Deficiency of AVP produces central diabetes insipidus. Resistance to AVP at the kidney level is termed nephrogenic diabetes insipidus. AVP is also called ADH (antidiuretic hormone).

8. **The correct answer is D.** The symptomatology of red eye, extreme pain, and blurred vision with halos around light is characteristic of narrow-angle glaucoma. This condition is most frequent in Asians and generally in individuals with narrow angles of the anterior chamber (1% of all people older than 35). It is an emergency to be promptly treated with drugs that lower intraocular pressure, such as acetazolamide or osmotic diuretics (glycerol or mannitol). Tonometric measurement of intraocular pressure confirms the diagnosis, but the affected eye even feels hard on palpation.

Direct ophthalmoscopy (**choice A**) to evaluate the retina, along with tonometry and visual field testing (**choice E**), is the mainstay for the diagnosis and management of open-angle glaucoma. Direct ophthalmoscopy allows examination of the optic disc for glaucomatous cupping. Visual field assessment documents loss of peripheral vision in open-angle glaucoma, which may result in "tunnel vision."

MRI of the head (**choice B**) would have no diagnostic value in this case.

Slit-lamp examination (**choice C**) is particularly useful in the evaluation of lens opacities (cataract) or other pathology in the anterior chamber.

9. **The correct answer is E.** The most common form of pneumonia in AIDS patients is bacterial pneumonia. The pneumococcus is the bacterial pathogen most likely to cause the acute onset of severe symptomatic pneumonia; systemic symptoms include fever, chills, rigors, and gastrointestinal complaints. Given this patient's presentation, *Streptococcus pneumoniae* is the most likely pathogen.

Isospora belli (**choice A**) is not a known pulmonary pathogen. It is known, however, to cause diarrhea in HIV-positive individuals.

Mycobacterium avium-intracellulare (**choice B**) causes a wasting systemic disease in HIV-positive patients and not a pneumonia-like picture. It is known, however, to colonize the airways of patients with chronic obstructive pulmonary disease.

Tuberculosis (TB), caused by *Mycobacterium tuberculosis* (**choice C**), usually presents as a chronic or subacute illness with cough, fever, drenching night sweats, malaise, and weight loss. Even in HIV-positive patients, TB rarely causes dyspnea. When it does, there is usually multilobar involvement or disseminated miliary TB.

Pneumocystis carinii (**choice D**) causes pneumonia (PCP) in patients with deficient cell-mediated immunity. It is the most common opportunistic infection in HIV-positive patients. It develops over weeks, with a dry cough, fever, and progressively worsening dyspnea, especially with exertion.

10. **The correct answer is G.** It is clear that this woman has severe nephrotic syndrome. *Membranous glomerulopathy* is the most common cause of nephrotic syndrome in adults (minimal change disease shares this distinction in children). This disease is immune complex-mediated, and subepithelial immune deposits can be demonstrated by ultrastructural studies. Although often idiopathic, many cases are associated with some underlying condition, infectious or noninfectious. Among infectious causes, hepatitis B is the most common (syphilis is second in frequency).

CD4 cell count less than 200 cells/mL (**choice A**) is a defining feature of AIDS. The most common renal complication of AIDS is *focal segmental glomerulosclerosis*.

Circulating C3 nephritic factor (**choice B**) refers to a circulating IgG that binds to C3 convertase, stabilizing this factor and promoting activation of the alternative pathway of complement. This pathogenetic mechanism has been observed in type 2 *membranoproliferative glomerulonephritis*, which manifests with nephritic or combined nephritic/nephrotic syndrome.

Elevated antistreptolysin levels (**choice C**) would be present in a patient with recent streptococcal infection, which may lead to acute *postinfectious glomerulonephritis*. This glomerulopathy manifests with nephritic syndrome. Proliferative glomerulonephritis would be seen in a renal biopsy.

Elevated serum IgA antibodies (**choice D**) are associated with 50% of cases of *Berger disease*, the most common form of glomerulonephritis. Berger disease manifests with recurrent hematuria and/or proteinuria, often in concomitance with an upper respiratory flu-like syndrome or intestinal infection. Mesangial expansion with deposition of IgA is found on biopsy.

Positive antineutrophil cytoplasmic antibodies (ANCA) (**choice E**) are characteristic of *pauci-immune glomerulonephritides*, which include Wegener granulomatosis, Churg-Strauss syndrome, and microscopic polyangiitis. All these conditions are associated with sites of involvement other than kidneys (e.g., lungs and skin).

A positive antinuclear antibody test (**choice F**) would be found in a patient with SLE or other collagen vascular diseases. The incidence of glomerulopathy is particularly high in SLE, in which renal impairment represents an important cause of morbidity and mortality.

11. **The correct answer is D.** The clinical presentation is consistent with *acromegaly*, due to overproduction of growth hormone (GH). This syndrome manifests when excessive production of GH occurs in adulthood after closure of the epiphyseal growth plates. Consequently, hypertrophy of acral bones and skeletal muscle results, leading to enlargement of the tongue, hands, feet, and craniofacial skeleton. Hypertrophy of pharyngeal and laryngeal tissues makes the voice deeper. Changes in facial morphology and voice are often not recognized by the patient or friends and relatives since they develop slowly, but are commonly recognized by people who have not seen the patient for many years. Often, the patient realizes that his hat, ring, or shoes do not fit any more. Secondary diabetes mellitus, arthritis, hyperhidrosis (with moist and doughy handshake), cardiomegaly, and hypertension are frequent manifestations. GH-producing pituitary adenomas are the usual cause. The diagnosis, once suspected, is confirmed by a glucose suppression test: serum levels of GH are assessed in a blood sample drawn after an overnight fast and following a challenge with 100 g oral glucose. A GH concentration higher than 2 ng/mL in men or 5 ng/mL in women is considered positive. The initial screening test (not an option) is a random IGF-1 level.

CT scans of the head (**choice A**) and MRI (**choice B**) of the head are used to reveal a pituitary adenoma following a positive GH-suppression glucose test. MRI is the method of choice for pituitary lesions.

Measurement of baseline growth hormone levels (**choice C**) is inadequate. Some patients may have normal baseline GH levels, but exercise, stress, hepatic or renal diseases, and a number of drugs may produce abnormally high levels.

Measurement of TSH levels (**choice E**) would be appropriate in case of suspected hyper- or hypothyroidism.

12. **The correct answer is E.** The most common cause of secondary amenorrhea is pregnancy. The woman is of child-bearing age, so the first possibility is that she is pregnant (consistent with a prolactin level of 200). Also, although prolactinoma is usually associated with prolactin levels greater than 200, it might be present in this patient. A CT scan (**choice B**) could be performed to rule this out, but first the physician should rule out the possibility of pregnancy.

A chest x-ray film (**choice A**) is unlikely to aid in the diagnosis, and, again, pregnancy should be ruled out first.

Hypothyroidism can increase prolactin levels moderately but would not be likely to produce such a marked elevation as that observed in this patient; therefore, measurement of thyroid hormone levels (**choice C**) is not necessary at this time. Some of the symptoms associated with hypothyroidism are fatigue, cold intolerance, slow movements, and weight gain.

A prolactin level of 200 is not normal and warrants further investigation (compare with **choice D**).

13. **The correct answer is D.** The triad of flank pain, hematuria, and abdominal mass is highly suggestive of renal cell carcinoma, although it represents the clinical presentation in only 20% of cases. Ultrasonography and CT scan studies are used for further diagnostic investigations. Most commonly, renal cell carcinoma presents with an isolated finding, such as painless hematuria (microscopic or macroscopic), weight loss, or flank

pain. Note the history of cigarette smoking, which is a recognized risk factor for this type of cancer.

Adult polycystic kidney disease (**choice A**) manifests with hypertension, microscopic hematuria, and bilateral kidney enlargement.

Angiomyolipoma (**choice B**) is a rare tumor composed of a mixture of adipose tissue, blood vessels, and smooth muscle. It is a hamartomatous lesion, most often found in association with tuberous sclerosis.

Hydronephrosis (**choice C**) may result in a palpable renal mass, but is usually preceded by a history of urologic problems resulting from obstructive uropathy. Among these, the most frequent are renal stones, prostatic hyperplasia, vesicoureteral reflux, and anomalies in the ureteropelvic junction.

Simple renal cyst (**choice E**) is probably the most common lesion found in the kidneys. Rarely, it presents as a palpable mass. It is usually an incidental finding in the course of investigations undertaken for other reasons. Once a renal lesion is discovered, the problem of whether it is a common renal cyst or a carcinoma must be addressed with further investigation. Ultrasonography is the method of choice.

14. **The correct answer is D.** The complex of fever, right upper abdominal pain, and jaundice is referred to as *Charcot triad*, which is diagnostic of acute cholangitis. This usually results from a small gallstone impacted within the common bile duct. Blockage of the common bile duct results in cholestatic jaundice: hence, elevated bilirubin (mostly direct) and high serum alkaline phosphatase. Gram-negative enteric bacteria then penetrate into the biliary ducts and cause ascending cholangitis, with resultant fever and neutrophilic leukocytosis. The pain is due to acute distention of the gallbladder. This condition must be urgently treated with cholecystectomy.

Acute cholecystitis (**choice A**) is associated with gallstones usually impacted within the cystic duct. Colicky pain is not associated with fever, but jaundice occurs in a minority of cases. This condition (as any other form of *symptomatic* cholelithiasis) must be treated with cholecystectomy.

Acute hepatitis (**choice B**) manifests with mild right upper abdominal pain, nausea, anorexia, and low-grade fever. Serum levels of AST and ALT are markedly elevated, helping to differentiate this condition from cholangitis.

Acute pancreatitis (**choice C**) manifests with extremely intense deep epigastric pain, usually radiating to the back. High serum levels of amylase and lipase support a diagnosis of acute pancreatitis. However, mild elevation of amylase may be seen with cholangitis, and mild jaundice may be present in acute pancreatitis.

The designation of cystic duct syndrome (**choice E**) is given to clinical conditions characterized by dyspeptic symptoms (e.g., upper abdominal discomfort, nausea, bloating, and flatulence) that manifest after meals and are caused by biliary dysfunction. There are two situations in which cystic duct syndromes may develop: *precholecystectomy*, resulting from obstruction of the cystic duct by fibrosis or kinking, and *postcholecystectomy*, due to incorrect diagnosis, neuroma of the cystic duct stump, foreign body granuloma, and common bile duct anomalies, for example.

15. **The correct answer is E.** The patient has indirect (unconjugated) hyperbilirubinemia. In adults, the causes include intravascular hemolysis (due to acquired and genetic causes of hemolytic anemia, such as sickle cell anemia, hereditary spherocytosis, glucose-6-phosphate dehydrogenase deficiency, and autoimmune hemolysis) and genetic deficiencies of liver glucuronyl transferase activity (Gilbert syndrome and Crigler-Najjar syndrome). In contrast, direct (conjugated) hyperbilirubinemia can be due to intrahepatic causes (notably hepatitis, drug toxicity, and alcoholic liver disease) or extrahepatic causes (notably common duct stone and pancreatic cancer).

Carcinoma of the ampulla of Vater (**choice A**) can cause direct hyperbilirubinemia.

Gallstone disease (**choice B**) involving the common bile duct can cause direct hyperbilirubinemia. Hemolytic anemias predispose for bile gallstones, rather than cholesterol stones.

Dubin-Johnson syndrome (**choice C**) is a hereditary disease with direct hyperbilirubinemia.

Hepatic cirrhosis (**choice D**) can cause direct hyperbilirubinemia.

16. **The correct answer is B.** This question tests your knowledge about the effectiveness of angiotensin converting enzyme (ACE) inhibitors in cardiac remodeling in diabetics. High-dose ACE inhibitors have been shown to have a mortality benefit in hypertensive patients. All the other medicines are good hypertensive alternatives, but captopril is the most effective in diabetics. ACE inhibitors also exert a protective effect on the kidneys in diabetics by inhibiting the actions of angiotensin II on renal afferent arterioles and by attenuating the stimulatory effect of angiotensin II on glomerular cell growth and mesangial matrix production. Of course if the creatinine were high, indicating renal insufficiency, then we would have to reevaluate our options.

Atenolol (**choice A**) would be the drug of choice in a patient with coronary artery disease. Beta blockers reduce mortality in such patients by decreasing chronotropy and exerting a protective effect.

Furosemide (**choice C**) is a loop diuretic used when diuresing a patient in congestive heart failure.

Hydrochlorothiazide (**choice D**) is a diuretic useful in the management of hypertension, especially in African Americans. It is the initial medication for isolated hypertension.

Isordil (**choice E**) belongs to the nitrate family of vasodilators and exerts its effects as a venodilator that decreases preload. It is used as an adjunct to first-line therapy in hypertension and coronary artery disease.

17. **The correct answer is D.** The constellation of high cholesterol level, MI at a young age, positive family history for early-onset MI, and multiple xanthomas is consistent with *familial hypercholesterolemia*. This autosomal dominant disorder is caused by mutations in the gene for the LDL receptor, resulting in cholesterolemia that is two to three times the normal level in heterozygotes and five to six times the normal level in homozygotes. The molecular defect leads to impairment in the ability of the liver and other tissues to take up LDL from the plasma. Homozygotes often die in their 20s or 30s because of myocardial or cerebral infarction.

Abnormalities in apolipoprotein CII (**choice A**) represent the molecular basis for the rare hyperlipoproteinemia type V, characterized by elevation of cholesterol *and* triglycerides. ApoCII is a major component of VLDL and is removed in the conversion of VLDL into IDL.

Inherited abnormalities of apolipoprotein E (**choice B**) lead to hyperlipoproteinemia type III, which is characterized by increased IDL and elevated levels of cholesterol *and* triglycerides. These patients manifest early atherosclerotic disease as well.

3-Hydroxy-3-methylglutaryl coenzyme A reductase (**choice C**) catalyzes the rate-limiting step in the biosynthesis of cholesterol. There is no known familial abnormality affecting this enzyme.

Lipoprotein lipase (**choice E**) is present in peripheral tissues (adipose tissue and skeletal muscle) and is involved in the uptake of triglycerides from chylomicrons and VLDL. Abnormalities in this enzyme result in hyperlipoproteinemia types I and IV, characterized by recurrent pancreatitis and hepatosplenomegaly. The atherogenic effects of these abnormalities is minimal, since cholesterol is minimally affected.

18. **The correct answer is F.** Trichinosis (trichinellosis) is due to the nematode *Trichinella spiralis*, whose larvae are acquired by ingestion of improperly cooked pork or other types of meat, including boar, bear, and horse. The invasive phase of trichinellosis preferentially affects the skeletal muscle, but also the myocardium, lungs, and brain. A transient intestinal stage (diarrhea and abdominal cramps for a few days) is followed by the muscle invasion stage. The muscles most commonly involved include the masseters, tongue, diaphragm, intercostals, extraocular muscles, laryngeal muscles, nuchal muscles, deltoids, and biceps. Pain and tenderness of involved muscles, periorbital edema, conjunctivitis, hoarseness, and dysphagia are the most characteristic manifestations. Blood eosinophilia, elevated creatine kinase, and a reversed ratio of albumin and globulin are highly characteristic. Serologic tests are available to confirm the clinical diagnosis.

Cysticercosis (**choice A**) develops following ingestion of *Tenia solium* eggs in undercooked pork. The brain is one of the preferred sites for cysticercosis, and cysticerci may develop within the brain parenchyma, ventricles, or subarachnoid space.

Trichinosis may simulate collagen vascular diseases, such as dermatomyositis (**choice B**), polyarteritis nodosa (**choice C**), and systemic lupus erythematosus (**choice D**). Eosinophilia, however, is consistent with a parasitic disease. Furthermore, collagen vascular diseases are associated with an elevated erythrocyte sedimentation rate, which is usually normal in trichinosis.

Toxoplasmosis (**choice E**) may affect skeletal muscles, in addition to the CNS, retina, lungs, and myocardium. The cat is the definitive host for *Toxoplasma gondii*. Primary infection results from ingestion of cysts in inappropriately cooked meat, contaminated vegetables, handling of cat litter, or transplacental infection. The acute infection in immunocompetent hosts is mild and self-limiting. Fever, malaise, myalgia, and cervical lymphadenopathy are characteristic manifestations.

Trypanosomiasis (**choice G**) causes *Chagas disease*, endemic in South America. It is transmitted from person to person by *triatomids* known as "kissing bugs." *Trypanosoma cruzi* is an intracellular protozoon that localizes mainly in the heart and nerve cells of the myenteric plexuses, leading to myocarditis, achalasia, megacolon, and megaureter.

19. **The correct answer is A.** This patient has a metabolic acidosis, due to the increase in ketone bodies, with respiratory compensation. (The P_{CO_2} of 32 is below the normal value of 40, indicating hyperventilation in agreement with the compensatory increased respiratory rate.)

Choice B represents metabolic acidosis with no respiratory compensation.

Choice C represents respiratory alkalosis, characterized by an isolated decrease in carbon dioxide.

Choice D represents metabolic alkalosis, as evidenced by the increased bicarbonate.

In **choice E** there is both metabolic acidosis and respiratory acidosis.

20. **The correct answer is A.** Hypophosphatemia is defined as a plasma phosphate less than 2.5 mg/dL. Clinically significant hypophosphatemia occurs in a relatively small number of clinical settings. One of these is a prolonged negative phosphate balance due to binding to aluminum-containing antacids. Other causes include hyperparathyroidism, other hormonal disturbances (Cushing syndrome, hypothyroidism), electrolyte disorders (hypomagnesemia, hypokalemia), theophylline intoxication, chronic diuretic administration, malabsorption, renal dialysis, and starvation.

Calcium carbonate (**choice B**) commonly causes constipation and can cause increased serum phosphate as part of the milk alkali syndrome.

Magnesium hydroxide (**choice C**) has a laxative effect and rarely causes hypermagnesemia.

Simethicone (**choice D**) is sometimes added to antacids to alleviate gas symptoms and is relatively free of side effects.

Sodium alginate (**choice E**) is sometimes added to antacids and makes a foam that allows smaller antacid doses to be used; it is relatively free of side effects.

21. **The correct answer is A.** Problem drinking is one of the most common problems coming to the attention of primary care physicians. It encompasses conditions of varying severity, ranging from alcohol dependence (the most serious), to alcohol abuse, and at-risk drinking. History is the key to detection of problem drinking. There are no specific laboratory tests that assist in the diagnosis. However, medical complications related to excessive alcohol consumption can be detected, or suspected, by using certain laboratory parameters. Of the ones listed above, the serum level of carbohydrate-deficient transferrin appears to correlate best with heavy alcohol consumption (more than five drinks daily). This is not a useful screening test, but it may be valuable in the follow-up of patients who enrolled in specialized programs for treatment of alcoholism.

Studies show that gamma-glutamyl transferase (GGT) levels (**choice B**) are elevated in more than 30% of problem drinkers, and that providing feedback information about GGT levels to problem drinkers results in a better treatment outcome.

Mean corpuscular red blood cell volume (**choice C**) is often elevated in chronic alcohol abusers because of frequent coexistence of vitamin deficiency. Vitamin B_{12} and folic acid deficiencies are the most frequent and cause megaloblastic anemia.

Serum triglycerides (**choice D**) are also frequently above normal levels (>180 mg/dL) in problem drinkers, who also exhibit high levels of uric acid (**choice E**) in the blood (>7 mg/dL). Neither test is useful in screening for problem drinking because of low sensitivity.

22. **The correct answer is C.** NSAIDs inhibit the production of prostaglandins, which are essential for protecting the stomach and duodenum from ulcers. In patients who absolutely require NSAIDs, misoprostol administration will decrease the incidence of peptic ulcer disease (PUD) and upper gastrointestinal bleeding. In patients with a history of these conditions, other agents should be used for pain control if possible.

Cimetidine (**choice A**) is an H2 blocker that has not proven beneficial for treating NSAID-induced ulcers.

Clarithromycin (**choice B**) is an antibiotic active against *Helicobacter pylori*, a known pathogen in PUD. The drug has not been proven beneficial in NSAID-induced ulcers.

Omeprazole (**choice D**) is a proton-pump blocker. It is not appropriate for treating NSAID-induced ulcers.

Sucralfate (**choice E**) is a viscous liquid that coats ulcer beds. It has not been proven beneficial in NSAID-induced ulcers.

23. **The correct answer is B.** Erythromycin is the treatment of choice for *Mycoplasma* pneumonia. Bullous myringitis, which occurs in a small percentage of patients with *Mycoplasma* infection, is characterized by the presence of erythematous and painful papules on the surface of the tympanic membranes. This patient also has cold agglutinins (classically associated with *Mycoplasma*), which precipitate on cooling and clear with warming. The IgM antibodies made against *Mycoplasma* agglutinate RBCs at low temperatures, causing hemolysis in less than 15% of cases. This patient has classic signs and symptoms of *Mycoplasma*: he is young and has headaches, nonproductive cough, low-grade fever, and infiltrate or atelectasis on chest x-ray.

24. **The correct answer is C.** This is Ménière disease, a disease of poorly understood pathophysiology in which a generalized dilation of the membranous labyrinth of the inner ear (endolymphatic hydrops) is associated with attacks of vertigo, tinnitus, and initially fluctuating and later progressive hearing loss. The clinical description illustrated in the question stem is typical. Ménière disease can affect any age or sex, with a (broad) peak in the fourth and fifth decades of life. Treatment is pharmacologic and often requires some experimentation before medications (e.g., anticholinergics, antihistamines, barbiturates, and diazepam) effective in a particular individual are found.

Benign paroxysmal positional vertigo (**choice A**) is characterized by violent vertigo induced by moving the head to certain positions.

Herpes zoster oticus (**choice B**) has prominent pain symptoms in addition to hearing loss, vertigo, and sometimes paralysis of the facial nerve.

Purulent labyrinthitis (**choice D**) is a bacterial infection of the inner ear and occurs as a complication of acute otitis media or purulent meningitis.

Vestibular neuronitis (**choice E**) presents with an initial, persistent, severe episode of vertigo that eventually fades to a paroxysmal form, which usually completely disappears within a year or two.

25. **The correct answer is E.** Sjögren syndrome is an autoimmune disorder resulting in dysfunction of exocrine glands, which leads to dryness of the eyes and mouth, dental caries, dysphagia, and parotid enlargement because of infiltration of these structures with lymphocytes and plasma cells. Dyspareunia may develop, as in this case, due to decreased vaginal lubricant. There is an association with systemic lupus erythematosus, rheumatoid arthritis, scleroderma, polymyositis, and autoimmune thyroid disease. Treatment is supportive, with artificial

tears and dental hygiene. The disease is usually benign, but lymphoma may develop.

CREST syndrome (**choice A**) differs from scleroderma (systemic sclerosis) in that there is a lower risk of renal involvement, a higher risk of pulmonary hypertension, and an overall better prognosis. CREST patients have thickened skin only on their hands and face, as opposed to the more diffuse skin involvement in scleroderma. Both diseases are characterized by an immune-mediated fibrosis of internal organs and skin.

Dermatomyositis (**choice B**) is a systemic disease of unknown etiology characterized by proximal muscle weakness and a "heliotrope" rash. It is associated with underlying malignancy.

Raynaud phenomenon (**choice C**) usually affects younger women. The peripheral vasculature exhibits an abnormal response to the cold. Patients experience painful cyanosis in the fingertips in response to cold or to emotions. Treatment includes keeping the patient's hands warm with gloves, having the patient refrain from smoking, and, in extreme cases, prescribing calcium channel blockers.

Scleroderma (**choice D**), or systemic sclerosis, causes hardening and contraction of the connective tissue. The skin is tough and thick and has patches of pigmentation.

26. **The correct answer is B.** The patient has reflux esophagitis that has become complicated by metaplasia of the squamous mucosa to intestinal-type mucosa (as indicated by the goblet cells). This change, called Barrett esophagus or Barrett mucosa, is considered premalignant since adenocarcinoma of the esophagus can arise in these areas. Recommended treatment of gastroesophageal reflux disease includes elevation of the head of the bed; avoidance of acid stimulators, such as coffee and alcohol; avoidance of agents that decrease lower esophageal sphincter pressure, such as anticholinergics, fats, and chocolate; use of antacids after meals and at bedtime; and use of H2 blockers, prokinetic agents, or proton-pump inhibitors, such as omeprazole. Once Barrett esophagus has been demonstrated, endoscopic surveillance to detect developing adenocarcinoma is recommended every one or two years.

Achalasia (**choice A**) would show aperistalsis and increased lower esophageal sphincter pressure on manometry.

Corrosive esophagitis (**choice C**) is seen after accidental or suicidal ingestion of caustic poisons, such as strong cleaning solutions.

Esophageal adenocarcinoma (**choice D**) is a major complication of Barrett esophagus, but it is not indicated here by the biopsy since the cells seen are regular and nonmalignant.

Zenker diverticulum (**choice E**) is a posterior outpouching of the esophageal mucosa and submucosa through the cricopharyngeal muscle.

27. **The correct answer is A.** The clinical presentation is consistent with *hypertrophic cardiomyopathy*, a frequently inherited disorder due to mutations in one of the genes encoding myofibrillary proteins. Left ventricular dysfunction is due to impaired diastolic filling. The septum is disproportionately thick compared with the free wall (asymmetric hypertrophy), resulting in outflow obstruction. The latter is the cause of the systolic murmur, which intensifies with decreased left ventricular filling, such as during the Valsalva maneuver. Beta blockers or calcium channel blockers should be the initial treatment.

Digitalis (**choice B**) is contraindicated in hypertrophic cardiomyopathy because it enhances myocardial contractility and, consequently, the degree of outflow obstruction secondary to increased septal contraction.

Long-acting nitrates (**choice C**) are used for treatment of angina and related coronary artery syndromes, but not for chest pain secondary to hypertrophic cardiomyopathy. The latter, in fact, is not due to vascular stenosis but to a combination of decreased left ventricular output and increased oxygen demands of the hypertrophic myocardium.

Aortic valve replacement (**choice D**) is indicated for treatment of aortic stenosis, but the aortic valve is normal in this condition. Outflow obstruction is the result of a thick septum that partially obstructs the outflow tract.

Partial excision of the myocardial septum (**choice E**) has been successful in some centers but should be reserved for severe cases in which pharmacologic therapy has failed.

28. **The correct answer is D.** This is central pontine myelinolysis, which is a feared complication of severe hyponatremia. This demyelinating condition of the pons often produces permanent damage, which may manifest as illustrated in the question stem. More severe cases can even cause a locked-in syndrome, in which the patient is in an awake and sentient state but has complete, generalized motor paralysis, leaving only perhaps a limited ability to communicate by coded eye movements. (Fiction aficionados may recall that the character Noirtier in *The Count of Monte Cristo* had this syndrome. He could communicate only with his granddaughter, who was the only person patient enough to talk to him and interpret his eye blinks.) Overly rapid correction of severe hyponatremia increases the chances that the complication will develop, possibly because of fluid shifts in the confined area of the pons. It is now recommended that plasma sodium be raised no faster that 1 mEq/L/hr, with an upper limit of 10 mEq/L/24 h.

Although demyelination can also involve other areas of the brain to much lesser degrees, the cerebellum (**choice A**), cerebral cortex (**choice B**), peripheral nerves (**choice C**), and spinal cord (**choice E**) are not usually as significantly damaged as the pons in this condition.

29. **The correct answer is D.** The most common cause of asymptomatic hypercalcemia is primary hyperpara-

thyroidism. In older women, 85% of cases are due to adenoma of a single gland, 15% are caused by hyperplasia of all four parathyroid glands, and about 1% are associated with carcinoma. Most patients have asymptomatic hypercalcemia that is found incidentally during a routine laboratory examination.

Excess vitamin D intake (**choice A**) is an uncommon cause of hypercalcemia.

Occult malignancies (**choice B**) are responsible for most cases of "in hospital" hypercalcemia. Underlying mechanisms include release of a PTH-like substance, local osteolytic hypercalcemia, cytokine release, and peripheral activation of 1,25-OH vitamin D.

Paget disease (**choice C**) is associated with an increase in alkaline phosphatase and normal calcium and phosphate.

Sarcoidosis (**choice E**) is associated with hypercalcemia due to increased production of $1,25\text{-}(OH)_2$ vitamin D_3 by alveolar macrophages, but it is less common. This phenomenon also occurs in other chronic granulomatous disorders, in lymphomas, and in idiopathic hypercalciuria.

30. **The correct answer is A.** The patient has erythema multiforme, which is an inflammatory eruption characterized by lesions showing a variety of morphologies that may involve both skin and mucous membranes. Erythema multiforme can occur idiopathically; as a complication of viral infections (notably herpes simplex viruses, but also coxsackievirus and echovirus), *Mycoplasma pneumoniae* infection, or fungal infections (histoplasmosis); or as reaction to a drug (penicillin, sulfonamides, barbiturates) or vaccine (BCG, vaccinia, poliomyelitis). Erythema multiforme tends to have a sudden onset, with a predilection for most severe involvement of the hands (notably palms), feet (notably soles), and face (notably near or involving mucous membranes). The most helpful lesion morphology is the target lesion, with an erythematous ring, midpallor, and central erythematous macule; it may, in practice, be necessary to look at a number of lesions before a target lesion is identified. Attacks of erythema multiforme tend to last two to four weeks; treatment is usually primarily directed against any underlying condition or drug that triggered the skin reaction.

Erythema nodosum (**choice B**) usually causes tender red nodules of the pretibial areas of the legs.

Granuloma annulare (**choice C**) causes a peripheral ring of nodules around normal to slightly depressed skin.

Pemphigus (**choice D**) causes flaccid blisters of skin and mucous membranes.

Toxic epidermal necrolysis (**choice E**) causes sheets of skin to peel off, analogous to the peeling skin of sunburn.

31. **The correct answer is A.** The most crucial step in beginning investigations on a jaundiced patient is to determine whether the jaundice is due to hemolytic disease, hepatocellular damage, or biliary obstruction. Generally, jaundice resulting from hemolysis or hepatocellular damage must be treated with medical measures, whereas obstructive jaundice requires surgical treatment. Obstructive jaundice is characterized by a high proportion of *direct* (conjugated) bilirubin, elevated serum alkaline phosphatase levels, and normal or mildly elevated aminotransferases. This case is therefore due to biliary obstruction. How to proceed? The most appropriate investigation is ultrasound examination to evaluate the hepatobiliary system and pancreas, determine whether extrahepatic bile ducts are dilated, establish the presence of gallstones, and identify hepatic or pancreatic masses.

CT or MRI scans (**choice B**) are also adequate but are more expensive; thus, ultrasound constitutes the most convenient initial diagnostic test.

Endoscopic retrograde cholangiopancreatography (ERCP; **choice C**) is the method of choice to study pancreatic and ampullary lesions, carry out stone extraction from the common bile duct, or insert a stent.

Percutaneous liver biopsy (**choice D**) is the definitive study for hepatocellular or infiltrative diseases. It is not used as an initial diagnostic procedure because of its invasiveness and potential adverse effects.

Percutaneous transhepatic cholangiography (**choice E**) can identify the location of biliary obstruction, but may be associated with serious complications such as bacteremia, bile peritonitis, and hemorrhage. At any rate, this procedure should follow other noninvasive radiologic methods.

32. **The correct answer is C.** From a primary care perspective, the great majority of cases of low back pain are due to degenerative joint disease. However, the primary care physician should be alert to "red flags" that may signal the presence of more serious pathology. A history of corticosteroid treatment may be associated with osteoporosis of the vertebral column, which predisposes patients to compression fractures of the vertebral bodies. This type of fracture may present with back pain without any apparent history of preceding trauma.

Ankylosing spondylitis (**choice A**) is characterized by onset before 40 years of age, progressive ankylosis of the vertebral column, and bilateral involvement of the sacroiliac joints. More than 90% of cases are associated with HLA-B27 histocompatibility antigen. This disease should be suspected in a young person complaining of chronic lower back pain, especially when the symptoms are worst at night.

Cauda equina syndrome (**choice B**) is an acute clinical picture of lumbar root compression. It is a surgical emergency due to acute herniation of an intervertebral disk or other anatomic abnormalities and is characterized by the sudden onset of pain, saddle anesthesia, and bowel/bladder incontinence.

A herniated intervertebral disk (**choice D**) manifests with the acute onset of low back pain, which radiates down the leg in the distribution of a spinal root. The most common sites of disk herniation are the intervertebral spaces between L4-L5 and L5-S1. Sensory and motor testing usually reveals neurologic deficits in a dermatomal distribution.

Infection (**choice E**) of the vertebral bodies or joints (spinal osteomyelitis) is most prevalent among IV drug abusers. Fever and constitutional symptoms are associated with back pain.

A neoplasm (**choice F**) should be suspected if there is concomitant weight loss or other constitutional symptoms (e.g., anorexia, malaise, or fatigue). Metastases (breast, lung, prostate, renal cell, colon) and multiple myeloma are the most common malignancies affecting the spinal column.

Spinal stenosis (**choice G**), an infrequent cause of low back pain, is more prevalent in the elderly population. Narrowing of the lumbar spinal canal by osteophytes is thought to account for the symptomatology. Pain due to compression of lumbar roots manifests while in the upright position or walking (pseudoclaudication), when the spinal canal becomes narrower. The pain is relieved by sitting or leaning forward, as the spinal canal widens.

33. **The correct answer is C.** This patient most likely has infective bacterial endocarditis. Ill-advised use of antibiotics, before samples for blood culture are obtained, is a serious problem in the diagnosis and treatment of infections and is a leading cause of the increase in drug-resistant pathogens.

Fungal infections (**choice A**) can cause endocarditis in patients with indwelling catheters, IV drug abusers, diabetics, and immunocompromised hosts, but bacterial infections are more frequent in IV drug abusers.

Blood cultures usually yield results (compare with **choice B**) if the samples are obtained under sterile conditions. With positive blood cultures, however, it is important to ensure that the cultures are not falsely positive because of contamination.

Prosthetic valve seeding (**choice D**) is relatively common. In fact prosthetic valves, bicuspid aortic valves, and mitral valve prolapse are risk factors for bacterial endocarditis, rather than the cause of negative cultures.

Right-sided endocarditis (**choice E**) should still yield positive blood cultures. Right-sided infection can lead to emboli to the lungs, causing hemoptysis, and right-sided cardiac failure.

34. **The correct answer is C.** Although steatosis (fatty liver) has a wide variety of causes, the three most commonly encountered in clinical medicine in the U.S. are alcohol use, obesity, and diabetes mellitus. Rarer causes include jejunal bypass surgery, malnutrition, and as a complication of some drugs (e.g., glucocorticoids, synthetic estrogens, amiodarone, tamoxifen). The specific etiology of the steatosis cannot be determined reliably by pathologic examination, so clinical correlation is necessary. Cases

may be picked up incidentally, as in this case, or during liver biopsy performed in patients for other reasons (e.g., in asymptomatic patients with a two- to threefold increase in AST or ALT).

Tamoxifen therapy of breast cancer (**choice A**) is an unusual cause of fatty liver.

Chronic pancreatitis (**choice B**) does not cause fatty liver, although both can coexist in alcoholics.

Peptic ulcer disease (**choice D**) does not cause fatty liver.

Glucocorticoid therapy in systemic lupus erythematosus (**choice E**) is an unusual cause of fatty liver.

35. **The correct answer is E.** The first step in solving this question is to recognize that the patient has severe PUD in the setting of markedly increased basal acid secretion by the stomach and markedly elevated levels of serum gastrin. This suggests Zollinger-Ellison syndrome, in which an endocrine tumor secretes gastrin. All Zollinger-Ellison patients have serum gastrin levels greater than 150 pg/mL. Markedly elevated levels (>1,000 pg/mL) in the setting of compatible clinical features and gastric acid hypersecretion (>60% of the amount of acid after a maximal stimulating dose of histamine) is considered diagnostic. In this case, the hypergastrinemia comes from a pancreatic endocrine tumor; other sites can include the duodenum, splenic hilum, mesentery, stomach, or even lymph nodes or ovary. More than 50% of gastrinomas are malignant. About half the patients with Zollinger-Ellison syndrome have multiple tumors, usually as part of multiple endocrine neoplasia type I (MEN I, or Wermer syndrome). In MEN I, pancreatic islet cell tumors are found in 30% to 75% of patients; parathyroid adenomas in more than 90%; and pituitary adenomas in 50% to 65%. MEN I patients may also rarely have duodenal gastrinomas.

MEN IIA, or Sipple syndrome, is characterized by medullary carcinoma of the thyroid (**choice B**; more than 90% of affected patients), pheochromocytomas (**choice D**; 50%), and parathyroid adenomas (25%).

MEN IIB, or mucosal neuroma syndrome, is characterized by mucosal neuromas (**choice C**; close to 100% of affected patients), Marfanoid habitus (**choice A**; close to 100%), medullary carcinoma of the thyroid (**choice B**; more than 90%), and rarely parathyroid adenomas. All of the MEN syndromes have unique dermatologic findings as well.

36. **The correct answer is A.** Be aware that ketoacidosis can be seen in conditions other than diabetes mellitus. The two most important are starvation and chronic alcoholism. The mechanism of ketone production in chronic alcoholics appears to be a combination of alcohol withdrawal and starvation with increased free fatty acid release. The typical history (when it can be obtained) is that of an alcoholic binge that ended with vomiting, after which the patient consumed neither food nor water for

24 hours or more. Abdominal pain is usually a prominent complaint. Many of these patients have pancreatitis, and impaired glucose tolerance or even mild type 2 diabetes mellitus are often demonstrated after the patients recover from their acute episode.

Congestive heart failure (**choice B**), emphysema (**choice C**), and rheumatoid arthritis (**choice E**) do not cause nondiabetic ketoacidosis.

Although severe inflammatory bowel disease (**choice D**) could in theory cause enough "starvation" to induce ketoacidosis, in practice this is not usually seen.

37. **The correct answer is E.** This patient has euvolemic hyponatremia, which means that her effective circulating volume is normal. Her euvolemic status is supported by her normal jugular venous pressure (JVP) of 7 cm H_2O, an indication of her intravascular status. Patients in congestive heart failure would have an elevated JVP. Furthermore, her lungs are clear, and she has no leg edema. Euvolemic hyponatremia can be caused by a glucocorticoid defect, hypothyroidism, or inappropriate secretion of arginine vasopressin (antidiuretic hormone; ADH). SIADH can be caused by many things, including trauma, infections, medications, and certain neoplasms (ectopic production), including lung cancer. Excess ADH secretion leads to retention of free water, producing hyponatremia. The first step in managing this would be to restrict the intake of water, producing a negative water balance that results in gradual, daily reduction in weight and a progressive rise in serum sodium.

Giving diuretics and water (**choice A**) is a therapeutic option for treating hypernatremia. The diuretic would lead to the removal of excess salt, which would not be desirable.

Administering isotonic saline (**choice B**) is the equivalent of giving more free water, which will be retained, and the salt will be excreted, thus worsening the hyponatremia.

Administering water (**choice C**) will worsen the hyponatremia since the patient is simply being given free water. This treatment would be appropriate in treating hypernatremia.

This patient is hyponatremic since her effective salt load is low. Restricting the salt intake would thus not help (**choice D**). In fact, allowing her to take salt is also not likely to be effective in controlling the hyponatremia since ADH leads to excess retention of free water at the cost of sodium excretion.

38. **The correct answer is D.** The radial nerve originates from C_5-T_1 and innervates the triceps, brachioradialis, wrists, and finger and thumb extensors. The lesion usually affects the spiral groove of the humerus. Clinical features include wrist drop and inability to extend the elbow and fingers because of severe denervation of the dorsolateral hand. Radial nerve palsy is sometimes known as "Saturday night palsy," since it is found in patients who have been drinking and fall asleep with an arm hanging over a chair. Patients on crutches may also pinch the nerve with their crutches, producing a similar palsy.

The axillary nerve, C_5-C_6 (**choice A**), innervates the deltoid muscle and teres minor. The symptoms of axillary nerve palsy include weakness in shoulder abduction. The injury usually occurs near the shoulder joint.

Dorsal scapular nerve (C_5) palsy (**choice B**) leads to dysfunction of the levator scapulae and rhomboid muscles.

Palsy of the median nerve, C_6-T_1 (**choice C**), which innervates the abductor pollicis brevis, forearm, pronator, and finger and thumb flexors, may be due to carpal tunnel syndrome (entrapment of the median nerve in the flexor retinaculum at the wrist). Patients classically are unable to make a circle with their thumb and index finger because of sensory paresthesias in the ventral aspect of the lateral 2 1/2 fingers. It is commonly seen in workers who spend hours at a time at a keyboard.

The ulnar nerve, C_8-T_1 (**choice E**), innervates the flexors of the wrist, the flexors of the fourth and fifth digits, and most intrinsic hand muscles. With ulnar nerve palsy, the injury usually occurs at the ulnar groove in the elbow. The patient may display "claw hand," with weakness of finger adduction and abduction, and thumb adduction and abduction.

39. **The correct answer is A.** The patient probably has primary biliary cirrhosis. This disorder of unknown etiology appears to involve an autoimmune response to mitochondrial antigens. Autoantibodies in these patients have been found that recognize mitochondrial inner membrane proteins, such as enzymes of the pyruvate dehydrogenase complex, the branched chain alpha-ketoacid dehydrogenase complex, and the alpha-ketoglutarate dehydrogenase complex. The antimitochondrial antibody assay is the best test to diagnosis primary biliary cirrhosis. An IgG autoantibody directed against mitochondrial antigens is present in 90% of affected patients.

Antismooth muscle antibody (**choice B**) is positive in some patients with autoimmune chronic hepatitis, but is not specific or highly useful in the diagnosis of primary biliary cirrhosis.

ERCP (**choice C**) is better used in the diagnosis and monitoring of secondary biliary cirrhosis due to prolonged biliary tract obstruction.

Serum protein electrophoresis (**choice D**) might show a diffuse increase in immunoglobulins, but this is nonspecific and may be found in many chronic liver diseases.

The sulfur colloid technetium (^{99m}Tc) scan (**choice E**) is useful for detecting portal hypertension and hypersplenism, but it is not specific.

40. **The correct answer is E.** With any invasive procedure, there are risks. One such risk is that of bleeding. Patients with liver disease have varying degrees of damage to their liver parenchyma and thus less synthetic ability. Liver

patients often exhibit coagulopathies for this reason; their prothrombin time (PT) can exceed 19 seconds. Although the risk of bleeding is not directly related to a prolonged PT, it is positively associated, so this number is crucial to know prior to performing any procedure on a patient. A number of studies indicate that paracentesis may be safely performed in patients with a PT international normalized ratio (INR) up to 5.0.

Bleeding time (**choice A**) is a marker of platelet function or number. This is not a laboratory value frequently obtained today since its utility is unclear.

Hematocrit (**choice B**) is not a necessary value to know prior to performing this procedure. It will not effect current management whether the value is increased or decreased.

Although the PTT (**choice C**) is also mildly prolonged in liver disease, this is not a risk factor for bleeding episodes associated with invasive procedures.

It is a generally accepted practice to order a platelet count (**choice D**) prior to a paracentesis. This is not the most useful hematologic value to obtain; however, profound thrombocytopenia (<10,000/mm^3) can be associated with an increased risk of bleeding after invasive diagnostic procedures.

41. **The correct answer is D.** There is actually no magic treatment to undo the neurologic damage done by prolonged cardiac arrest, but there is some evidence that moderate hypothermia improves the chances for a better outcome.

Anticoagulation (**choice A**) has nothing to offer in this setting.

Steroids (**choice B**) are used often in neurologic situations. There is some evidence that they may help patients with spinal cord injury, and there is well-documented dramatic benefit in lowering intracranial pressure in patients with brain tumors, but in this particular setting there is no indication for using them.

Hyperventilation (**choice C**) has been used in the past in a prophylactic way, in situations in which brain edema is expected. The current consensus is that it should not be used until increased intracranial pressure has been diagnosed.

Sedation (**choice E**) has been used as a last-resort measure in cases of increased intracranial pressure, with the idea of decreasing the metabolic needs of the brain at a time when the oxygen supply might be compromised. Currently, hypothermia is preferred to achieve the same objective.

42. **The correct answer is E.** The history of hypertension punctuated by paroxysmal episodes of hypertensive crises is highly suggestive of *pheochromocytoma*, a tumor of the adrenal medulla or paraganglia that secretes large amounts of epinephrine and/or norepinephrine, resulting in hypertension. These hormones also cause hyperglycemia and, consequently, glycosuria. Note the orthostatic hypotension and tachycardia (due to vasodilation and dehydration), which are frequent manifestations of pheochromocytoma. The most appropriate initial diagnostic test is to measure

catecholamines and vanillylmandelic acid (a metabolic product of catecholamines) in the urine. An overnight urine collection is generally sufficient for this purpose.

CT and/or MRI studies of the abdomen (**choice A**) should be performed for localization of pheochromocytoma once the diagnosis has been supported by the previous test.

Measurement of epinephrine and norepinephrine in the blood (**choice B**) is the most sensitive test, but needs to be carried out during paroxysmal episodes of hypertension.

Measurement of fasting glucose levels in plasma or serum (**choice C**) represents an ancillary test that is not indispensable for a diagnosis of pheochromocytoma. It is certainly mandatory in suspected cases of diabetes mellitus.

Pharmacologic provocative tests (**choice D**) are no longer recommended. These are based on drugs that provoke release of catecholamines, raising blood pressure, or block adrenergic receptors, lowering blood pressure.

43. **The correct answer is D.** The clinical picture is that of malignant hyperthermia that is often triggered in susceptible patients by succinylcholine. The intrinsic problem is sustained muscular contracture.

Bacteremia (**choice A**) could account for rapid temperature rise, but would not produce hypertension and hyperkalemia.

Catecholamine release (**choice B**) in a patient not previously diagnosed with pheochromocytoma is most impressive for the amounts of arterial hypertension that rapidly develop. Massive temperature elevation is not a prominent feature.

A thyroid storm (**choice C**) can produce altered mental states, tachycardia and hyperthermia, but the setting would typically be that of a known patient with hyperthyroidism who is subjected to stress.

Adrenal insufficiency (**choice E**) would produce hyperkalemia, but the other manifestations include hyponatremia and hypotension. Temperature elevation is not a feature.

44. **The correct answer is K.** Takayasu arteritis, also known as *pulseless disease* because of the frequent absence of pulses in the upper extremities, was first described in Asian countries but has been reported in the U.S. as well. This inflammatory arteritis affects the main branches originating from the aortic arch, causing signs and symptoms of ischemia to the brain and upper extremities. Young women are most commonly affected.

45. **The correct answer is M.** Patients with Wegener granulomatosis are young (usually younger than 40 years) and have a history of chronic upper respiratory symptoms due to such conditions as otitis media, sinusitis, and pharyngitis. Later, the lungs (with hemoptysis and respiratory difficulties), as well as the kidneys (hematuria is the most frequent manifestation), become involved. ESR is elevated; fever, malaise, and weight loss are frequent. The presence

of circulating autoantibodies of c-ANCA type supports a diagnosis of Wegener granulomatosis.

Aortic dissection (**choice A**) manifests with chest pain of sudden onset radiating to the back, signs of shock, and severe distress.

Atherosclerotic disease (**choice B**) would not explain any of these clinical presentations.

Churg-Strauss syndrome (**choice C**) is a vasculitis affecting small vessels of lungs, kidneys, skin, and other organs. It is usually associated with eosinophilia and p-ANCA antibodies.

Cryoglobulinemic vasculitis (**choice D**) results from deposition of immune complexes composed of immunoglobulins that precipitate at cold temperatures in capillaries and venules. The skin is frequently involved.

Giant cell arteritis (**choice E**) most commonly affects the branches of the external carotid artery, especially the temporal artery. It manifests in middle-aged or elderly persons with headache, fever, and malaise. It may lead to blindness if not promptly treated.

Henoch-Schönlein purpura (**choice F**) is associated with deposition of immune complexes containing IgA in the skin (purpura), gastrointestinal tract (abdominal pain and melena), joints (arthralgia), and glomeruli (hematuria).

Kawasaki syndrome (**choice G**) predominantly affects children. Cervical lymphadenopathy, inflammation of conjunctiva and oral mucous membranes, a desquamative rash typically involving the palms, and fever are the most typical manifestations. Vasculitis of coronary arteries occurs in 80% of cases and is the most common cause of death.

Microscopic polyangiitis (**choice H**) is a vasculitis similar to polyarteritis nodosa but results from an immune response to circulating agents, such as drugs (antibiotics) or infectious agents. Circulating p-ANCA are frequently found.

Polyarteritis nodosa (**choice I**) may affect medium-sized arteries of kidneys, heart, gastrointestinal tract, joints, muscles, and central and peripheral nervous systems. It is not associated with circulating ANCA.

Syphilitic aortitis (**choice J**) is a complication of the tertiary stage of syphilis. It results from endarteritis obliterans involving the vasa vasorum of the ascending aorta, which undergoes scarring and dilatation with consequent aortic regurgitation.

Thromboangiitis obliterans (**choice L**) occurs almost exclusively in young male smokers. It is an inflammatory condition affecting the neurovascular bundles in the limbs and causing ischemia, venous thrombosis, and pain due to nerve involvement.

46. **The correct answer is B.** The history of this case outlines the characteristic clinical features of one of the most common disorders of infants and young children: *atopic dermatitis.* Although its pathogenesis is not entirely clear, a pathologic predisposition to abnormal immune reac-

tions plays a crucial role, which is emphasized by the frequent occurrence of allergic diseases in family members (e.g., allergic rhinitis, asthma, food intolerance). The manifestations of atopic dermatitis vary with age. Infants and children up to two years present with a scaly, erythematous, itchy rash distributed mainly on the face and dorsal hands and feet. Dry skin and accentuation of skin markings are additional frequent features. As the child grows, the distribution changes, involving predominantly flexural areas. The course is punctuated by periods of remission and exacerbation, but often the disease resolves spontaneously in late childhood. In a few unfortunate individuals, it persists into adulthood. Topical application of steroids affords temporary improvement, but cases of widespread skin involvement may require short-term systemic treatment. Systemic steroids, however, are associated with growth retardation.

47. **The correct answer is H.** As the name suggests, nummular eczema is characterized by coin-shaped lesions, which are covered by a uniform scaly crust. Itching may or may not manifest. It usually affects adult individuals without any apparent predisposing condition, except for a long-lasting tendency for dry skin. It is not caused by fungi, and microscopic examination of KOH-treated skin scrapings thus fails to reveal hyphae or spores. In contrast to fungal infections, the lesions of nummular eczema are homogeneous and do not show central clearing. The pathogenesis of nummular eczema is obscure and appears unrelated to allergic mechanisms. Fortunately, the lesions undergo spontaneous resolution in most of the cases without any need for therapy, except for symptomatic treatment if pruritus is present.

48. **The correct answer is K.** The most typical presentation of seborrheic dermatitis is a scaly, oily, dandruff-like rash on the scalp and eyebrows of infants (*cradle cap*), which is well known to all mothers. Adult patients with a congenital tendency for seborrhea may develop seborrheic dermatitis in a typical distribution, involving forehead, nasolabial folds, chin, beard area, chest, and anterior chest. Up to 50% of AIDS patients develop widespread seborrheic dermatitis, often in unusual locations. Other patients prone to this skin condition are those with Parkinson disease and those who are elderly and acutely ill.

Allergic contact dermatitis (**choice A**) is mediated by a type IV hypersensitivity reaction to a variety of allergens. Thousands of substances have been identified that can trigger this condition. Soaps, cosmetics, plastic compounds, glues, and fabrics are just a few examples of common allergens. The distribution of eczematous lesions and the clinical history are the most helpful elements for the diagnosis.

Hypothyroidism (**choice C**) should be considered as a possible cause of skin manifestations that may mimic eczematous reactions. Pretibial myxedema and loss of hair in the lateral eyebrows are the most typical cutaneous manifestations of hypothyroidism.

Immunodeficiency states (**choice D**) are associated with a wide range of cutaneous lesions, including chronic eczema and erythroderma. However, other signs of immune depression are usually present, including recurrent infections, diarrhea, and failure to thrive.

Irritant contact dermatitis (**choice E**) is caused by the irritating action of chemicals on the skin. It is not due to an allergic (i.e., immune-mediated) mechanism, but the skin manifestations are virtually indistinguishable from those of allergic contact dermatitis. Erythematous patches of itchy eczema develop in the areas in contact with the causative irritant. Again, distribution of lesions and clinical history are the most important clues to a correct diagnosis.

Langerhans cell histiocytosis (**choice F**) may manifest with three different syndromes. The systemic form (*Letterer-Siwe disease*) is the least frequent but most severe and affects infants and young children. It manifests with innumerable papules that may be mistaken for eczema. The child, however, appears acutely ill, with fever and severe systemic symptoms. The other forms affect older children or adults and manifest with localized formation of granuloma-like collections of Langerhans cells in skin, bone, and other organs.

Lupus erythematosus (**choice G**), both in its systemic form and skin-limited (*discoid*) variants, results in a classic erythematous rash that involves predominantly the face in a "butterfly-like" pattern. The lesions are exacerbated by exposure to sunlight.

Psoriasis (**choice I**) may be confused with seborrheic dermatitis since its characteristic silvery scaly lesions develop in the scalp as well. Indeed, there seems to be a "continuum" of clinical expressions encompassing seborrheic dermatitis, common dandruff, and psoriasis.

Scabies (**choice J**) is a disease due to *Sarcoptes scabiei* that manifests with a papulovesicular rash in a linear distribution. The preferred sites are inguinal, axillary, and finger webs. Linear burrows can be seen on close examination. The mite can be identified by applying a drop of mineral oil on suspected lesions, obtaining scrapings from these areas, and examining the scrapings under a magnifying lens or a ten-power objective.

Tinea corporis (**choice L**) is due to dermatophytes, fungal organisms that colonize the most superficial layers of the epidermis. The most characteristic appearance of skin lesions associated with tinea corporis is a *ring-like* pattern, due to central clearing as the infection spreads in a radial fashion. KOH-treated skin scrapings examined under a microscope allow identification of spores or hyphae.

A number of vitamin deficiencies (**choice M**) may cause skin alterations. Among these are deficiencies of vitamins A, B, C, and K.

49. **The correct answer is E.** Uncomplicated cases of systemic hypertension are associated with few or no laboratory abnormalities. Some laboratory tests are recommended depending on the clinical history. If there is no clinical evidence of secondary hypertension, the following tests are generally considered satisfactory: fasting glucose to exclude diabetes; serum electrolytes to exclude hyperaldosteronism; creatinine and urinalysis to detect signs of renal impairment; plasma lipids (**choice E**) to identify additional risk factors for atherosclerosis; and ECG to identify signs of left ventricular hypertrophy (LVH). ECG is not very sensitive in detecting LVH, however, and some authors recommend performing M-mode echocardiography on all patients with newly diagnosed hypertension. However, the management would not be affected by the finding of mild degrees of LVH on echocardiography.

50. **The correct answer is G.** In this case, the patient presents with hypertension associated with signs and symptoms highly suggestive of hyperthyroidism. Thus, more focused laboratory testing is warranted to confirm the underlying condition. Measurement of thyroid hormone and TSH (**choice G**) will allow a diagnosis of hyperthyroidism. ECG is necessary to check for the presence and type of arrhythmia. Hyperthyroidism often causes not only sinus tachycardia, but also atrial fibrillation. Note that the patient has systolic hypertension, but the diastolic pressure is low.

Chest x-ray films (**choice A**) are usually useless in diagnostic work-up of hypertension.

The dexamethasone suppression test (**choice B**) is specific for hypercortisolism (Cushing disease).

A growth hormone (GH) glucose suppression test (**choice C**) is performed after an overnight fast to confirm/rule out acromegaly. Oral administration of 100 g glucose normally suppresses plasma levels of GH. This response is not observed in the presence of abnormal GH production.

Measurement of urinary catecholamines (**choice D**) is a highly specific test for pheochromocytoma, which manifests with attacks of headache, anxiety, palpitations, and other "sympathetic" symptoms. Hypertension may be paroxysmal or sustained. Thyroid function tests are usually normal, but hyperglycemia and glycosuria are often detected.

Plasma renin level (**choice F**) is an additional test to perform if there are clinical or laboratory signs of hyperaldosteronism. This condition (usually due to an isolated adrenal adenoma) is associated with hypokalemia and low plasma renin activity.

Two-dimensional echocardiogram (**choice H**) is too expensive for the initial diagnostic work-up of hypertension. It is definitely more sensitive than ECG for early detection of LVH, but no more so than M-mode echocardiography.

Internal Medicine: **Test Six**

1. A 50-year-old man with progressive renal failure over four years presents with recent onset of numbness of his feet and hands. He is on a dietary regimen of water and salt restriction. Examination shows decreased sensation to pinprick and vibration stimuli below the knee and in the hands, and absence of ankle reflexes. Blood studies show:

Hematocrit	35%
Sodium	140 mEq/L
Potassium	5.0 mEq/L
Urea nitrogen	98 mg/dL
Creatinine	8.5 mg/dL
Bicarbonate	20 mEq/L

Which of the following is the most appropriate next step in management?

(A) Treatment with vitamin B_{12}
(B) Administration of bicarbonate supplements
(C) Arterial blood gas analysis
(D) Treatment with recombinant erythropoietin
(E) Preparation for nonurgent dialysis
(F) Sural nerve biopsy

2. A 56-year-old woman is brought to the emergency department by her husband because she attempted suicide two hours ago by ingesting some unknown medication. Her husband says that she is taking medications for depression, anxiety, and hypertension, but he cannot name the drugs. He also says that his wife has "drinking problems." The patient appears mildly confused. Her temperature is 38.3° C (101° F), blood pressure is 120/85 mm Hg, pulse is 130/min, and respirations are 22/min. ECG reveals prolonged QRS complexes. On examination, dilated pupils, flushed skin, and muscle twitching are noted. Hepatic transaminases are normal, and blood gas analysis shows a normal pH. Which of the following is the most likely cause of this patient's symptoms?

(A) Alcohol
(B) Benzodiazepines
(C) Clonidine
(D) Monoamine oxidase (MAO) inhibitors
(E) Specific serotonin reuptake inhibitors (SSRIs)
(F) Tricyclic antidepressants

3. An otherwise healthy 28-year-old man comes to the physician because of recent onset of chest pain. He started an active exercise program of weight lifting one week prior to the onset of symptoms. The pain began 24 hours ago and has been constant in intensity. It is sharp, localized to the precordial region, and exacerbated by movement. His temperature is 37° C (98.6° F), blood pressure is 124/78 mm Hg, pulse is 70/min, and respirations are 12/min. There is tenderness on palpation of the chest wall muscles in the precordial region. Which of the following is the most appropriate next step in management?

(A) Mental health screening tests

(B) Oral anti-inflammatory treatment and prevention of future muscle overuse

(C) Administration of an oral "GI cocktail" containing xylocaine and antacid

(D) Performance of a Bernstein test

(E) ECG at rest and during exercise

(F) Chest x-ray examination

(G) Upper gastrointestinal endoscopy

4. A 50-year-old man is evaluated in the emergency department following an automobile accident. An x-ray film of his leg fails to reveal an accident-related fracture, but does show a variety of abnormal features of the femur and tibia, including microfractures, increased bone density, cortical thickening, bowing, and overgrowth. Follow-up studies show marked cortical thickening of the bones of the head. Laboratory findings include normal serum calcium, normal serum phosphate, and elevated serum alkaline phosphatase with increased urinary excretion of pyridinoline cross links. Which of the following is the most likely diagnosis?

(A) Bone metastasis from prostate cancer

(B) Fibrous dysplasia

(C) Hyperparathyroidism

(D) Multiple myeloma

(E) Paget disease

5. A 45-year-old man, who recently immigrated from Sudan, presents with painful and frequent urination for several months. He reports recurrent episodes of blood in the urine in the past year. Microhematuria is found on a urinary dipstick test. Blood tests reveal mild anemia. Which of the following would be most likely to yield the correct diagnosis?

(A) Examination of urine for eggs

(B) Ultrasound examination of the urinary tract

(C) Plain x-ray film of the lower abdomen

(D) Intravenous pyelography (IVP)

(E) Cystoscopy

6. A 33-year-old man has AIDS and a CD4 cell count of 180/mL. He has a history of *Pneumocystis carinii* pneumonia and Kaposi sarcoma of the small bowel. He is currently on combination therapy consisting of two nucleoside analogs (zidovudine and didanosine) and a protease inhibitor (saquinavir). He also receives prophylactic treatment with trimethoprim-sulfamethoxazole and an antimycobacterial medication. At present, his condition is stable. Which of the following vaccinations may be safely administered to this patient?

(A) Bacillus of Calmette-Guerin (BCG)

(B) Influenza

(C) Measles

(D) Mumps

(E) Oral polio vaccine

(F) Rubella

(G) Yellow fever

7. A 78-year-old man is admitted to the hospital because of the acute onset of dysuria, frequent, profound malaise, and shaking chills. His temperature is 39.8° C (104° F), blood pressure is 105/62 mm Hg, pulse is 120/min, and respirations are 28/min. Examination reveals pronounced tenderness in the right costovertebral angle. Urinalysis shows:

Red blood cells	10/hpf
White blood cells	100/hpf
Protein	2+
Casts	None

    A urine sample is sent for cultures. Pending urine culture results, which of the following is the most appropriate next step in management?

    (A) Single-dose administration of cephalexin

    (B) Single-dose administration of trimethoprim-sulfamethoxazole

    (C) Infusion of Ringer's lactate solution

    (D) Treatment with intramuscular ceftriaxone plus oral doxycycline

    (E) Treatment with IV ampicillin and gentamicin

8. A 25-year-old woman presents with increasing weakness. She reports that she has had a history of menorrhagia and easy bruising. She has no other prior medical history. She has no family history of bleeding disorders and denies a history of substance abuse. On physical examination she is tachycardic and pale, with multiple bruises on her body. Laboratory studies show a low iron level and decreased mean corpuscular volume. Coagulation studies are notable for a normal prothrombin time (PT), a prolonged partial thromboplastin time (PTT), a normal platelet count, and a prolonged bleeding time. Which of the following is the most likely diagnosis?

    (A) Aspirin ingestion

    (B) Factor VII deficiency

    (C) Factor IX deficiency

    (D) Hemophilia A

    (E) Von Willebrand disease (vWD)

9. A healthy 26-year-old man is brought to the emergency department after a motor vehicle accident in which he sustained an open fracture of his left tibia and fibula. Physical examination fails to disclose any signs of trauma to the head, neck, or abdomen. The next morning, the patient develops acute dyspnea, confusion, and a diffuse rash. His temperature is 37.7° C (99.9° F), blood pressure is 105/65 mm Hg, and pulse is 100/min. There is no jugular venous distension. Scattered rales are heard bilaterally in multiple lung fields. He has a rapid and regular S2 and S3. A repeat chest x-ray film reveals diffuse pulmonary edema. Arterial blood gas determination (on room air) shows a pH of 7.52, a P_{CO_2} of 29 mm Hg, and a P_{O_2} of 70 mm Hg. Which of the following is the most likely diagnosis?

    (A) Aspiration pneumonia

    (B) Asthma

    (C) Cardiac contusion

    (D) Congestive heart failure

    (E) Fat embolism

10. A 22-year-old woman with type 1 diabetes presents to the emergency department with anorexia, nausea, vomiting, and abdominal pain. She is recovering from pneumonia and has had much difficulty regulating her blood sugars lately. On arrival to the emergency department, her blood glucose is 760 mg/dL, sodium is 125 mEq/L, potassium is 3.0 mEq/L, bicarbonate is 12 mEq/L, chloride is 92 mEq/L, and her blood is positive for ketones by acetone screening. Which of the following is the most appropriate initial step in management?

    (A) Broad coverage antibiotic therapy

    (B) IV glucose and insulin

    (C) IV hypertonic saline

    (D) IV potassium

    (E) IV saline

11. A 50-year-old man presents to his physician after an absence of 5 years. The physician notices that the man's facial features have changed, with protrusion of the mandible and malocclusion of the teeth. On questioning, the patient reports that he has had to buy larger shoes and have his wedding ring enlarged because of trouble taking it off. Physical examination demonstrates fairly coarse body hair, prominent sweating, and irregularity of the surface of the nose and forehead related to enlarged sebaceous glands. The voice is deep and husky. This patient most likely has a tumor involving which of the following?

   (A) Adrenal gland

   (B) Parathyroid gland

   (C) Pituitary gland

   (D) Testes

   (E) Thyroid gland

12. A 36-year-old woman presents with a 16-year history of severe rheumatoid arthritis. She has had progressive difficulty walking for the past three months and is now virtually bedridden. Involved joints include proximal small joints of the hands, wrists, shoulders, knees, and ankles, with erosions and moderate deformities. Current medications include naproxen, methotrexate, and prednisone. Clinical examination shows mildly swollen and tender joints in the noted areas. Neurologic examination is notable for increased tone in both lower limbs, bilateral pathologically brisk reflexes in the upper and lower limbs, ankle clonus, positive Babinski sign, and minimal patchy sensory loss in the hands and feet. Grip strength is about 70% of normal. Which of the following is the most likely diagnosis?

   (A) Atlantoaxial dislocation

   (B) Cervical spondylotic myelopathy

   (C) Osteoporotic spinal fractures and cord compression

   (D) Peripheral neuropathy

   (E) Spinal epidural lipomatosis

13. A 70-year-old man with amyotrophic lateral sclerosis living in a nursing home is transported to the emergency department because of cough productive of foul-smelling sputum and breathing difficulties for one week. His temperature is 38.5° C (101.3° F), blood pressure is 140/84 mm Hg, pulse is 90/min, and respirations are 18/min. Inspection of his oral cavity reveals poor dental hygiene. A chest x-ray film shows a cavity with an air-fluid level within the left lower lobe in association with a mild pleural effusion. Which of the following is the most likely pathogen?

   (A) *Escherichia coli*

   (B) *Klebsiella pneumoniae*

   (C) *Legionella pneumophila*

   (D) Mixed anaerobic bacteria

   (E) *Pseudomonas aeruginosa*

   (F) *Staphylococcus aureus*

   (G) *Streptococcus pneumoniae*

14. A 71-year-old woman is admitted to the hospital for dehydration. She has a history of coronary artery disease, rheumatoid arthritis, hyperthyroidism, hypertension, and renal artery stenosis, but has been well over the past few months. She was brought to the hospital by her daughter, who found her weak and nauseated. The patient reports that, with the onset of summer, she had been feeling quite fatigued and has had significantly decreased oral intake and progressive nausea. Current medications include digoxin, atenolol, aspirin, acetaminophen, prednisone, fluoxetine, levothyroxine, and nifedipine. Admission laboratory tests show:

Sodium	132 mEq/L
Potassium	3.4 mEq/L
Bicarbonate	30 mEq/L
Chloride	98 mEq/L
Urea nitrogen	52 mg/dL
Creatinine	1.9 mg/dL
Leukocytes	5,300/μm^3
Hematocrit	48%

Her last set of laboratory data, obtained seven months ago, revealed completely normal values. On the basis of these admission laboratory values, which of her medications requires dosing adjustment?

(A) Acetaminophen

(B) Atenolol

(C) Digoxin

(D) Fluoxetine

(E) Levothyroxine

15. A 75-year-old man comes to the physician because of bleeding gums and increasing malaise for several months. He lives alone in poor economic conditions. Examination reveals numerous petechiae, which are mostly perifollicular on closer examination, on his legs. Several ecchymoses are also noted on the arms and legs, and splinter hemorrhages are seen in the nail beds. His hair is brittle. Laboratory studies show:

Hematocrit	30%
Mean corpuscular volume	90 mm^3
Mean corpuscular hemoglobin	30 pg/cell
Prothrombin time (PT)	12 sec
Partial thromboplastin time (PTT)	80 sec

Which of the following is most likely deficient in this patient's diet?

(A) Iron

(B) Vitamin A

(C) Vitamin B_1 (thiamin)

(D) Vitamin B_6 (pyridoxine)

(E) Vitamin B_{12} or folate

(F) Vitamin C (ascorbic acid)

(G) Vitamin K

16. A 52-year-old woman with type 1 diabetes mellitus presents with increasingly severe right otalgia and foul purulent discharge from the ear canal. Examination reveals granulations in the right ear canal associated with extreme edema and erythema of the canal skin. The tympanic membrane cannot be visualized. Paresis of the right abducens nerve is also appreciated. A CT scan of the head demonstrates bone erosion around the ear canal, extending into the middle fossa. Which of the following is the most likely pathogen?

(A) *Haemophilus influenzae*

(B) Mixed anaerobic flora

(C) *Pseudomonas aeruginosa*

(D) *Staphylococcus aureus*

(E) *Streptococcus pneumoniae*

(F) *Moraxella catarrhalis*

17. A 48-year-old man with a long history of smoking presents to the emergency department with a chief complaint of difficulty breathing for the past two days. His temperature is 38.3° C (101° F), blood pressure is 120/70 mm Hg, and pulse is 103/min. Dullness to percussion and decreased breath sounds are noted over the right lower lung field. An upright chest x-ray film reveals a significant right-sided pleural effusion. Decubitus films show layering of the effusion. A diagnostic thoracentesis is performed. The following results are obtained:

Pleural fluid:

pH	7.18
Glucose	40 mg/dL
Protein	3.8 g/dL
LDH	220 IU/L

Serum:

Protein	7.0 g/dL
LDH	320 IU/L

Which of the following is the most likely etiology of the effusion?

(A) An exudate of infectious etiology

(B) An exudate of malignant etiology

(C) A transudate of infectious etiology

(D) A transudate of noninfectious etiology

18. A 55-year-old man comes to medical attention because of progressive tightness of the skin over his hands and face. He also reports difficulties swallowing solid foods. Laboratory studies show elevated titers of antinuclear and anti-DNA-topoisomerase antibodies. Which of the following autoantibodies would be consistent with the CREST variant of this condition?

(A) Anticentromere

(B) Anti-DNA topoisomerase 1

(C) Anti-double stranded DNA

(D) Antiphospholipid

(E) Anti-ribonucleoprotein (anti-U1-RNP)

(F) Anti-Smith antigen

19. A 45-year-old woman presents to the emergency department complaining of acute abdominal pain. She has a history of a peptic ulcer for several years that has been treated with an H2 blocker. She denies diarrhea, nausea, or vomiting, and states that she does not use alcohol or nonsteroidal anti-inflammatory medications. The pain is constant and nonradiating. On examination, she is tachycardic, but does not have a fever. Abdominal examination is remarkable for rigidity and rebound tenderness. Rectal examination produces dark stool that is guaiac positive. Which of the following is the most appropriate next step in management?

(A) Abdominal CT scan

(B) Upright chest x-ray film

(C) Upper endoscopy

(D) Laparoscopic exploration

(E) Exploratory laparotomy

20. A 56-year-old man presents with a ten-month history of increasing dyspnea on exertion and occasional dry cough. He has been smoking half a pack of cigarettes daily for 40 years and has a history of rheumatoid arthritis. Chest examination reveals mild hyperresonance in all lung fields and diminished breath sounds. Lung volume measurements show increased total lung capacity (TLC) and residual volume (RV), with an elevated RV:TLC ratio. Which of the following is the most likely diagnosis?

(A) Asthma

(B) Bronchiectasis

(C) Chronic bronchitis

(D) Emphysema

(E) Interstitial lung disease

21. A 62-year-old man presents with complaints of severe pain in his left wrist, which he says is episodic and has increased in frequency over the past year. He says that he cannot move the wrist when this happens. His father had similar problems before he died of kidney problems due to diabetes. The patient is also diabetic and is taking insulin. His physical examination is normal except for the limitation of motion of the left wrist. A CBC is normal, and serum chemistry findings are as follows:

Sodium   139 mEq/L

Potassium   3.9 mEq/L

Chloride   98 mEq/L

Calcium   9.2 mEq/L

Uric acid   4 mg/dL

Aspiration of the joint fluid shows rhomboidal positively birefringent crystals under polarized light. Which of the following is the most likely diagnosis in this patient?

(A) Degenerative joint disease

(B) Gout

(C) Pseudogout

(D) Rheumatoid arthritis

(E) Septic arthritis

22. A 40-year old man complains of symptoms of an upper respiratory infection. He has a sore throat and reports cervical adenopathy. He has previously been healthy and has not taken any medications. Family history is negative. On physical examination, he has a low-grade fever and a blood pressure of 105/70 mm Hg. He has left anterior cervical adenopathy, measuring 2.5 × 3 cm, that is nontender and immobile. No other adenopathy is palpable. The patient is sent home with instructions to take fluids and advised that symptoms should resolve within a week. He is reevaluated over six months for recurrent respiratory tract infections. Although the lymph node has regressed, it has not disappeared. The patient reports that it has waxed and waned in response to antibiotics. The patient undergoes a lymph node biopsy. Which of the following is the most likely diagnosis?

(A) Burkitt lymphoma

(B) Diffuse large cell lymphoma

(C) Follicular mixed lymphoma

(D) Follicular small cleaved cell lymphoma

(E) Immunoblastic lymphoma

23. A 35-year-old man presents with a 5-year history of low back pain. The pain is severe enough to interfere with daily activities and is associated with prominent stiffness of the lower back. The pain lasts for two to three hours following awakening and persists (though in a less severe form) for most of the day. He has mild pain and swelling in both knees and was recently treated with local glucocorticoid injections for pain and tenderness in both heels. Two years ago, he had a self-limited episode of pain in the right eye associated with photophobia and visual blurring, which resolved spontaneously over four weeks. Physical examination is notable for bilateral tenderness over the sacroiliac joints, reduction in spinal flexion movements, and mild bilateral knee effusions. Cardiac auscultation is notable for a barely audible murmur, suggesting aortic regurgitation. The erythrocyte sedimentation rate (ESR) is 46 mm/hr, and a complete blood count (CBC) and biochemistry are normal. Which of the following is the most likely diagnosis?

(A) Ankylosing spondylitis

(B) Lumbar canal stenosis

(C) Lumbar degenerative arthritis

(D) Pseudogout

(E) Rheumatoid arthritis

24. A 35-year-old man comes to the emergency department because of the acute onset of colicky pain in his right upper abdominal quadrant and jaundice. He had been working as an engineer in a Middle East country for two years and returned to the U.S. two months ago. On admission, his temperature is 37.2° C (99° F). The liver is slightly tender and palpable 2 cm below the costal arch. A CT scan of the abdomen reveals a 15-cm cyst in the right hepatic lobe, compressing the common bile duct. The cyst contains smaller cysts, and its wall is focally calcified. Which of the following is the most likely diagnosis?

(A) Amebic abscess

(B) Bacterial abscess

(C) Carcinoma

(D) Echinococcosis

(E) Hemangioma

25. A 55-year-old Caucasian man consults a physician because of weight loss. He has also had chronic epigastric pain, nausea, and diarrhea. On physical examination, the weight loss is evident and 3+ ankle edema is noted. A complete blood count is unremarkable. Clinical chemistry studies are notable only for a serum albumin of 1.5 g/dL. Endoscopy demonstrates marked thickening of gastric folds in the body of the stomach. Gastric biopsy demonstrates a markedly thickened mucosa, with atrophy of glands accompanied by marked foveal hyperplasia with mucous gland metaplasia in many areas. Which of the following is the most likely diagnosis?

    (A) Deep gastritis

    (B) Gastric lymphoma

    (C) Linitis plastica

    (D) Ménétrier disease

    (E) Pernicious anemia

26. A 56-year-old woman undergoes neurologic evaluation for recent onset of seizures and a gradually worsening tingling sensation in her right arm. Examination reveals mild loss of strength in the right upper extremity. CT scan and MRI show a 5-cm dural-based mass in the left frontoparietal region. The mass is well demarcated and compresses the underlying parenchyma. T_1-weighted MRI scans after gadolinium enhancement show marked contrast enhancement within the lesion associated with a characteristic "dural tail." There is prominent thickening of the overlying calvarial bone. Which of the following is the most likely diagnosis?

    (A) Glioblastoma multiforme (GBM)

    (B) Langerhans cell histiocytosis

    (C) Meningioma

    (D) Metastasis

    (E) Paget disease

    (F) Schwannoma

    (G) Tuberculoma

27. A 36-year-old woman who has worked as a hospital nurse for the past ten years comes to the physician because of fatigue, weight loss, cough with blood-tinged sputum, and night sweats for four months. She has had evening temperatures up to 38.5° C (101.3° F). Prior to this, she had been in good health. Chest examination is remarkable for bilateral rhonchi and coarse crackles in the upper lung fields. A chest x-ray film reveals bilateral pulmonary infiltrates and cavitary lesions in the upper lobes. Her records show that she became positive to the tuberculin skin test in her first year of work as a nurse but was not treated. Which of the following interventions at that time would most likely have prevented her current condition?

    (A) Annual chest x-ray examination

    (B) BCG vaccination

    (C) Close observation only

    (D) Isoniazid for six months

    (E) Rifampin for six months

28. A 33-year-old man is brought to the local health clinic with an acute attack of what he calls "podagra." He says that his father, who died at age 65 in a car accident, had the same disease. On examination, his right great toe is swollen, red, and extremely tender to touch. His temperature is 38.7° C (101.7° F). The patient is otherwise healthy and does not take any medications. Laboratory studies show leukocytosis and a serum uric acid level of 9.8 mg/dL. Which of the following is the most appropriate treatment at this time?

    (A) Allopurinol and nonsteroidal anti-inflammatory drugs (NSAIDs)

    (B) Aspirin

    (C) Colchicine

    (D) Intra-articular administration of corticosteroids

    (E) NSAIDs alone

    (F) Parenteral administration of corticosteroids

29. A 25-year-old man develops malaise with high fevers and rigors, followed several hours later by abdominal pain, vomiting, jaundice, and itching. His girlfriend brings him to the emergency department. Physical examination is remarkable for right upper-quadrant tenderness and slight icterus. A urine sample is dark, and a fecal sample is pale. Liver function tests show marked elevations of serum bilirubin and alkaline phosphatase, as well as modest elevations of the transaminases. Blood cultures later show *Escherichia coli*. The patient undergoes emergency endoscopic sphincterotomy, which fails to improve drainage of the biliary tract. An endoscopic cholangiogram demonstrates many bulbous dilations of the intrahepatic bile ducts with a relatively normal appearing extrahepatic biliary tree. Which of the following is the most likely diagnosis?

    (A) Caroli disease
    (B) Crigler-Najjar syndrome
    (C) Dubin-Johnson syndrome
    (D) Gilbert syndrome
    (E) Rotor syndrome

30. A 74-year-old woman suddenly became delirious one hour ago. She was well until five days ago, when she tripped and injured her right leg; she has been bedridden since the accident. On examination, her temperature is 37.2° C (99° F), blood pressure is 110/70 mm Hg, pulse is 110/min, and respirations are 32/min. Her heart, lungs, and abdomen are normal, and there are no focal motor or sensory deficits. Passive flexion of her right hip causes obvious pain. Pulse oximetry shows an oxygen saturation of 80%, and a chest x-ray is normal. An ECG shows sinus tachycardia. Which of the following is the most likely diagnosis?

    (A) Acute cerebral hemorrhage
    (B) Acute cerebral infarction
    (C) Myocardial infarction
    (D) Pulmonary infarction
    (E) Pulmonary thromboembolism

31. A 35-year-old man comes to the physician because of recurrent bouts of high fever with shaking chills for one week. He was on a safari trip in sub-Saharan Africa one month ago. Each attack begins with shaking chills lasting a few hours, followed by fever up to 41.0° C (106° F), which resolves with profuse sweating. These attacks have occurred every other day. The patient feels slightly tired between episodes of fever but otherwise is well. Examination reveals mild splenomegaly. The liver is not palpable. A blood smear at this time is negative for parasites. Which of the following is the most appropriate next step in diagnosis?

    (A) Blood cultures
    (B) Repeat blood smear every eight hours for three days
    (C) Repeat blood smear during an attack
    (D) Repeat blood smear once more
    (E) Start treatment with chloroquine

32. A 42-year-old alcoholic presents to the emergency department complaining of 12 hours of epigastric pain radiating to the back. One and a half hours ago he began to experience nausea and vomiting. His temperature is 38.4° C (101.2° F), pulse is 100/min, blood pressure is 110/70 mm Hg, and respirations are 18/min. Abdominal examination reveals mid-epigastric tenderness without guarding, rebound tenderness, or distension. Laboratory tests show a serum amylase of 1,050 U/L, AST of 300 U/L, and a white blood cell count of 18,000/mm^3. A plain film of the abdomen shows several small bowel air-fluid levels. Which of the following is the most likely diagnosis?

    (A) Acute cholecystitis
    (B) Acute gastritis
    (C) Acute pancreatitis
    (D) Intestinal obstruction
    (E) Perforated peptic ulcer

33. A 50-year-old woman with a history of breast cancer treated with mastectomy develops multiple metastases. As her disease progresses, she also develops anemia accompanied by a decreased white blood cell count and platelet count. The possibility of a myelophthisic anemia is considered. Which of the following features on peripheral blood smear would most strongly support this diagnosis?

    (A) Hypochromic macrocytes

    (B) Nucleated red cells

    (C) Ringed sideroblasts

    (D) Schistocytes

    (E) Sickled cells

34. A 45-year-old woman comes to the emergency department because of the sudden onset of abdominal pain that radiates from the right hypochondrium to the shoulder. The pain is steady, with periodic exacerbations. The patient is afebrile. Ultrasound examination reveals a stone in the cystic duct. Which of the following is the most appropriate next step in management?

    (A) Cheno- or ursodeoxycholic acid treatment

    (B) Lithotripsy with bile salt treatment

    (C) Endoscopic sphincterotomy with stone extraction

    (D) Laparoscopic cholecystectomy

    (E) Open cholecystectomy

35. A 45-year-old white man presents to his physician because of difficulty with defecation and fresh blood on his stool. He has no other complaints. Vital signs and most of the physical examination are unremarkable. Rectal examination demonstrates a 4-cm papillary mass at the anal verge. No mass lesions in the liver or lungs are visible on CT. Wide local excision of the tumor demonstrates well-differentiated nonkeratinizing squamous carcinoma arising in condyloma acuminatum. This lesion is most closely associated with which of the following viruses?

    (A) Herpes simple I

    (B) Herpes simplex II

    (C) HIV

    (D) Human papilloma virus (HPV)

    (E) Molluscum contagiosum

36. A 24-year-old man with no significant past medical history is brought to the emergency department (ED) by his friends after two days of unusual behavior. His friends report that the patient has made unwanted advances toward several women at work and that he seemed unconcerned when confronted by his boss. They also note that he had forgotten to attend two engagements in the past two days. The ED visit was prompted by a prolonged spell during which the patient seemed "in a daze," picking at his clothes for several minutes while a friend was trying to talk to him. In the ED, he is awake and alert but slightly disoriented. There is no meningismus. He has poor short-term memory, but the neurologic examination is otherwise nonfocal. Vital signs are remarkable for a temperature of 38.1° C (100.5° F). A CT scan of the brain with and without contrast is read as normal. A lumbar puncture is performed with the following results:

Opening pressure	18 cm
Glucose	80 mg/dL
Protein	75 mg/dL
WBCs	25/mm^3 with a lymphocytic predominance
RBCs	8/mm^3

Which of the following is the most likely diagnosis?

    (A) Bacterial meningitis

    (B) Brain abscess

    (C) Creutzfeldt-Jakob disease

    (D) Hemorrhagic infarct

    (E) Viral encephalitis

37. A 55-year-old Caucasian man presents to a physician with complaints of fatigue and weakness. On physical examination, the man is pale, but no other abnormalities are noted. A complete blood count demonstrates a severe microcytic anemia. Stool is positive for occult blood. Esophagogastroduodenoscopy is negative. Colonoscopy demonstrates a large fungating mass of the cecum. CT scans of the chest and abdomen do not reveal metastatic disease. Prior to surgery, measurement of serum levels of which of the following substances would provide a baseline to assess the possibility of recurrent cancer later in life?

    (A) Alpha fetoprotein (AFP)

    (B) Carcinoembryonic antigen (CEA)

    (C) Human chorionic gonadotropin (hCG)

    (D) Prostate-specific antigen (PSA)

    (E) Thyroid-stimulating hormone (TSH)

38. A 20-year-old male college student comes to the physician because of dry cough, fever, headache, and muscle pains for two weeks. He reports that other residents of his fraternity house have recently developed similar symptoms. He denies the use of illicit drugs. His temperature is 38.2° C (100.8° F), pulse is 90/min, and respirations are 18/min. On chest examination, no rhonchi or bronchial breathing is appreciated. A chest x-ray film shows multifocal interstitial opacities throughout the lung parenchyma. Blood studies show mild leukocytosis and a positive cold agglutinin test. Which of the following is the most likely pathogen?

    (A) Influenza virus

    (B) Mixed anaerobic bacteria

    (C) *Mycoplasma pneumoniae*

    (D) *Pneumocystis carinii*

    (E) *Streptococcus pneumoniae*

39. A 53-year-old man with chronic alcoholism presents to a community clinic with complaints of fatigue and weakness. Screening blood chemistry studies demonstrate hypocalcemia and hypokalemia. Depletion of the body stores of which of the following minerals is also likely in this patient?

    (A) Iodine

    (B) Iron

    (C) Magnesium

    (D) Selenium

    (E) Zinc

40. A 50-year-old man presents with arthralgias, hepatomegaly, and increased skin pigmentation for three months. Examination reveals a bronze color of the skin. The liver is palpable 3 cm below the right costal arch, but there is no splenomegaly. Moderately advanced testicular atrophy is appreciated. An S_3 sound is heard on cardiac auscultation. Laboratory studies show:

AST	80 U/L
ALT	70 U/L
Alkaline phosphatase	120 U/L
Bilirubin, total	1.5 mg/dL
Ferritin	400 ng/dL
Transferrin saturation	60%
Glucose, fasting	180 mg/dL

Serologic tests for hepatitis virus antibodies are negative.

Which of the following investigations would be the most appropriate next step in diagnosis?

    (A) CT or MRI studies of the liver

    (B) Measurement of serum alpha 1-antitrypsin

    (C) Measurement of urinary copper excretion

    (D) Serum titers of antinuclear and antimitochondrial antibodies

    (E) Determination of hepatic iron content in a liver biopsy

41. A 23-year-old nun has a six-month history of amenorrhea and galactorrhea. She is very concerned that others may believe that she is pregnant, and she vehemently denies such a possibility. Physical examination confirms that milk can indeed be expressed from both breasts, but it is otherwise unremarkable. The pelvic examination is also unremarkable, showing no uterine enlargement or ovarian masses. Visual fields are normal. A pregnancy test is negative. Once the diagnosis is confirmed, which of the following is the most appropriate management?

    (A) Bilateral mastectomy

    (B) Bromocriptine

    (C) Streptozocin

    (D) Systemic chemotherapy

    (E) Tamoxifen

42. A 65-year-old man is brought to the emergency department 30 minutes after the acute onset of headache, nausea, and sudden loss of balance. The patient is unable to stand or walk, but there is no loss of muscular strength or sensory deficits. Consciousness is preserved, and the patient is oriented to person, space, and time. He says that he had hypertension for a long time but has not taken any antihypertensive therapy. His blood pressure is now 166/98 mm Hg, and his pulse is 65/min. A CT scan of the head reveals an acute intracranial hematoma. Which of the following is the most likely location of the hematoma?

    (A) Cerebellum
    (B) Cerebral white matter
    (C) Epidural space
    (D) Pons
    (E) Putamen
    (F) Thalamus

43. A previously healthy 37-year-old woman is brought to the emergency department complaining of lethargy and fever. Her husband reports she has been increasingly somnolent. The patient is complaining of discomfort in her left thigh. She denies obvious trauma, although reports removing a splinter from her left calf two days ago while bringing firewood into the house. Her temperature is 40.0° C (104° F), blood pressure is 85/50 mm Hg, and pulse is 130/min. On examination, she has exquisite tenderness to palpation. There is mild edema and erythema over her left thigh. Laboratory studies show an elevated creatinine kinase, liver function tests, and white count. Bedside debridement reveals that soft tissue has started to necrose. One blood culture bottle turns positive five hours after being drawn. The cultures are positive for group A streptococci. The patient is given a diagnosis of necrotizing fasciitis. Which of the following is the appropriate management at this time?

    (A) Administration of clindamycin
    (B) Administration of erythromycin
    (C) Administration of penicillin G
    (D) Emergent surgery
    (E) Initiation of vasopressor agents

44. A 45-year-old woman comes to the clinic for a new-patient visit. A physician last evaluated her six years ago. She denies chest pain, shortness of breath, or palpitations. She is not taking any medications and denies any prior medical problems. On physical examination, she is noted to have a lesion on her left earlobe. She first noticed the lesion six months ago, and mentions that it has doubled in size. It is painless. She works as a gardener and is exposed to the sun. She denies wearing a hat. The lesion is fixed, with an ulcerated center with glistening, heaped-up edges. Which of the following is the most likely diagnosis?

    (A) Basal cell carcinoma
    (B) Erythema nodosum
    (C) Leukoplakia
    (D) Melanoma
    (E) Squamous cell carcinoma

45. A 44-year-old man presents complaining of lethargy, morning weakness and somnolence, and an inability to concentrate at work. He notes that these symptoms have become progressively worse over the last three years. This started about six months after a devastating breakup with his fiancée, when he decided to begin binge eating. He denies any other medical problems. He no longer complains of depression and is involved in a positive relationship. He denies substance use. Vital signs are within normal limits. He is 65 inches tall and weighs 308 pounds, which represents a 118-lb weight gain over the last three years. The rest of the physical examination is unremarkable. Which of the following is the most appropriate next diagnostic step?

    (A) Empiric trial of weight loss and exercise
    (B) Laboratory tests for hypothyroidism
    (C) Mask continuous positive airway pressure (CPAP)
    (D) MRI of the head and neck for soft tissues
    (E) Overnight oxygen saturation/apnea monitoring

The response options for items 46-47 are the same. You will be required to select one answer for each item in the set.

(A) Aminoglycoside toxicity

(B) Analgesic toxicity

(C) Cardiogenic shock

(D) Goodpasture syndrome

(E) Henoch-Schönlein purpura

(F) Hyperuricemia

(G) Hypovolemic shock

(H) Malignant hypertension

(I) Multiple myeloma

(J) Myoglobinuria

(K) Postinfectious glomerulonephritis

(L) Prostatic hyperplasia

(M) Radiographic contrast toxicity

(N) Sickle cell disease

(O) Unilateral ureteral stone

For each patient with oliguria/anuria, select the most likely underlying cause.

46. A 30-year-old man is admitted to the hospital because of extensive burn injuries involving 45% of the total body surface. Twenty-four hours following admission, he develops oliguria. Laboratory studies show elevated BUN and serum creatinine, with a BUN:creatinine ratio of 30. Urine osmolality is 800 mOsmol/kg H_2O, and fractional excretion of sodium is 0.5%.

47. A 70-year-old man is admitted to the hospital because of the acute onset of anuria, nausea, vomiting, and malaise. Recent medical history is remarkable for intravenous pyelography (IVP) performed two weeks ago and treatment with tricyclic antidepressants started one week ago. Insertion of a Foley catheter yields 700 mL of concentrated urine. Laboratory studies show high urine osmolality and low urine sodium.

The response options for items 48-50 are the same. You will be required to select one answer for each item in the set.

(A) Acute cholecystitis

(B) Acute pericarditis

(C) Acute pleuritis

(D) Angina pectoris

(E) Aortic dissection

(F) Aortic regurgitation

(G) Aortic stenosis

(H) Costochondritis

(I) Esophageal carcinoma

(J) Esophageal spasm

(K) Herpes zoster

(L) Mitral valve prolapse

(M) Myocardial infarction

(N) Myocarditis

(O) Pneumonia

(P) Prinzmetal angina

(Q) Psychological chest pain

(R) Pulmonary thromboembolism

(S) Reflux esophagitis

(T) Secondary pneumothorax

(U) Spontaneous pneumothorax

(V) Thoracic outlet syndrome

For each patient with chest pain, select the most likely diagnosis.

48. A 52-year-old man presents with episodic precordial pain and dyspnea on exertion. His blood pressure is 110/85 mm Hg, pulse is 85/min, and respirations are 16/min. Examination reveals a harsh systolic murmur along the left sternal border radiating to the neck. ECG changes are consistent with left ventricular hypertrophy.

49. A previously healthy 25-year-old man comes to the physician because of left chest pain that began suddenly two days ago at rest. He drinks alcohol on social occasions and does not smoke. His height is 186 cm (73 in), and his weight is 70 kg (154 lb). His temperature is 36.8° C (98.2° F), blood pressure is 120/80 mm Hg in both arms, pulse is 80/min and regular, and respirations are 22/min. Chest examination reveals decreased tactile fremitus, hyperresonance, and diminished breath sounds in the left hemithorax.

50. A 54-year-old woman comes to the physician because of recurrent substernal pain that manifests after meals and on reclining. She reports transient relief from taking antacids or drinking milk. Examination is otherwise unremarkable, but the patient is extremely anxious, fearing that she may have heart problems like her father, who died at age 84 of a "heart attack."

Internal Medicine Test Six:
Answers and Explanations

ANSWER KEY

1.	E	26.	C
2.	F	27.	D
3.	B	28.	E
4.	E	29.	A
5.	A	30.	E
6.	B	31.	B
7.	E	32.	C
8.	E	33.	D
9.	E	34.	D
10.	E	35.	D
11.	C	36.	E
12.	A	37.	B
13.	D	38.	C
14.	C	39.	C
15.	F	40.	E
16.	C	41.	B
17.	A	42.	A
18.	A	43.	D
19.	B	44.	A
20.	D	45.	E
21.	C	46.	G
22.	D	47.	L
23.	A	48.	G
24.	D	49.	U
25.	D	50.	S

1. **The correct answer is E.** This patient with chronic renal failure is manifesting typical signs and symptoms of uremic peripheral neuropathy. Sensorimotor neuropathy in a "stocking and glove" distribution is the most common form. Usually, peripheral neuropathy develops when the glomerular filtration rate falls below 10% of normal values. This is one of the indications for starting renal replacement therapy (i.e., dialysis). Parenthetically, uremic manifestations that warrant urgent initiation of dialysis treatment include pericarditis, coagulopathy, fluid overload not responsive to diuresis, hyperkalemia resistant to dietary restriction, severe acidosis (pH <7.20), and neurologic complications (e.g., encephalopathy, seizures, and neuropathy).

Peripheral neuropathy of renal failure is not due to vitamin B_{12} deficiency; thus, treatment with vitamin B_{12} (**choice A**) is not helpful in this case. Vitamin B_{12} deficiency may play a role in some cases of anemia associated with chronic renal failure.

Administration of bicarbonate supplements (**choice B**) may help in correcting acid-base disorders, but serum bicarbonate levels of 20 mEq/L are considered satisfactory and do not need any further intervention.

Arterial blood gas analysis (**choice C**) would be appropriate if metabolic acidosis were suspected.

Treatment with recombinant erythropoietin (**choice D**) is used to obviate insufficient production by the kidneys and correct anemia of renal failure. This treatment is started when the hematocrit falls below 30% to 35% in the absence of other causes of anemia (blood loss, vitamin B_{12} deficiency, or iron deficiency). In any case, it would not be beneficial for peripheral neuropathy.

Sural nerve biopsy (**choice F**) is rarely necessary in a clinical setting of chronic renal failure, since the underlying etiology is quite clear.

2. **The correct answer is F.** Tricyclic compounds (e.g., amitriptyline and imipramine) are among the drugs most commonly used by depressed patients in suicide attempts. Their toxic effects are mostly attributable to peripheral anticholinergic activity and "quinidine-like" action (sodium channel block) on the heart. Mild overdose is principally associated with anticholinergic effects, such as mydriasis, tachycardia, impaired sweating with flushed skin, dry mouth, constipation, and muscle twitching. More severe intoxication leads to cardiac arrhythmias, namely ventricular tachyarrhythmias and bradycardia. Prolongation of the QRS complex (> 0.1 sec) is typical and constitutes a more sensitive indicator of toxicity than serum drug levels. Seizures, severe hypotension, and coma are the most severe manifestations. Hyperthermia may result from impaired sweating and/or status epilepticus. Gastric lavage in the first hour following ingestion, supportive care, anticon-

vulsants, and appropriate antiarrhythmic drugs (e.g., sodium bicarbonate bolus, lidocaine, and phenytoin) are the recommended treatments. None of the other choices cause EKG abnormalities.

Severe intoxication with alcohol (**choice A**) manifests with respiratory depression, hypothermia, and coma. Ethanol levels greater than 300 mg/dL produce coma in persons who are not chronic abusers, but regular drinkers can tolerate even higher levels.

Benzodiazepines (**choice B**), like alcohol, depress the activity of the cerebral cortex, cerebellum, and brainstem reticular activating system. Thus, acute benzodiazepine intoxication produces stupor, coma, and respiratory depression.

Clonidine (**choice C**) is an antihypertensive agent with sympatholytic properties. Thus, clonidine overdose results in bradycardia, hypotension, miosis, and respiratory depression. Similar signs are produced by ingestion of topical nasal decongestants.

Monoamine oxidase (MAO) inhibitors (**choice D**) represent a second-line treatment for major depression. Overdose induces ataxia, excitement, hypertension, and tachycardia. These toxic reactions can be triggered by concomitant ingestion of *tyramine*-containing foods and beverages (aged cheese and red wine). *Serotonin syndrome*, characterized by fatal hyperthermia, may develop in patients on MAO inhibitors who take serotoninergic drugs, such as fluoxetine, meperidine, tryptophan, and dextromethorphan.

Specific serotonin reuptake inhibitors (SSRIs) (**choice E**), such as fluoxetine, are the "newer" generation of antidepressant drugs and are devoid of the anticholinergic effects of tricyclic compounds. Overdose with these drugs may, however, cause seizures.

3. **The correct answer is B.** Most cases of chest pain occurring in young patients are of noncardiac origin. In particular, chest pain arising in patients aged 18-45 is usually due to one of three causes: muscular chest pain, costochondritis (Tietze syndrome), or gastroesophageal reflux. Factors supporting a diagnosis of chest pain of muscular origin, in this case, include exacerbation with movement, tenderness on palpation, and onset following strenuous physical exercise. When the clinical picture is clear, no further diagnostic tests are necessary (or cost-effective). The patient should receive symptomatic treatment, which may include administration of anti-inflammatory drugs, rest, and appropriate instructions to avoid future overuse of chest wall muscles.

Mental health screening tests (**choice A**) are indicated when chest pain is suspected to be of psychological origin, usually anxiety-related.

Administration of an oral "GI cocktail" containing xylocaine and antacid (**choice C**) is an appropriate diagnostic measure when chest pain is thought to result from gastroesophageal reflux or spasm. Such cocktails usually contain a mixture of viscous xylocaine and antacids in varying concentrations. Prompt relief of symptoms following ingestion supports a diagnosis of chest pain of esophageal origin.

Performance of a Bernstein test (**choice D**) is based on the administration of diluted HCl (0.1 N solution) into the esophagus. An esophageal origin of chest pain (reflux or spasm) is supported if this maneuver reproduces the patient's symptoms.

An ECG at rest and during exercise (**choice E**) is not necessary in patients with a clear clinical picture of non-cardiac chest pain.

Chest x-ray examination (**choice F**) would be useless in this case. X-ray films are necessary when there are indications of pulmonary pathology, such as pneumonia or pleuritis.

Upper gastrointestinal endoscopy (**choice G**) is the most sensitive test for gastroesophageal reflux or peptic ulcer disease.

4. **The correct answer is E.** This patient has Paget disease of bone, which is characterized by localized areas of hyperactive bone. The etiology is unknown. Most patients are older than 40, with a 3:2 male predominance. Histologic examination of affected bone shows both heavy osteoclastic and heavy osteoblastic activity, resulting in coarsely woven, thick trabeculae that are heavily calcified but structurally weak. The radiologic findings illustrated in the question stem are typical. Some patients, such as this one, are picked up incidentally when x-ray films are performed for other reasons. Other patients may come to medical attention because of symptoms related to peripheral nerves compressed at cranial ostia (including hearing loss and increasingly severe pain) or pathologic fractures, or because an alert physician notices bitemporal skull enlargement (frontal bossing), a hobbling gait, or bowing of the legs or thighs. Drug therapy (etidronate disodium and related compounds, calcitonin) is now available to influence calcium and phosphate metabolism and thus at least partially control the disease process.

Bone metastasis from prostate cancer (**choice A**) usually occur in men older than 60. There are typically fewer bony lesions unless very advanced, and it is usually associated with a highly elevated prostate-specific antigen (PSA).

Fibrous dysplasia, as seen in secondary hyperparathyroidism, (**choice B**) produces cystic bone lesions.

Hyperparathyroidism (**choice C**) may cause bone lesions similar to those of Paget disease, but would be accompanied by hypercalcemia.

Multiple myeloma (**choice D**) causes cystic bone lesions.

5. **The correct answer is A.** These manifestations are highly suggestive of vesical *schistosomiasis*, which is endemic in the Middle East and many parts of Africa. It is due to *Schistosoma haematobium*, the adult form of which lives in the venules of the bladder. The eggs passed in the urine develop into the larval form, which infects snails. Infective larvae are excreted by the snails into water and penetrate through intact skin or mucous membranes into exposed persons. The larvae reach the portal circulation, where they mature, mate, and migrate to terminal venules. *S. haematobium* reaches the vesical plexus, whereas *Schistosoma japonicum* and *Schistosoma mansoni* reach the venules of the bowel, causing vesical and intestinal schistosomiasis, respectively. Cystitis caused by chronic schistosomiasis manifests with recurrent hematuria and predisposes to squamous cell carcinoma of the bladder. Search for ova in the urine is the fundamental diagnostic test.

Ultrasound examination of urinary tract (**choice B**) is the imaging method of choice when there are signs and symptoms of ureteral obstruction and hydronephrosis. Because nephrolithiasis is quite common, even in areas in which schistosomiasis is endemic, ultrasound is often performed first, but definitive diagnosis of schistosomiasis rests on finding the eggs in the urine.

A plain x-ray film of the lower abdomen (**choice C**) may show calcifications of the ureters and/or vesical wall.

Intravenous pyelography (IVP; **choice D**) may be useful in demonstrating blockage of the urinary tract but does not help in establishing a specific etiologic diagnosis.

Cystoscopy (**choice E**) may show alterations of the bladder mucosa, ulcers, and areas of squamous metaplasia in advanced disease.

6. **The correct answer is B.** Influenza vaccination should be administered yearly to persons at increased risk of severe complications. Among such groups are AIDS patients, elderly persons, and patients with chronic pulmonary or cardiac diseases. Although recent studies have shown that HIV viremia may be transiently increased by influenza vaccination, this effect seems to have no clinical significance. Thus, influenza vaccination is currently recommended for AIDS patients. Immunosuppressed patients, however, may have a poor antibody response to vaccinations.

Vaccinations based on live attenuated viruses or microorganisms should not be used in AIDS patients or otherwise immunocompromised individuals since they can bring about serious postvaccinal infections. These vaccinations include BCG (**choice A**), measles (**choice C**), mumps (**choice D**), oral polio vaccine (**choice E**), rubella (**choice F**), and yellow fever (**choice G**).

7. **The correct answer is E.** The clinical picture is consistent with acute pyelonephritis (upper urinary tract infection), a severe condition that should be promptly treated with wide-spectrum antibiotic therapy without waiting for

the culture results to be available. Patients usually need to be admitted to the hospital. Blood and urine are cultured to identify the agent and determine susceptibility to antibiotics. Meanwhile, treatment with IV ampicillin and an aminoglycoside (usually gentamicin) is started. This combination affords a wide-spectrum coverage that is usually effective against the most common pathogens associated with urinary tract infections, in particular *Escherichia* and *Proteus*.

Single-dose administration of cephalexin (**choice A**) or trimethoprim-sulfamethoxazole (**choice B**) is used to treat uncomplicated episodes of cystitis in women. Men with cystitis usually have some underlying condition that needs to be investigated. Cystitis manifests with dysuria, frequency, and suprapubic discomfort, but the patient is generally afebrile.

Infusion of Ringer's lactate solution (**choice C**), as well as any other supportive measure, although necessary, is not adequate treatment for such a severe infection.

Intramuscular ceftriaxone plus oral doxycycline (**choice D**) is used to treat sexually transmitted infections, such as acute epididymitis, in which both gonococcus and *Chlamydia* may be involved.

8. **The correct answer is E.** Von Willebrand disease (vWD) is a genetic defect with variable transmission that results in the deficiency or derangement of the antigenic portion of factor VIII (von Willebrand factor). This antigen is involved in the intrinsic coagulation pathway and facilitates platelet-endothelium interaction. In vWD, there is prolongation of the PTT, which is indicative of a defect in the intrinsic pathway, and of the bleeding time, which is indicative of a defect in the factor VIII antigen and endothelium interaction. This patient is menorrhagic and iron deficient because of the bleeding diathesis.

Aspirin (**choice A**) permanently inhibits platelet adhesion by suppressing platelet prostaglandin synthesis, which results in defective platelet function. It should not cause an increase in prolonged partial thromboplastin time (PTT) since it does not affect the coagulation factors.

Factor VII (**choice B**) is in the extrinsic arm of the coagulation pathway, and deficiency of this factor should increase only the prothrombin time (PT).

Factor IX (**choice C**) causes hemophilia B, which affects males because of sex linkage of the genes. Isolated prolongation of PTT is expected in such a situation.

Similarly, hemophilia A (**choice D**) is due to a deficiency in factor VIII, not in the von Willebrand factor as seen in vWD. Hemophilia A affects males, given the X-linked recessive inheritance, and prolongs the PTT.

9. **The correct answer is E.** Fat emboli occur after the introduction of neutral fat into the venous circulation, occur-

ring most commonly after bone trauma or fracture. The clinical scenario described is classic. After a latent period of 12-36 hours, during which the patient is asymptomatic, cardiopulmonary and neurologic deterioration occurs. Dyspnea, tachypnea, and tachycardia occur with radiographic findings of diffuse bilateral infiltrates, consistent with adult respiratory distress syndrome (ARDS) and a self-limiting petechial rash. Reduction in arterial oxygen content is consistent with widespread lung injury. Treatment is supportive, and mortality is high.

Aspiration pneumonia (**choice A**) develops after the inhalation of virulent microbial flora or foreign bodies. It occurs more frequently in patients with an impaired level of consciousness (e.g., those using alcohol or drugs or those experiencing seizures) or in patients with swallowing or mechanical impediments (e.g., nasogastric tube). Pneumonia is characterized by the sudden onset of fever, purulent sputum, and cough. Aspiration of foreign bodies is usually through the right bronchus, with unilateral changes on chest x-ray. Aspirated organisms may originally produce an infiltrate on chest x-ray, but ultimately tissue necrosis and pulmonary cavitation may occur.

Asthma (**choice B**) is a disease of the airway characterized by increased responsiveness of the tracheobronchial tree to multiple stimuli. It is an episodic disease associated with dyspnea, cough, and wheezing. Acute exacerbation results in hypoxia, along with hypocapnia and respiratory alkalosis. The chest x-ray is usually normal, but may show hyperinflation.

Cardiac contusion (**choice C**) is the most common injury following blunt heart trauma. The major cause of contusion is direct impact force applied to the intact pericardium, usually occurring without fracture of the bony thorax. The contusion results in a discrete or disseminated hemorrhage of the myocardium. Damage may be confined to the myocardium, or be complicated by lacerations of the endo- or epicardial surfaces. Pericardial effusions occur in more than 50% of patients. A fibrinous reaction of the contusion site may cause pain and a friction rub. Pain is usually immediate, retrosternal, or anginal, simulating that of coronary thrombosis. It is responsive to oxygen. The patient may develop tachycardia and arrhythmias, with all types of ECG changes noted.

Congestive heart failure (**choice D**) occurs when the heart cannot provide sufficient output to satisfy the metabolic needs of the body. It is commonly termed "congestive" heart failure because of increased venous pressure (pulmonary congestion with left heart failure and peripheral edema with right heart failure). Failure is usually the result of chronic disease, including atherosclerotic coronary artery or valvular disease, or renal disease resulting in fluid imbalance. It is rare in healthy young adults, but may occur acutely following cardiac trauma. The most common symptom of left heart failure is shortness of breath. Though there are no ECG changes specific for heart failure, typical findings may reflect underlying disease. Chest x-ray films demonstrate cardiomegaly and pulmonary vascular congestion.

10. **The correct answer is E.** The management of diabetic ketoacidosis (DKA) requires a basic understanding of three concepts: the patient has some underlying trigger for the DKA, the patient is very volume depleted, and the patient has severe electrolyte abnormalities. The management therefore focuses on these issues. This patient has an anion gap acidosis (gap >20) and elevated blood glucose. The first step in the care of all DKA patients is prompt restoration of their volume status. This is the priority, as the ongoing diuresis from the elevated glucose will only worsen their acidosis.

Administration of broad coverage antibiotic therapy (**choice A**) would be appropriate if the patient has an underlying infection. However, this intervention has no place in the acute management of DKA.

Administration of IV glucose and insulin (**choice B**) is appropriate once the blood glucose falls below 250 mg/dL. It is important at all times to have insulin on board for diabetic patients. Once the glucose falls below 250 mg/dL during therapy, glucose must be given with the insulin to prevent hypoglycemia and assist with clearance of the ketone bodies.

Hypertonic saline should not be administered (**choice C**), since this patient's corrected sodium is 133 mEq/L (any extra glucose in the sample of blood used to calculate serum electrolytes will decrease the measured serum sodium by 2.6 mEq/L per 100 mg/dL of glucose), which is acceptable.

Administration of IV potassium (**choice D**) will be needed as the patient's acidosis begins to correct and serum potassium begins to decline. In DKA patients, total body potassium becomes depleted as a result of cellular shifts and diuresis.

11. **The correct answer is C.** The features illustrated are typical of acromegaly, which is due to excess growth hormone produced by a pituitary adenoma. Other clinical features that may be seen include thickened, sometimes darkly pigmented skin, a barrel chest, tongue enlargement, and an increase in hat size. Joint symptoms, which may include a crippling degenerative arthritis, are frequent. Other problems include peripheral neuropathies due to nerve compression, headaches, visual changes (related to the pituitary tumor), cardiac disease, hypertension, and increased cancer risk (particularly colorectal). The diagnosis is usually made clinically and then substantiated with plasma IGF-1 levels.

Adrenal tumors (**choice A**) can cause hypo- or hypersecretion of mineralocorticoids, glucocorticoids, and epinephrine/norepinephrine.

Parathyroid tumors (**choice B**) can alter calcium and phosphorus metabolism.

Testicular tumors (**choice D**) can secrete androgens, estrogens, or other steroid hormones.

Thyroid tumors (**choice E**) are almost always nonfunctional; they rarely cause hyperthyroidism or hypothyroidism.

12. **The correct answer is A.** There is clear clinical evidence of corticospinal tract disease. Inflammation and destruction of the atlantoaxial joints is a crucial clinical diagnosis to make in the management of patients with severe rheumatoid arthritis. Local pain may be minimal, and the progression may be so slow that dysfunction and disability are attributed to peripheral arthritis. Episodes of deficit progression may occur and may be precipitated by unusual neck movements. Any kind of manipulation is absolutely contraindicated. Management requires urgent neuroradiologic (MRI) and neurosurgical evaluations.

Though cervical spondylotic myelopathy (**choice B**) is statistically the most common cause of cervical spinal cord compression in an adult, onset is typically after the age of 50. The clinical features may be indistinguishable, but radiologic examination is diagnostic. The atlantoaxial articulation is not a site for degenerative arthritis.

The patient is at risk for severe osteoporosis because of long-term use of prednisone. Osteoporotic spinal fractures (**choice C**) are associated with back pain and loss of vertebral height and predominantly involve the thoracic spine. Cervical level compression cannot occur in this situation.

There is no convincing clinical evidence of peripheral neuropathy (**choice D**). A mild glove-and-stocking sensory neuropathy is relatively common in rheumatoid arthritis; however, this neuropathy is usually benign and does not imply inflammation of the nerves. Patchy distinct sensory loss may also be due to spinal cord compression, carpal/tarsal tunnel syndromes, or mononeuritis multiplex. Reflexes are usually hypoactive or absent, rather than hyperactive.

Epidural fat (**choice E**), especially at the thoracic level, may increase sufficiently during chronic use of glucocorticoids to result in spinal cord compression. It should always be considered if bony compression is not documented and spinal cord symptoms remain unexplained. MRI is the diagnostic modality of choice. It is a rare condition.

13. **The correct answer is D.** Cough productive of foul-smelling sputum should immediately suggest a pulmonary infection involving anaerobic bacteria. This is often associated with poor dental hygiene and/or

conditions favoring aspiration, such as neurologic disorders, depressed level of consciousness, or tracheal/nasogastric tubes. *Prevotella melaninogenica, Fusobacterium nucleatum*, and anaerobic streptococci are among the most common pathogens. In this case, the patient has developed a pulmonary abscess, as the x-ray finding of a "cavity with air-fluid level" strongly suggests.

Escherichia coli (**choice A**) is a common cause of *nosocomial* pneumonia, defined as pneumonia occurring in hospitalized patients more than 48 hours after admission.

Klebsiella pneumoniae (**choice B**) is particularly associated with *community-acquired* pneumonia in patients with alcohol abuse or diabetes mellitus. It may also cause nosocomial (hospital-acquired) pneumonia.

Legionella pneumophila (**choice C**), one of the most common causes of community-acquired pneumonia, preferentially affects immunocompromised patients, heavy smokers, and patients with chronic obstructive pulmonary disease (COPD). Outbreaks of legionellosis result from exposure to contaminated sources, such as air conditioning towers or shower heads.

Pseudomonas aeruginosa (**choice E**) is frequently isolated in cases of nosocomial pneumonia, as well as in pneumonia occurring in cystic fibrosis patients.

Staphylococcus aureus (**choice F**) is one of the pathogens associated with nosocomial pneumonia.

Streptococcus pneumoniae (**choice G**) is the most common cause of community-acquired pneumonia. Pneumococcal pneumonia typically causes lobar consolidation and frequently follows an upper respiratory tract infection.

14. **The correct answer is C.** All medications are cleared either by the liver, the kidney, or the lung. The majority are cleared by one of the first two routes, whereas inhalational anesthetics are largely cleared by the third. Many patients, especially inpatients on current day medical and surgical wards, have impaired renal function, liver function, or both, and very careful consideration to dosing adjustments must be made. In fact, most house-staff manuals have lists of drugs that commonly have altered dosing in renal failure. The importance of altering dosing regimens depends on both the drug in question and its therapeutic index. Some drugs have a very close overlap between therapeutic dosing and toxic dosing. Digoxin is a perfect example of a drug that highlights both of these points and is VERY commonly seen on inpatient drug lists. The difference between a therapeutic and toxic dose for this drug can result from an increase in creatinine of only 0.5 mg/dL or an increased dose of 125 μg per day. Since this patient has impaired renal function, as evidenced by the increased blood urea nitrogen and creatinine, the dose of digoxin should be lowered.

Acetaminophen (**choice A**) is an example of a drug that is cleared almost entirely by the liver and also has a very

narrow therapeutic index. In cases of liver disease, acetaminophen toxicity is very common.

Atenolol (**choice B**) is a long-acting formulation of a beta-1 selective antagonist used for treatment of hypertension and ischemic heart disease. It is largely cleared by the liver.

Fluoxetine (**choice D**) is a selective serotonin uptake inhibitor that is used as an antidepressant medication. It is cleared primarily by the liver.

Levothyroxine (**choice E**) is a thyroid hormone that is cleared primarily by uptake to the liver and normal endocrine pathway utilization.

15. **The correct answer is F.** The clinical picture is consistent with *scurvy* due to vitamin C deficiency. Nowadays, this is an infrequent disorder, but it may be occasionally seen in alcoholic patients or in elderly people who do not eat enough fresh vegetables and fruits. The most important known function of ascorbic acid is to act as an essential cofactor in the hydroxylation of collagen. Deficiency of ascorbic acid leads to defective collagen synthesis, which results in capillary fragility, petechiae, ecchymoses, poor wound healing, and abnormal hair. Small hemorrhages in a perifollicular distribution are highly characteristic of scurvy. Gingival bleeding is also frequent but does not occur in edentulous patients.

Iron deficiency (**choice A**) results in hypochromic microcytic anemia. Dietary deficiency is rare in industrialized countries. Iron deficiency is usually caused by chronic blood loss.

Vitamin A deficiency (**choice B**) causes night blindness and xerophthalmia. This dietary deficit is most frequent in patients with malabsorption who do not receive appropriate vitamin supplementation. It may develop in people who abuse mineral oil laxatives.

Vitamin B_1 (thiamin) deficiency (**choice C**) is frequent in alcoholics and manifests with myopathy and neurologic deficits, including paresthesias, footdrop, wristdrop, and absence of ankle and knee reflexes. In its most severe form, it will cause high-output cardiac failure and Wernicke-Korsakoff syndrome.

Vitamin B_6 (pyridoxine) deficiency (**choice D**) is rare since this factor is present in virtually all foods. Subclinical forms, however, seem to be relatively frequent. Secondary deficiency due to drugs that act as pyridoxine antagonists (e.g., isoniazid, penicillamine, and estrogens) should be kept in mind. Overt pyridoxine deficiency manifests with hypotonia, seborrheic dermatitis, glossitis, cheilosis, peripheral neuropathy, and sometimes seizures.

Deficiency of vitamin B_{12} or folate (**choice E**) leads to similar hematologic consequences, namely megaloblastic anemia. However, neurologic deficits due to degeneration of the posterior and lateral columns of the spinal cord are associated with vitamin B$_{12}$, but not with folate deficiency. Vitamin K deficiency (**choice G**) can result in bleeding diathesis. This, however, is accompanied by an elevated prothrombin time caused by impaired synthesis of clotting factors VII, IX, X, and prothrombin.

16. **The correct answer is C.** Physical examination shows the features of *external otitis*, an infectious disease of the ear canal that is most commonly caused by gram-negative rods or fungi. In diabetic persons, this infection typically follows a particularly aggressive course and leads to osteomyelitis of the cranial base if not promptly treated. Cranial nerve palsies, especially involving the sixth nerve, may develop. CT scan in this case confirms the presence of bone involvement. This severe form, which is also known as *malignant external otitis*, is most often due to *Pseudomonas aeruginosa*. Ciprofloxacin is the treatment of choice for *Pseudomonas* infections.

    Haemophilus influenzae (**choice A**), *Streptococcus pneumoniae* (**choice E**), and *Moraxella catarrhalis* (**choice F**) represent the most common etiologic agents of *acute otitis media*. This is often preceded by an upper respiratory viral infection that blocks the auditory tube, allowing accumulation of fluid and bacterial proliferation within the middle ear. Otalgia is severe, and the tympanic membrane appears opaque and bulging outward. Amoxicillin or erythromycin plus sulfonamide is the treatment of choice.

    Mixed anaerobic flora (**choice B**) and *Staphylococcus aureus* (**choice D**), as well as *Proteus* and *Pseudomonas*, are the bacterial species most frequently involved in *chronic otitis media*. This manifests with chronic purulent discharge, little or no pain, and a perforated tympanic membrane. With time, conductive hearing loss develops unless appropriate medical and surgical therapy are established.

17. **The correct answer is A.** This is an exudative effusion by definition. The pleural fluid LDH to serum LDH ratio is <0.6, and the pleural fluid protein to serum protein ratio is >0.5, so **choices C and D** can be eliminated. Determining whether this is infectious or malignant is tricky. In malignant effusions (**choice B**), very rarely is the pleural fluid glucose level less than 60 mg/dL (15%). The subacute clinical scenario (2 days of symptoms) and the temperature to 38.5° C (101.3° F) generally indicate an infectious etiology. The low pH is seen in both complicated parapneumonic effusions and cancer and does not help in the diagnosis. Further testing, including Gram stain, cultures, and cytology, should be done on this fluid.

18. **The correct answer is A.** Skin changes, arthralgia, Raynaud phenomenon, and dysphagia are among the most common presenting symptoms of *scleroderma* (*progressive systemic sclerosis*, PSS). This immune-mediated fibrosing condition affects the skin, gastrointestinal tract, lungs, kidneys, and myocardium, leading to severe functional damage. The exact pathogenetic mechanism is unclear, but the fibrosing reaction is probably mediated by T-lymphocytes, with production of cytokines that stimulate fibroblastic growth and collagen synthesis. Anticentromere antibodies are specifically associated with the CREST variant of systemic sclerosis. This affects specific body sites and has a more favorable clinical course. *C*alcinosis, *R*aynaud phenomenon, *e*sophageal dysmotility, *s*clerodactyly, and *t*elangiectasia are the defining features.

    Antinuclear antibodies (ANAs) of various types are found in PSS, but the most specific (although not highly sensitive) is *anti-DNA topoisomerase 1*, also known as *SCL-70* (**choice B**). This is present in up to one-third of patients with scleroderma.

    Anti-double stranded DNA (**choice C**) and anti-Smith antigen (**choice F**) are ANAs specifically correlated with *systemic lupus erythematosus* (SLE).

    Antiphospholipid antibodies (**choice D**) may be found in association with other collagen vascular diseases, especially SLE, but may occur as an isolated manifestation (*antiphospholipid antibody syndrome*). It leads to recurrent arterial and venous thrombosis.

    Anti-ribonucleoprotein (anti-U1-RNP) (**choice E**) is an antibody specifically correlated with a form of autoimmune disease encompassing features of SLE, scleroderma, and polymyositis, known as *mixed connective tissue disease*.

19. **The correct answer is B.** This patient most probably is suffering from a perforated ulcer and has free air in the peritoneum. Such patients often present with a rigid abdomen and rebound tenderness. The best way to detect this is to look for free air under the diaphragm, which is best achieved with an upright chest x-ray.

    A CT scan may be useful if the upright film is negative and no diagnosis has been made yet (**choice A**).

    Upper endoscopy may be needed if the diagnosis is not made with initial radiologic studies, but this is an emergency and laparotomy may be considered first (**choice C**).

    Laparoscopic exploration might not be viable if the surgery needs to be done emergently (**choice D**).

    Exploratory laparotomy (**choice E**) may be needed to correct the perforation, but the upright x-ray film should be obtained first to confirm the diagnosis.

20. **The correct answer is D.** Most cases of emphysema are associated with long exposure to cigarette smoking. Emphysema manifests with progressive respiratory difficulty and a characteristic increase in the anteroposterior diameter of the chest (barrel chest). Hyperresonance and diminished breath sounds are present on chest examination, whereas chest x-ray shows hyperinflation and frequent parenchymal bullae (especially subpleural). The most characteristic changes in pulmonary function tests

include increased TLC and RV, with an elevated RV:TLC ratio, which indicates that there is a predominant expansion of RV at the expense of functioning lung parenchyma.

Asthma (**choice A**) is associated with a typical history of paroxysmal episodes of breathing difficulties with wheezing.

Bronchiectasis (**choice B**) refers to abnormal progressive enlargement of a bronchial segment, with resultant accumulation of secretions and recurrent bronchopneumonia. Bronchiectasis typically presents with cough productive of copious amounts of purulent, often foul-smelling sputum.

Chronic bronchitis (**choice C**) is clinically defined as productive cough occurring for at least 3 months in 2 or more consecutive years. This patient did not have a history of productive cough. Asthma, bronchiectasis, and chronic bronchitis are often associated with emphysema in a clinicopathologic picture referred to as *chronic obstructive pulmonary disease* (COPD).

Interstitial lung disease (**choice E**) is due to diffuse diseases of the interstitium, leading to decreased expansion of the lung parenchyma and, consequently, reduced TLC and RV. This picture is known as *restrictive lung disease* and is associated with sarcoidosis, pneumoconioses, idiopathic pulmonary fibrosis, and collagen vascular diseases (including rheumatoid arthritis).

21. **The correct answer is C.** The presence of rhomboidal, positively birefringent crystals in the joint aspirate is diagnostic of pseudogout. This type of crystal arthropathy usually occurs in persons older than 60 years. The crystals consist of calcium pyrophosphate and tend to deposit on the joint cartilage. Pseudogout is associated with a variety of metabolic disorders, such as diabetes, hypothyroidism, hyperparathyroidism, and Wilson disease. Management consists of NSAID administration for acute episodes. Colchicine can be used for prophylaxis.

Degenerative joint disease (**choice A**) tends to cause continuous, rather than episodic, pain, and there are no crystals in the joint fluid.

Gout (**choice B**) typically presents with pain in the first metatarsophalangeal joint or in the knee joint. The uric acid might be increased, and the joint aspirate would show negatively birefringent needle-shaped crystals.

Rheumatoid arthritis (**choice D**) usually presents with pain in small joints and morning stiffness; it is associated with rheumatoid factor.

Septic arthritis (**choice E**) is associated with evidence of microorganisms in the joint aspirate or elsewhere in the body, and there are large numbers of neutrophils in the joint fluid.

22. **The correct answer is D.** Follicular small cleaved cell lymphoma is among the most common indolent non-Hodgkin lymphomas. It accounts for approximately 40% of all cases. Even without treatment, patients have waxing and waning lymphadenopathy. Over time, the disease will progress, necessitating chemotherapy. This is a low-grade malignant lymphoma.

Burkitt lymphoma (**choice A**) has been associated with the Epstein-Barr virus and is usually found in Africa. In the U.S., patients present with intra-abdominal tumors. In Africa, patients present with large extranodal tumors of the jaws and abdominal viscera.

Diffuse large cell lymphoma (**choice B**) is characterized by large malignant lymphocytes and is less common than follicular small cleaved lymphomas. It is among the more aggressive lymphomas.

Follicular mixed lymphomas (**choice C**) account for approximately 30% of patients. Follicular mixed lymphomas consist of large cell and small cleaved cell populations. This subtype is indolent, but is more aggressive than follicular small cleaved cell lymphoma.

Immunoblastic lymphoma (**choice E**) is a high-grade non-Hodgkin lymphoma and is rapidly fatal unless effective treatment is administered promptly.

23. **The correct answer is A.** This patient is exhibiting most of the typical features of ankylosing spondylitis, one of the members of the seronegative spondyloarthropathies. Other members of this group include the inflammatory arthritis and enthesitis (inflammation of the junction of ligaments and bone) associated with inflammatory bowel disease, psoriasis, and Reiter disease. Clinical features include male sex, young adult age group, sacroiliitis, large-joint arthritis, iritis, aortic regurgitation, and pain/tenderness at bone-ligament junctions. Low back pain and stiffness are usually the dominant symptoms. Treatment is symptomatic and usually involves nonsteroidal anti-inflammatory agents.

Lumbar canal stenosis (**choice B**) is characterized by local or lumbosacral radicular pain in an older person that is induced and worsened by standing. Posture is crucial, as keeping the spine flexed relieves pain. For example, bicycling may be well tolerated, whereas walking is not. Ankylosing spondylitis may be a cause of this syndrome, although the most common cause is degenerative arthritis, typically in the setting of a congenitally narrow bony canal.

Trauma and degenerative disease of the lumbar spine (**choice C**) are the most common causes of low back pain. Severe and prolonged stiffness does not occur, nor does sacroiliitis.

Pseudogout (**choice D**) due to deposition of calcium pyrophosphate or hydroxyapatite comes in several clinical forms: acute inflammatory monarthritis, incidental radiologic abnormality, symmetric polyarthritis, and deforming-mutilating arthritis. Axial involvement is exceptional. Sacroiliitis does not occur, nor do the other inflammatory associations.

Rheumatoid arthritis (**choice E**) is a symmetric poly-arthritis of the proximal small joints and large axial joints. Low back pain and sacroiliitis are not features. Appendicular involvement is limited to the midcervical spine or the atlantoaxial joints.

24. **The correct answer is D.** Echinococcosis or *hydatid disease* is caused by *Echinococcus granulosus* and is endemic in Mediterranean countries and throughout the Middle East. The sheep is the intermediate host, whereas the dog is the definitive host. Humans become infected by ingesting the eggs in dog feces. The eggs hatch in the duodenum and reach the liver, where they develop into hydatid cysts, which are found in the liver, but some may also be found in the lungs and rarely in other organs. After approximately 6 months, the primary cyst will produce daughter cysts, and the daughter cysts may generate third-generation cysts. The fluid in the cysts can produce anaphylactic shock if the cyst ruptures into a serosal cavity or the blood stream. Usually, hydatid cysts remain asymptomatic for long periods until they reach the size of a palpable mass in the liver, compress the bile ducts producing cholestatic jaundice, undergo secondary infection, or break into the biliary tree. Radiologically, the characteristic features include a large cyst enclosing smaller cysts and calcifications within the wall, allowing differentiation from abscesses, hemangioma, or cancer.

Amebic abscess (**choice A**) is a complication of *Entamoeba histolytica* infection, which is endemic in tropical and subtropical countries. The patient presents with a 1- to 2-week history of right upper quadrant pain, fever, and marked liver tenderness on palpation. CT scan allows differentiating this condition from *Echinococcus* cysts. The pus is classically described as "anchovy paste."

Bacterial abscess (**choice B**) is most commonly due to ascending cholangitis caused by a stone, stricture, or neoplasm. Insidious onset of right upper quadrant pain and fever are the presenting symptoms. CT and MRI are the diagnostic techniques of choice.

Carcinoma (**choice C**) of the liver is the most common cancer in African and Asian countries in association with hepatitis B. In the U.S., alcoholic and hepatitic cirrhosis are the most common predisposing conditions. CT and MRI studies are able to differentiate cancer from hepatic abscesses or cysts.

Hemangioma (**choice E**) is the most common benign hepatic neoplasm and often represents an incidental finding. MRI is most useful in establishing the diagnosis.

25. **The correct answer is D.** This is Ménétrier disease, an uncommon gastric disorder characterized by markedly

thickened gastric folds. The disorder is idiopathic, with the gross and microscopic features illustrated in the question stem. Ménétrier disease can cause decreased acid secretion (hypochlorhydria) and a protein-losing enteropathy with weight loss and edema secondary to decreased serum albumin that may clinically mimic cancer. Medical treatments are typically ineffective, and some patients require partial or complete gastric resection to control severe hypoalbuminemia.

Deep gastritis (**choice A**) is a common form of nonerosive gastritis, usually related to *Helicobacter pylori* infection.

Gastric lymphoma (**choice B**) can also produce markedly thickened rugae, but the microscopic description would mention large numbers of atypical lymphocytes.

Linitis plastica (**choice C**) is a term used for an aggressive form of adenocarcinoma in which individual abnormal mucous cells (sometimes with "signet-ring" morphology) penetrate the wall of the stomach and trigger a marked fibrotic reaction. It can also cause thickened rugae.

Pernicious anemia (**choice E**) is characterized by marked gastric mucosal atrophy, rather than thickening.

26. **The correct answer is C.** Meningiomas are benign neoplasms of meningothelial origin. They grow from the dura ("dural-based") toward the cerebral parenchyma, pushing without infiltrating the brain. This pushing pattern of growth, resulting in "well-demarcated" borders, is highly characteristic of any benign neoplasm. An additional MRI/CT feature pointing to meningioma is the presence of a "dural tail" following contrast enhancement. Meningioma is the most frequent of benign CNS tumors and is two times as common in women than in men. Surgical excision is usually easy when located in the cerebral convexities. Rarely, meningiomas may have malignant features, invade the brain, and even result in extracranial metastasis. Meningioma frequently expands into the skull, inducing reactive bone condensation, but this is not a sign of malignancy.

Glioblastoma multiforme (GBM) (**choice A**) is the most frequent of primary malignant tumors of the brain. It is an *intraaxial* tumor (i.e., grows within the brain) and thus can be easily ruled out in this case. GBM is at the most malignant end of the spectrum of *astrocytomas*, tumors of astrocytic origin. It has a very poor prognosis.

Langerhans cell histiocytosis (**choice B**), in its most frequent monostotic form, produces a single osteolytic lesion within a bone, commonly in the calvarium.

A metastasis (**choice D**) may involve any brain structure, including dura mater, but most commonly metastatic disease manifests as multiple brain masses located preferentially at the gray-white matter junction.

Paget disease (**choice E**) is a common disease that produces marked thickening and irregularities of bones, especially the calvarium. Pain is a common symptom. It is not associated with an intracranial mass.

Schwannoma (**choice F**), like meningioma, is an extraaxial tumor. The great majority of schwannomas originate from the eighth cranial nerve in the cerebellopontine angle. Note that several synonyms are used to designate this tumor (acoustic neuroma or neurinoma is probably the most common).

Tuberculoma (**choice G**) is a large aggregate of granulomas due to mycobacterial infection. Rarely, a tuberculoma may develop in the dura mater and simulate a meningioma, but this is definitely an unlikely occurrence.

27. **The correct answer is D.** The patient is exhibiting typical symptomatology of active tuberculosis, which preferentially affects the posterior segments of the upper lobes. Isoniazid (300 mg/day) prevents active disease in most individuals who are recent "skin test converters," defined as persons with a prior documented negative tuberculin test within 2 years of a newly positive test. Isoniazid prophylaxis is also recommended for all HIV-positive or immunocompromised patients and for close contacts of patients with active TB.

Annual chest x-ray examination (**choice A**) is not an adequate measure to prevent skin converters from developing active tuberculosis and exposes the patient to significant levels of radiation.

BCG vaccination (**choice B**) refers to immunization with live attenuated strains of mycobacteria. BCG vaccination is currently recommended in some countries for tuberculin-negative persons, including health professionals, who are repeatedly exposed to patients with tuberculosis.

Close observation (**choice C**) would be insufficient to prevent active tuberculosis in a skin test converter. It may be used in the follow-up of close contacts of patients with tuberculosis due to isoniazid-resistant strains.

Rifampin for 6 months (**choice E**) is also indicated for close contacts of patients with isoniazid-resistant tuberculosis.

28. **The correct answer is E.** The patient's self-diagnosis of gout is confirmed by his clinical signs and symptoms, family history, and elevated serum uric acid levels. Treatment of the acute attack of gout relies on NSAIDs. Indomethacin has been traditionally used for this purpose, but any of the NSAIDs are equally effective. The treatment should be continued until the symptoms have completely subsided (usually for 1 week).

It would be a mistake to begin treatment for acute gout and hyperuricemia at the same time with allopurinol and NSAIDs (**choice A**). If treatment for hyperuricemia is necessary, it should be started after all the acute symptoms have resolved. Rapid reduction of serum uric acid levels can precipitate or worsen acute attacks of gout.

Allopurinol acts by inhibiting xanthine oxidase. It is usually administered at an initial dose of 100 mg/day and is increased until the urate level is within normal limits.

Aspirin (**choice B**) is contraindicated in gout because it increases serum urate concentration.

Colchicine (**choice C**) is effective but causes significant gastrointestinal side effects, such as abdominal cramps and diarrhea. It is therefore reserved for patients who should avoid NSAIDs because of allergies, peptic ulcer disease, or impaired renal function.

Intra-articular administration of corticosteroids (**choice D**) may be used to provide prompt relief in acute attacks of monoarticular gout. This treatment is reserved for patients unable to take NSAIDs. The same is true for parenteral administration of corticosteroids (**choice F**), such as IV methylprednisolone, which is otherwise used for polyarticular gout.

29. **The correct answer is A.** This is Caroli disease, complicated by ascending cholangitis. The question stem illustrates a typical presentation of this congenital cystic malformation syndrome of the intrahepatic biliary tree. The disease may also present in early childhood. Associated ascending cholangitis may be difficult to treat; it may also recur and cause hepatic abscesses. Caroli disease strongly predisposes for biliary cirrhosis, and about 10% of these patients develop cholangiocarcinoma (bile duct cancer). About half the patients with Caroli disease also have congenital hepatic fibrosis.

Crigler-Najjar syndrome (**choice B**) is an inherited enzymatic abnormality of the liver that causes serious unconjugated hyperbilirubinemia.

Dubin-Johnson syndrome (**choice C**) is an inherited enzymatic abnormality that causes a dark gray liver and conjugated hyperbilirubinemia.

Gilbert syndrome (**choice D**) is a benign inherited enzymatic disease with asymptomatic unconjugated hyperbilirubinemia.

Rotor syndrome (**choice E**) is similar to Dubin-Johnson syndrome, but without the liver discoloration.

30. **The correct answer is E.** This patient has classic risk factors for pulmonary thromboembolism (PTE): leg injury and bedridden state. Her tachycardia, tachypnea, decreased O_2 saturation on pulse oximetry, and low-grade fever are also consistent with the diagnosis. The chest x-ray is often normal in cases of PTE, as in this patient. Her presenting symptom, delirium, is most likely due to her hypoxic state. Sinus tachycardia is the most sensitive finding on EKG.

Note that PTE is one of the diagnoses the physician is likely to miss if he or she does not actively think about it; this can be fatal to the patient. Shortness of breath is the most common symptom of PTE, and tachypnea is the most frequent sign. In young patients, the common signs and symptoms (cardiac and respiratory) of PTE may mimic anxiety, especially when other corroborating signs are absent. In older patients whose primary complaint is vague chest discomfort, the symptoms might be confused with those of myocardial infarction (MI) (**choice C**), causing the patient to be discharged without further pulmonary work-up after MI is ruled out. At the very least, always suspect PTE when a patient presents with tachycardia and tachypnea and consider ordering a high-resolution CT scan or a ventilation-perfusion (V/Q) scan if suspicions are high.

Acute cerebral hemorrhage and acute cerebral infarction (**choices A and B**) might also produce delirium, but one would expect other accompanying neurologic symptoms and signs as well. In addition, a cerebral insult would be less likely to produce this patient's cardiopulmonary symptoms.

The diagnosis of MI (**choice C**) requires satisfying two of the following criteria: history of prolonged chest discomfort, evidence of ischemia or necrosis on ECG (e.g., ST or T wave changes, Q waves), or elevated cardiac enzymes.

Pulmonary infarction (**choice D**) usually signifies the presence of a small PTE and typically causes severe pleuritic pain.

31. **The correct answer is B.** The recent travel history to a *malaria*-endemic region, and especially the sequential occurrence of typical febrile attacks every other day, should alert the physician to the possibility of *Plasmodium* infection. This parasite should be looked for in peripheral blood smears. Thick blood films are used for detection, whereas thin blood films are used for identification of the *Plasmodium* species. The number of parasites varies considerably during the course of the disease, and *Plasmodium falciparum* (the most dangerous) is particularly difficult to detect. Thus, to establish the diagnosis, blood smears should be examined every 8 hours during and between febrile attacks for at least 3 days.

Blood cultures (**choice A**) are not useful in this case since *Plasmodium* parasites cannot be cultured. An ELISA test for *P. falciparum* has recently become available.

Repeating blood smears during an attack (**choice C**) or just once (**choice D**) may not be sufficient to demonstrate *Plasmodium* parasites in red blood cells.

Starting treatment with chloroquine (**choice E**) before establishing diagnosis is not appropriate, although chloroquine is the agent of choice for prophylaxis and therapy of malaria. However, chloroquine-resistant strains of *P. falciparum* are present throughout the world, including Africa. Patients with *falciparum* malaria should be hospitalized. In addition, before starting treatment for acute malaria, it is essential to establish whether the

patient has received any other antimalarial medication in the previous days to avoid the risk of overdose.

32. **The correct answer is C.** Acute pancreatitis is most often associated with gallstones and excessive alcohol ingestion. Patients usually present with epigastric pain that radiates to the back, nausea, and vomiting. Examination is significant for fever and tachycardia. Abdominal examination is variable. The diagnosis is established by demonstrating an increase in serum amylase. Serum lipase is also elevated. Leukocytosis and elevated liver enzymes are usually present.

Acute cholecystitis (**choice A**) usually begins with colicky pain that progresses and becomes generalized in the right upper quadrant. The classic triad of right upper quadrant pain, fever, and leukocytosis suggests the diagnosis. The patient usually presents with anorexia, nausea, and vomiting. Abdominal examination is significant for right upper quadrant rebound and guarding, as well as distention resulting from a paralytic ileus. Leukocytosis and liver enzyme abnormalities are usually present. The amylase level is normal.

Acute gastritis (**choice B**) is usually associated with illness or drugs. The presentation is variable, but patients generally complain of upper abdominal or epigastric pain, nausea, and vomiting. Physical examination is usually normal. Laboratory abnormalities are rare. Guaiac-positive stools may be present if hemorrhage occurs.

Intestinal obstruction (**choice D**) usually presents with colicky pain, abdominal distention, and bilious vomiting. Abdominal x-ray films demonstrate distended loops of bowel, air fluid levels, and a paucity of air in the distal colon.

Perforated peptic ulcer (**choice E**) presents with severe epigastric pain. Laboratory abnormalities are rare. The diagnosis is easily made by the presence of free intraperitoneal air on abdominal x-ray films.

33. **The correct answer is D.** Schistocytes are small, fragmented, red cells that are formed when red cells squeeze through spaces too small for them and are fragmented. This can happen in myelophthisic anemia, which occurs when tumor, fibrosis, or granulomatous disease obliterates large areas of the marrow cavity. Myelophthisic anemia can be very difficult to treat unless the underlying disease process is controlled, since the marrow simply does not have the necessary volume to produce enough blood cells. Some of these patients will have erythropoiesis in extra-marrow sites such as the spleen or liver. Patients with severe disease are often transfusion dependent.

Hypochromic macrocytes (**choice A**) are seen in folate deficiency anemia, vitamin B_{12} deficiency anemia, and the thalassemias.

Nucleated red cells (**choice B**) are immature forms that are seen as a nonspecific finding in many forms of anemia.

Ringed sideroblasts (**choice C**) are a feature of sideroblastic anemia, which is a problem with erythrocyte maturation and utilization of iron.

Sickled cells (**choice E**) are a feature of sickle cell anemia, and may superficially resemble schistocytes, but are of normal size.

34. **The correct answer is D.** This patient manifests the classic symptomatology of biliary colic, characterized by pain in the right hypochondrium, which often radiates to the right shoulder. Patients are most often anicteric and afebrile. Virtually all of these cases are due to a gallstone obstructing the cystic duct. If the stone is in the common bile duct, obstructive jaundice becomes a prominent sign. Laparoscopic cholecystectomy is the intervention of choice since the patients can be discharged within 48 hours after surgery, and the procedure is associated with minimal trauma to the abdominal wall.

Cheno- or ursodeoxycholic acid treatment (**choice A**) may help dissolve small cholesterol stones and represents an alternative therapy for asymptomatic patients or patients who decline surgery. This treatment is effective only when the gallbladder is functioning.

Endoscopic sphincterotomy with stone extraction (**choice C**) may be used for choledocholithiasis, especially in those patients who have already undergone cholecystectomy. Lithotripsy with bile salt treatment (**choice B**) is also an alternative under similar circumstances.

Open cholecystectomy (**choice E**) is not the preferred treatment since it is associated with more severe abdominal trauma and longer convalescence compared with the laparoscopic method. However, if any complication should arise during a laparoscopic procedure, the surgeon may easily switch to a more conventional open cholecystectomy.

35. **The correct answer is D.** Approximately 3% to 5% of the distal large bowel cancers are epidermoid carcinoma, with either a nonkeratinizing squamous cell or a basaloid histologic pattern. They can arise in condyloma acuminata (genital warts), which are virally induced proliferations of warts due to infection by HPV. HPV can be transmitted with sexual contact. The more superficial of the epidermoid carcinomas can often be treated with wide excision alone. A combination of chemotherapy and radiation therapy is often successful for somewhat deeper lesions.

Herpes simplex I (**choice A**) and II (**choice B**) do not cause cancer.

HIV (**choice C**), when it produces clinical AIDS, may predispose to growth of condyloma, but is not itself directly carcinogenic, so HPV is a better answer.

The lesions of molluscum contagiosum (**choice E**) are volcano-like skin lesions that do not predispose for cancer. The disorder is caused by a poxvirus.

36. **The correct answer is E.** Herpes simplex virus can produce a fulminant encephalitis that has a tendency to begin in the inferior frontal and medial temporal lobes. This location often leads to behavioral abnormalities as the presenting symptoms, followed by seizures that may be complex partial, as in this case, or generalized tonic-clonic. Imaging may be initially normal, but MRI subsequently demonstrates inflammation in the medial temporal and inferior frontal lobes. The CSF profile shows a lymphocytic pleocytosis with some evidence of a hemorrhagic component. EEG may show periodic focal spikes on a background of slow or low-amplitude ("flattened") activity.

Bacterial meningitis (**choice A**) typically causes meningismus and should show a neutrophil-predominant CSF profile with a decreased glucose.

Brain abscess (**choice B**) typically presents with high fever, headaches, focal neurologic complaints, and seizures. A head CT with contrast should demonstrate a ring-enhancing lesion with edema and mass effect.

Creutzfeldt-Jakob disease (**choice C**), a degenerative dementia caused by infective prion proteins, can present with behavioral symptoms but follows a more subacute course. The CSF is usually unremarkable.

Infarcts may rarely present with behavioral symptoms and no focal features, but a 2-day-old hemorrhagic infarct (**choice D**) would be apparent on a CT.

37. **The correct answer is B.** The patient has colon cancer. It is important before many cancer surgeries to measure serum levels of appropriate tumor markers, since elevation of these markers before surgery indicates that they can then be used for monitoring disease recurrence. In the case of colon cancer, appropriate markers include CEA, CA 19-9, and CA 125. CEA is actually a nonspecific marker for many solid tumors, but is particularly useful in colon cancer, where it is commonly elevated.

AFP (**choice A**) is a marker for liver, ovary, and testicular cancer.

hCG (**choice C**) is produced by many tumors but is not as good as CEA for colon cancer.

PSA (**choice D**) is a marker for prostate cancer, although it is increased in benign prostatic hyperplasia as well.

TSH (**choice E**) is produced by some choriocarcinomas.

38. **The correct answer is C.** This is the typical clinical presentation of *primary atypical pneumonia*, which is most frequently caused by *Mycoplasma pneumoniae*, and less frequently by viruses (influenza, respiratory syncytial virus, adenovirus, rhinoviruses, rubeola, and varicella virus), *Chlamydia*, or *Coxiella burnetii*. What differentiates

primary atypical pneumonia from other forms of acute pneumonia is the predominantly interstitial, rather than intra-alveolar, inflammation and scarcity of "localizing" symptoms. *M. pneumoniae* infections are often associated with circulating *cold agglutinins*. Small outbreaks within close communities are characteristic of pneumonia due to this microorganism. Erythromycin is the drug of choice.

Influenza virus (**choice A**) causes infection in an epidemic pattern. The symptoms begin rapidly, with sore throat, nasal stuffiness, fever, chills, and muscle aches. Leukopenia is commonly seen. Superimposed bacterial pneumonia is frequent in chronically ill individuals and the elderly. In young people, influenza is usually a self-limiting disease that lasts approximately 1 week.

Mixed anaerobic bacteria (**choice B**) are responsible for cases of pneumonia associated with lung cavitation (abscess) and clinically manifesting with cough productive of foul-smelling sputum. There are usually predisposing conditions, such as poor dental hygiene or situations favoring aspiration.

Pneumocystis carinii (**choice D**) is a fungus that causes pneumonia in severely immunocompromised hosts, especially AIDS patients. The clinical picture is severe. Symptoms begin abruptly, with high fever, chills, malaise, and shortness of breath. Acute respiratory failure ensues if appropriate therapy (trimethoprim-sulfamethoxazole) is not instituted.

Streptococcus pneumoniae (**choice E**) is the most common etiologic agent of community-acquired pneumonia, resulting in consolidation of a single lobe and high fever with rigors, productive cough, and profound malaise.

39. **The correct answer is C.** Magnesium deficiency usually results from inadequate intake coupled with defective renal or gut absorption. Chronic alcoholism is an important clinical cause of magnesium deficiency in the U.S., probably because of both inadequate intake and excessive renal excretion. Alcoholism may also affect calcium and potassium metabolism. Hypomagnesemia may also be seen in malabsorption, kwashiorkor, parathyroid disease (particularly after removal of a parathyroid tumor), and chronic diarrhea. Manifestations include anorexia, nausea, vomiting, lethargy, weakness, seizures, and tetany.

Iodine deficiency (**choice A**) can cause thyroid dysfunction with goiter.

Iron deficiency (**choice B**) can cause microcytic anemia, glossitis, and esophageal webs.

Selenium deficiency (**choice D**) is very rare but can cause cardiomyopathy.

Zinc deficiency (**choice E**) can cause growth retardation, night blindness, and skin and hair changes.

40. **The correct answer is E.** Hepatomegaly, arthralgias, and skin hyperpigmentation (which may give the characteristic "bronze" color) are among the most common initial signs of *hemochromatosis*. Testicular atrophy is often present as well. Hemochromatosis leads to iron overload affecting the whole organism, but the liver, heart, pancreas, and endocrine glands bear the most injurious effects of iron deposition. Thus, cardiomyopathy and diabetes frequently manifest because of myocardial and pancreatic damage. A gallop rhythm, with associated S_3 sound, is evidence of cardiomegaly. Note the high ferritin levels and elevated transferrin saturation, indicating systemic iron overload. This disease is due to an autosomal recessive mutation of a gene (named *HFE*) encoding a protein that interacts with beta-2 microglobulin. The ensuing pathogenetic steps are still unclear. When hemochromatosis is suspected, the definitive diagnostic confirmation relies on determination of iron content in liver biopsies. Histologic evaluation of iron deposition is not sufficiently accurate.

CT or MRI studies of the liver (**choice A**) may demonstrate iron overload in the liver, but these radiologic methods are not sensitive.

Measurement of serum alpha-1 antitrypsin (**choice B**) is undertaken when alpha-1 antitrypsin deficiency is suspected. In this case, liver damage and other signs and symptoms indicate iron overload as the most likely underlying etiology.

Measurement of urinary copper excretion (**choice C**) is the initial diagnostic method of choice, together with ceruloplasmin serum levels, in the diagnosis of *Wilson disease*, because of excessive copper accumulation in liver and other organs.

Serum titers of antinuclear and antimitochondrial antibodies (**choice D**) are elevated in 90% to 95% of patients with primary biliary cirrhosis. These patients usually present with generalized pruritus, presumably secondary to retention of bile salts.

41. **The correct answer is B.** This is one of those "higher cognitive level" questions that bypasses the diagnosis and goes directly to management, on the logical assumption that unless you have made a tentative diagnosis, you cannot select the appropriate treatment. Here the clinical diagnosis is prolactinoma, from a pituitary microadenoma (too small to produce visual field defects). The first line of treatment is bromocriptine or cabergoline. Pituitary surgery can be performed if needed.

Bilateral mastectomy (**choice A**) would indeed wipe out milk production, but it would do so in a mutilating, totally unnecessarily radical way. The breasts are normal, all we need to do is stop their stimulation by prolactin.

Streptozocin (**choice C**) is the chemotherapeutic agent of choice when the islands of Langerhans have to be destroyed. Thus, it is indicated for inoperable tumors producing gastrin, insulin, or glucagon.

Choices D and E are offered for those who mistakenly assumed that abnormal milk production is a sign of advanced breast cancer. It is not.

42. **The correct answer is A.** Among hypertensive intracerebral bleeds, cerebellar hematomas merit special consideration. A hematoma within a cerebellar hemisphere manifests with sudden onset of headache and ataxia in an otherwise lucid patient. This highly characteristic presentation warrants immediate medical attention because of the possibility of full recovery if properly treated.

An intracerebral hematoma in the cerebral white matter (**choice B**) is usually accompanied by lateralized motor and/or sensory deficits.

Epidural hemorrhage (**choice C**) is always of traumatic origin and manifests with the characteristic *talk-and-die syndrome*. There is a lucid interval between trauma and coma.

Following hemorrhages in the pons (**choice D**), the patient falls into immediate coma with quadriparesis and usually dies of cardiorespiratory arrest.

The putamen (**choice E**) is the most frequent site of hypertensive bleeding. Putamenal hemorrhage usually involves the adjacent internal capsule, leading to contralateral hemiparesis, hemianesthesia, and hemianopia.

Bleeding into the thalamus (**choice F**) may be suspected when the patient manifests hemianesthesia that precedes hemiparesis.

43. **The correct answer is D.** With the progress of necrotizing fasciitis, the tenderness may evolve to anesthesia, as cutaneous nerves are infarcted. Surgery for debridement and fasciotomy is needed for diagnosis and treatment because the infection is extensive and rapidly progressive. Once the surgery is complete, antibiotics must be continued.

This patient has a shock-like syndrome that is the result of the pyrogenic exotoxin A produced by the bacteria. Clindamycin (**choice A**) arrests the production of the exotoxin. Surgery is of paramount importance, however.

Erythromycin (**choice B**) may be used if the patient had a penicillin allergy.

Penicillin G (**choice C**) is also adjunctive therapy because surgery is of paramount importance.

If the patient becomes progressively hypotensive and risks hemodynamic collapse, vasopressors may be needed (**choice E**). But, fluid resuscitation should be attempted first.

44. **The correct answer is A.** Given this patient's extensive sunlight exposure, she most likely has a basal cell carcinoma. This is the most common form of skin cancer. Risk factors include sun exposure and ultraviolet radiation. Excision may be needed to avoid metastasis.

Erythema nodosum (**choice B**) is a vascular disorder. Skin manifestations include erythematous and nodular lesions, typically on the anterior aspect of the tibia.

Leukoplakia (**choice C**) is caused by the Epstein-Barr virus. It is found on the lateral aspects of the tongue and is white in appearance.

Melanoma (**choice D**) has the maximum metastatic potential and may be nodular or radial. It may have irregular borders, may be of variegated coloration, be >4 mm in size, and be on any aspect of the body.

Squamous cell carcinoma (**choice E**) is the second most common form of skin cancer. They commonly occur on the lower lip.

45. **The correct answer is E.** This patient has the signs and symptoms of obstructive sleep apnea. This condition is characterized by poor nighttime sleeping resulting in daytime somnolence and the psychological consequences of prolonged sleep deprivation. Patients tend to be irritable, have difficulty concentrating on daytime tasks, and have an inappropriate lack of energy given their activity level. Although only 50% of obstructive sleep apnea patients are obese, obese patients tend to have an increased amount of redundant nasal and nasopharyngeal tissue, which makes their upper airway more likely to obstruct in the supine position. Diagnosis of obstructive sleep apnea is initially made by the appropriate history and symptoms and is confirmed by polysomnography, or sleep study, which documents apnea or hypopnea in addition to oxygen desaturations during these obstructive episodes.

Empiric trial of weight loss and exercise (**choice A**) is part of the treatment plan in patients who have obstructive sleep apnea, but it does not confirm the diagnosis. Also, anatomic abnormalities independent of the increase in soft tissues associated with obesity may be the source of the problem, which would not resolve with weight loss or exercise.

Laboratory tests for hypothyroidism (**choice B**) are not indicated at this time, given the lack of other symptoms consistent with a diagnosis of hypothyroidism.

Mask continuous positive airway pressure (CPAP) (**choice C**) should not be administered unless the patient has been evaluated clinically for the presence of obstructive sleep apnea, either with polysomnography or continuous oxygen saturation measurements. In addition, CPAP administration will not be funded without documented evidence of sleep apnea.

An MRI of the head and neck for soft tissues (**choice D**) is not indicated and may not provide any information regarding the pathology of the insomnia. In addition, obstructive sleep apnea is a dynamic process that would need to be viewed radiologically in real time. The presence of redundant soft tissues in the nasopharynx and oropharynx does not necessarily confirm the diagnosis of obstructive sleep apnea.

46. **The correct answer is G.** In this case, oliguria and other signs of acute renal failure may result from either sustained hypotension (secondary to fluid loss) or acute tubular necrosis. The latter may result from hypoxic/ischemic damage to the tubular cells in the setting of shock or sepsis. Thus, prerenal azotemia is due to decreased renal perfusion, whereas renal azotemia is due to intrinsic damage to renal tubules. The treatment differs depending on the underlying cause. The parameters that allow the differential diagnosis between prerenal and renal azotemia are principally the fractional excretion of sodium (FR_{Na}) and the ratio between BUN and serum creatinine. Renal failure due to hypovolemic shock, as in this case, will manifest with prerenal azotemia, associated with FR_{Na} <1% and BUN:Cr ratio >20. Usually, urine is hyperosmolar compared with plasma. Cardiogenic shock (**choice C**) may also give rise to acute renal failure because of prerenal azotemia (hypoperfusion). In this case, however, the most likely mechanism is hypovolemic shock secondary to loss of fluid.

47. **The correct answer is L.** The clinical picture is consistent with acute urinary retention secondary to prostatic hyperplasia, which is an example of *postrenal azotemia*. Acute onset of anuria is usually accompanied by signs of acute renal failure: nausea and vomiting, malaise, and obtunded sensorium. This acute clinical picture is usually preceded by a long history of urinary symptoms due to prostatic hyperplasia, namely progressively increasing hesitancy, decreased force of stream, and postvoid dribbling. Use of drugs with anticholinergic properties, such as tricyclic antidepressants, may precipitate acute urinary retention. The recent history of intravenous pyelography (IVP) should not mislead you. Radiologic contrast media may act as direct nephrotoxins. However, acute renal failure secondary to radiographic contrast toxicity (**choice M**) develops within 24 hours after administration of IV radiocontrast. Further, it is obvious that anuria in this case is due to obstruction, not to intrinsic renal damage.

Aminoglycoside toxicity (**choice A**) is a common cause of acute renal failure due to acute tubular necrosis, in which case FR_{Na} is >1% since damaged tubular cells are unable to reabsorb sodium. In addition, the BUN:Cr ratio is <20, and urine osmolality approaches that of the plasma (250-300 mOsmol/kg).

Analgesic toxicity (**choice B**) is due to chronic ingestion of large amounts of such agents as NSAIDs, aspirin, and acetaminophen. It may result in papillary necrosis and progressive renal interstitial damage. Such damage will eventually lead to chronic interstitial nephritis, manifesting with chronic renal failure. Polyuria due to inability of the kidneys to concentrate urine is a typical early sign.

Goodpasture syndrome (**choice D**) is a chronic inflammatory disorder affecting the lungs and kidneys. It is mediated by antibodies against the collagen of the basement membranes of the lungs and glomeruli. Hemoptysis and nephritic syndrome often progressing to renal failure are its clinical manifestations.

Henoch-Schönlein purpura (**choice E**) is a disease of children. Purpura, hematuria, abdominal pain, melena, and arthralgias constitute its clinical picture, and IgA-mediated vasculitis its pathologic substrate.

Hyperuricemia (**choice F**) may cause acute renal failure, which develops in patients with rapid cell turnover, namely patients with leukemia or lymphoma who are undergoing chemotherapy.

Malignant hypertension (**choice H**) may cause hematuria, proteinuria, and loss of renal function because of arteriolar damage. Blood pressure is very high, usually >220/120 mm Hg.

Multiple myeloma (**choice I**) is a plasma cell neoplasia associated with production of a monoclonal immunoglobulin. Fragments of this immunoglobulin (usually dimers of light chains) are filtered through the glomerulus and may precipitate in the tubules. This will result in proteinuria, hypertension, and progressive renal failure.

Myoglobinuria (**choice J**) may produce acute tubular necrosis in the setting of extensive crush injuries that cause necrosis of skeletal muscle.

Postinfectious glomerulonephritis (**choice K**) usually follows pharyngitis or impetigo due to group A *Streptococcus* and manifests with typical nephritic syndrome. Rarely, this condition may manifest with rapidly progressive glomerulonephritis (i.e., crescentic type), leading to acute rheumatic fever.

Sickle cell disease (**choice N**) is one of the causes of renal papillary necrosis. Other causes include analgesic toxicity, obstructive uropathy with recurrent urinary tract infections, and diabetes.

Unilateral ureteral stone (**choice O**) would manifest with acute onset of colicky flank pain, associated with gross or microscopic hematuria. Acute renal failure does not ensue in this situation, unless the contralateral kidney is already impaired.

48. **The correct answer is G.** These clinical manifestations, especially the characteristics of the systolic murmur, are consistent with aortic stenosis, which is often associated with anginal pain. The patient also shows signs of impeding left ventricular failure, namely exertional dyspnea and left ventricular hypertrophy. Aortic stenosis manifesting in younger individuals (<50 years) is usually due to a

congenitally abnormal aortic valve. In the elderly, calcification of aortic valve cusps is the most common cause.

49. **The correct answer is U.** The clinical history and objective findings are highly characteristic of spontaneous (primary) pneumothorax, which often affects tall, thin men between 20 and 40 years of age. Chest pain and respiratory distress begin suddenly, usually at rest and often during sleep. Patients often seek medical attention days after the onset of symptoms. If the pneumothorax is large, diminished breath sounds, reduced tactile fremitus, and hyperresonance are present. The condition is thought to arise from spontaneous rupture of subpleural bullae in otherwise normal lungs.

50. **The correct answer is S.** Despite the vague familial history of heart problems, the clinical symptomatology is classic for gastroesophageal reflux or reflux esophagitis. The onset of pain in the recumbent position and soon after meals, along with the relief provided by antacids or milk, is virtually diagnostic. Upper endoscopy is the diagnostic procedure of choice to establish a definitive diagnosis and to obtain biopsy specimens of the esophageal mucosa.

Acute cholecystitis (**choice A**) manifests with abdominal pain in the right upper quadrant radiating to the back and right shoulder, fever, and leukocytosis. Occasionally, it may present with precordial pain.

Acute pericarditis (**choice B**) is associated with precordial pain, fever, and evidence of pericardial effusion (e.g., a pericardial rub). If pericardial effusion is abundant, cardiac tamponade may ensue.

Acute pleuritis (**choice C**) is characterized by lateralized chest pain that intensifies with deep breathing. Objective signs of pleural effusion, as well as a pleuritic rub, are usually present.

Angina pectoris (**choice D**), in its most common form, manifests with precordial pain that has a crushing or squeezing quality. The pain is triggered by exercise or emotional stress and relieved by rest or vasodilators.

Aortic dissection (**choice E**) is an emergency manifesting with excruciating chest pain radiating to the back, pulse and pressure discrepancies, onset of aortic regurgitation, and shock. A history of hypertension is often present.

Aortic regurgitation (**choice F**) is associated with a diastolic murmur and a wide differential between systolic and diastolic pressure.

Costochondritis (**choice H**), also known as Tietze syndrome, is due to inflammation of the chondrocostal junctions, which are swollen and sore.

Esophageal carcinoma (**choice I**) may produce chest pain but usually manifests with progressive dysphagia, anorexia, and weight loss. Alcohol and smoking habits are often present in the history.

Esophageal spasm (**choice J**) is a rare cause of chest pain, but it is usually associated with swallowing difficulties. An x-ray after barium may show evidence of spasm.

Herpes zoster (**choice K**) is characterized by a vesicular eruption along a dermatome, which may be followed by chronic burning pain, especially in elderly patients.

Mitral valve prolapse (**choice L**) is due to myxomatous degeneration of mitral valve leaflets. It results in a characteristic midsystolic click followed, in the more severe cases, by a regurgitation murmur.

Myocardial infarction (**choice M**) usually results in extremely severe chest pain radiating to the left shoulder. The pain typically lasts longer than 30 minutes and is not relieved by rest or vasodilators. Many exceptions exist to this classic presentation, such as painless infarction, pain with unusual localization or radiation, or in women or diabetics.

Myocarditis (**choice N**) may be asymptomatic, or it may lead to the acute onset of arrhythmias and acute heart failure or the late onset of slowly progressive congestive heart failure.

Pneumonia (**choice O**) may cause chest pain along with cough, sputum production, and fever. Pulmonary infiltrates are present on chest x-ray.

Prinzmetal angina (**choice P**) characteristically manifests with precordial pain in the early morning and results from coronary vasospasm without atherosclerotic stenosis.

Psychological chest pain (**choice Q**) is commonly associated with underlying depressive, anxiety, or panic disorders. It is a diagnosis of exclusion.

Pulmonary thromboembolism (**choice R**) usually occurs in the setting of predisposing conditions and manifests with chest pain, respiratory distress, tachypnea, and tachycardia. These symptoms, however, may be mild and difficult to interpret. Chest x-ray films and ventilation-perfusion scans are mandatory in any patient with suspicious signs.

Secondary pneumothorax (**choice T**), in contrast to the spontaneous form, develops in lungs with preexisting alterations, most commonly in chronic obstructive pulmonary disease (COPD). COPD leads to formation of subpleural bullae that may rupture. Abrupt onset of pain and worsening of dyspnea develop.

Thoracic outlet syndrome (**choice V**) originates from anatomic or inflammatory alterations of the thoracic outlet (a cervical rib, for example), which may result in compression or irritation of the neurovascular bundle. Pain is triggered by movements of the upper extremity or shoulder and is associated with paresthesias and muscle weakness.

Internal Medicine: **Test Seven**

1. A 55-year-old man with a history of chronic alcohol dependence presents with fever and cough productive of mucopurulent sputum for 2 days. His temperature is 39.0° C (102.0° F), blood pressure is 120/75 mm Hg, pulse is 110/min, and respirations are 26/min. Auscultation of the chest reveals rales and decreased breath sounds in the left lower lung field. Chest x-ray films show a pulmonary infiltrate in the lower left lobe. Which of the following is the most likely pathogen?

   (A) Influenza virus

   (B) *Klebsiella pneumoniae*

   (C) *Legionella pneumophila*

   (D) *Mycoplasma pneumoniae*

   (E) *Pneumocystis carinii*

   (F) *Staphylococcus aureus*

2. A 45-year-old man presents to the emergency department, complaining of the sudden onset of left substernal chest pain. He describes this as a chest pressure that rates 8 on a scale of 1 to 10. He has never had these symptoms before. He has a history of hypercholesterolemia, for which he takes a lipid lowering drug. On physical examination, he appears anxious and is diaphoretic. His blood pressure is 100/90 mm Hg, and his pulse is 110/min. The remainder of the physical examination is unremarkable. He undergoes an ECG, which reveals ST elevation in leads II, III, and aVF. He is diagnosed with an acute myocardial infarction. On cardiac catheterization, which of the following vessels will most likely be occluded?

   (A) Circumflex artery

   (B) Left anterior descending artery

   (C) Left coronary artery

   (D) Posterior descending artery

   (E) Right coronary artery

3. A 37-year-old woman presents to the emergency department with emesis. She states that she has fibromyalgia syndrome and uses a number of "pain killers" to control her pain. On waking this morning, she promptly vomited "coffee grounds." On examination, she is cool but well perfused. Her blood pressure is 120/70 mm Hg, and her pulse is 110/min, with no orthostasis. The remainder of her physical examination is unremarkable. A nasogastric tube is passed, which returns 200 mL of coffee ground material that eventually clears with normal saline lavage. The patient is sent for endoscopy. Which of the following is the most likely diagnosis?

   (A) Esophagitis

   (B) Esophageal varices

   (C) Gastric neoplasm

   (D) Gastric ulcers

   (E) Mallory-Weiss tears

4. Twenty-five guests at an outdoor wedding party are abruptly stricken with severe symptoms, including cramping abdominal pain, nausea, vomiting, and non-bloody diarrhea. Approximately 3 hours earlier, they had eaten refreshments that had been sitting in the sun for several hours, including pastries filled with whipped cream. Within 12 hours, everyone is feeling much better. Which of the following was the most likely cause of the abdominal distress?

   (A) *Campylobacter*

   (B) *Clostridium botulinum*

   (C) *Clostridium perfringens*

   (D) *Escherichia coli* O157:H7

   (E) *Staphylococcus aureus*

5. A 55-year-old man presents with a 2-day history of hemoptysis. He reports an acute onset of eight episodes of coughing bright blood. He has coughed a teaspoon worth of blood on average in each instance. He reports no other symptoms, except for a cough productive of 5-10 mL of sputum each morning. He has a history of chronic obstructive pulmonary disease, for which he takes bronchodilators. He has smoked 30 cigarettes daily for the past 30 years. Physical examination is normal, and an x-ray film is clear. Which of the following is the most likely cause of this man's hemoptysis?

   (A) Alpha-1 antitrypsin deficiency

   (B) Bronchiectasis

   (C) Bronchogenic carcinoma

   (D) Chronic bronchitis

   (E) Pulmonary tuberculosis

6. A 30-year-old man is recovering from abdominal trauma and now develops multiple bruises all over his body. He has completed a 2-week course of antibiotics and has also been receiving nutrition parenterally for 21 days. He is otherwise healthy and has never been on medications prior to this admission. On physical examination, his vital signs are stable. He has multiple ecchymoses on his abdomen. The heart is regular in rate and rhythm. His prothrombin time is elevated. His hematocrit and platelet count are normal. Which of the following is the most likely cause of his easy bruising?

   (A) Calcium deficiency

   (B) Disseminated intravascular coagulation (DIC)

   (C) Magnesium deficiency

   (D) Sepsis

   (E) Vitamin K deficiency

7. A 27-year-old woman comes to her physician because of weakness, weight loss, and amenorrhea for 6 months. Her blood pressure is 100/65 mm Hg. On examination, increased skin pigmentation is seen, especially around the nipples and over the knees, elbows, and knuckles. Laboratory analysis shows:

Sodium	125 mEq/L
Potassium	6.3 mEq/L
Chloride	100 mEq/L
Calcium	10 mEq/L

   Complete blood count shows mild lymphocytosis with eosinophilia. Low plasma levels of cortisol and high levels of ACTH are detected on a blood sample drawn at 8 A.M. Which of the following is the most common cause of this disease in the U.S.?

   (A) Adrenoleukodystrophy

   (B) Autoimmune destruction

   (C) Bilateral adrenal hemorrhage

   (D) Fungal infection

   (E) Metastatic disease

   (F) Tuberculosis

8. A 46-year-old woman complains of dyspnea on exertion and orthopnea that started 7 months ago. She has a prior history of pericarditis, which had been treated with indomethacin. An ECG shows low voltage in the limb leads. A chest radiograph reveals pericardial calcification, and echocardiography shows pericardial thickening. Cardiac catheterization reveals equal pressures in the four cardiac chambers during diastole with all pressures elevated. Which of the following findings on her physical examination would be consistent with a diagnosis of constrictive pericarditis?

   (A) Increased neck vein distention on inspiration

   (B) Exaggerated first and second heart sounds (S1 and S2)

   (C) Extra third heart sound (S3)

   (D) Extra fourth heart sound (S4)

   (E) Predominance of left-sided symptoms over right-sided symptoms

9. A healthy 29-year-old woman comes to the physician for a health maintenance examination. Palpation of the neck reveals a firm, 0.5-cm nodule in the right thyroid lobe. The remainder of the gland is normal. The physical examination is otherwise unremarkable. The patient denies any symptoms attributable to hyperthyroidism. The results of thyroxine and TSH immunoassays are within normal limits. Which of the following is the most appropriate next step in diagnosis?

   (A) MRI scan of the neck

   (B) CT scan of the neck

   (C) Radioactive iodine scan

   (D) Fine needle aspiration

   (E) Excision

10. A 40-year-old IV drug addict complains of right-sided weakness and headache over the past week. He has been previously healthy and is on no prescribed medications. On physical examination, he is afebrile, cachectic, and in mild distress. His neck is supple, and his lungs and skin are clear. Cardiac examination reveals no murmur. He has a mild right hemiparesis. He is tested for HIV and found to be negative. An echocardiogram reveals no valve vegetation. Which of the following is the most likely diagnosis?

    (A) Bacterial endocarditis

    (B) Bacterial meningitis

    (C) Brain abscess

    (D) Cryptococcal meningitis

    (E) Foreign body embolus

11. A 75-year-old woman is brought to the emergency department after being found unconscious by a neighbor. The woman has a history of type 2 diabetes. A stat blood draw demonstrates a plasma glucose of 975 mg/dL. Which of the following additional findings would be most consistent with the patient's probable diagnosis?

    (A) Blood urea nitrogen 5 mg/dL

    (B) Plasma strongly positive for ketones

    (C) Serum creatinine 0.3 mg/dL

    (D) Serum osmolality 380 mOsmol/kg

    (E) Serum sodium 132 mEq/L

12. An elderly woman complains to her physician of chronic constipation. Her physician performs a full physical examination, including a rectal examination to exclude masses. A complete blood count, thyroid-stimulating hormone, fasting glucose, and electrolyte studies are also ordered. Neither the physical examination nor the laboratory tests reveal any abnormalities that might suggest serious disease. Which of the following is the most appropriate next step in management?

    (A) Docusate

    (B) Lactulose

    (C) Magnesium phosphate

    (D) Mineral oil

    (E) Psyllium

13. A 22-year-old woman is seen by a physician because she feels poorly. Physical examination demonstrates waxy pallor of her skin and mucous membranes. She also has multiple purpura on her extremities that she attributes to minor trauma, such as hitting her hand accidentally on a drawer. Blood studies are performed, demonstrating a red cell count of 1.5 million/μL, white count of 1,300/μL (80% lymphocytes), and platelet count of 40,000/μL. Reticulocytes are absent. All blood cells seen have normal morphology. Bone marrow biopsies obtained from the hips bilaterally show predominately fat, with markedly diminished precursors in all blood cell lines. Which of the following is the most likely diagnosis?

    (A) Aplastic anemia

    (B) Iron deficiency anemia

    (C) Folate deficiency anemia

    (D) Myelophthisic anemia

    (E) Vitamin B_{12} deficiency anemia

14. An 8-year-old girl is brought to the physician's office by her parents because of 2 days of progressive left-sided facial weakness. On physical examination, a left facial droop is noted. Vesicular eruptions are seen in the left external auditory canal, as well as on the left side of the pharynx. Which of the following is the most likely diagnosis?

    (A) Bell's palsy

    (B) Guillain-Barré syndrome

    (C) Horner syndrome

    (D) Ménière disease

    (E) Ramsay Hunt syndrome

15. A 25-year-old man consults a dermatologist because of a rash. He states that the rash started with a single lesion on his chest, which grew larger; other lesions then developed. He thinks he might have ringworm. Physical examination demonstrates multiple scaly lesions on his chest and back. The largest of these, which the patient says was his first, is 5 cm in diameter, oval, and rose colored. A slightly raised border (collarette) is seen around the edge of the lesion. Many small plaques, about 1 cm in diameter with a similar appearance, are also seen. Which of the following is the most likely diagnosis?

    (A) Molluscum contagiosum

    (B) Pityriasis rosea

    (C) Pityriasis rubra pilaria

    (D) Rosacea

    (E) Scabies

16. Four hours after repairing a dissected aortic aneurysm, a patient develops paraplegia below the T10 level. He is nonresponsive to pain or temperature but has preserved proprioception. Which of the following arteries is most likely affected?

    (A) Anterior cerebral

    (B) Middle cerebral

    (C) Posterior cerebral

    (D) Thalamostriate

    (E) Ventral spinal

17. A 24-year-old woman comes to the emergency department because of abdominal pain, nausea, and anorexia for 24 hours. She is sexually active but does not take oral contraceptives. Her last menstrual period was 2 weeks ago. Her temperature is 38.0° C (100.4° F). The pain is constant and localized in the right lower abdomen, where palpation elicits guarding and rebound tenderness. Pain in the right lower quadrant of the abdomen is also provoked by palpation of the left lower quadrant. Bowel sounds are absent. Pelvic examination is normal. Laboratory investigations show moderate neutrophilic leukocytosis and beta-hCG within normal limits. Urinalysis shows two erythrocytes per high power field. Which of the following is the most appropriate next step in management?

    (A) Antibiotic therapy

    (B) Barium enema

    (C) Ultrasonography of urinary tract

    (D) Dilatation and curettage

    (E) Appendectomy

18. A 33-year-old woman complains of diplopia in the early evening every day for the past month, which resolves following sleep. She also complains of jaw weakness after eating large meals. She has no significant past medical history. Physical examination is normal, except repeated blinking elicits a ptosis that resolves following the administration of IV edrophonium. Which of the following is the most likely diagnosis?

    (A) Botulism

    (B) Eaton-Lambert syndrome

    (C) Guillain-Barré syndrome

    (D) Multiple sclerosis

    (E) Myasthenia gravis

19. A previously healthy 50-year-old woman presents with progressive muscle pain and weakness for 3 weeks. The symptoms are localized mainly to the proximal muscle groups, affecting the deltoid and the pelvic muscles. On physical examination, there is tenderness on palpation of affected muscles and objective loss of strength. Laboratory investigations reveal a serum creatine kinase level of 2,000 U/L. Electromyography demonstrates myopathic changes. A biopsy of the deltoid muscle reveals atrophy and necrosis of scattered myofibers with endomysial inflammatory infiltration mostly composed of lymphocytes. Which of the following is the most likely diagnosis?

    (A) Denervation atrophy

    (B) Dermatomyositis

    (C) Inclusion body myositis

    (D) Polymyositis

    (E) Systemic lupus erythematosus

20. During a health maintenance examination, an otherwise healthy 50-year-old man has a blood pressure reading of 150/94 mm Hg supine and 145/92 mm Hg standing. Physical examination does not disclose any abnormalities. Which of the following is the most appropriate next step in management?

    (A) Evaluate or refer within 1 week

    (B) Evaluate or refer within 1 month

    (C) Recheck within 2 months

    (D) Recheck in 1 year

    (E) Recheck in 2 years

    (F) Start treatment with diuretics

21. Thirty-six hours after surgical removal of a large parathyroid adenoma, a 50-year-old man becomes irritable and develops a tingling sensation around his mouth and in his hands. Facial spasm can be easily triggered by tapping in front of the ear. Laboratory studies show:

Blood, serum:

Albumin	4.0 g/dL
Bicarbonate	25 mEq/L
Calcium	7.1 mg/dL
Phosphorus	7.5 mg/dL
Magnesium	1.8 mEq/L

Arterial blood (room air):

pH	7.40
PO2	90 mm Hg
P_{CO_2}	42 mm Hg

Which of the following is the most likely cause of this condition?

    (A) Atrophy of the remaining parathyroids

    (B) Hungry bone syndrome

    (C) Hyperventilation syndrome

    (D) Magnesium deficiency

    (E) Metastatic parathyroid carcinoma

22. A 69-year-old man presents with the chief complaint of difficulty remembering things. His family states that he also has episodes of confusion and disorientation. A complete physical examination is unrevealing. His score on a mini-mental status examination is 18 of 30. Laboratory results show an RPR reactive titer of 1:4 and a positive fluorescent treponemal antibody absorption (FTA-ABS) test. A CT scan of the brain is unremarkable. Lumbar puncture reveals 3 red cells and 2 white cells/mm^3 of CSF. A CSF VDRL is negative. The patient had a previous anaphylactic reaction to penicillin. Which of the following is the most appropriate management for this patient?

    (A) Azithromycin

    (B) Ceftriaxone

    (C) Chloramphenicol

    (D) Doxycycline

    (E) No treatment is necessary

23. A 52-year-old man presents with a 6-month history of slowly progressive exertional dyspnea and swelling of his legs. He admits to heavy alcohol abuse for the past 20 years. His blood pressure is 135/84 mm Hg, pulse is 103/min, and respirations are 18/min. Chest examination shows bilateral rales at the lung base and a gallop rhythm with an S_3. The liver margin is palpable 3 cm below the costal margin, and there is mild splenomegaly. Pitting edema is present in the lower extremities. A chest x-ray film reveals dilatation of the veins in the upper pulmonary lobes and cardiac biventricular enlargement. ECG shows low QRS voltage and occasional premature ventricular beats. Blood studies show:

Alanine aminotransferase (ALT)	60 U/L
Aspartate aminotransferase (AST)	76 U/L
Bilirubin, total	1.0 mg/dL
Albumin, serum	4.2 g/dL
Prothrombin time (PT)	14 sec
Ferritin, serum	100 ng/mL

Endocrine studies of pituitary and thyroid functions are within normal limits. Which of the following is the most likely diagnosis?

(A) Alcoholic cirrhosis

(B) Dilated cardiomyopathy

(C) Hemochromatosis

(D) Hypertrophic cardiomyopathy

(E) Restrictive cardiomyopathy

24. A previously healthy 47-year-old woman comes to medical attention because of loss of sensation in her right hand for 2 days. Physical examination is unremarkable other than confirming the presence of right hand hypoesthesia. CT and MRI scans demonstrate a focal lesion in the left parietal cortex. Laboratory investigations show high levels of antiphospholipid antibodies, prolonged activated partial thromboplastin time (aPTT), and normal prothrombin time (PT). Which of the following complications is most likely to develop?

(A) Glomerulonephritis

(B) Lymphoma

(C) Pulmonary fibrosis

(D) Recurrent bleeding

(E) Recurrent thrombosis

25. A 50-year-old woman is admitted for urinary tract infection, complicated by profound weakness, abdominal pain, vomiting, and diarrhea. Her temperature is 40.0° C (104° F), blood pressure is 90/60 mm Hg, pulse is 110/min, and respirations are 18/min. Examination reveals signs of dehydration and skin hyperpigmentation over the elbows and knees. Urinalysis shows pyuria. Laboratory studies show hyponatremia, hyperkalemia, and hypoglycemia. Complete blood count is remarkable for eosinophilia. While waiting for the results of urine and blood cultures, intravenous corticosteroids, broad-spectrum antibiotics, and volume replacement therapy is instituted. In addition to such treatment, which of the following is the most appropriate next step?

(A) Cortisol level

(B) Cosyntropin stimulation test

(C) IV mineralocorticoids

(D) Oral corticosteroids

(E) Renal ultrasonography

26. A 62-year-old man with a long history of cigarette smoking goes to a physician because of a drooping right eyelid. The patient denies headache or weight loss. He complains of an occasionally productive cough but is otherwise in good health. Examination shows right ptosis and a small pupil. Extraocular movements and visual acuity are normal. The right side of his face appears warm and dry. Which of the following is the most appropriate step in diagnosis?

(A) Chest x-ray examination

(B) Laboratory testing for syphilis

(C) MRI scan of the head

(D) Ophthalmologic referral

(E) Tonometric measurement

27. A 60-year-old white man is evaluated by a physician because of weight gain and increasing abdominal girth of several months' duration, despite no change in diet. His temperature is 37.1° C (98.8° F), blood pressure is 70/40 mm Hg, pulse is 120/min, and respirations are 18/min. Head and neck examination is remarkable for "bags" under the eyes and jugular venous distension. Chest examination demonstrates pulmonary rales and a third heart sound. Abdominal examination reveals an enlarged, tense abdomen with a palpable fluid wave; abdominal organ palpation is inadequate because of the tension. Examination of the extremities demonstrates pitting edema at the ankles. Which of the following is the most likely diagnosis?

    (A) Alcoholic cirrhosis

    (B) Chronic hepatitis B infection

    (C) Congestive heart failure

    (D) Gastric carcinoma

    (E) Hypothyroidism

28. A 65-year-old man comes to the physician because of progressive severe shortness of breath, weight loss, and left chest pain. Chest examination reveals dullness to percussion and diminished breath sounds over the left hemithorax. A chest x-ray film shows irregular nodular thickening of the visceral pleura, with partial obliteration of the pleural sac and modest pleural effusion. The underlying lung parenchyma is minimally involved. Cytologic examination of the pleural effusion is positive for malignant cells. Which of the following is the most likely predisposing factor for this patient's condition?

    (A) Cigarette smoking

    (B) Occupational asbestos exposure

    (C) Occupational coal exposure

    (D) Occupational silica exposure

    (E) Prior radiation therapy

29. A 60-year-old woman consults a physician because of recurrent nose bleeds. Physical examination of the nose demonstrates no obvious mucosal abnormalities or masses, but the mild trauma of the examination causes a nosebleed that persists for 10 minutes. A complete blood count is performed, showing a platelet count of 600,000/μL. Which of the following additional findings would most strongly support essential thrombocythemia as the cause of this woman's elevated platelet count?

    (A) Giant platelets

    (B) Increased bone marrow fibrosis

    (C) Increased RBC mass

    (D) Positive Philadelphia chromosome

    (E) Tear drop-shaped RBCs

30. A 50-year-old alcoholic woman is brought to the emergency department 24 hours following a suicide attempt by ingestion of 5 g acetaminophen and 80 mg diazepam. A patient's neighbor relates that she had been drinking heavily for the past week. The patient is drowsy and difficult to arouse. Her temperature is 36.5° C (98° F). Physical examination reveals mild jaundice, fetor hepaticus, and gingival bleeding. Laboratory studies show:

AST	2,500 U/L
ALT	3,000 U/L
Bilirubin, total	2.5 mg/dL
Prothrombin time	23 sec

    Which of the following is (are) the most important factor(s) leading to this patient's hepatic disease?

    (A) Acetaminophen alone

    (B) Alcohol alone

    (C) Alcohol and acetaminophen

    (D) Diazepam alone

    (E) Diazepam and alcohol

31. An otherwise healthy 20-year-old man is referred for genetic counseling because of a family history of multiple endocrine neoplasia (MEN) type IIa. He elects to undergo genetic testing. He is found to have a mutation of the *RET* proto-oncogene. Which of the following is the most appropriate next step in management to prevent morbidity and mortality?

    (A) Periodic calcitonin level measurements

    (B) Periodic screening with imaging studies

    (C) Periodic screening for latent pheochromocytoma

    (D) Prophylactic parathyroidectomy

    (E) Prophylactic total thyroidectomy

32. A 24-year-old woman consults a physician because of difficulty swallowing both solid foods and liquids. She first noted occasional difficulty with swallowing 3 years ago, but states that the problem is now much more severe and persistent and is accompanied by regurgitation. Often the food she regurgitates 1 to 2 hours after a meal still tastes like "normal food." She has lost approximately 10 pounds, which she relates to uncomfortable feelings in her chest when she eats. Barium x-ray demonstrates a strikingly dilated esophagus with marked narrowing at the lower esophageal sphincter. Esophageal manometry shows aperistalsis. The lower esophageal sphincter pressure is increased, and there is often incomplete relaxation on swallowing. Which of the following is the most likely diagnosis?

    (A) Achalasia

    (B) Esophageal cancer

    (C) Esophageal web

    (D) Lower esophageal ring

    (E) Symptomatic diffuse esophageal spasm

33. A patient consults a physician because of chronic nasal congestion and nosebleeds over the past 2 years. He has tried numerous over-the-counter medications, but nothing has helped. He has also felt chronically ill, with low-grade fever, malaise, and anorexia. Nasal examination demonstrates a friable mucosa with a red, raised granular appearance that bleeds easily. A small area of nasal septal perforation is seen. Chest x-ray film demonstrates pulmonary infiltrates with associated cavitation in one case. Which of the following is the most appropriate next step in diagnosis?

    (A) Abdominal CT scan

    (B) Liver enzymes

    (C) Pancreatic enzymes

    (D) Urinalysis

    (E) Bladder biopsy

34. A 55-year-old woman with hypertension presents to her primary care physician with 3 weeks of worsening headaches and language difficulty. She reports severe headaches that waken her from sleep and are worse in the morning, frequently associated with nausea. She complains of slowness of speech and difficulty with word-finding. She is afebrile. A neurologic examination is remarkable for slow, effortful speech with poor repetition, and a right pronator drift. The physician refers her to the emergency department for an urgent MRI study, which shows a diffusely enhancing intra-axial abnormality in the left frontal region. Which of the following is the most likely diagnosis?

    (A) Astrocytoma

    (B) Brain abscess

    (C) Cerebral infarct

    (D) Complicated migraine

    (E) Meningioma

35. A 22-year-old woman presents with an 8-month history of bilateral and symmetric polyarthritis affecting the proximal small joints of the hands, wrists, elbows, knees, hips, and ankles. Morning stiffness is prominent. Marginal bony erosions are noted on radiologic examination. The erythrocyte sedimentation rate (ESR) is 66 mm/hr, and rheumatoid factor is positive. She has been treated with paracetamol and ibuprofen (600 mg, two to three times a day) with minimal relief. Clinical examination confirms the presence of fluid and swelling of the joints. Which of the following is the most appropriate management strategy?

    (A) Anti-inflammatory doses of nonsteroidal anti-inflammatory drugs (NSAIDs)

    (B) NSAIDs and a disease-modifying antirheumatic drug (DMARD)

    (C) NSAIDs with low-dose narcotic analgesics

    (D) NSAIDs and low-dose prednisone

36. A 55-year-old alcoholic man is brought to the emergency department by the police after being found wandering and mumbling to himself. The man is unable to give a coherent history. The initial impression is of an emaciated, jaundiced, and confused man who appears older than his stated age. Vital signs are stable and within normal limits. The breath has a musty, sweet odor. Abdominal examination shows ascites and marked nodularity of the liver edge. A "caput medusa" is seen near the umbilicus. Neurologic examination is notable for asterixis. A toxicology screen is negative. Aspartate aminotransferase (AST), alanine aminotransferase (ALT), and blood ammonia are all moderately increased. The man is admitted to the hospital and given an extremely low protein diet with oral carbohydrate supplementation. The bowels are cleared with an enema. Which of the following is the most appropriate pharmacotherapy?

    (A) Ampicillin, oral

    (B) Benzathine penicillin, intramuscular

    (C) Ceftriaxone, oral

    (D) Neomycin, oral

    (E) Penicillin G, IV

37. A 69-year-old man with history of congestive heart failure secondary to hypertension and atrial fibrillation comes to the physician because of increasing nausea, headache, and blurred vision in both eyes over the past 3 days. He also complains of seeing "yellow halos around lights." His medications include hydrochlorothiazide, enalapril, and digoxin. His blood pressure is 132/84 mm Hg, pulse is 56/min with irregular rhythm, and respirations are 16/min. Which of the following is the most likely cause of these symptoms?

    (A) Acute narrow-angle glaucoma

    (B) Digoxin toxicity

    (C) Diuretic-induced hypokalemia

    (D) Enalapril overdose

38. A 45-year-old white woman consults a physician because of chronic weakness, fatigue, and dizziness on standing. The patient frequently feels nauseous and sometimes vomits and has diarrhea. Physical examination demonstrates diffuse tanning of the skin, even in areas not exposed to sun, which is most pronounced over bony prominences. Scattered black freckles are seen on the head and neck, as are occasional patches of vitiligo. The areola and the mucous membranes of the mouth and vagina have bluish-black discoloration. Which of the following is the most likely diagnosis?

    (A) Addison disease

    (B) Conn disease

    (C) Cushing disease

    (D) Graves disease

    (E) Hashimoto disease

39. A 26-year-old woman presents to her physician after noticing a neck mass. Physical examination reveals a large thyroid gland that is firm, multilobular, and mobile. Her serum thyroid-stimulating hormone (TSH) is elevated, but her serum triiodothyronine (T3) and thyroxine (T4) are low. Her serum antithyroglobulin titer is positive. A thyroid scan reveals nonuniform uptake. A biopsy of the thyroid mass is most likely to show which of the following?

    (A) Fibrosis

    (B) Granulomas

    (C) Lymphocytic infiltration

    (D) Neutrophilic infiltration

    (E) Parafollicular ("C") cell hyperplasia

40. A 43-year-old woman who has recently moved to the United States from Greece goes to the local clinic for her annual physical examination. She suffers from anemia which was diagnosed during her first pregnancy at the age of 19, for which she has taken an iron pill on and off throughout her entire adult life. She says her hemoglobin levels have never been less than 10 g/dL and she has never needed any blood transfusion. She reports that she has not taken her iron pills in over a year and she feels well. She had a hysterectomy about 3 years ago but her anemia continued the same even after her menses stopped. On examination, the patient's vital signs are all within normal limits and the rest of her examination is unremarkable. A Pap smear and routine mammogram are ordered. Laboratory studies show:

Hemoglobin	10.8 g/dL
Platelet count	250,000/mm^3
MCH	28 g/dL
MCV	69 fL
RDW	13.9%
Leukocytes	5,600/mm^3

Two weeks later the patient comes in for a follow-up visit and to review the results of her lab tests. Which of the following management options is of the greatest diagnostic value at this time?

(A) Order a hemoglobin electrophoresis

(B) Order a bone marrow biopsy

(C) Prescribe oral ferrous sulfate

(D) Order vitamin B$_{12}$ and folate levels

(E) Order iron, ferritin, and total iron binding capacity

41. A 40-year-old man with type 1 diabetes mellitus for 10 years was recently found to have mild hypertension (stage 1) and microalbuminuria. Renal function tests are otherwise normal. There is evidence of mild left ventricular hypertrophy on ECG and echocardiographic studies. Blood lipids are within normal limits. Which of the following is the most appropriate pharmacologic treatment for this case of hypertension?

(A) ACE inhibitors

(B) Beta blockers

(C) Calcium channel blockers

(D) Central alpha-agonist, e.g., clonidine

(E) Thiazide diuretics

42. A 28-year-old African American woman comes to the emergency department complaining of chest and abdominal pain that is rated an 8 out of 10. The pain is severe enough to cause her to vomit repeatedly. She tells you that she has had episodes such as this in the past that are associated with her sickle cell disease, and that she thinks this pain is similar. For the last year, however, she has been fairly healthy, aside from a respiratory infection that she just got over a few days ago. Her vital signs are: temperature 37.8° C (100° F), blood pressure 158/90 mm Hg, pulse 110/min, and respirations 28/min. Examination reveals a woman in pain but without any specific findings. A complete blood count with a manual slide review reveals a hematocrit of 29%, a white blood cell count of 12,000 cells/mm^3, and platelets of 400,000/mm^3. Numerous crescent-shaped red blood cells, red blood cells with eccentrically located ovoid granules, red blood cells with a dark center surrounded by a light band that again is encircled by a darker ring, and nucleated red blood cells are present. An electrocardiogram reveals sinus tachycardia, and a set of cardiac enzymes drawn in the emergency department is normal. This patient is most likely to benefit from which of the following therapies?

(A) Acetaminophen

(B) Aspirin

(C) Broad-spectrum antibiotics

(D) Narcotics and hydration

(E) Plasma exchange

43. A previously healthy 25-year-old man comes to medical attention because of generalized edema and a sensation of abdominal fullness. Family and personal medical history are unremarkable. Examination reveals diffuse edema and signs of ascites. Laboratory investigations show:

Blood, serum:

Albumin	1.7 g/dL
Triglycerides	260 mg/dL
Cholesterol, total	280 mg/dL
Erythrocyte sedimentation rate	50/min
Glucose	110 mg/dL
BUN	15 mg/dL
Creatinine	1.0 mg/dL

Urine:

Protein (24-hour collection)	5 g
Sediment	Occasional nonspecific casts
Leukocytes	None
Glucose	None

Which of the following is a frequent complication in this setting?

(A) Acute pyelonephritis

(B) Acute renal failure

(C) Hemorrhages

(D) Hypertension

(E) Venous thrombosis

44. A 19-year-old woman is evaluated because of a 6-week history of intermittent low-grade fever, weight loss, and night sweats. On physical examination she is found to have enlarged lymph nodes on both jugular chains and supraclavicular areas, and chest CT scan shows a large mediastinal mass. One of the most accessible cervical nodes is excised surgically for biopsy; the pathologist reports the presence of Reed-Sternberg cells. Abdominal CT scan is nondiagnostic and bone marrow biopsy is positive. Which of the following is the most appropriate next step in management?

(A) Bilateral neck dissections and surgical mediastinal exploration

(B) Bone marrow transplant

(C) Radiation therapy to the affected areas

(D) Staging laparotomy

(E) Systemic chemotherapy

The response options for items 45-46 are the same. You will be required to select one answer for each item in the set.

(A) Anemia of chronic disease

(B) Aplastic anemia

(C) Chronic lymphocytic leukemia

(D) Glucose-6-phosphate dehydrogenase deficiency

(E) Hairy cell leukemia

(F) Hereditary spherocytosis

(G) Iron-deficiency anemia

(H) Megaloblastic anemia

(I) Microangiopathic anemia

(J) Myelodysplastic syndrome

(K) Myelofibrosis

(L) Sickle cell anemia

(M) Thalassemia

For each patient with anemia, select the most likely diagnosis.

45. Six hours after starting treatment with sulfonamides for acute otitis, a 25-year-old man from southern Italy presents to the emergency department because of acute onset of headache, malaise, and cola-colored urine. He says that he had two similar episodes in Italy: one after eating fava beans, another following treatment with acetylsalicylic acid. Blood and serum studies are significant for:

Red blood cells	1.5 million/mm^3
Hemoglobin	7.5 g/dL
Reticulocytes	6%
Indirect bilirubin	5.2 mg/dL

46. A 10-year-old African American boy has had jaundice, splenomegaly, and chronic ulcers over his lower legs since his first year of life. Recurrent episodes of bone pain manifest periodically, especially in concomitance with infectious illnesses.

The response options for items 47-48 are the same. You will be required to select one answer for each item in the set.

(A) Acute cholangitis

(B) Acute cholecystitis

(C) Acute pancreatitis

(D) Adenoma of the liver

(E) Alcoholic hepatitis

(F) Amebic liver abscess

(G) Focal nodular hyperplasia

(H) Gilbert syndrome

(I) Hemochromatosis

(J) Hepatocellular carcinoma

(K) Pancreatic carcinoma

(L) Primary biliary cirrhosis

(M) Primary sclerosing cholangitis

(N) Rotor syndrome

(O) Viral hepatitis

(P) Wilson disease

For each patient with jaundice, select the most likely diagnosis.

47. A 65-year-old man with a history of cholelithiasis presents with jaundice for 1 week, a 5-kg weight loss for 1 month, and deep epigastric pain for 2 months. He also reports dark urine and clay-colored stools. A palpable distended gallbladder is noted on physical examination. Serum chemistry tests show:

Bilirubin

Total	5.0 mg/dL
Direct	3.5 mg/dL
Alkaline phosphatase	800 U/L
ALT	45 U/L
AST	40 U/L
Amylase	150 U/L
Glucose (fasting)	150 mg/dL

48. A 10-year-old boy comes to medical attention because of jaundice and right upper abdominal tenderness for 2 days. Laboratory studies show elevated serum aminotransferases, hyperbilirubinemia, and prolonged prothrombin time. A gray-green ring is found in the Descemet membrane of the cornea on slit-lamp examination. The urinary copper level is high.

The response options for items 49-50 are the same. You will be required to select one answer for each item in the set.

(A) Accumulation of uremic toxins

(B) Hyperkalemia

(C) Platelet dysfunction

(D) Salt and water retention

(E) Secondary hyperparathyroidism

(F) Shunting of blood through arteriovenous fistula

For each patient with chronic renal failure, select the factor involved in the pathogenesis of the described findings.

49. A 66-year-old man on long-term hemodialysis for chronic renal failure presents with bone pains and proximal muscle weakness. The glomerular filtration rate (GFR) is less than 25% of normal. X-ray films reveal generalized osteopenia, particularly pronounced in the phalanges and distal clavicle, and ectopic calcifications in soft tissues around joints.

50. A 54-year-old woman with progressive renal failure secondary to diabetes mellitus is found to have a blood pressure of 160/95 mm Hg during a routine follow-up examination. Her blood pressure was previously within normal limits. She is on peritoneal dialysis and dietary management with restriction of protein, water, and salt intake. Treatment with subcutaneous injections of recombinant erythropoietin for anemia was recently started.

Internal Medicine Test Seven:
Answers and Explanations

ANSWER KEY

1.	B	26.	A
2.	E	27.	C
3.	D	28.	B
4.	E	29.	A
5.	D	30.	C
6.	E	31.	E
7.	B	32.	A
8.	A	33.	D
9.	D	34.	A
10.	C	35.	B
11.	D	36.	D
12.	E	37.	B
13.	A	38.	A
14.	E	39.	C
15.	B	40.	A
16.	E	41.	A
17.	E	42.	D
18.	E	43.	E
19.	D	44.	E
20.	C	45.	D
21.	A	46.	L
22.	D	47.	K
23.	B	48.	P
24.	E	49.	E
25.	A	50.	D

1. **The correct answer is B.** In this case, productive cough of recent onset, fever, auscultatory findings, and radiologic evidence of a pulmonary infiltrate are consistent with acute bronchopneumonia. *Klebsiella pneumoniae* is the most common organism causing community-acquired pneumonia in chronic alcoholics.

   Influenza virus (**choice A**) may result in respiratory symptoms mimicking pneumonia, but chest x-ray films do not reveal lobar pulmonary infiltrates, unless there is a superimposed bacterial infection.

   Legionella pneumophila (**choice C**) is one of the most common causes of community-acquired pneumonia. It usually affects individuals with some degree of immune impairment or respiratory damage, especially heavy smokers and patients with chronic obstructive pulmonary disease (COPD). Outbreaks of legionellosis result from exposure to contaminated sources, such as air conditioning towers or shower heads.

   M. pneumoniae (**choice D**) is the most frequent etiologic agent of *atypical pneumonia*, characterized by dry cough, low-grade fever, and relatively few localizing symptoms. Small outbreaks within close communities are characteristic of pneumonia due to this microorganism.

   Pneumocystis carinii (**choice E**) causes pneumonia in severely immunocompromised patients. The clinical picture consists of high fever and subacute respiratory compromise, which may progress to acute respiratory failure.

   Staphylococcus aureus (**choice F**) causes pneumonia most often in hospitalized patients or as a complication of influenza. It is characterized by necrotizing inflammation and frequent development of cavitation.

2. **The correct answer is E.** The right coronary artery supplies the inferior and posterior segments of the heart. ST changes would be seen in II, III, and aVF.

   The circumflex artery (**choice A**) supplies the anterolateral regions of the heart and would affect leads V5-V6 and I-aVL.

   The left anterior descending (LAD) artery (**choice B**) supplies the anteroseptal and anteroapical regions, and a lesion would be represented by ST changes in V1-V4.

   Left coronary artery occlusion (**choice C**) would encompass regions supplied by the LAD and circumflex and would affect V1-V6 and I, and aVL.

   The posterior descending artery (**choice D**) supplies the posterior aspect of the heart and would show tall R waves in V1-V2.

3. **The correct answer is D.** The most common causes of upper gastrointestinal (UGI) bleeds are peptic ulcer disease (PUD, 45% to 50%), gastritis (30%), varices (10%), and then the remainder of causes such as Mallory-Weiss tears, esophagitis, and neoplasms. In any patient with a his-tory of "pain killer" use, especially women with rheumatologic conditions, the diagnosis of gastritis or gastric ulcers secondary to NSAID use must be suspected. The most common cause of these two conditions is NSAID use.

   Esophagitis (**choice A**) is usually due to acid reflux disease and is not a significant cause of UGI bleeding.

   Esophageal varices (**choice B**) are a very common cause of UGI bleeds in patients with cirrhosis. In the U.S., the most common causes of cirrhosis are alcohol and hepatitis virus infection. Worldwide, schistosomiasis is the most common cause. Since this patient has none of the above diseases, the likelihood of her having varices is almost zero.

   Gastric neoplasm (**choice C**), although accounting for a small percentage of patients with UGI bleeding, requires other associated findings of cancer to be suspected. Gastric cancer in particular is associated with early satiety, epigastric pain, a palpable abdominal mass, and certain nitrate-containing foods.

   Mallory-Weiss tears (**choice E**) are small esophageal tears induced by acute acid erosion secondary to vomiting. It should be suspected in patients who have the triad of hematemesis, alcohol abuse, and vomiting. It is not a cause of severe, prolonged, or recurrent UGI bleeding.

4. **The correct answer is E.** The toxin of coagulase positive *Staphylococcus* characteristically produces food poisoning with abrupt onset of severe gastrointestinal symptoms 2-8 hours after ingestion of contaminated custards, cream-filled pastry, milk, processed meat, or fish. The diarrhea is characteristically nonbloody because the toxin does not produce mucosal ulceration. Most patients recover spontaneously within 12 hours; a few develop sufficiently severe acid-base and electrolyte imbalance to cause shock and even death, particularly among infants, the elderly, and the chronically ill.

   Campylobacter (**choice A**) is the most common bacterial cause of infectious diarrhea in the U.S., typically producing illness lasting several days.

   Clostridium botulinum toxin (**choice B**) produces botulism, characterized by a flaccid paralysis.

   Clostridium perfringens (**choice C**) causes usually relatively mild gastroenteritis 6-24 hours after ingestion of contaminated food, notably meats.

   Escherichia coli O157:H7 (**choice D**) causes acute bloody diarrhea due to a toxin similar to that of *Shigella*.

5. **The correct answer is D.** This patient most likely has chronic bronchitis, as evidenced by his cough and sputum production. Bronchitis involves excessive mucus production in the bronchial tree, leading to a productive cough for at least 3 months during each of 2 successive years. It is among the most common causes of hemoptysis in

adults. However, lung cancer must be high on the differential diagnosis list.

Alpha-1 antitrypsin deficiency (**choice A**) is a genetic factor predisposing to emphysema. This should not cause hemoptysis. It would certainly lead to wheezing and symptoms seen in chronic obstructive pulmonary disease.

A normal chest x-ray film does not necessarily rule out bronchiectasis (**choice B**). Bronchiectasis is a pathologic, irreversible dilatation of the bronchi that is caused by destruction of the bronchial wall, usually resulting from suppurative infection of an obstructed bronchus. Symptoms may occasionally include hemoptysis.

Bronchogenic carcinoma (**choice C**) must be considered in someone with a long smoking history and hemoptysis. Statistically, bronchitis is still more common. Chest x-ray films can be clear in lung cancer; if there is clinical suspicion, this patient must get a chest CT to rule out a mass.

Chest x-ray films can be clear in a patient with pulmonary tuberculosis (**choice E**). Radiographic signs, if present, include apical granulomas on lung chest x-ray. Other symptoms may include cough, weight loss, and hemoptysis. Acid fast bacilli (AFB) smear and cultures may be positive for *Mycobacterium tuberculosis*. Pulmonary tuberculosis is less likely than chronic bronchitis in this smoker.

6. **The correct answer is E.** Antibiotics can suppress normal gut flora that produce vitamin K. In addition, most total parenteral nutrition (TPN) preparations do not include vitamin K. This vitamin is essentially in the normal functioning of coagulation factors II, VII, IX, and X; deficiency frequently leads to coagulation defects, manifested by easy bruising and prolonged prothrombin time (PT).

Calcium is a cofactor in the coagulation pathway, but deficiency is generally not associated with easy bruisability (**choice A**).

Disseminated intravascular coagulation (DIC) (**choice B**) can lead to a coagulopathy as a result of the consumption of coagulation factors. However, the patient would also have reduced platelets.

Magnesium deficiency (**choice C**) can lead to cardiac arrhythmias but not a bleeding diathesis.

Sepsis (**choice D**) can result in DIC and generalized shock. The patient, however, would be pressor dependent and have elevated PT and partial thromboplastin time (PTT) and reduced platelets.

7. **The correct answer is B.** This patient manifests a classic syndrome of hypocortisolism, the most common manifestations of which include chronic weakness, menstrual disturbances, skin melanosis, hypotension, hyponatremia, and hyperkalemia. Eosinophilia and relative lymphocytosis are also frequent findings. The most frequent cause of *Addison disease* (the designation given to this clinical picture) in the U.S. is autoimmune destruction of the adrenal glands, evidenced by lymphocytic infiltration and progressive atrophy of the adrenal cortex. High ACTH levels represent a compensatory response of the anterior pituitary gland. High ACTH levels, skin hyperpigmentation, and hyperkalemia are absent in cases secondary to hypopituitarism. The disease is more frequent in women.

Adrenoleukodystrophy (**choice A**) is a rare X-linked hereditary disorder resulting in accumulation of very long chain fatty acids in the adrenals, testes, and CNS. Thus, adrenal insufficiency, neurologic deficits, and hypogonadism constitute the predominant manifestations. This condition accounts for one-third of cases of adrenal insufficiency in male children.

Bilateral adrenal hemorrhage (**choice C**) may cause adrenal insufficiency and occurs as a complication of anticoagulation therapy, major traumas, or open heart surgery.

Fungal infection (**choice D**) was a very rare cause of adrenal insufficiency until the AIDS epidemic. Disseminated histoplasmosis is probably the most common fungal infection causing adrenal insufficiency in AIDS patients. Coccidioidomycosis and CMV infections are other possible etiologies of Addison disease in immunocompromised patients.

Metastatic disease (**choice E**) may result in adrenal insufficiency if both glands are significantly affected. Metastatic carcinomas have a peculiar propensity to involve the adrenal gland despite the small size of this organ.

Tuberculosis (**choice F**) was once the most common cause of adrenal insufficiency, and is still the most common cause in areas in which tuberculosis is endemic.

8. **The correct answer is A.** Constrictive pericarditis is diffuse thickening of the pericardium in reaction to prior inflammation, resulting in reduced distensibility of the cardiac chambers. Cardiac output is limited, and filling pressures are increased to match the external constrictive force placed on the heart by the pericardium. In both constrictive pericarditis and cardiac tamponade, the diastolic pressures are equal in all four chambers of the heart. Jugular veins are distended, indicating systemic venous hypertension. This neck vein distention increases with inspiration and is called Kussmaul's sign.

The first and second heart sounds (S1 and S2) are reduced in intensity because of reduced sound transmission through the thickened pericardium (**choice B**).

Patients with congestive heart failure have an extra, third sound (**choice C**). This occurs during rapid filling of the left ventricle.

The fourth heart sound (**choice D**) is heard in patients in sinus rhythm and with heart failure. In elderly patients, it may indicate reduced compliance of the stiff ventricle.

In most cases of constrictive pericarditis, the clinical findings of right-sided failure are more prominent than those of left-sided failure (**choice E**). Thus ascites, jaundice, and edema will be commonly seen.

9. **The correct answer is D.** An isolated thyroid nodule is a frequent finding in asymptomatic adults, and most of such are benign. Fine needle aspiration allows a diagnosis in most cases. The material aspirated with a needle is smeared on a slide and stained. In only 15% of cases is the aspirated material "nondiagnostic." Suspicious cases are followed with repeated fine needle aspiration. Malignant nodules are usually large (>3 cm) and/or fixed to the surrounding parenchyma. Papillary carcinoma is the most common malignant thyroid neoplasm.

Ultrasonography may also be of value in distinguishing solid from cystic nodules and is preferred to MRI scan (**choice A**) or CT scan (**choice B**) because of its high sensitivity and lower cost. However, CT and MRI are valuable in defining the extent of malignant tumor, once the diagnosis is made.

Radioactive iodine scan (**choice C**) is needed when a solitary thyroid nodule is associated with symptoms of thyrotoxicosis. Radioactive iodine scan helps to distinguish a toxic adenoma from Graves disease, in which high uptake is seen in the whole gland.

Excision of a thyroid nodule (**choice E**) is performed if it proves to be malignant, or in case of a *hot* (i.e., hyperfunctioning) nodule causing thyrotoxicosis.

10. **The correct answer is C.** IV drug users are prone to developing bacteremia, which can lead to a brain abscess. Patients with brain abscesses are typically afebrile and can exhibit progressive neurologic dysfunction.

IV drug abusers are prone to developing bacterial endocarditis (**choice A**), but they are typically febrile. This patient's echocardiogram and physical examination lead away from the diagnosis. However, in the management of this patient, blood cultures should be drawn, and suspicion of endocarditis must be high.

Patients with bacterial meningitis (**choice B**) are typically toxic appearing and febrile and have positive signs of meningeal irritation. They also often exhibit nuchal rigidity. Elevated WBC in the CSF, decreased glucose level, elevated protein, and a predominance of neutrophils are indicative of this diagnosis.

HIV meningitis causes a headache and meningeal irritation. Focal neurologic deficits do not occur. Cryptococcal meningitis (**choice D**) typically presents with altered behavior and a headache. Stroke-like events are rare.

IV drug use can lead to a foreign body embolus (**choice E**) and apoplectic neurologic problems. An embolus may reach the brain via a right-to-left cardiac shunt or pulmonary arteriovenous malformation if the injection is venous. Embolic phenomena are more common in the setting of endocarditis.

11. **The correct answer is D.** This woman is in a nonketotic hyperglycemic hyperosmolar coma, a feared complication of type 2 diabetes mellitus that is associated with a 50% mortality rate. The basic problem is when extreme hyperglycemia occurs, glucose spills into the urine and can cause profound dehydration since the glucose acts as an osmotic diuretic. Features of this syndrome include CNS alterations, extreme hyperglycemia (typical values in the range of 1,000 mg/dL), and dehydration. These features lead to hyperosmolality (the correct choice in this case; normal values are less than about 290 mOsmol/kg), mild metabolic acidosis, no ketonemia to minimal hyperketonemia, and prerenal azotemia. Diabetic ketoacidosis, the other diagnosis that should be considered, is uncommon in type 2 diabetics and is associated with lower blood glucose levels than nonketotic hyperglycemic hyperosmolar coma.

Blood urea nitrogen (**choice A**) and serum creatinine (**choice C**) are usually elevated (owing to prerenal azotemia) rather than decreased in nonketotic hyperglycemic hyperosmolar coma.

Strongly positive ketones in blood (**choice B**) are a feature of diabetic ketoacidosis. Minimally elevated ketones in the blood are sometimes seen in nonketotic hyperglycemic hyperosmolar coma.

Serum sodium (**choice E**) is usually normal to increased in nonketotic hyperglycemic hyperosmolar coma.

12. **The correct answer is E.** Chronic constipation is a common problem in the elderly; however, before reassuring the patient, the physician has an obligation to exclude serious disease such as colon cancer. Once the physician is reasonably convinced that there is no serious underlying pathology, the next steps are to suggest increasing fiber in the diet and to discontinue any medications that may be causing the constipation. If these steps fail, then the addition of bulking agents (bran, psyllium, calcium polycarbophil, or methylcellulose) and hydration are warranted. Long-term use of other types of laxatives is not recommended.

Docusate (**choice A**) is a wetting agent (detergent laxative) that softens stools by increasing their water content.

Lactulose (**choice B**) and magnesium phosphate (**choice C**) are osmotic agents sometimes used to prepare patients for diagnostic bowel procedures.

Mineral oil (**choice D**) softens fecal matter but is not recommended for long-term use because it may decrease absorption of fat soluble vitamins.

13. **The correct answer is A.** This patient has aplastic anemia. A characteristic feature of this condition is that the growth of erythrocyte, granulocyte, and megakaryocyte precursors is markedly impaired. The marrow is usually replaced by adipose tissue. Aplastic anemia typically develops insidiously, but may have a more rapid course. In about half of cases, no cause is ever identified. In the remainder, causes may include chemical exposures (e.g., benzene and inorganic arsenic), radiation, or drug reactions (e.g., antineoplastic agents, antibiotics, anticonvulsants, and NSAIDs), and parvovirus B19 in patients with hemoglobinopathies or spherocytosis. Historically, the condition has required marrow transplantation, but this therapy is now reserved for patients who fail to improve with equine antithymocyte globulin or cyclosporine therapy.

    Iron deficiency anemia (**choice B**) produces a microcytic anemia.

    Folate deficiency anemia (**choice C**) and vitamin B_{12} deficiency anemia (**choice E**) produce a megaloblastic anemia.

    Myelophthisic anemia (**choice D**) can clinically resemble aplastic anemia, but bone marrow studies would demonstrate tumor, granulomatous disease, or fibrosis replacing the normal marrow.

14. **The correct answer is E.** This question asks you to differentiate between different types of peripheral motor neuropathies. Ramsay Hunt syndrome, caused by herpes zoster infection of the geniculate ganglion, results in facial palsy. It differs from the other neuropathies in that there is usually a vesicular eruption, typical of herpes infections.

    Bell's palsy (**choice A**), the most common form of facial paralysis, is idiopathic. The onset is abrupt, with maximal weakness in the first 48 hours. Eighty percent of patients fully recover in a few weeks.

    Guillain-Barré syndrome (**choice B**) is an acute inflammatory polyradiculoneuropathy, causing bilateral facial palsy and usually producing areflexic motor paralysis. A viral illness often precedes the onset of neuropathy.

    Horner syndrome (**choice C**) affects the oculosympathetic nerves, usually ipsilaterally, specifically causing unilateral miosis and ptosis, with normal pupillary response to light. Hemianhidrosis of the face also occurs.

    Ménière disease (**choice D**) manifests with recurrent vertigo and is associated with tinnitus and progressive deafness. There is no facial paralysis.

15. **The correct answer is B.** The patient has pityriasis rosea, and the large lesion is known as the "herald patch." Any description of this disease in a question will probably either use this term or describe the initial, larger lesion. The scaly lesions tend to involve the trunk and may be either oval or circinate (increasing an initial impression of ringworm). The lesions on the back may follow the lines of cleavage of the skin, producing a "Christmas tree" appearance of the lesion distribution. The condition is self-limited, but may persist more than 2 months. It is suspected to be infectious in nature, with potential causative species including a picornavirus, herpes virus 7, and *Mycoplasma*.

    Molluscum contagiosum (**choice A**) causes multiple small papules with umbilicated centers.

    Pityriasis rubra pilaria (**choice C**) has a predilection for involving the hands and soles and does not produce a herald patch.

    Rosacea (**choice D**) causes telangiectasia, erythema, papules, and pustules of the nose and cheeks.

    Scabies (**choice E**) would be suggested in a question stem if the physician found small skin burrows in addition to papules. Also, itching is prominent with scabies.

16. **The correct answer is E.** This patient has a bilateral loss of pain and temperature sensation, with preserved proprioception, below the T10 dermatome. This implies damage at the spinal, rather than the brainstem, level. The ventral (anterior) spinal artery's course begins in the anterior median sulcus of the spinal cord, with branches supplying the ventral and lateral funiculi and most of the spinal cord gray matter. Damage to the ventral spinal artery produces bilateral loss of pain and temperature sensation below the level of the lesion as a result of injury to the spinothalamic tracts on both sides.

    Damage to the anterior cerebral artery (**choice A**) would be expected to produce paresis of the contralateral lower extremity resulting from injury to the paracentral lobule.

    Damage to the middle cerebral artery (**choice B**) would be expected to result in some degree of contralateral hemiparalysis, primarily of the face and upper extremity. If the dominant hemisphere were affected, aphasia would be expected as well.

    Damage to the posterior cerebral artery (**choice C**) would diminish blood flow through the calcarine artery, resulting in contralateral homonymous hemianopia. Lack of blood flow through the thalamic branches of the posterior cerebral artery would produce hemiplegia with varying degrees of contralateral sensory loss. Thalamic pain (constant excruciating pain in the hemiplegic extremities) might appear later.

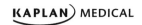

The thalamostriate arteries (**choice D**) are small branches of the middle cerebral arteries that supply the internal capsule and portions of the basal ganglia. They are particularly susceptible to rupture and hemorrhage in patients with hypertension or arteriosclerosis. In such cases, complete contralateral paralysis usually ensues.

17. **The correct answer is E.** This patient has the classic symptomatology of *acute appendicitis.* Pain in the right lower quadrant provoked by palpation of other areas of the abdominal wall is known as *Rovsing sign.* Presence of rebound tenderness is a sign of early peritoneal involvement. The pain usually begins in the periumbilical region and then moves to its characteristic location. Anorexia is the second most frequent symptom and usually precedes or accompanies pain. Vomiting is often present and usually *follows* the onset of pain. Fever, if present, is usually modest. Moderate neutrophilic leukocytosis is often detected. A few RBCs may be seen on urinalysis because of secondary involvement of the adjacent ureter. Pelvic exam should be performed in all women with acute abdominal pain to rule out intrauterine or ectopic pregnancy, pelvic inflammatory disease, ovarian cysts, or malignancies. A normal pelvic examination and negative assay for beta-hCG makes pregnancy a highly unlikely cause of this patient's symptomatology. In the presence of this classic picture, laparotomy and appendectomy are mandatory, but surgery is often performed when less than typical symptomatology is observed. It is, in fact, preferable to remove a few normal appendices than to leave untreated a potentially life-threatening condition.

Antibiotic therapy (**choice A**) is inadequate treatment for appendicitis. Antibiotics, however, are used pre- and postoperatively to decrease the incidence of wound infections.

No radiologic investigation can confirm a clinical diagnosis of appendicitis. Barium enema (**choice B**) may be helpful in uncertain cases, but is often unnecessary. A filling defect in the cecum is highly suggestive of appendicitis.

Ultrasonography of urinary tract (**choice C**) is warranted in cases of abdominal pain attributable to urolithiasis or other urologic conditions. As mentioned, the presence of few erythrocytes in the urine is frequently seen in association with appendicitis and does not indicate urinary tract disease.

Dilatation and curettage (**choice D**) would not be appropriate in a woman with suspected appendicitis.

18. **The correct answer is E.** Myasthenia gravis is an autoimmune disease caused by circulating antibodies that bind to acetylcholine receptors on the postsynaptic membrane. The disease is characterized by weakness and fatigue. The weakness usually begins in the extraocular muscles with ptosis and diplopia. The symptoms may be localized to the ocular muscles or generalized. The weakness usually becomes more prominent toward the end of the day or following continuous use of affected muscles. Other bulbar muscles may be involved, causing difficulty in swallowing, chewing, or speaking. Closing the eyes or relaxing makes the symptoms disappear. Ocular weakness can be induced with repetitive blinking, with the patient developing ptosis. Administration of edrophonium causes a transient resolution of symptoms.

Botulism (**choice A**) is caused by the exotoxin of *Clostridium botulinum* and occurs following the ingestion of contaminated food. The toxin interferes with the release of acetylcholine at the neuromuscular junction. Symptoms usually appear several days after ingestion and include blurry vision, diplopia, and difficulty swallowing. Gastrointestinal symptoms may develop, and the weakness spreads rapidly to cause paralysis of limb, cranial, and respiratory muscles. Administration of edrophonium will not reverse symptoms.

Eaton-Lambert syndrome (**choice B**) is a presynaptic disorder of the neuromuscular junction, usually associated with an underlying malignancy. Multiple muscle groups, most commonly the proximal muscles of the lower limbs, are affected. Diplopia and ptosis may also be present. Eaton-Lambert is readily differentiated from myasthenia gravis, as patients with Eaton-Lambert syndrome have markedly depressed or absent reflexes, autonomic changes, and slow incremental responses with repetitive nerve stimulation. Treatment with edrophonium does not improve symptoms.

Guillain-Barré syndrome (**choice C**) is an acute polyneuropathy characterized by a rapidly progressive, predominantly motor neuropathy that may paralyze all voluntary muscles, including those supplied by cranial nerves. Pain is common, along with some degree of autonomic dysfunction. Bilateral facial paralysis is also common and helps to differentiate the syndrome from other polyneuropathies. Onset is usually 2-3 weeks after a respiratory infection. On examination, the weakness usually progresses from the lower to upper extremities, and finally to the face. Deep tendon reflexes are absent, and symmetric weakness of all extremities is noted.

Multiple sclerosis (**choice D**) is the most common immune demyelinating disorder of the CNS. It usually presents between the ages of 20 and 40 and is characterized by remissions and exacerbations of neurologic dysfunction. It usually involves several different sites of the CNS and progresses over many years. The typical presentation is that of an otherwise healthy woman developing an acute loss of vision, diplopia, vertigo, incontinence, or paralysis. Resolution of symptoms will generally occur over several weeks and do not resolve with rest or edrophonium and cannot be elicited with repetitive use.

19. **The correct answer is D.** Polymyositis presents with the described clinical picture (i.e., proximal muscle weakness and pain). Because of ongoing destruction of myofibers, the levels of creatine kinase are often strikingly elevated. The disease is thought to arise from an abnormal T-lymphocyte-mediated response targeting myofiber antigens. This condition is not associated with underlying malignancies.

Denervation atrophy (**choice A**) results from loss of innervation of skeletal muscle (e.g., after traumatic nerve transection or axonal degeneration). Inflammation is minimal or absent, while myofibers undergo progressive shrinkage without necrosis. Myopathic changes seen with electromyographic studies, proximal muscle involvement, and histopathologic changes argue against a diagnosis of denervation atrophy.

Dermatomyositis (**choice B**) may mimic polymyositis on muscle biopsy, but skin involvement is absent in the latter. In dermatomyositis, muscle biopsy often shows characteristic perifascicular atrophy, with the atrophic fibers mainly distributed at the periphery of fascicles. A significant number of cases (up to 30%) are associated with some form of visceral malignancy.

Inclusion body myositis (**choice C**) has a predilection for the distal musculature and presents histologically with modest degrees of inflammation. *Rimmed vacuoles* are the specific morphologic changes that allow a pathologic diagnosis on biopsy.

Systemic lupus erythematosus (**choice E**) may involve skeletal muscles. However, this systemic disease is usually accompanied by multiorgan involvement, especially the skin, kidneys, and serosal membranes. Inflammatory infiltration in the muscle would be more conspicuous around the vessels.

20. **The correct answer is C.** According to the recommendations issued in 1997 by the Joint National Committee on Detection, Education, and Treatment of High Blood Pressure, normal adult values of blood pressure are systolic <130 and diastolic <85 mm Hg. *Stage 1* (mild) hypertension is defined as a systolic pressure in the range of 140 to 159 mm Hg, or a diastolic pressure in the range of 90 to 99 mm Hg. If stage 1 hypertension is detected, the diagnosis should be confirmed within 2 months. Currently, hypertension is diagnosed as elevation of either the systolic *or* the diastolic value above the normal level.

A systolic pressure >180 mm Hg or a diastolic pressure >110 mm Hg is defined as *stage 3* (severe) hypertension. According to the above recommendations, a patient presenting with these values should be evaluated again or referred within 1 week (**choice A**).

Patients with *stage 2* (moderate) hypertension are those who have a systolic pressure of 160 to 179 mm Hg or a diastolic pressure of 100 to 109 mm Hg. The current recommendation is to evaluate or refer within 1 month (**choice B**).

A systolic pressure of 130 to 139 mm Hg or a diastolic pressure of 85 to 90 mm Hg is defined as "high normal." In this case, the recommendation is to recheck in 1 year (**choice D**) to determine whether a condition of hypertension has developed.

Blood pressure should be rechecked within 2 years (**choice E**) if the values fall within normal limits, that is, systolic <130 mm Hg and diastolic <85 mm Hg.

Stage 1 hypertension does not necessarily require pharmacologic treatment, such as diuretics (**choice F**). Nonpharmacologic approaches, such as exercise, weight loss, and changes in diet or lifestyle, may be sufficient.

21. **The correct answer is A.** Low calcium and high phosphorus levels, combined with the characteristic manifestations of hypocalcemia (muscle spasms and perioral paresthesias), are characteristic of hypoparathyroidism. This often occurs as a transient postoperative manifestation following removal of a large parathyroid adenoma, which had previously caused atrophy of the remaining normal glands. Symptomatic hypocalcemia must be treated with IV calcium gluconate, followed by oral calcium and vitamin D administration.

Hungry bone syndrome (**choice B**) develops days or weeks following resection of a parathyroid adenoma because of avid calcium uptake by a previously demineralized bone. However, since PTH returns to normal levels as the normal glands become functional again, hypocalcemia is *not* associated with hyperphosphatemia, as in this case. Hungry bone syndrome is the main reason patients require calcium and vitamin D supplementation for months after surgery.

Hyperventilation syndrome (**choice C**) may produce symptoms mimicking hypocalcemia, such as paresthesias, agitation, and spasms. CO_2 levels are decreased, and pH is increased (respiratory alkalosis).

Magnesium deficiency (**choice D**) may lead to hypocalcemia and hyperphosphatemia mimicking hypoparathyroidism. It is indeed mediated by impairment of PTH secretion and peripheral resistance to PTH action. But the normal levels of magnesium reported above exclude this cause.

Metastatic parathyroid carcinoma (**choice E**) would be associated with persistent hyperparathyroidism. Parathyroid carcinoma is a rare cause of hyperparathyroidism.

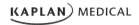

22. **The correct answer is D.** This patient has late latent syphilis. He has no physical signs of syphilis, with positive serologic tests and a negative lumbar puncture. Treatment is usually with benzathine penicillin G. In a patient who has a penicillin allergy, alternatives include tetracycline or doxycycline.

Azithromycin (**choice A**) is used for penicillin-allergic patients with primary syphilis.

Ceftriaxone (**choice B**) and chloramphenicol (**choice C**) are used in the treatment of late (tertiary) syphilis.

Because the diagnosis of syphilis has been confirmed with a FTA-ABS, it is important to determine the stage of the disease. As described above, the patient has late latent syphilis and is at risk for developing tertiary syphilis in the future. Therefore, the patient should be treated, which makes **choice E** an incorrect answer.

23. **The correct answer is B.** The clinical picture is that of biventricular failure, with evidence of pulmonary congestion and peripheral edema. Hepatomegaly is the result of passive congestion, not the effect of primary liver disease. ALT and AST are mildly elevated, and other liver function tests (bilirubin levels, prothrombin time [PT], and serum albumin) are within normal limits. The enlargement of the heart detected on chest x-ray is indicative of dilated cardiomyopathy, a condition that may result from chronic alcohol abuse or previous myocarditis (among numerous other causes).

Alcoholic cirrhosis (**choice A**) is the most frequent form of cirrhosis in the U.S. Liver function tests would be markedly impaired, with reduced serum albumin and prolonged PT. Ascites is usually present, and the liver may not be palpable in the cirrhotic stage.

Hemochromatosis (**choice C**) may manifest with congestive heart failure because of myocardial involvement by iron accumulation. However, normal serum ferritin values and the absence of other signs of hemochromatosis (e.g., skin hyperpigmentation, cirrhosis, and pancreatic dysfunction) exclude this hypothesis.

Hypertrophic cardiomyopathy (**choice D**) does not result in cardiomegaly. Indeed, the heart size may be within normal limits on chest x-ray. The most important finding is thickening of the interventricular septum on echocardiography, which results in stenosis of the outflow tract and a systolic murmur.

Restrictive cardiomyopathy (**choice E**) is clinically similar to hypertrophic cardiomyopathy. The cardiac silhouette is usually normal on chest x-ray. The underlying hemodynamic deficit is impaired diastolic filling (similar to hypertrophic cardiomyopathy) in contrast to the impaired contractility of dilated cardiomyopathy.

24. **The correct answer is E.** Prolongation of aPTT in patients with *antiphospholipid antibody syndrome* is related to an *in vitro* reaction of such antibodies with phospholipids present in the reaction test. Surprisingly, these patients are not prone to developing recurrent bleeding (**choice D**), but instead have *hypercoagulability*. The resultant propensity to develop thrombosis, both in the arterial and in the venous channels, may lead to fatal cerebral, myocardial, and intestinal infarcts, as well as to recurrent venous thrombosis. This syndrome may be associated with specific collagen vascular diseases (most commonly with systemic lupus erythematosus) or occur as an isolated condition. Other manifestations include renal disease due to microangiopathy, and repeated miscarriage.

Glomerulonephritis (**choice A**) is not a feature of antiphospholipid antibody syndrome. Systemic lupus erythematosus causes glomerulonephritis of varying forms and severity in up to 90% of patients.

Lymphoma (**choice B**) is not a complication of antiphospholipid antibody syndrome. An autoimmune-mediated disease leading to increased risk of lymphoma is *Sjögren syndrome*.

Pulmonary fibrosis (**choice C**) may develop in association with several immune-mediated collagen vascular diseases, especially rheumatoid arthritis and progressive systemic sclerosis.

25. **The correct answer is A.** This patient probably has *acute adrenal insufficiency,* or *adrenal crisis.* Measurement of serum cortisol will verify the likely diagnosis (cortisol levels would normally be increased following the stress of surgery). Adrenal insufficiency occurs in patients with latent Addison disease who have stress due to events such as surgery, infections, or severe trauma. Other common situations that may precipitate an adrenal crisis include bilateral adrenalectomy, removal of a cortical adenoma that has suppressed the normal gland, and abrupt cessation of exogenous corticosteroid therapy. Withdrawal of corticosteroid treatment should be carried out by gradually tapering the doses. Acute adrenal insufficiency is characterized by signs and symptoms similar to Addison disease, but manifesting with dramatic severity. Indeed, this is a life-threatening condition requiring emergency administration of IV hydrocortisone (100-300 mg), lest the patient develop irreversible shock. Naturally, fluid infusion should be concomitantly administered, and treatment of the underlying cause (in this case, infection) carried out.

The cosyntropin stimulation test (**choice B**) is used to confirm a diagnosis. However, when the clinical picture is so severe, as in this example, hydrocortisone treatment takes precedence over diagnostic confirmation.

IV mineralocorticoids (**choice C**) are not necessary when such large doses of hydrocortisone are administered, as glucocorticoids also have mineralocorticoid activity.

Oral corticosteroids (**choice D**) would not be appropriate in a medical emergency such as adrenal crisis. They are used once the patient's condition has stabilized. Further, patients in adrenal crisis most often are unable to take anything by mouth because of nausea and vomiting.

Renal ultrasonography (**choice E**) is used to study the kidney and collecting system to screen for such conditions as hydronephrosis and renal masses. It would be hardly justifiable in the present case.

26. **The correct answer is A.** This patient is exhibiting the signs of *Horner syndrome*, resulting from damage to the cervical sympathetic plexus that contains presynaptic fibers to the superior cervical ganglion. This results in deficient sympathetic innervation to the iris and the tarsal muscles of the eye, as well as to the sweat glands and vessels in the ipsilateral face. This deficit leads to miosis and ptosis in the ipsilateral eye, and anhidrosis and redness of the ipsilateral hemiface. The most common cause of this syndrome is pulmonary cancer of the apex, which may spread to the sympathetic plexus by contiguity. A patient presenting with Horner syndrome, especially if a smoker, should undergo radiologic investigations to exclude a lung tumor.

Laboratory testing for syphilis (**choice B**) would be appropriate in the presence of other neurologic signs of syphilitic involvement of the nervous system, such as impaired proprioception and vibration sense. *Argyll-Robertson pupil* is a manifestation of tabes dorsalis. The pupils are small and poorly reactive to light but normally reactive to accommodation.

There is no indication that any type of intracranial pathology is responsible for the ocular changes seen in this case; thus, MRI scan of the head (**choice C**) would not be a useful diagnostic method.

Ophthalmologic referral (**choice D**) would certainly be appropriate for more complex symptomatology, but classic Horner syndrome is an easy diagnosis, which should, without delay, prompt a search for the underlying cause.

Tonometric measurement (**choice E**) is appropriate in the presence of signs suggesting narrow-angle (acute) *glaucoma*, including severe unilateral eye pain, redness, a dilated and fixed pupil, and blurring of vision.

27. **The correct answer is C.** Although cirrhosis usually comes to mind first when you think of ascites, you should remember that ascites can have a variety of causes, both hepatic and nonhepatic. Hepatic causes include cirrhosis (especially alcoholic), chronic hepatitis, severe alcoholic hepatitis without cirrhosis, and Budd-Chiari syndrome (hepatic vein obstruction). Nonhepatic causes include generalized fluid retention (heart disease, nephrotic syndrome, severe hypoalbuminemia, renal failure), intra-abdominal disease (cancer or tuberculosis involving the peritoneum; rarely pancreatitis), and, rarely, hypothyroidism. A useful rule of thumb is that ascites isolated from or disproportionate to peripheral edema is usually due to liver or intra-abdominal disease, whereas systemic diseases such as congestive heart failure tend to produce both peripheral edema and ascites. The clinical findings illustrated in the question stem are typical of congestive heart failure.

Alcoholic cirrhosis (**choice A**) is the most common form of cirrhosis, but it is not usually accompanied by severe peripheral edema.

Chronic hepatitis B infection (**choice B**), even in the absence of cirrhosis, can cause ascites, but it is not usually accompanied by severe peripheral edema.

Intra-abdominal cancers (**choice D**) that have spread to the peritoneum can cause an ascites that is usually not accompanied by severe peripheral edema.

Hypothyroidism (**choice E**) is a rare cause of significant ascites that is usually accompanied by other stigmata of hypothyroidism, such as coarse hair and facial puffiness with periorbital edema and eyelid droop.

28. **The correct answer is B.** The clinical picture is consistent with *mesothelioma*, a cancer of mesothelial origin that manifests as a diffuse plaque-like thickening of the pleura. Peritoneal mesotheliomas are much more uncommon. Most mesotheliomas coming to clinical attention nowadays result from prior occupational exposure to asbestos, which was associated with shipyard work, insulation, brake lining, building and roof work, and mining, among others. Inhalation of asbestos fibers is also a risk factor for other cancers, including bronchogenic, laryngeal, and colon carcinoma. The main differential diagnosis is with bronchogenic carcinoma, which may spread to the pleura but is usually accompanied by one or more intrapulmonary nodules.

Cigarette smoking (**choice A**) does not seem to predispose to the development of mesotheliomas. However, it does increase the risk of bronchogenic carcinoma in persons exposed to asbestos.

Occupational exposures to coal (**choice C**) and silica (**choice D**) are associated with coal-worker pneumoconiosis and silicosis, respectively, but not mesotheliomas.

Prior radiation injury (**choice E**) to the lungs may be followed by two conditions: acute radiation pneumonitis (occurring 2-3 months after radiation) and interstitial fibrosis (manifesting 6-12 months after exposure).

Radiation is not a predisposing factor for either broncho-genic carcinoma or mesothelioma.

29. **The correct answer is A.** An increased platelet count is more formally called thrombocythemia. Thrombocythemia can occur in primary form (essential thrombocythemia), as part of other myeloproliferative disorders (e.g., polycythemia vera, chronic myelogenous leukemia, and idiopathic myelofibrosis), or secondary to other processes such as acute infection, chronic inflammatory disorders (rheumatoid arthritis, inflammatory bowel disease, tuberculosis, sarcoidosis, Wegener granulomatosis), hemorrhage, iron deficiency, or tumors (cancers and lymphomas). Essential thrombocythemia is a clonal abnormality of a hemopoietic stem cell that is seen most often in patients between 50 and 70 years of age. The platelet count may reach 1,000,000/μL or higher, but may also be in a more ambiguous range down to about 500,000/μL. Helpful clinical clues on the peripheral smear are platelet aggregates, giant platelets, and megakaryocyte fragments.

Increased bone marrow fibrosis (**choice B**) and tear-drop shaped RBCs (**choice E**) are features of idiopathic myelofibrosis, which can also have elevated platelet counts.

Increased RBC mass (**choice C**) is a feature of polycythemia vera, which can also show elevated platelet counts.

The Philadelphia chromosome (**choice D**) is a feature of chronic myelogenous leukemia, which can also show elevated platelet counts.

30. **The correct answer is C.** This patient manifests signs and symptoms of fulminant hepatic failure. Infectious hepatitis due to hepatitis B virus (HBV) is responsible for half the cases of fulminant hepatitis in the U.S. Fulminant hepatic failure carries a 60% mortality rate. Drugs are the most frequent nonviral causes of fulminant hepatic failure. Acetaminophen produces liver injury in a dose-dependent fashion. Acute acetaminophen overdose usually manifests with doses higher than 7 g in adults, but concomitant alcohol abuse lowers the threshold of hepatic toxicity. Patients with chronic alcohol abuse may develop acute diffuse liver necrosis (the pathologic substrate of fulminant hepatic failure) after taking as little as 4 g acetaminophen within a 24-hour period. The synergistic effect between alcohol and acetaminophen is mediated by the activating action of alcohol on cytochrome P-450, which converts acetaminophen into a highly toxic intermediate. This intermediate depletes hepatic glutathione stores, resulting in increasing concentration of free radicals and consequent cellular toxicity.

Acetaminophen alone (**choice A**) is also capable of producing significant hepatotoxicity, especially in children. The patient's history suggests, however, that alcohol played a contributing role.

Alcohol alone (**choice B**) is also a hepatotoxic drug and in large amounts may cause acute alcoholic hepatitis. However, fulminant hepatic failure exclusively related to alcohol toxicity is exceedingly rare.

Diazepam alone (**choice D**) does not explain the clinical and laboratory signs of hepatic failure. Diazepam overdose results in prolonged sedation, which usually resolves with supportive measures. Respiratory depression is the most significant and potentially life-threatening consequence. This is particularly likely when diazepam (or similar benzodiazepine) is ingested in association with alcohol (**choice E**).

31. **The correct answer is E.** Genetic screening for MEN type II is available to persons with a family history of this condition. Mutations of the *RET* proto-oncogene make these patients more likely to develop all the endocrine conditions associated with MEN type IIa, including *pheochromocytoma, parathyroid hyperplasia/adenoma,* and *medullary carcinoma* of the thyroid. Medullary carcinoma of the thyroid is an aggressive cancer arising from calcitonin producing cells (C cells) in the thyroid. Although penetrance of this autosomal dominant genetic mutation is incomplete, the risk of developing medullary carcinoma warrants prophylactic thyroidectomy. Recall that MEN IIb is similar to MEN IIa, except for the additional presence of mucosal neuromas and a Marfan-like body habitus.

If persons with family history of MEN type II decline genetic testing, they may be offered the possibility of screening for early medullary carcinoma by calcitonin measurements (**choice A**) following pentagastrin stimulation. Peaks greater than 190 pg/mL in males or 80 pg/mL in females are consistent with medullary carcinoma.

Periodic screening with imaging studies (**choice B**) is not a valuable option to detect early medullary carcinoma, since an early lesion may be too small to be seen on CT or MRI scans.

Periodic screening for latent pheochromocytoma (**choice C**) is not cost-effective, since pheochromocytomas develop less frequently than medullary carcinomas and are usually benign. However, screening for latent pheochromocytoma (urinary catecholamine levels) should be carried out before performing any major surgical procedure to avoid a hypertensive crisis.

Prophylactic parathyroidectomy (**choice D**) is not indicated. Hyperplasia or adenoma of the parathyroids may lead to hyperparathyroidism, in which case parathyroidectomy may be performed.

32. **The correct answer is A.** This is a classic presentation of achalasia, which is an esophageal disorder characterized by impaired esophageal peristalsis and impaired relaxation of the lower esophageal sphincter. It is thought to be due to

malfunction of the esophageal myenteric plexus. Achalasia can occur at any age, but most frequently presents in the third or fourth decade. Achalasia can be complicated by (usually nocturnal) pulmonary aspiration of regurgitated food, life-threatening esophageal rupture, and a questionably increased incidence of esophageal cancer. Treatment of achalasia is by forceful dilation of the lower esophageal sphincter. Sublingual nitroglycerin before meals and calcium channel blockers are sometimes used to prolong the times between lower esophageal forced dilation. More aggressive therapies, such as injection of botulinum toxin in the lower esophageal sphincter or myotomy of the lower esophageal sphincter, are reserved for patients who do not respond to other therapies.

Esophageal cancer (**choice B**) would produce an area of ulceration or a mass in the esophagus, which would have been picked up on the barium swallow.

An esophageal web (**choice C**) is a thin mucosal web that grows across the lumen of the esophagus, typically in the upper esophagus. It would have been detected on the barium studies.

A lower esophageal (Schatzki) ring (**choice D**) is a 2- to 4-mm mucosal ring near the squamocolumnar junction that is probably of congenital origin and usually causes only relatively mild difficulty with swallowing of solids.

Symptomatic diffuse esophageal spasm (**choice E**) differs from achalasia in that there are strong, but poorly coordinated and ineffective, painful esophageal contractions, rather than aperistalsis. Over many years, it may evolve into achalasia, but the disorders are clinically considered distinct.

33. **The correct answer is D.** The patient has both significant nasal disease and significant pulmonary disease. This should suggest the possibility of Wegener granulomatosis (WG), which is a granulomatous inflammation of the upper and/or lower respiratory tract that can also destroy the kidneys. Nasal or pulmonary biopsy confirms the clinically suspected diagnosis by showing granulomas and a perivascular inflammatory infiltrate. If renal damage has occurred, urinalysis typically shows proteinuria, hematuria, and red cell casts. The clinical presentation illustrated is a common variant. Other patients may present with systemic symptoms mimicking cancer (malaise, fever, weight loss, anorexia), migratory polyarthritis, granulomatous skin lesions, or ocular manifestations. WG formerly had a dismal prognosis, but now can be well controlled with immunosuppressive cytotoxic drugs.

Abdominal CT scan (**choice A**) would probably not show anything of significance.

Liver (**choice C**) or pancreatic (**choice D**) enzymes would not be expected to be altered in this condition.

Bladder biopsy (**choice E**) would probably not show anything of significance; however, a renal biopsy might be very helpful.

34. **The correct answer is A.** Astrocytoma typically presents in the 40- to 60-year age range with headaches, focal neurologic symptoms, and seizures. Headaches from tumors may waken patients from sleep and are worse in the morning, presumably from increased intracranial pressure after being supine over night. High-grade astrocytomas tend to enhance diffusely on imaging.

Brain abscesses (**choice B**) may present with headache and focal findings but typically progress more rapidly. Fever is a prominent component. Imaging shows a ring-enhancing lesion.

Cerebral infarcts (**choice C**) rarely cause headaches. The clinical course would not be progressive but would begin acutely and then stabilize. Infarcts may show diffuse enhancement after several weeks.

Complicated migraine (**choice D**) refers to migraine headache with a focal but transient neurologic deficit, which may include language difficulty or hemiparesis. Migraine headaches do not typically waken people from sleep. Patients with complicated migraine have an increased risk of stroke, but imaging studies during a complicated migraine are usually normal.

Meningiomas (**choice E**) are more common in women and may present with headaches and focal features from mass effect. The course tends to be more chronic, however, and imaging will demonstrate an extra-axial structure compressing the underlying brain.

35. **The correct answer is B.** This patient seems to have aggressive erosive disease and requires a disease-modifying (slow-acting antirheumatic) drug (DMARD). There are numerous choices, including methotrexate, cyclosporine, minocycline, and anticytokine (tumor necrosis factor) therapies. Anti-inflammatory doses of NSAIDs are also generally required. Short-term use of prednisone may be of use to control inflammation rapidly, but only in conjunction with disease-modifying therapy. Longer term, low-dose (less than 10 mg) use is common in as many as one-fourth of patients seen in hospital-based clinics because of inadequately controlled inflammation. Anti-inflammatory therapy alone can allow progression of erosive joint disease.

NSAIDs alone (**choice A**) are inappropriate in this case because of the reasons noted above.

Pain relief should occur through control of inflammation, rather than the use of narcotics (**choice C**). The efficacy of narcotics alone in inflammatory arthritic pain is limited.

KAPLAN) MEDICAL

NSAIDs with prednisone (**choice D**) may be very effective for controlling overt symptoms but not for preventing disease progression.

36. **The correct answer is D.** This patient has hepatic encephalopathy (hepatic coma, portal-systemic encephalopathy), a neuropsychiatric syndrome caused by liver disease. It is usually associated with portal-systemic shunting of venous blood, which can cause esophageal varices and dilation of veins near the umbilicus ("caput medusa"). The diagnosis is usually made on clinical, rather than laboratory, grounds, liver function tests correlate poorly. Serum ammonia level is usually elevated, but specific values correlate poorly with clinical status. Therapy is based on removing sources of nitrogen (e.g., protein) in the gut by enema, restriction of dietary protein, and reduction of bacterial load (since some bacteria produce ammonia). Two different strategies are often used for reducing the bacterial load: oral lactulose, which acts as an osmotic cathartic to "wash the bacteria out," and oral neomycin (a poorly absorbed aminoglycoside), which can be used to kill most of the bacteria while minimizing significant systemic side effects. (Oral neomycin is also sometimes used as part of bowel preparation prior to abdominal surgery.) Other types and routes of administration of antibiotics are not usually used in this setting. In some hospitals, oral neomycin is initially used for bacterial load reduction. Patients are then switched to longer term lactulose, thereby limiting the potential nephrotoxicity and ototoxicity of the neomycin.

Oral ampicillin (**choice A**) is a commonly used antibiotic in outpatient settings.

Benzathine penicillin (**choice B**) is an intramuscular, depot form of penicillin that is used most often for syphilis and for month-long prophylaxis against recurrent rheumatic fever.

Oral ceftriaxone (**choice C**) is a commonly used third-generation cephalosporin.

IV penicillin G (**choice E**) is reserved for treatment of patients with sensitive organisms in a hospital setting.

37. **The correct answer is B.** The symptoms (particularly xanthopsia/verdopsia = a yellow-green cast to the vision) are characteristic of digitalis toxicity. Bradycardia and different types of arrhythmias are also effects of excess digitalis. The medication should be immediately discontinued in these cases.

Acute narrow-angle glaucoma (**choice A**) manifests with unilateral severe eye pain and redness, accompanied by blurred vision and halos around lights.

Diuretic-induced hypokalemia (**choice C**) is a potential risk with thiazide and loop diuretics. Intravascular volume depletion, with resultant prerenal azotemia, hyperglycemia, hyperuricemia, and hepatic dysfunction, can also occur.

Enalapril overdose (**choice D**) would manifest with hypotension, which is not present in this case. ACE inhibitors have been shown to improve survival and are a mainstay in the treatment of congestive heart failure. They decrease ventricular preload by causing venous dilatation and diminishing venous return.

38. **The correct answer is A.** This is an example of Addison disease, which can occur in all ages and both sexes and is caused by the destruction of the adrenal cortexes due to processes such as autoimmune disease, tuberculosis, infarction, and cancer. Although the symptoms of Addison disease (chronic adrenocortical insufficiency) are very nonspecific and can easily resemble other endocrine disorders (notably hypothyroidism), significant hyperpigmentation can be a helpful diagnostic clue. With the exception of adrenal insufficiency due to pituitary failure, pigmentation is usually increased because of large amounts of ACTH, which has some activity in stimulating melanocytes. Other symptoms and signs of Addison disease that are not mentioned in the question stem include a decreased tolerance to cold, ECG changes (decreased voltage and prolonged PR), EEG changes (generalized slowing of alpha rhythm), and, in later stages, weight loss, dehydration, hypotension, and small heart size. Adrenal crises, characterized by severe abdominal pain and cardiovascular collapse, may complicate septicemia, trauma, and operative procedures. Vitiligo is likely manifesting another autoimmune disease; autoimmunity increases the likelihood of further autoimmune disease.

Conn disease (**choice B**) is primary aldosteronism. It is characterized by episodic weakness, paresthesias, transient paralysis, tetany, and diastolic hypertension.

Cushing disease (**choice C**) is hypercortisolism due to a pituitary adenoma. It is characterized by rounded facies, buffalo hump, muscle wasting, thin skin, abdominal striae, hypertension, glucose intolerance, and reduced resistance to infection.

Graves disease (**choice D**) is an autoimmune cause of hyperthyroidism, with heat intolerance, palpitations, tachycardia, tremor, and ophthalmopathy.

Hashimoto disease (**choice E**) is an autoimmune cause of (usually) hypothyroidism, with cold intolerance, rubbery goiter, facial puffiness, and sparse, coarse hair.

39. **The correct answer is C.** This patient most likely has Hashimoto thyroiditis, which is the most common cause of thyroiditis in the U.S., with a predominance in women. Patients notice a goiter but are initially euthyroid. Needle biopsy will reveal a lymphocytic infiltration, and serum analysis typically shows antibodies directed against thyroglobulin.

Fibrosis (**choice A**) is seen in Riedel struma, also known as Riedel fibrosing thyroiditis. This disorder is associated with intense fibrosis of the thyroid, leading to induration of neck tissues. The principal importance of this disorder is that it requires differentiation from thyroid neoplasia.

Granulomas (**choice B**) with multinucleate giant cells are seen in subacute granulomatous (de Quervain) thyroiditis.

Neutrophils (**choice D**) would be seen in subacute granu-lomatous (de Quervain) thyroiditis, which usually follows an upper respiratory infection. Symptoms include malaise and pain over the thyroid gland referred to the lower jaw. Patients have a high erythrocyte sediment rate (ESR). Serum T3 and T4 are high and TSH is undetectable.

Parafollicular hyperplasia (**choice E**) is associated with medullary thyroid cancer. Primary thyroid carcino-mas may be classified into two varieties, depending on whether the lesions arise from the thyroid follicular epithelium or from the parafollicular, or C, cells. The mainstay of therapy is surgical excision; external radia-tion and chemotherapy have a palliative role for excision for recurrent or residual disease.

40. **The correct answer is A.** This patient clearly has an anemia that is long-standing and is not related to her menses, considering that she had a hysterectomy and the anemia persists, plus this patient is of Mediterranean descent. The most likely cause of her anemia is an abnormal hemoglobin, such as thalassemia, because her RDW is less than 15%. Therefore, the most appropriate diagnostic option for this patient would be a hemoglobin electrophoresis.

Bone marrow biopsy (**choice B**) in patients with micro-cytic anemia is indicated only if sideroblastic anemia were suspected; in this patient, the diagnosis of sidero-blastic anemia is not considered.

Prescribing oral ferrous sulfate (**choice C**) or ordering iron, ferritin, and total iron binding capacity (**choice E**) would be incorrect. If this patient had iron deficiency anemia her RDW would be above 15%. If iron deficiency anemia were suspected, then iron studies would be of diagnostic value.

Ordering B_{12} and folate levels (**choice D**) is not indicated because this is a *microcytic* anemia; B_{12} and folate defi-ciency would produce a *macrocytic* anemia.

41. **The correct answer is A.** The most appropriate pharma-cologic treatment of hypertension in diabetic patients is an ACE inhibitor, especially if there is concomitant evidence of diabetic glomerulopathy (i.e., microalbu-minuria). Studies have shown that ACE inhibitors exert a beneficial effect on diabetic nephropathy by lowering the intraglomerular capillary pressure. Thus, ACE inhibitors

are also used to slow the progression of asymptomatic diabetic glomerulonephropathy, even in the absence of systemic hypertension.

Most studies have suggested that monotherapy with either a beta blocker (**choice B**) or a thiazide diuretic (**choice E**) is the most appropriate initial treatment for uncomplicated hypertension (i.e., hypertension without detectable end-organ damage).

Calcium channel blockers (**choice C**) are frequently used as first-line antihypertensive agents. These drugs are also beneficial in case the patient has asthma, migraine, or urinary incontinence. However, recent studies have sug-gested an association between use of calcium channel blockers and cardiac complications.

Central alpha-agonists (e.g., clonidine [**choice D**]), are seldom used as first-line agents for treatment of hypertension because of their undesirable side effects. Methyldopa is frequently used in pregnancy.

42. **The correct answer is D.** This patient has a sickle cell pain crisis, a condition caused by microvascular occlusive events. The pain is severe and often requires admission for pain control with narcotic level analgesics and rehy-dration.

Acetaminophen (**choice A**) and aspirin (**choice B**) can be adjunct pain medications but are not likely to provide adequate control for a sickle cell pain crisis.

Broad-spectrum antibiotics (**choice C**) are inappropriate. Mild infections often can cause a sickle cell crisis. Low-grade fevers, anemia, and leukocytosis are common in a sickle cell crisis and do not indicate sepsis.

Plasma exchange (**choice E**) may be used if a sickle cell crisis progresses to multiorgan failure. It is not indicated for an acute pain episode.

43. **The correct answer is E.** What is illustrated here is a clas-sic example of nephrotic syndrome: abundant urine loss of proteins, which constitutes the *first* pathophysiologic event in the chain leading to hypoproteinemia; edema due to reduced oncotic pressure; and hyperlipidemia sec-ondary to a compensatory increase in hepatic lipoprotein synthesis. Alterations in plasma proteins often result in an elevated erythrocyte sedimentation rate (ESR). Loss of plasma globulins increases susceptibility to infection. Finally, loss of antithrombin III, protein C, and protein S (circulating anticoagulants) results in predisposition for venous thrombosis. Renal venous thrombosis is particu-larly dangerous in this setting.

Acute pyelonephritis (**choice A**) is not a complication of nephrotic syndrome or any of the diseases associated with it. Infections in the setting of nephrotic syndrome usually involve the respiratory tract and are sustained by gram-positive organisms.

KAPLAN) MEDICAL

Acute renal failure (**choice B**) does not constitute an immediate threat for patients with nephrotic syndrome. Depending on the underlying glomerular disease, progression to chronic renal failure occurs more or less frequently.

Hemorrhages (**choice C**) do not frequently occur. Nephrotic syndrome results in abnormal hypercoagulability.

Hypertension (**choice D**) is a manifestation of nephritic syndrome, along with hematuria and mild proteinuria (<3 g/day).

44. **The correct answer is E.** We already know that this woman has Hodgkin lymphoma with disease in her cervical nodes, mediastinum, and bone marrow (stage IV). The standard initial treatment for her is chemotherapy.

Surgical excision of affected nodes (**choice A**) is not indicated for Hodgkin lymphoma. The role of the surgeon in this disease is limited to diagnosis. In visceral lymphoma, on the other hand, surgical resection may be part of the overall therapeutic plan.

Bone marrow transplant (**choice B**) may be used in selected patients who have failed standard therapy, but it would not be first-line treatment.

Radiation therapy (**choice C**) often is used for localized disease. This woman has systemic, advanced disease that is best treated with chemotherapy. In selected cases both modalities may be combined.

Staging laparotomy (**choice D**) is a vanishing tool, rarely used nowadays. When radiation therapy was the main modality and CT scans were not readily available, it was important to know if abdominal disease was present to select the best treatment. Although the abdominal CT scan in this case was nondiagnostic, we already have enough information from the chest CT and the bone marrow biopsy to choose chemotherapy. Abdominal exploration is not needed.

45. **The correct answer is D.** This presentation and past medical history are suggestive of hemolytic anemia due to glucose-6-phosphate dehydrogenase (G6PD) deficiency. This X-linked genetic defect makes erythrocytes vulnerable to oxidative damage, which may be triggered by infections, drugs, or naturally occurring substances. About 1 million people are affected by this disorder throughout the world, with the highest prevalence in some Mediterranean regions (Sardinia, Sicily, Greece, and Turkey) and western Africa. In the U.S., G6PD deficiency affects 10% to 15% of African Americans. The clinical symptomatology is characterized by recurring episodes of acute hemolysis. A more severe Mediterranean variant results in chronic hemolysis with prominent reticulocytosis, as well as classic hemolytic crises. Dark-colored urine is due to severe hemoglobinuria. Severe hemolytic episodes may be life-threatening and require urgent blood transfusion.

46. **The correct answer is L.** Sickle cell anemia results from an autosomal recessive mutation of the beta-globin chain of hemoglobin, resulting in an abnormal form of hemoglobin (HbS). Chronic hemolytic anemia, painful episodes due to vaso-occlusive crises, splenomegaly, chronic ulcers of the legs, and susceptibility to infection by the pneumococci and other bacteria are among its most common manifestations. Hematocrit lower than 30%, sickle-shaped erythrocytes, reticulocytosis, and *Howell-Jolly bodies* are characteristic hematologic features. Approximately 8% of African Americans are carriers of the HbS gene. The diagnosis rests on electrophoretic demonstration of HbS in peripheral blood.

Anemia of chronic disease (**choice A**) may complicate any chronic disorder, such as rheumatoid arthritis, collagen vascular diseases, cancer, and liver disease. It is a normocytic and normochromic anemia, usually of mild-to-moderate degree. It results from iron sequestration in the bone marrow.

Aplastic anemia (**choice B**) is due to bone marrow suppression. Usually, it is seen in conjunction with neutropenia and thrombocytopenia (pancytopenia). Most cases are idiopathic, but drugs are among the most common identifiable causes.

Chronic lymphocytic leukemia (CLL; **choice C**) is an indolent form of leukemia that affects middle-aged and elderly individuals. It is characterized by marked lymphocytosis in the blood and bone marrow, resulting from progressive accumulation of monoclonal (but well-differentiated) B lymphocytes. Anemia and thrombocytopenia eventually manifest as a result of bone marrow replacement.

Hairy cell leukemia (**choice E**) is a rare form of leukemia due to neoplastic transformation of a subset of B lymphocytes. The designation derives from the characteristic hair-like cytoplasmic projections of leukemic cells. Pancytopenia and massive splenomegaly are consistently present.

Hereditary spherocytosis (**choice F**) is characterized by spherocytes (small round erythrocytes lacking central pallor) and reticulocytosis on peripheral blood smears. Such abnormal spherocytes are prone to lysis. Chronic hemolysis ensues, with secondary splenomegaly. The underlying abnormality is a defect in *spectrin*, a cytoskeletal protein forming the scaffolding of the erythrocytic membrane.

Iron-deficiency anemia (**choice G**) is characterized by small, hypochromic erythrocytes (microcytic and hypochromic anemia) and usually results from chronic blood loss.

Megaloblastic anemia (**choice H**) is so designated because of the presence of megaloblasts in the bone marrow. Megaloblasts are abnormally large red blood cell precursors. Their counterparts in peripheral blood are macrocytes, large red blood cells having a mean corpuscular volume of up to 130 fL. Macrocytic (megaloblastic) anemia is due to vitamin B_{12} or folate deficiency.

Microangiopathic anemia (**choice I**) is a form of hemolytic anemia due to "mechanical" causes, usually resulting from the presence of widespread small thrombi in the microcirculation or prosthetic cardiac devices. Fragmentation of red blood cells is the crucial pathophysiologic event, which leads to the appearance of characteristic *schistocytes* in peripheral blood smears. DIC and thrombotic thrombocytopenic purpura are examples of diseases leading to this form of anemia.

Myelodysplastic syndrome (**choice J**) is a heterogeneous set of disorders characterized by abnormal maturation of bone marrow stem cells. Cytopenias (affecting at least two blood cell lines) associated with hypercellular bone marrow are characteristic. Myelodysplastic syndromes affect elderly persons, who may come to medical attention because of chronic fatigue or bleeding diatheses. Some subsets of myelodysplastic syndromes have a propensity to leukemic transformation.

Myelofibrosis (**choice K**) is characterized by progressive bone marrow fibrosis and resultant pancytopenia. As the spleen takes over hematopoietic functions, massive splenomegaly develops. *Teardrop*-like erythrocytes are the most peculiar morphologic abnormalities on peripheral blood smears.

Thalassemia (**choice M**) is a group of hereditary disorders due to deficient production of one of the globin chains (either alpha or beta, or both). Microcytosis is prominent. Positive family history is usually present. Alpha-thalassemia is seen most frequently in people from southeast Asia, whereas beta-thalassemia is seen most commonly in Mediterranean people. Both forms are found in African Americans. The clinical manifestations depend on whether the individual is heterozygous or homozygous. In the most severe forms, manifestations appear after 6 months of age, with growth failure, jaundice, hepatosplenomegaly, and bone and facial deformities. In carriers of thalassemia trait, microcytosis is often the only sign.

47. **The correct answer is K.** The type of jaundice manifested by this patient is obstructive, as evidenced by mostly conjugated hyperbilirubinemia, high serum levels of alkaline phosphatase, and clay-colored stools. Concomitant weight loss and deep epigastric pain are highly suggestive of pancreatic malignancy. The presence of a distended gallbladder associated with jaundice, known as *Courvoisier sign,* is also suggestive of cancer. Infiltration of the pancreas may also lead to insulin deficiency and glucose intolerance (hence, the hyperglycemia detected in this patient). Although relatively rare, this cancer represents the fifth most common cause of cancer-related deaths in the U.S., since it comes to medical attention in advanced, usually inoperable, stages.

48. **The correct answer is P.** Wilson disease should be suspected in any case of cirrhosis or chronic hepatitis manifesting in children or young adults. The presence of *Kayser-Fleischer rings* in the cornea is pathognomonic of this condition. Neuropsychiatric manifestations may precede or follow hepatic involvement. Wilson disease is an autosomal recessive disorder caused by mutations of a gene that codes for a copper-transporting protein in the hepatocytes (not ceruloplasmin). The diagnosis is confirmed by low serum ceruloplasmin levels, high urinary copper excretion, and high copper content in liver biopsy.

Acute cholangitis (**choice A**) is usually secondary to a gallstone in the common bile duct. In this case, pain and obstructive jaundice are associated with fever, since enteric bacteria gain access to the biliary system and cause infection (*ascending cholangitis*).

Acute cholecystitis (**choice B**) manifests with the classic picture of biliary colic, characterized by pain in the right hypochondrium radiating to the right shoulder. It is usually related to a small gallstone that becomes impacted in the cystic duct, resulting in blockage of bile outflow and acute distention and inflammation of gallbladder.

Acute pancreatitis (**choice C**) is an emergency condition manifesting with extremely severe deep abdominal pain and frequently associated with shock. Elevated amylase and lipase levels in the serum support the diagnosis.

Adenoma of the liver (**choice D**) is most commonly asymptomatic and may be discovered incidentally. However, severe intraperitoneal hemorrhage due to rupture may constitute a life-threatening presentation. Use of oral contraceptives and anabolic steroids are predisposing conditions.

Alcoholic hepatitis (**choice E**) is similar to any other form of acute hepatitis in its clinical manifestations and laboratory findings. Abdominal pain, nausea, mild jaundice, low-grade fever, and malaise are associated with elevated serum transaminase levels.

Amebic liver abscess (**choice F**) presents with right upper quadrant pain and fever. Usually, the patient comes to medical attention after several weeks of symptoms. A recent travel history to tropical countries is often elicited. Liver tests are mildly abnormal. Ultrasonography, CT, or MRI demonstrates the location and size of the lesion. The aspirated fluid is often described as "anchovy paste."

Focal nodular hyperplasia (**choice G**) is a nodular lesion consisting of hepatocytes and a stellate-shaped fibrous stroma (a sort of "focal cirrhosis"). It is usually asymptomatic. It is most commonly associated with chronic alcohol abuse.

Gilbert syndrome (**choice H**) is a form of hereditary jaundice due to *glucuronyl transferase* deficiency. Bilirubin is thus mostly of the indirect (unconjugated) type. The condition is benign and asymptomatic (except for jaundice).

Hemochromatosis (**choice I**) is an autosomal recessive hereditary disorder caused by excessive intestinal absorption of iron. Iron deposition results in cirrhosis, cardiomyopathy, pancreatic damage with diabetes, and skin hyperpigmentation (due to melanin overproduction, not iron itself).

Hepatocellular carcinoma (**choice J**) is most often associated with cirrhosis in industrialized countries. Its development may be unsuspected until the cirrhotic patient manifests rapid deterioration and weight loss.

Primary biliary cirrhosis (**choice L**) is characteristic of middle-aged women and is associated with high titers of circulating antimitochondrial autoantibodies.

Primary sclerosing cholangitis (**choice M**) is a rare disorder affecting patients with some underlying disease, most commonly ulcerative colitis. It is due to a chronic inflammatory reaction of probable autoimmune origin, which results in sclerosis and obliteration of the extrahepatic bile ducts. Progressively severe obstructive jaundice is the presenting picture.

Rotor syndrome (**choice N**) is another hereditary form of jaundice caused by deficient liver excretion of conjugated bilirubin. Since activity of glucuronyl transferase is normal, most circulating bilirubin is of the direct (conjugated) type. The condition is benign.

Viral hepatitis (**choice O**) manifests with an acute syndrome characterized by right upper abdominal pain, nausea, malaise, low-grade fever, and laboratory signs of hepatocellular necrosis. This picture is shared by all forms of viral hepatitis, but acute infection due to HCV is usually asymptomatic.

49. **The correct answer is E.** When GFR falls below 25%, phosphorus excretion becomes impaired, leading to hyperphosphatemia. Hyperphosphatemia results in hypocalcemia, triggering increased release of parathyroid hormone (PTH; **choice E**). High PTH levels increase phosphaturia and normalize serum calcium levels, but at the expense of bone calcium. Concomitantly, renal failure results in decreased hydroxylation of 25-hydroxycholecalciferol to 1,25-dihydroxycholecalciferol (the metabolically active form of vitamin D_3), leading to decreased intestinal absorption of calcium. Loss of renal function causes metabolic acidosis, and the excess hydrogen ions in the blood are buffered by calcium salts deriving from bone. Finally, aluminum, used in chronic renal failure as a phosphorus binder, may itself deposit in the bone, contributing to bone damage. All these factors, in varying degrees, result in renal osteodystrophy, which manifests with rarefaction of bone (osteomalacia) on x-ray films, bone pains, muscle weakness, and pathologic fractures. On x-ray films, the phalanges and the distal third of the clavicles appear more severely affected.

50. **The correct answer is D.** Hypertension is an inevitable consequence, and the most common complication, of chronic renal failure. Control of hypertension is crucial in the management of renal failure as high blood pressure accelerates renal damage. While fluid and salt retention (**choice D**) plays the most important pathogenetic role, other factors may contribute. Recombinant erythropoietin, used to treat anemia, causes hypertension in about 20% of cases. Hypertension may develop abruptly at the beginning of treatment.

Accumulation of uremic toxins (**choice A**) has deleterious effects on many tissues and organs. It is thought responsible for the development of uremic *encephalopathy* (obtunded sensorium), *peripheral neuropathy*, and uremic *pericarditis*. The occurrence of any of these complications warrants initiation of renal replacement therapy to eliminate uremic toxins.

Hyperkalemia (**choice B**) usually develops when GFR falls below 10% of normal, but many endogenous and exogenous factors may hasten its appearance. Hyperkalemia interferes with neuromuscular junctions and causes *muscle weakness*, abdominal distention, and diarrhea. It also affects cardiac fiber excitability, resulting in *arrhythmias*. Chronic hyperkalemia is treated with dietary restriction and, if necessary, oral administration of an ion exchange resin such as sodium polystyrene sulfonate.

Platelet dysfunction (**choice C**) is thought to be the principal mechanism of *coagulopathy* associated with chronic renal failure. While platelet number might be only slightly decreased, platelet adhesiveness and aggregation are impaired, which manifests with prolonged bleeding time. Patients with chronic renal failure, therefore, frequently develop purpura and petechiae.

Shunting of blood through arteriovenous fistula (**choice F**) occurs in patients treated with hemodialysis in which vascular access is guaranteed by establishing a permanent arteriovenous fistula. Shunting of blood through such fistula may contribute to the development of *congestive heart failure*. Other factors include anemia and salt and fluid retention.

Internal Medicine: **Test Eight**

1. A 57-year-old man is noted on a pre-employment physical to have "moon facies" and truncal obesity with a "buffalo hump." Muscle wasting and abdominal striae are also noted. The man is referred to an internal medicine specialist for further evaluation. Early morning plasma cortisol is 35 mg/dL. A screening dexamethasone suppression test is then ordered, in which 1 mg of oral dexamethasone is given at 11:30 P.M. The following morning, a 7:00 A.M. plasma cortisol is 6 mg/dL. No dexamethasone is given for 1 week. Then a repeat study is performed in which oral dexamethasone 0.5 mg every 6 hours is given for 2 days. Urinary free cortisol on the second day is 30 mg/24 hours. The oral dose of dexamethasone is then increased to 2 mg every 6 hours for 2 days, and urinary free cortisol is 10 mg/24 hours on the fourth day. These findings are most consistent with which of the following?

    (A) Exogenous cortisol administration

    (B) Hypersecretion of ACTH by an adrenal tumor

    (C) Hypersecretion of ACTH by the pituitary gland

    (D) Hypersecretion of ACTH by a small cell carcinoma

    (E) Hypersecretion of cortisol by an adrenal tumor

2. A 57-year-old man is referred for a neurologic consultation because of a 10-week history of rapidly progressive impairment of memory, increasing drowsiness, and abnormal jerking movements. The neurologist observes that myoclonic jerks can be elicited by sudden acoustic stimuli, such as hand clapping. Routine blood studies are within normal limits, and CSF shows no alterations. EEG studies reveal periodic complexes of slow waves occurring at intervals of 1 to 2 seconds. MRI shows hyperintense signals bilaterally in the caudate-putamen, but no brain atrophy, ventricular dilatation, or focal intracranial lesions. Which of the following is the most common epidemiologic form of this disorder?

    (A) Acquired by occupational exposure

    (B) Acquired from cadaveric growth hormone

    (C) Acquired from ingestion of beef

    (D) Familial

    (E) Sporadic

3. A 23-year-old man who moved to the U.S. from a southern province of China comes to medical attention because of a right serous otitis media for 4 months. The patient denies recent upper respiratory infections or previous history of allergies. General examination is unremarkable. There is swelling of the nasopharyngeal mucosa, resulting in obstruction of the right auditory tube. Inspection of the ear canal reveals a dull tympanic membrane and air bubbles in the middle ear. No cervical lymphadenopathy is found. Which of the following is the most appropriate next step in management?

    (A) Blind (random) biopsies of nasopharyngeal mucosa

    (B) Measurement of serum IgG antibodies to Epstein-Barr virus (EBV)

    (C) MRI scans of the head and neck

    (D) Placement of a ventilation tube through the tympanic membrane

    (E) Short course of oral corticosteroids

    (F) Treatment with oral antibiotics

4. Two months after a full course of radiation therapy for carcinoma of the right lung, a 64-year-old man develops increasing shortness of breath, dry cough, and temperatures to 38.5° C (101.3° F). Chest examination reveals inspiratory crackles over the right lung. Laboratory studies show a leukocyte count of 11,500/mm^3 and an erythrocyte sedimentation (ESR) rate of 88 mm/hour. A chest x-ray film shows a sharply demarcated infiltrate with a ground-glass appearance in the right lung. Which of the following is the most likely diagnosis?

    (A) Bacterial pneumonia

    (B) Cytomegalovirus (CMV) pneumonia

    (C) Pulmonary radiation fibrosis

    (D) Radiation pneumonitis

    (E) Recurrence of primary carcinoma

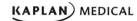

5. A medical consultant for a managed care organization receives a call from a hospital administrator who is concerned about the health care dollars spent on patients with lung cancer over the past 5 years. The administrator wants to reduce the expenditures for treatment by implementing a screening test for lung cancer. What should the consultant advise the administrator?

    (A) Annual chest x-ray after age 50

    (B) Annual chest x-ray after age 40 for all smokers

    (C) Annual physical exam with pulmonary function tests

    (D) Annual questionnaire to look for high risk behaviors

    (E) No effective screening program is available

6. An obese, premenopausal, 41-year-old woman with a 30+ year smoking history presents complaining of malaise, weakness, anorexia, constipation, and back pain. She reports having been told that she has high blood pressure but does not take any medication. The patient states that her mother died of cancer, and her father died in a farming accident. During the course of the interview, the physician notes the presence of an intermittent cough. A chest x-ray film shows a solitary, coin-shaped lesion in the right upper lobe of the lung. Laboratory studies reveal the following:

Albumin	3.2 mg/dL
Calcium	14 mg/dL
Phosphorus	2.6 mg/dL
Chloride	110 mg/dL
BUN	45 mg/dL
Creatinine	2.0 mg/dL

    On physical examination, the patient is generally lethargic. Her lungs are clear to auscultation bilaterally with no wheezes. Bowel sounds are hypoactive, but she does not complain of any pain on palpation of her abdomen. Which of the following is the most appropriate next step in management?

    (A) Administration of IV bisphosphonates

    (B) Administration of IV normal saline

    (C) Administration of thiazide diuretics

    (D) Bronchoscopy

    (E) Collection of sputum samples

7. A 27-year-old Hispanic man presents complaining of cough for the past 4 days. He has been coughing up yellow sputum for the past 2 days and has had a temperature of up to 38.0° C (100.5° F). The man admits to smoking an average of one pack of cigarettes daily for the past 10 years. He denies prior illnesses similar to the present one, stating that he has always been "healthy as a horse." Physical examination is remarkable for diffuse rhonchi bilaterally, with no areas of consolidation. Which of the following is the most likely diagnosis?

    (A) Acute bronchitis

    (B) Chronic bronchitis

    (C) Cystic fibrosis

    (D) Pneumonia

    (E) Sinusitis

8. A 72-year-old woman comes to the physician because of persistent left lower abdominal pain and frequency of urination for 2 days. In the past year, she had similar episodes accompanied by mild fever, which resolved spontaneously. Her temperature is 38.5° C (101.3° F). Tenderness is noted on palpation of the left lower quadrant of the abdomen. Bowel sounds are absent. Complete blood count shows 12,000 leukocytes/mm^3, with 85% neutrophils. Microscopic urinalysis shows 5 leukocytes/high power field. A test of stool is positive for occult blood. Which of the following is the most appropriate next step in evaluation?

    (A) Plain abdominal x-ray film

    (B) CT scan of the abdomen

    (C) Barium enema

    (D) Colonoscopy

    (E) Intravenous pyelography

9. A 32-year-old woman comes to the physician because of sudden onset of palpitations and fatigue. She says that she has been in good health until a couple of months ago, when she began to lose weight despite an apparent increase in appetite. She also has insomnia and increasing anxiety. She is 168 cm (66 in) tall and weighs 50 kg (110 lb). Her temperature is 37.2° C (100.0° F), blood pressure is 140/65 mm Hg, and pulse is 120/min and irregular. Her lungs are clear to auscultation. An ECG reveals atrial fibrillation. Which of the following is the most appropriate next step in diagnosis?

   (A) Chest x-ray

   (B) Complete blood count

   (C) Echocardiogram

   (D) Neuropsychiatric referral

   (E) Thyroid-stimulating hormone (TSH) assay

10. A 32-year-old nurse complains of sporadic episodes of feeling lightheaded and dizzy. Laboratory analysis shows persistently low glucose levels of less than 50 mg/dL during the episodes. Insulin levels are elevated, but C-peptide levels are low. Insulin antibodies are present. Which of the following is the most likely diagnosis?

    (A) Alimentary hypoglycemia

    (B) Insulinoma

    (C) Surreptitious insulin administration

    (D) Surreptitious oral sulfonylurea administration

11. An Alabama gardener consults a physician about lesions on his hand and forearm. The initial lesion had been a small, nontender papule that slowly expanded and developed a necrotic central area. About a week later, the patient noticed several subcutaneous nodules in his forearm. He didn't think they had been there before, but he wasn't absolutely sure. These nodules continued to enlarge, and he sought medical care when one of them started to ulcerate. Throughout this entire period, the patient had no systemic symptoms. At the time of the physician's examination of the arm, the patient had lesions for approximately 1 month. The physician's examination confirms the patient's observations. It is also noted that the draining nodules are arranged as a chain running proximally up the arm with the most distal lesion being the initial one. Which of the following is the most likely diagnosis?

    (A) Aspergillosis

    (B) Candidiasis

    (C) Cryptococcosis

    (D) Mucormycosis

    (E) Sporotrichosis

12. A 23-year-old woman consults a physician because she has just learned that her sexual partner has chronic hepatitis B infection. She is not clinically ill, but she is very worried that she may have been exposed to the virus. Which of the following offers the first evidence of acute hepatitis B infection?

    (A) Anti-HBc

    (B) Anti-HBs

    (C) HBcAg

    (D) HBeAg

    (E) HBsAg

13. A 45-year-old woman undergoes thyroid surgery to remove a nodular goiter. Afterward, the surgeon returns daily to lightly tap the facial nerve just anterior to the exterior auditory meatus to see whether this causes the patient's facial muscles to twitch. This physical sign is a marker for which of the following electrolyte disturbances?

    (A) Hyperchloremia

    (B) Hyperkalemia

    (C) Hypernatremia

    (D) Hypocalcemia

    (E) Hypophosphatemia

14. A pregnant woman complains to her obstetrician of changes on her face. Examination demonstrates areas of hyperpigmentation on the woman's forehead, temples, and cheeks. The lesions are brown, sharply marginated patches of skin several inches across. The skin texture in these areas is normal. Which of the following is the most likely diagnosis?

    (A) Actinic keratosis

    (B) Melasma

    (C) Miliaria

    (D) Nevus flammeus

    (E) Seborrheic keratosis

15. A 32-year-old African American man has a routine physical examination with blood studies for life insurance purposes. Serum chemistries are notable for a serum calcium level of 12.1 mg/dL; other values are within normal limits. If parathyroid disease is excluded, which of the following is the most likely cause of this man's hypercalcemia?

    (A) Bartter syndrome

    (B) Crohn disease

    (C) Pancreatitis

    (D) Sarcoidosis

    (E) Systemic lupus erythematosus

16. A 52-year-old woman comes to the physician because of generalized itching. Her vital signs are within normal limits. Examination reveals jaundiced sclerae, mildly enlarged liver, and small xanthomas around the eyelids. Serum chemistry shows:

ALT	200 U/L
AST	150 U/L
Alkaline phosphatase	700 U/L
Bilirubin	
Total	3.8 mg/dL
Direct	2.1 mg/dL
Cholesterol	240 mg/dL

    High titers of circulating antimitochondrial autoantibodies are found. Which of the following is the most likely diagnosis?

    (A) Alcohol-related liver disease

    (B) Autoimmune hepatitis

    (C) Hemochromatosis

    (D) Primary biliary cirrhosis

    (E) Wilson disease

17. A 40-year-old obese woman consults a gynecologist because of chronic vaginal discharge. Gynecologic examination demonstrates cheesy, curd-like, white vaginal discharge. Culture of this material demonstrates *Candida albicans*. The patient's infection clears with oral itraconazole but recurs 1 month later. During the recurrence, she also develops candidiasis of the skin beneath her breasts and of her oral cavity. Which of the following screening blood biochemistry tests would be most appropriate at this point?

    (A) Bicarbonate

    (B) Calcium

    (C) Glucose

    (D) Iron

    (E) Sodium

18. A 52-year-old man with a history of psoriasis, hypertension, and alcohol abuse has a diet that consists mainly of beer and potato chips. For the past few months he has had a tingling sensation in his hands and legs. On examination, he is mildly obese and has numerous spider angiomata on his chest. There is diminished proprioception and vibratory sensation in all four extremities distally. Distal strength and deep tendon reflexes are also symmetrically diminished. A Romberg sign and bilateral Babinski signs are present. Which of the following is the most likely diagnosis?

    (A) Niacin deficiency

    (B) Protein deficiency

    (C) Vitamin B_{12} deficiency

    (D) Vitamin C deficiency

    (E) Zinc deficiency

19. A surgeon performing a needle liver biopsy sustains an accidental needle stick during the procedure. Three months later, the physician has newly developed anti-HCV antibodies. What is the chance of developing chronic hepatitis C infection, once infection is documented?

    (A) 10%

    (B) 20%

    (C) 45%

    (D) 75%

    (E) 98%

20. A 35-year-old African American woman consults a physician because of patches of pale skin that have been developing over the past several years. Once a patch develops, it never seems to get dark again, and it burns easily when she goes into the sun. Physical examination demonstrates a half dozen hypopigmented patches of skin on the neck and trunk that vary in size from 1 to 6 cm. The involved skin appears otherwise normal, with no erythema or irregularities of texture noted. Which of the following is the most likely diagnosis?

(A) Albinism

(B) Keloid

(C) Lentigo

(D) Melasma

(E) Vitiligo

21. A 70-year-old woman with a history of diabetes mellitus, hypertension, chronic obstructive lung disease, and congestive heart failure is admitted to the hospital for a deep vein thrombosis of the right lower extremity. Heparin is started at the time of admission. Her outpatient medications include NPH insulin, furosemide, albuterol, enalapril, and metoprolol. Admission laboratories show an elevated potassium level (6.0 mEq/L), which is confirmed on repeat testing. Which of the following medications should be discontinued?

(A) Albuterol

(B) Enalapril

(C) Furosemide

(D) Heparin

(E) NPH insulin

22. A 25-year-old woman consults a physician because of a persistent "sore throat." Approximately 3 weeks earlier, she had an upper respiratory infection, which never seemed to completely resolve. She was still experiencing fevers, and the pain in her throat, particularly on swallowing, seemed to be getting worse. Her temperature is 38.1° C (100.6° F), blood pressure is 110/60 mm Hg, pulse is 60/min, and respirations are 12/min. No erythema, exudates, or swelling are seen on examination of the pharynx. However, the thyroid gland is asymmetrically enlarged, firm, and exquisitely tender. Which of the following is the most likely diagnosis?

(A) Graves disease

(B) Medullary carcinoma

(C) Nontoxic goiter

(D) Papillary carcinoma

(E) Subacute thyroiditis

23. A 73-year old man presents with a chief complaint of three episodes of fainting over the past month. He also relates several episodes of left-sided chest pain that occurred with exertion and resolved on resting. Furthermore, he has noticed increasing leg edema and orthopnea. He has no prior cardiac history and is not on any medications. His blood pressure is 130/70 mm Hg, and his pulse is 70/min. Pitting edema is present in both lower extremities. The carotid upstroke is delayed. Cardiac examination is remarkable for a normal S1 and a soft, single S2. A harsh, late peaking systolic ejection murmur is heard in the right upper sternal border. An ECG shows signs of left ventricular hypertrophy. Which of the following is the most likely diagnosis?

(A) Aortic insufficiency

(B) Aortic stenosis

(C) Mitral insufficiency

(D) Mitral stenosis

(E) Tricuspid insufficiency

24. An 81-year-old woman is admitted to the hospital for worsening depression and questionable dementia. She has a past medical history of type 1 diabetes mellitus, hypertension, and an anterior wall myocardial infarction 10 years ago. She takes nifedipine, atenolol, insulin, aspirin, furosemide, simvastatin, multivitamins, and Colace, and was recently started on methylphenidate (Ritalin) for depression by her primary care physician. She lives at home, and her family reports that she has become increasingly withdrawn and confused over the past few months. On examination, she is obese and in no distress, and has normal vital signs. Her neck is supple, with a normal thyroid, clear lungs, and 1+ nonpitting lower extremity edema. She is alert to person and month but not to date or location. She has poor concentration. In addition to evaluation of her medication list for potential causes of confusion, which of the following is the most appropriate next step in diagnosis?

    (A) Calcium level
    (B) Diffusion weighted MRI of brain
    (C) Head CT scan with contrast
    (D) Rapid plasma reagin test
    (E) Thyroid stimulating hormone level

25. A 25-year-old, apparently healthy man undergoes a complete physical as part of screening for health insurance. The physical is negative, but chemistry screening shows plasma bilirubin of 2.1 mg/dL as the only abnormal finding. The man is referred to an internist for further evaluation. The internist notes that all the serum liver enzymes are within normal limits and that there is no evidence on complete blood count of anemia or reticulocytosis. The urine is negative for bile compounds. Fractionation of the plasma bilirubin demonstrates a predominance of unconjugated bilirubin. Which of the following is the most likely diagnosis?

    (A) Alcoholic hepatitis
    (B) Crigler-Najjar syndrome
    (C) Gilbert syndrome
    (D) Hepatitis A infection
    (E) Hepatitis B infection

26. A 46-year-old man comes to medical attention because of slowly progressive dyspnea on exertion over a 6-month period. His blood pressure is 110/75 mm Hg, pulse is 106/min, and respirations are 18/min. The patient underwent radiation therapy for a mediastinal neoplasm 10 years ago. On examination, the liver is palpable 3 cm below the right costal margin. Heart sounds are decreased in intensity, and jugular veins appear distended, especially during inspiration. Bibasilar crackles that clear with coughing are detected on chest auscultation. A chest x-ray film shows calcifications around the heart, which appears of normal size. Echocardiography reveals a thickened pericardial sac, but the ventricular wall appears normal. Which of the following is the most likely diagnosis?

    (A) Dilated cardiomyopathy
    (B) Hypertrophic cardiomyopathy
    (C) Pericardial tamponade
    (D) Restrictive pericarditis
    (E) Tricuspid regurgitation

27. A fair-skinned, 53-year-old woman comes to her physician because of a nodule behind the right ear, which has been growing very slowly for years. She is worried, however, because the nodule recently developed a scab. Examination reveals a 2-cm nodular lesion, with rolled-up edges and central erosion. The rest of the physical examination is otherwise normal. Which of the following would a biopsy likely show?

    (A) Actinic keratosis
    (B) Basal cell carcinoma
    (C) Hemangioma
    (D) Keratoacanthoma
    (E) Melanoma
    (F) Psoriasis
    (G) Seborrheic keratosis

28. A 46-year-old woman presents with a chief complaint of chest pain on inspiration. She states that the pain is on the left side and is lessened when she sits up and leans forward. She has a history of chronic renal failure from diabetes, and usually undergoes hemodialysis three times a week but has missed her last four appointments. On auscultation, there is a scratchy, leathery sound heard during both systole and diastole. An ECG shows diffuse S-T segment elevation and P-R segment depression. The QRS amplitude is low. Which of the following is the most appropriate next step in this patient's management?

    (A) Beta blockers

    (B) Morphine

    (C) Nitroglycerin

    (D) Nonsteroidal anti-inflammatory drugs

    (E) Steroids

29. A 29-year-old woman arrives at the emergency department complaining of nausea, vomiting, anorexia, and fatigue. She reports that she ate raw oysters that she had collected while on vacation 2 weeks ago. Physical examination is remarkable for jaundice. Serum chemistry studies shows marked elevations of aspartate aminotransferase (AST) and alanine aminotransferase (ALT). Which of the following is the most likely pathogen?

    (A) Hepatitis A

    (B) Hepatitis B

    (C) Hepatitis C

    (D) Hepatitis D

    (E) Hepatitis G

30. A 40-year-old man is brought to the emergency department because he is vomiting large quantities of bright red blood. His temperature is 37.0° C (98.6° F), blood pressure is 65/25 mm Hg, pulse is 110/min, and respirations are 20/min. Which of the following is the most appropriate initial step in patient care?

    (A) Coagulation studies and liver function tests

    (B) Complete physical examination

    (C) Detailed history

    (D) Endoscopy

    (E) Transfusion

31. A 60-year-old man with a history of alcoholic cirrhosis has had repeated episodes of bleeding from esophageal varices, which have become increasingly refractory to standard sclerotherapy or endoscopic ligation. Transjugular intrahepatic portosystemic shunt (TIPS) is being considered as a therapeutic option until a liver is available for transplantation. Which of the following is the most important factor affecting long-term success of shunting procedures or liver transplantation?

    (A) Abstinence from alcohol

    (B) Coexistence of infection with hepatitis C virus

    (C) Lactulose treatment

    (D) Low-protein diet

    (E) Severity of ascites

32. A 55-year-old Asian woman is brought to the emergency department in very severe abdominal pain. She is asked whether anything seems to make the pain better, and she replies that lying quietly helps a great deal. On the basis of the available information, which of the following is the most likely diagnosis?

    (A) Cholelithiasis

    (B) Peptic ulcer disease

    (C) Peritonitis

    (D) Pyelonephritis

    (E) Rupturing aortic aneurysm

33. A 31-year-old woman presents with a chief complaint of amenorrhea for the past 4 months. She has no significant past medical history and had menarche at 12 years of age. She has had menstrual periods every 4 to 5 weeks since. Over the past few months, she has noticed a decrease in her menses and then cessation of her periods. She performed a home pregnancy test, which she says was negative. On review of systems, she says that her eyesight has been "bothering" her and that she has occasional problems seeing objects far to the left or right. She has also been having headaches over the past few months that have required daily self-medication with acetaminophen. After confirming that she is not pregnant, which of the following is the most appropriate next step in diagnosis?

    (A) Serum 17-beta-estradiol level

    (B) Serum LH and FSH

    (C) Serum prolactin level

    (D) Head MRI scan

    (E) Visual evoked potentials

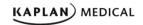

34. A 27-year-old man presents with complaints of 2 weeks of a dry cough, low-grade fever, and dyspnea on exertion. He smokes one pack of cigarettes per day and recently returned from a camping trip in the Southwest. Lung auscultation reveals fine dry rales. The remainder of the physical examination is normal. A chest radiograph shows diffuse infiltrates, and sputum Gram stain shows multiple hyphae. Which of the following is the most likely causal organism?

(A) *Candida albicans*

(B) *Coccidioides immitis*

(C) *Cryptococcus neoformans*

(D) *Histoplasma capsulatum*

35. An 82-year-old man is brought to the physician by his son because of increasing confusion, disorientation in his own home, and urinary incontinence. The son notes that his father's gait has become increasingly broad-based and hesitant over the past several months. The patient scores 18/30 on a mini-mental status examination, and lower extremity deep tendon reflexes are brisk. No other focal abnormalities are noted on neurologic examination. Which of the following is the most likely diagnosis?

(A) Alzheimer disease

(B) Huntington disease

(C) Multiple infarct dementia

(D) Normal pressure hydrocephalus

(E) Pick disease

36. A 38-year-old woman has a 6-month history of atrial fibrillation resistant to any pharmacologic treatment. She denies anginal pain. She has been hospitalized twice for pharmacologic and electrical cardioversion, but each time atrial fibrillation recurred shortly thereafter. Cardiac echocardiography has failed to reveal any structural abnormalities. She is currently being treated with a beta blocker and aspirin, 325 mg/day. Which of the following is the most appropriate next step in management?

(A) Maintain the patient on the same medications

(B) Measure serum levels of TSH and free T_4

(C) Perform a dexamethasone suppression test

(D) Start anticoagulation with warfarin

(E) Perform coronary arteriography

37. A 20-year-old man comes to medical attention because of recurrent bone fractures since childhood. Examination reveals blue sclerae, misshapen blue-yellow teeth, and kyphoscoliosis. Audiologic evaluation demonstrates conductive hearing loss. A positive family history of similar bone fragility and hearing loss is present on his father's side. Serum chemistry tests are normal. Which of the following is the most likely abnormal gene product?

(A) Fibrillin

(B) Fibroblast growth factor (FGF) receptor 3

(C) Procollagen I

(D) Procollagen III

(E) Mucopolysaccharides

38. A 28-year-old man with AIDS and a CD4 count of 84 cells/mL is brought to the emergency department 12 hours after the onset of headache, vomiting, and delirium. On arrival, he appears acutely ill and confused. His temperature is 39.5° C (103.1° F), blood pressure is 110/70 mm Hg, pulse is 100/min, and respiratory rate is 18/min. There is mild resistance to passive flexion of the neck. There are no focal neurological symptoms. Following a funduscopic examination to exclude papilledema, a lumbar puncture is performed. The opening pressure is elevated, and the CSF reveals mild lymphocytosis and mildly increased protein. The CSF titer of cryptococcal antigen is greater than 1:500,000. Which of the following is the most appropriate drug treatment?

(A) Amphotericin B

(B) Clarithromycin-rifabutin

(C) Fluconazole

(D) Sulfadiazine-pyrimethamine

(E) Trimethoprim-sulfamethoxazole

39. On a routine medical checkup, an 18-year-old man is found to have a midsystolic click followed by a murmur. His height is 195 cm (77 in), arm span is 205 cm (81 in), and weight is 80 kg (175 lb). Examination shows pectus excavatum, bossing of frontal eminences, and laxity of ligaments. The thumb can be extended to the wrist. He says that his father died at the age of 40 because of heart problems. Which of the following is the most likely diagnosis?

    (A) Ehlers-Danlos syndrome

    (B) Klinefelter syndrome

    (C) Marfan syndrome

    (D) McCune-Albright syndrome

    (E) Osteogenesis imperfecta

40. A 45-year old man is brought to the intensive care unit after a motor vehicle accident in which he sustained severe crush injury. He is increasingly short of breath and in respiratory distress. On physical examination, he appears tachypneic and cyanotic. Lungs exhibit diffuse crackles. He is emergently intubated for airway protection. He has been previously healthy and is on no medications. His family indicates that he has never smoked. Given his respiratory distress, it is determined that, as a sequelae of the crush injury, the patient is exhibiting signs of adult respiratory distress syndrome (ARDS). Which of the following findings will most likely be seen in this patient?

    (A) Increased arterial P_{CO_2}

    (B) Localized mass on chest x-ray films

    (C) Normal oxygenation with impaired ventilation

    (D) Pulmonary embolism

    (E) Reduced lung compliance

41. A 48-year-old woman complains of difficulty walking up stairs and rising from chairs for the past 3 months. She has no headaches or scalp pain. Physical examination reveals bilateral weakness of her proximal legs and arms. Laboratory studies reveal a markedly elevated creatinine phosphokinase (CPK) level and a normal erythrocyte sedimentation rate. Which of the following is the most appropriate initial step in management?

    (A) Intravenous fluid replacement

    (B) Plasma exchange

    (C) Corticosteroid administration

    (D) Neostigmine administration

    (E) Azathioprine administration

42. A 32-year-old man has been diagnosed with congenital hemolytic anemia (spherocytosis). A sonogram of his right upper quadrant demonstrates the presence of multiple small gallstones, although he has not had any symptoms referable to his gallbladder. Which of the following is the most likely type of stone?

    (A) Black pigment stones

    (B) Brown pigment stones

    (C) Calcium stones

    (D) Mixed stones, with a high proportion of cholesterol

    (E) Pure cholesterol stones

43. A 45-year-old man presents with complaints of flushing, diarrhea, and wheezing associated with food intake. He admits to intermittent abdominal distention and pain. Physical examination is remarkable for an apical systolic cardiac murmur, increased bowel sounds, mild abdominal distention, and scattered telangiectasias. Which of the following is most likely to confirm the diagnosis?

    (A) Calcitonin levels

    (B) Serum gastrin levels

    (C) Upper gastrointestinal tract endoscopy

    (D) Urinary 5-hydroxyindoleacetic acid (5-HIAA)

    (E) Urinary vanillylmandelic acid (VMA)

44. A 27-year-old woman is referred from an outlying primary care clinic because of severe headache that has been present for approximately 4 months and has been increasing in severity. The headache is constant, is worse in the mornings, and the patient points to the center of her head to describe its location. For the past 3 weeks, she has also experienced blurred vision and forceful vomiting. When examined now she is somewhat obtunded and she has bilateral papilledema, but her neurologic examination shows no focal findings. She has no history of recent head trauma. Which of the following diagnostic tests is most likely to provide the diagnosis?

    (A) MRI of the head
    (B) Skull x-rays
    (C) Spinal tap
    (D) Urinary catecholamines
    (E) Visual fields

45. A 25-year-old woman presents with complaints of lightheadedness and excessive thirst and urination. She states that she recently had a cold. She has a history of type 1 diabetes mellitus, for which she takes subcutaneous insulin. On physical examination, she appears anxious and has a supine blood pressure of 110/70 mm Hg and a pulse of 100/min, which change to 90/60 mm Hg and 140/min on sitting up. She is diaphoretic and breathing rapidly at 35 respirations/min. Her skin shows tenting, and her lungs are clear. Laboratory results show:

    Blood chemistries:

Sodium	140 mEq/L
Potassium	4.8 mEq/L
Chloride	100 mEq/L
Bicarbonate	10 mEq/L
Glucose	1,000 mEq/L

    Urinalysis:

    3+ glucose and ketones

    Arterial blood gases:

pH	7.27
P_{CO_2}	23 mm Hg
PO_2	100 mm Hg

    Which of the following is the most appropriate step in management?

    (A) Continuous infusion of isotonic fluid
    (B) Continuous infusion of modified (NPH) insulin
    (C) Continuous infusion of regular insulin
    (D) Continuous infusion of regular insulin and isotonic fluid
    (E) Subcutaneous injection of regular insulin every 4 hours

46. A 62-year-old woman has been complaining of constant back pain for 3 weeks. The pain is localized to the upper back and it bothers her more at night. On physical examination she is tender to direct palpation and percussion over the fourth thoracic vertebra. Neurologic examination reveals very mild weakness of the lower extremities, together with mild hyperreflexia. X-rays show a lytic lesion with an absent pedicle on T4, without collapse of the vertebral body. Three years earlier, the patient had a modified radical mastectomy for a T2, N1, Mo, infiltrating ductal carcinoma of the breast. She declined chemotherapy and was not placed on tamoxifen because her tumor was not estrogen receptor-positive. Further evaluation will best be done with which of the following?

    (A) Lumbar puncture
    (B) Mammogram of the contralateral breast
    (C) MRI of the thoracic area
    (D) Radionuclide bone scan of the thoracic area
    (E) Spiral CT scan of the chest

47. A 45-year-old man has several months of heartburn and indigestion. He denies dysphagia or weight loss. Furthermore, the patient denies chronic diarrhea, fever, chills, or shakes. The patient has no other medical issues. He has been placed on antireflux medications including omeprazole, 20 mg daily. This regimen has not cured the patient's symptoms, however. As a result, the patient undergoes an esophagoduodenoscopy. Endoscopy reveals nonspecific gastritis. Random biopsies done during the procedure reveal mucosa-associated lymphoid tissue (MALT) lymphoma. Which of the following is the appropriate management?

    (A) Chemotherapy
    (B) Eradication of *Helicobacter pylori*
    (C) Observation
    (D) Radiation therapy
    (E) Radiation therapy and chemotherapy

48. A 70-year-old man is being evaluated for progressive shortness of breath and fatigue. Since the symptoms began insidiously a few months ago, the patient has suffered progressive, nondescript fatigue and lethargy. Initially he attributed these symptoms to mild depression associated with a particularly cold and gloomy winter. However, over the past month he has been having episodes of dark urine and shaking chills. Before this he has been healthy; he has never had any major respiratory or cardiac illness. Physical exam is remarkable for scleral icterus and an enlarged spleen. Additionally, there is acral cyanosis and a livedo reticularis pattern on the patient's legs. Laboratory work is remarkable for a hemoglobin level of 10 g/dL (normal red blood cell indices), elevated indirect bilirubin level and lactate dehydrogenase (LDH) level, and a reduced amount of serum haptoglobin. A direct Coombs test is positive. Given this presentation, which of the following is the most appropriate test to diagnose this patient's anemia?

    (A) Bone marrow biopsy
    (B) Cold agglutinin titration
    (C) Ferritin and iron binding capacity
    (D) Indirect Coombs test
    (E) Mycoplasma pneumonia titers

The response options for items 49–50 are the same. You will be required to select one answer for each item in the set.

(A) Botulism

(B) Charcot-Marie-Tooth disease

(C) Diabetic neuropathy

(D) Guillain-Barré syndrome

(E) Lead neuropathy

(F) Ménière syndrome

(G) Neurofibromatosis

(H) Otosclerosis

(I) Polyarteritis nodosa

(J) Presbyacusis

(K) Schwannoma of eighth cranial nerve

(L) Traumatic neuroma

(M) Vertebrobasilar insufficiency

For each patient with neurologic deficits, select the most likely diagnosis.

49. An otherwise healthy 52-year-old man comes to the physician because of progressive hearing loss on the right, which is especially noticeable when he is using the telephone. He also complains of tinnitus on the same side but has no headache or vertigo. No gait ataxia, nystagmus, or other neurologic deficits are found on physical examination. The sound seems louder on the left side when the physician performs a Weber test.

50. A 38-year-old woman comes to medical attention because of a 2-week history of progressive muscle weakness. Initially, the patient had increasing difficulty climbing stairs. Subsequently, she noticed progressive reduction in arm strength. Physical examination confirms pronounced symmetric weakness in both upper and lower extremities, associated with mild impairment of joint, vibration, and pain sensation in the feet and hands. Tendon reflexes are markedly decreased. Vision is normal. Lumbar puncture reveals the following CSF values:

Opening pressure	Normal
Cells	35 cells/mL (mostly lymphocytes)
Protein	70 mg/dL
Glucose	50 mg/dL

Internal Medicine Test Eight:
Answers and Explanations

ANSWER KEY

1.	C	26.	D
2.	E	27.	B
3.	A	28.	D
4.	D	29.	A
5.	E	30.	E
6.	B	31.	A
7.	A	32.	C
8.	A	33.	C
9.	E	34.	B
10.	C	35.	D
11.	E	36.	B
12.	E	37.	C
13.	D	38.	A
14.	B	39.	C
15.	D	40.	E
16.	D	41.	C
17.	C	42.	A
18.	C	43.	D
19.	D	44.	A
20.	E	45.	D
21.	B	46.	C
22.	E	47.	B
23.	B	48.	B
24.	E	49.	K
25.	C	50.	D

1. **The correct answer is C.** The physical presentation illustrated in the question stem is typical for Cushing syndrome, in which the body responds to excess cortisol. Cushing syndrome is a clinically defined constellation, which has a variety of underlying etiologies. Consequently, unless there is an obvious cause, such as high levels of exogenous cortisone administration (as in deliberate medical immune suppression for transplantation cases or therapy of autoimmune diseases), there is a need to develop information that further defines the etiology. One of the most widespread tests used is the dexamethasone suppression test. Dexamethasone can inhibit ACTH secretion by the pituitary. In its simplest form, a single 1-mg oral dose is given at night; the following morning, a single plasma cortisol is taken, which in normal individuals will suppress to less than 5 mg/dL. Most patients with nonpituitary Cushing syndrome will not have a suppression of cortisol in this setting, and the morning plasma cortisol level is typically at least 9 mg/dL. In this patient, the morning level after the 1-mg dose was at an intermediate level, which was difficult to interpret; therefore, a more elaborate version of the dexamethasone test was then given. In this more elaborate test, "low-dose" dexamethasone is given for 2 days, which will inhibit ACTH secretion in normal subjects, but not in patients with an ACTH secreting pituitary tumor. These patients can, however, be suppressed with the higher dose given on the last 2 days of the test, unlike patients with either ACTH secretion by other tumors (such as small cell carcinoma) or primary adrenal disease producing the cortisol.

Exogenous cortisol administration (**choice A**) would not suppress with dexamethasone therapy.

Adrenal tumors (**choice B**) secrete cortisol, not ACTH.

A small cell tumor producing ACTH (**choice D**) would not be suppressed by dexamethasone, even at high doses.

An adrenal tumor secreting cortisol (**choice E**) would not be suppressed by dexamethasone, no matter what the dose.

2. **The correct answer is E.** The clinical vignette presents all the characteristic clinical, MRI, and EEG manifestations of Creutzfeldt-Jacob disease (CJD). Note the *startle myoclonus*, which is characteristic of CJD. This is a spongiform encephalopathy resulting from inherited or acquired alterations of prion protein (PrP), a normal neuronal protein of unknown function. The incidence is 1 in 1 million. Approximately 85% of cases are sporadic and occur without any apparent association with risk factors. The condition is contagious, although the mechanisms of transmission are unclear. The disease can be produced in monkeys by inoculation of a brain suspension from CJD patients.

Only rare cases of CJD acquired by occupational exposure (**choice A**) have been reported, for example in laboratory technicians. The fact that there is no increased incidence of CJD among physicians and patients' family members suggests that respiratory, enteric, or sexual transmission does not play a role.

Some cases of CJD have been reported in patients who received growth hormone (**choice B**), corneal transplants, or dural grafts from infected cadavers.

A recent outbreak of spongiform encephalopathy pathologically and clinically similar to CJD has been related to ingestion of beef (**choice C**), deriving from cows affected by *bovine spongiform encephalopathy*. Patients are younger and exhibit a milder clinical form without the typical EEG findings.

Approximately 15% of cases are familial (**choice D**), due to inherited mutations of PrP gene.

3. **The correct answer is A.** However perplexing the attributes of "blind" and "random" may appear, such biopsies may well disclose nasopharyngeal carcinoma in this case. This cancer, also known as *lymphoepithelioma*, is composed of poorly differentiated squamous epithelium admixed with a florid lymphocytic infiltrate (hence the alternative designation). Latent EBV infection is associated with this disease, and EBV genome can be detected in most cases. Nasopharyngeal carcinoma is endemic in Southeast Asia, especially in southern regions of China. It often manifests with serous otitis media (secondary to obstruction of the auditory tube) and cervical lymph node metastasis. Early in its course, this carcinoma may result only in subtle and nonspecific macroscopic alterations of the nasopharynx. Serous otitis media results from obstruction of the auditory tube; it is more common in children because of the anatomic features of this organ. In adults, serous otitis media usually follows an upper respiratory infection or barotrauma.

Measurement of serum IgG antibodies to EBV (**choice B**) has been proposed as an adjunct diagnostic test for detection of nasopharyngeal carcinoma, but it is not sensitive enough. The titers of anti-EBV antibodies will decrease in the serum after radiation treatment (which is the treatment of choice).

MRI scans of the head and neck (**choice C**) are used for staging purposes: to determine the extent of cancer spread to contiguous regions.

Placement of a ventilation tube through the tympanic membrane (**choice D**) may be used to relieve the symptomatology secondary to serous otitis media if pharmacologic treatment has been unsuccessful.

A short course of oral corticosteroids (**choice E**) and/or treatment with oral antibiotics (e.g., amoxicillin [**choice F**]), can be used to provide relief in serous otitis media. Further investigations should be carried out to search for the underlying cause of chronic serous otitis media, especially in adults.

4. **The correct answer is D.** Radiation therapy to the chest may result in radiation lung injury. The rate of symptomatic radiation lung injury varies depending on several parameters, but it is approximately 10% following treatment of lung carcinoma. Acute radiation pneumonitis develops on average 2-3 months after exposure and manifests with insidious onset of shortness of breath and chest pain. Fever may be present, and leukocytosis and elevated ESR are usually seen. The sharp demarcation of pulmonary infiltrate on chest x-ray and its close correspondence to the previously irradiated area are highly characteristic of acute radiation injury to the lung.

   Bacterial pneumonia (**choice A**) manifests with multifocal alveolar pulmonary infiltrates or lobar consolidation.

   CMV pneumonia (**choice B**) presents in immunocompromised hosts, such as patients with AIDS, organ transplantation, and hematologic malignancies. CMV pneumonia may give rise to radiographic evidence of multinodular or diffuse interstitial infiltrates.

   Pulmonary radiation fibrosis (**choice C**) is a delayed complication of radiation injury and manifests 6-12 months following radiation exposure. If the volume of lung irradiated is extensive, radiation fibrosis may result in respiratory insufficiency.

   Recurrence of primary carcinoma (**choice E**) would be highly unlikely within such a short period.

5. **The correct answer is E.** There is currently no effective screening program for lung cancer. Tests that allow early detection do not have an impact on overall mortality because of the high rate of metastasis (which can be clinically silent) in the most patients, even when primary tumors are detected at a very early stage.

6. **The correct answer is B.** This patient presents with cough, an abnormal chest x-ray, and symptoms of hypercalcemia (malaise, anorexia, and constipation). Her clinical picture is suspicious for a squamous cell carcinoma of the lung that is releasing a parathyroid hormone-like substance. The question requires you to know the management of hypercalcemia. The first principle of treatment is to restore normal volume status. Many hypercalcemic patients are dehydrated because of vomiting, decreased oral intake, and calcium-induced dysfunction in renal concentrating ability. Restoring euvolemia increases the glomerular filtration rate and increase renal tubular calcium clearance. Normal saline is used because increasing sodium excretion increases calcium clearance even further.

Giving bisphosphonate (**choice A**) is a possible treatment but can be toxic. Hydration should be restored first.

Thiazide diuretics (**choice C**) can actually cause hypercalcemia and are therefore not an appropriate therapy.

Although bronchoscopy (**choice D**) and sputum cytology (**choice E**) may be helpful in diagnosing the underlying pulmonary malignancy, it is more appropriate to first address and treat the patient's symptomatic hypercalcemia.

7. **The correct answer is A.** The patient's clinical picture (cough, fever, and yellow sputum in an otherwise healthy young man) is most consistent with acute bronchitis.

   Chronic bronchitis (**choice B**) might develop later on in this smoker, as symptoms usually begin in middle age.

   Cystic fibrosis (**choice C**) presents much earlier than 27 years of age.

   Pneumonia (**choice D**) would be associated with purulent sputum, consolidation on chest x-ray, and probably a higher fever.

   Sinusitis (**choice E**) is associated with a purulent nasal discharge. Note that postnasal discharge could also cause cough, but bilateral diffuse rales would not be expected on physical examination.

8. **The correct answer is A.** *Diverticular disease* with diverticulitis should be suspected in this case. This condition is extremely frequent in industrialized countries, but more than two-thirds of cases remain asymptomatic. The sigmoid colon is the most commonly affected segment. Complications of diverticulosis may include one or more of the following clinical syndromes: occult or obvious bleeding, acute hematochezia, or diverticulitis. Abdominal pain, fever, and neutrophilic leukocytosis suggest diverticulitis in the appropriate clinical setting. How should the physician proceed from this point? Barium enema (**choice C**) is certainly the most sensitive study to visualize colonic diverticula, but perforation, ileus, or bowel obstruction should be ruled out before undertaking further diagnostic studies. Plain abdominal x-rays in the flat and erect positions are necessary to identify radiologic signs of perforation (free air in the abdomen) or bowel obstruction.

CT scan of the abdomen (**choice B**) is useful to define the extent of extracolonic spread of diverticular inflammation, presence of paracolic abscesses, and coexistence of other anomalies (tumors).

Colonoscopy (**choice D**) is less sensitive than barium enema in visualizing diverticula and is not indicated during the acute phase of diverticulitis.

Frequent urination and mild leukocyturia result from inflammation of the left ureter due to the adjacent inflamed colonic diverticula. Urinary symptoms and leukocyturia and/or microscopic hematuria are sometimes associated with diverticulitis and should not suggest the need for intravenous pyelography (**choice E**).

9. **The correct answer is E.** The three most common causes of atrial fibrillation are myocardial ischemia, mitral valve disease, and hyperthyroidism. In some cases, atrial fibrillation may be the first manifestation of hyperthyroidism. In this case, atrial fibrillation is associated with additional signs and symptoms of exaggerated thyroid function, including loss of weight, increased appetite, insomnia, and anxiety. Another characteristic hemodynamic alteration of hyperthyroidism is a hyperdynamic (high output) circulation, which leads to a wide differential between systolic and diastolic pressures. Therefore, triiodothyronine (T_3), thyroxine (T_4), and thyroid resin uptake would all be elevated in this patient. Measurement of the TSH level is an even more sensitive test for thyrotoxicosis. TSH secretion is suppressed, except in those very rare cases due to increased hypothalamic TRH secretion, or to an equally rare TSH-releasing pituitary tumor.

Chest x-ray (**choice A**) or complete blood count (**choice B**) would not reveal any significant or specific change in this case.

An echocardiogram (**choice C**) is useful for identifying structural cardiac etiologies of atrial fibrillation. In this case, however, there are enough other data to suggest hyperthyroidism as the most likely cause of the atrial fibrillation.

Neuropsychiatric referral (**choice D**) is sometimes sought for patients with early signs of thyrotoxicosis because of increasing anxiety, sleeplessness, mood changes, and other psychologic symptoms. In this case, it is obvious that the condition has an organic etiology.

10. **The correct answer is C.** Since the patient is a nurse, she has access to insulin or oral diabetes medications. The insulin levels are elevated, but the C-peptide levels are low and insulin antibodies are present, all of which suggests an exogenous source for the insulin. When insulin is released naturally from the body, both insulin and C-peptide levels are elevated.

Alimentary hypoglycemia (**choice A**) causes postprandial hypoglycemia because of rapid gastric emptying and absorption of nutrients with heightened insulin release and decreased substrate available. Since these episodes are sporadic and not postprandial, alimentary hypoglycemia is unlikely.

Insulinoma (**choice B**) would increase insulin and C-peptide levels.

Oral sulfonylurea administration causes insulin release, resulting in elevated levels of insulin as well as C-peptide.

Since C-peptide levels are suppressed in this patient, surreptitious oral sulfonylurea administration (**choice D**) is an inadequate explanation for the observed findings.

11. **The correct answer is E.** This is a classic presentation of sporotrichosis, which is caused by the saprophytic mold *Sporothrix schenckii*. The organism is present on rose bushes, barberry bushes, sphagnum moss, and other mulches, and is typically introduced into the skin at a site of minor trauma. Helpful diagnostic clues are an exposure to gardens or forests; a chain of lesions, some of which may be ulcerated; and a rather striking absence of any systemic symptoms. The subcutaneous nodules are actually involved lymph nodes. The organism can be difficult to demonstrate in the lesions, so a careful history is the most helpful diagnostic maneuver. Rarely, hematogenous dissemination can occur. Treatment is with oral itraconazole; potassium iodide solution was formerly used.

Aspergillosis (**choice A**) usually involves the lungs, from which it may spread to other sites.

Candidiasis (**choice B**) can cause systemic disease or local involvement of mucous membranes and moist skin.

Cryptococcosis (**choice C**) usually starts as a pulmonary infection, although it can later spread to skin.

Mucormycosis (**choice D**) usually involves the rhinocerebral area, but can also develop in the skin, usually under occlusive dressings.

12. **The correct answer is E.** HBsAg is associated with the viral surface coat and is usually the first evidence that an acute hepatitis B infection is under way. It characteristically appears during the incubation period, typically during a period of 1-6 weeks before either liver enzymes rise or the patient develops jaundice. It usually disappears during convalescence; demonstrable persistence after that time indicates chronic infection.

Anti-HBc (**choice A**) is the antibody to the core antigen and generally appears at the onset of clinical illness and then declines slowly. Roughly 80% to 90% of patients will develop antibodies to the surface antigen, anti-HBs (**choice B**), usually weeks to months after HBsAg appears. Patients who do not develop the antibody are likely to have chronic infection.

HBcAg (**choice C**) is the core antigen and is usually not detectable in serum, except by special techniques that disrupt the infectious particles.

HBeAg (**choice D**) is the e antigen. It appears to be a peptide from the viral core, whose presence suggests active viral replication, with greater likelihood of progression to chronic liver disease, and with greater infectivity risk.

13. **The correct answer is D.** The facial muscle twitching described in the question is called the Chvostek sign and is frequently used as a marker for the tendency to tetany that is produced by hypocalcemia. Although it is still used with some frequency clinically, you should be aware that this sign is positive in up to 10% of healthy people and is often negative in chronic hypocalcemia. Thyroid surgery can damage the blood supply to the parathyroid glands (leading to decreased parathyroid hormone and hypocalcemia), and the Chvostek sign is an easy clinical marker for this complication.

Serum chloride levels (**choice A**), potassium levels (**choice B**), and sodium levels (**choice C**) would not be affected by parathyroid damage.

Hypophosphatemia (**choice E**) is seen in hyperparathyroidism, rather than hypoparathyroidism.

14. **The correct answer is B.** The patient has melasma, which produces patchy hyperpigmentation of otherwise normal skin. It is seen most frequently during pregnancy and in women on birth control pills. The hyperpigmentation tends to fade slowly once estrogen levels diminish because of completion of the pregnancy or discontinuation of hormonal therapy. The condition has no particular medical significance, although its cosmetic effects may be distressing to patients. Hydroquinone cream coupled with rigorous photoprotection (e.g., use of high SPF sun creams) may speed fading of the lesions.

Actinic keratoses (**choice A**) are small precancerous keratotic skin lesions that are usually pink and have a scaly or crusted surface.

Miliaria (**choice C**) are pruritic sweat gland inflammations.

Nevus flammeus (**choice D**) is a congenital, purplish skin lesion.

Seborrheic keratoses (**choice E**) are small, pigmented, superficial epithelial lesions that usually have a warty surface.

15. **The correct answer is D.** The most obvious cause of hypercalcemia is hyperparathyroidism, but you should be aware that hypercalcemia can be seen in a wide variety of other conditions and is sometimes the initial finding. These other causes include tumors with or without bone metastases, sarcoidosis and other granulomatous diseases, bone diseases, vitamins A and D toxicity, endocrine states (myxedema, Addison disease, postoperative Cushing disease, hyperthyroidism), thiazide diuretics, milk-alkali syndrome, and aluminum and lithium toxicity.

Bartter syndrome (**choice A**) can cause renal potassium and sodium wasting.

Crohn disease (**choice B**) and other causes of malabsorption can cause vitamin D deficiency with hypocalcemia.

Pancreatitis (**choice C**) can cause hypocalcemia as the calcium precipitates with fats altered by pancreatic enzymes.

Systemic lupus erythematosus (**choice E**) does not usually cause electrolyte disturbances, unless associated with renal dysfunction.

16. **The correct answer is D.** Primary biliary cirrhosis is characterized by chronic granulomatous inflammation leading to destruction of intrahepatic bile ducts. A cholestatic picture develops with conjugated hyperbilirubinemia. Increased alkaline phosphatase is a lab finding associated with cholestasis. Itching is due to elevated levels of circulating bile salts. The disease predominantly affects middle-aged women and progresses to cirrhosis. Ninety percent of patients have circulating antimitochondrial autoantibodies, which may play a pathogenetic role.

Alcohol-related liver disease (**choice A**) may manifest with acute alcoholic hepatitis, liver steatosis, or cirrhosis. In none of these conditions are antimitochondrial autoantibodies found.

Autoimmune hepatitis (**choice B**) occurs most frequently in young women and is associated with two types of autoantibodies: antinuclear and antismooth muscle (*type I* most common) and antimicrosomal (*type II* less common in the U.S.). Autoimmune hepatitis was also known as *lupoid hepatitis* because of its frequent association with ANAs similar to systemic lupus.

Hemochromatosis (**choice C**) is a hereditary disorder due to abnormal accumulation of iron in the liver, heart, and endocrine glands. Cirrhosis, cardiomegaly, skin hyperpigmentation, and diabetes are the most typical features. The diagnosis is suspected when there are elevated levels of serum iron and ferritin, with high transferrin saturation (>50%). Otherwise, there is no specific serologic marker for this condition.

Wilson disease (**choice E**) is an inherited condition characterized by accumulation of copper in the liver, brain, and eye. Elevated hepatic copper content and increased urinary excretion of copper are diagnostically important findings.

17. **The correct answer is C.** Recurrent candidiasis may simply indicate a resistant or poorly treated strain, but the severity of this patient's infection should raise the possibility of immunosuppression. Diabetes mellitus is a particularly likely candidate, since the combination of immunosuppression and glucose-rich secretions (the same process that spills glucose into urine will spill glucose into vaginal and other secretions) very much favors fungal infection. In some adult-onset diabetic

patients, recurrent candidiasis is the presenting complaint. Hence, the appropriate choice of tests is to screen blood glucose.

Bicarbonate (**choice A**), calcium (**choice B**), iron (**choice D**), and sodium (**choice E**) would not be markers for anything that might cause significant immunosuppression.

18. **The correct answer is C.** This patient has signs of vitamin B_{12} deficiency due to his poor diet. Patients first complain of paresthesias in the hands or legs (tingling, numbness, and "pins and needles" sensations). Later, symmetric distal impairment of vibratory sensation occurs, usually first in the legs but eventually reaching the trunk and arms. Position sense is affected less prominently, although a Romberg sign may be present. There may be diminished reflexes. Symmetric weakness in the legs (associated with spasticity, clonus at the knees and ankles, and extensor plantar responses) follows. Treatment is replacement of vitamin B_{12} by intramuscular injection. Early neurologic changes may be reversed if treatment is begun promptly within the first weeks or months of the disorder.

Niacin deficiency (**choice A**) or pellagra is characterized by the three D's: diarrhea, dementia, and dermatitis.

The clinical manifestations of protein deficiency (**choice B**) are variable. Kwashiorkor or marasmus may occur. In adults, symptoms and signs are dependent on the nutritional status of the patient prior to illness. Patients may have weight loss or depletion of fat stores, which presents as temporal wasting or interosseous wasting. The skin is dry with decreased turgor. Low serum proteins may result in dependent edema or anasarca.

Vitamin C deficiency (**choice D**) leads to scurvy, characterized by ecchymoses and purpura that may develop at areas of trauma, irritation, or pressure. Joints, muscles, and subcutaneous tissues may become sites of hemorrhage. Swollen, bleeding gums are characteristic of advanced deficiency. Wounds heal poorly, and healed wounds may open up again.

Zinc deficiency (**choice E**) may be classified as acute or chronic. Acute deficiency can occur in patients receiving parenteral nutrition and is characterized by diarrhea; disturbance of the CNS with mental irritability and depression; skin lesions of the face, perineum, limbs, and skin folds; and alopecia. Patients with AIDS, diabetes, uremia, or inflammatory bowel disease can develop chronic zinc deficiency.

19. **The correct answer is D.** Most initial infections with hepatitis C are subclinical. However, the infection has a 75% rate of chronicity (compared with 5% to 10% for hepatitis B), which can go on over a period of years to over a decade to develop cirrhosis. A rule of thumb about needle-stick exposures to known infectious patients is that the AIDS virus has a 3 in 1000 rate of being transmitted by this route; the hepatitis C virus has a 3 in 100 rate of being transmitted; and the hepatitis B virus has a 3 in 10 rate of being transmitted. However, we have available a vaccine against hepatitis B that virtually all medical workers have received, and no vaccine is yet available that is directed against the hepatitis C virus. Also, therapy for hepatitis C infection is very problematic. Interferon shows some activity against the virus; however, interferon therapy is extremely expensive and toxic and may need to be given for long periods or indefinitely. The addition of oral ribavirin significantly improves clinical response rates and is now the standard treatment for hepatitis C. Hemolytic anemia may occur during ribavirin therapy.

20. **The correct answer is E.** This is vitiligo, a common form of patchy hypopigmentation seen in 1% to 2% of the population. All races are affected, although the lesions appear more prominent in dark-skinned individuals. (The patches of hypopigmentation can be seen more easily in light-skinned individuals with use of Wood's light.) The condition is still considered idiopathic, although an autoimmune basis is suspected in at least some individuals. The possibility of coexisting autoimmune disease (e.g., Addison disease, diabetes mellitus, pernicious anemia, or thyroid dysfunction) in these patients should also be considered, since vitiligo can be associated with these conditions. Although therapy with oral or topical psoralens, coupled with ultraviolet A illumination, is often attempted in patients with vitiligo, treatment results are frequently unsatisfactory, and camouflaging cosmetics may give a more acceptable result.

Albinism (**choice A**) is an inherited condition characterized by a complete lack of melanin pigmentation of the skin, hair, and eyes.

Keloids (**choice B**) are hypertrophic scars that are frequently nonpigmented but produce a raised mass.

Lentigo (**choice C**) is a uniformly pigmented, brown to black, flat macule with sharp margins.

Melasma (**choice D**) produces facial hyperpigmentation in pregnant women.

21. **The correct answer is B.** All angiotensin converting enzyme (ACE) inhibitors produce varying degrees of hyperkalemia because of their effect on reducing aldosterone release.

Beta agonists, such as albuterol (**choice A**); loop diuretics, such as furosemide (**choice C**); heparin (**choice D**); and insulin (**choice E**) all cause potassium shifts into cells, which decrease the serum levels of potassium. These medications can be continued because they are not worsening the hyperkalemia, and may in fact help to control the hyperkalemia.

22. **The correct answer is E.** Subacute thyroiditis is unusual among thyroid diseases in that it produces an exquisitely tender thyroid gland. A preceding history of upper respiratory infection is common, and this inflammatory disease of the thyroid is probably caused by a virus. The pain may be interpreted as throat, dental, or ear pain. The condition may cause transient hypertension secondary to rupture of follicles. Biopsies of an involved thyroid gland typically demonstrate giant cell infiltration, neutrophils, and follicular disruption. Most cases are self-limiting, with resolution in a few months. Uncommonly, sufficient destruction of the thyroid gland occurs to produce permanent hypothyroidism.

Graves disease (**choice A**) is usually not painful, and characteristic features include the signs of hyperthyroidism (e.g., palpitations, heat intolerance, and nervousness), pretibial myxedena, and infiltrative ophthalmopathy.

Cancers of the thyroid, such as medullary (**choice B**) and papillary (**choice D**) carcinomas, are characteristically painless in the earlier stages.

Nontoxic goiter (**choice C**) is characteristically painless and is often multinodular.

23. **The correct answer is B.** The patient is showing signs of aortic stenosis (AS). Significant AS complications include angina, syncope, and congestive heart failure. This patient's symptoms seem critical, and he should be advised to undergo an aortic valve replacement. In AS, carotid upstrokes are delayed in timing and reduced in volume. The ejection murmur is loudest at the aortic head. The murmur also may be reflected to the mitral area, producing the false impression that mitral insufficiency is also present. This is called the Gallavardin phenomenon. The reduction in the motion of the aortic valve causes the A component of S2 to be reduced or silent. The ECG shows signs of left ventricular hypertrophy, since the ventricle contracts against the stenosed aortic valve.

Aortic insufficiency (**choice A**) can be caused by aortic root dilation, rheumatic heart disease, and Marfan syndrome. Chronic insufficiency will ultimately lead to left ventricular dysfunction and congestive heart failure. Symptoms include dyspnea and orthopnea. Physical signs include a high-pitched, blowing diastolic murmur heard along the left sternal border. Other signs include Quincke's pulse, which is a systolic blushing and diastolic blanching of the nailbed when gentle pressure is placed on the nail.

Mitral insufficiency (**choice C**) may also be caused by rheumatic heart disease, ruptured chordae tendineae,

and mitral valve prolapse. The insufficiency will cause increased left atrial pressure and decreased forward cardiac output, ultimately leading to left ventricular failure. The point of maximal intensity will be hyperdynamic. The carotid upstrokes will be brisk but reduced in volume. The murmur will be a holosystolic apical murmur radiating to the axilla. An S3 is usually heard.

Mitral stenosis (**choice D**) in adults is almost always due to rheumatic heart disease. Symptoms include orthopnea, dyspnea, ascites, hemoptysis, and fatigue. Signs include rales, increased S1, loud P2, opening snap, and a diastolic rumble. Diuretics, digoxin, anticoagulants, and mitral valve replacement may be needed.

Tricuspid regurgitation (**choice E**) is often caused by infective endocarditis, particularly in IV drug users. Symptoms include edema, ascites, right upper quadrant pain from hepatic congestion, a holosystolic murmur that increases with inspiration, and a large v wave in the jugular veins during systole. The liver may be pulsatile as well.

24. **The correct answer is E.** Hypothyroidism is an uncommon cause of confusion. However, in the elderly, especially women, hypothyroidism or subclinical hypothyroidism is extremely common, seen in up to 20% of all medical inpatients in some series. Given this, the evaluation of new confusion or suspected dementia should always include a thyroid stimulating hormone level when the patient is in this age group.

Calcium level (**choice A**) is included in the initial laboratory evaluation. However, interpretation of this test is difficult, primarily because asymptomatic hypercalcemia is very common in the elderly, with as much as a 50% prevalence rate. Given this, even the finding of elevated total serum calcium is without obvious significance, and hypothyroidism is still a much more common cause of altered mental status despite its lower prevalence.

Diffusion weighted MRI of brain (**choice B**) allows visualization of areas of acute infarction and is used only in special circumstances when an evolving infarct is suspected.

Head CT scan with contrast (**choice C**) is not indicated unless there is clinical suspicion for old infarcts or a bleed.

Rapid plasma reagin test (**choice D**) is the screening test for syphilis. Although this test is routinely sent with the panel of tests for the evaluation of dementia, tertiary syphilis is exceedingly rare and not a very common cause of dementia in any age group in the U.S.

25. **The correct answer is C.** As many as 3% to 5% of the general population has Gilbert syndrome, which is a completely benign condition (not even really a disease) in which there is a deficit in the liver's rate of conjugation

of bilirubin due to a slightly low glucuronyl transferase activity. No true clinically significant liver disease is present, but there is a risk of being misdiagnosed with chronic hepatitis.

Alcoholic hepatitis (**choice A**) would be accompanied by elevated liver transaminases with the aspartate aminotransferase (AST) about twice as high as the alanine aminotransferase (ALT).

Crigler-Najjar syndrome (**choice B**) is a true liver disorder characterized by a more severe glucuronyl transferase deficiency. It occurs in an autosomal recessive form that is fatal by age 1 and in a somewhat milder autosomal dominant form that permits survival into adulthood.

Infection with hepatitis A (**choice D**) or hepatitis B (**choice E**) would be accompanied by elevated serum liver enzymes.

26. **The correct answer is D.** The clinical picture is that of a patient with progressive congestive heart failure. The specific manifestations leading to the correct diagnosis include increased jugular pressure, especially during inspiration, and the calcific deposits in the pericardial sac. Restrictive pericarditis is due to a fibrocalcific transformation of the pericardium, which encases the heart and impairs ventricular filling. In the past, the most common etiology was tubercular pericarditis; nowadays, radiation therapy, cardiac surgery, and prior viral pericarditis represent the most frequent causes.

Dilated cardiomyopathy (**choice A**) is associated with cardiomegaly, resulting in an enlarged cardiac silhouette on chest x-ray. Impaired inotropism is the principal pathophysiologic mechanism of congestive heart failure due to dilated cardiomyopathy.

Hypertrophic cardiomyopathy (**choice B**) may not be associated with an enlarged heart, but a thickened left ventricular wall, especially the interventricular septum, would be demonstrated by echocardiography.

Pericardial tamponade (**choice C**) results from accumulation of fluid within the pericardial sac and consequently impaired diastolic filling. The course is acute or subacute, and concomitant symptomatology (e.g., precordial pain in case of pericarditis, or history of penetrating trauma or infarction in case of hemorrhage) is present.

The clinical manifestations of tricuspid regurgitation (**choice E**) may simulate restrictive pericarditis or cardiomyopathy, but this valvular defect would be associated with right ventricular enlargement and a pansystolic murmur, which are not present in this case.

27. **The correct answer is B.** Basal cell carcinomas are the most frequent skin malignancies. They develop on sun-exposed areas, often in fair-skinned individuals, grow slowly for years, and finally develop a central ulceration.

Although nearly entirely devoid of metastatic potential (the cases of proven metastatic basal cell carcinoma are publishable), they may erode into adjacent structures, resulting in cosmetic and/or functional alterations. In fact, the designation of these tumors in the old literature was *ulcus rodens* ("erosive or destructive ulcer").

Actinic keratosis (**choice A**) is related to ultraviolet sun damage and thus occurs in sun-exposed skin of fair individuals. It appears as small, flesh-colored or slightly pigmented papules that have a characteristic sandpaper-like surface. Actinic keratosis is a premalignant lesion, which may transform into squamous cell carcinoma in 1 of 1,000 cases.

Hemangioma (**choice C**) is a benign vascular tumor, of which the *capillary* type is the most frequent. Capillary hemangiomas appear in infancy, grow rapidly in the first year of life, and undergo spontaneous regression by age 5-7. These tumors are bright red to blue and are covered by intact skin.

Keratoacanthoma (**choice D**) is histologically extremely similar to squamous cell carcinoma but grows rapidly over a period of weeks and regresses spontaneously within 4-6 weeks. Usually, it presents a central, crater-like ulceration, which is keratin-filled.

Melanoma (**choice E**) manifests *de novo* or on a pre-existing mole as a pigmented lesion with asymmetric and irregular borders and variegated color. Ulceration is an infrequent feature.

Psoriasis (**choice F**) presents as silvery plaques on typical locations such as knees, elbows, and scalp. Lesions tend to occur frequently on sites of repetitive trauma.

Seborrheic keratosis (**choice G**) is an extremely common form of benign tumor of the elderly. The lesions of seborrheic keratosis are brown to black plaques with a velvety or warty surface. The lesions appear as if "stuck on" the epidermal surface, and indeed they can be easily lifted off the skin.

28. **The correct answer is D.** This patient's physical examination and history are suggestive of pericarditis. The ECG finding of PR depression alone nearly confirms this diagnosis. A triphasic pericardial friction rub may be heard on cardiac auscultation. Causes of pericarditis include uremia, viral infection, lupus, drugs such as hydralazine and isoniazid, and malignancy. This patient has missed her dialysis sessions and is probably uremic. Nonsteroidal anti-inflammatory drugs (NSAIDs), such as indomethacin, are useful for decreasing the inflammation. Ultimately, this patient will require dialysis.

Beta blockers (**choice A**) have no value in the acute management of pericarditis. This patient's chest pain is probably not from an ischemic event.

Morphine (**choice B**) can be given to patients in heart failure to act as a sedative. It decreases the sensation of drowning, thus suppressing the adrenergic drive that can worsen ischemia.

Nitroglycerin (**choice C**) is a vasodilator. It relieves acute chest pain by preload reduction and coronary artery dilation. Since the patient does not appear to be having cardiac ischemia, nitroglycerin will not be helpful.

Steroids (**choice E**) may be used in pericarditis if NSAIDs are not effective. However, NSAIDs should be the first-line therapy despite their association with increased risk of developing chronic restrictive pericarditis.

29. **The correct answer is A.** Hepatitis viruses known to be spread orally, thereby potentially causing epidemics, include A and E. Outbreaks of hepatitis E have been identified only in developing countries, so you are unlikely to encounter this form of hepatitis in the U.S. Hepatitis A virus is usually spread by fecal-oral contamination, although blood and secretions can also be infectious. Fecal shedding is particularly significant since it typically occurs during the prodromal period when the patient has undiagnosed disease. Water- and foodborne (including raw shellfish) epidemics occur most frequently in undeveloped countries with poor sanitation. Subclinical infections are common during epidemics, again favoring the spread of the virus. Hepatitis A causes acute hepatic disease but does not cause chronic infection and cirrhosis.

Hepatitis B (**choice B**) and C (**choice C**) are spread by blood and do not cause conventional epidemics, although they are becoming widely distributed through needle use and, especially for hepatitis B, sexual contact.

Hepatitis D (**choice D**) is a defective bloodborne virus, requiring coinfection with hepatitis B.

Hepatitis G (**choice E**) is a rare form of viral hepatitis that has been identified in a few cases of hepatitis transmitted by blood.

30. **The correct answer is E.** One of the basic principles of emergency medicine is that you stabilize a crashing patient as rapidly as possible, even if that causes some delay in doing other reasonable things. In this case, the patient's blood pressure is dangerously low, and he is obviously bleeding. Starting an IV line with saline and then getting appropriately typed blood into him as fast as possible is the best way to begin.

Coagulation studies and liver function tests (**choice A**) are appropriate in helping to define the basis of the patient's bleeding (coagulopathy or bleeding varices), but should not interfere with getting the blood (or other fluids if the blood is delayed) started.

Complete physical examination (**choice B**) is also important but should be done after stabilizing the patient.

A detailed history (**choice C**) is also important but should be done after stabilizing the patient.

Endoscopy (**choice D**) may be necessary to identify the site of bleeding and stop it; however, this procedure is much easier and safer to do when the patient is stabilized.

31. **The correct answer is A.** Total abstinence from alcohol is a fundamental prerequisite for the success of any therapeutic measure for cirrhosis. Transjugular intrahepatic portosystemic shunt (TIPS) is a frequently used alternative to surgical portosystemic shunting procedures in cases of recurrent variceal bleeding refractory to conventional treatments. Liver transplantation has a success rate as high as 80% in specialized centers, but patients must abstain from alcohol for at least 6 months before the procedure. TIPS has a lower success rate in patients with concomitant renal insufficiency (*hepatorenal syndrome*).

Coexistence of infection with hepatitis C virus (**choice B**) does not affect the outcome of either TIPS or the majority of liver transplants. In fact, hepatitis C recurs in virtually all HCV-positive patients receiving a liver transplant, but the effects appear to be negligible in the majority, at least for the first 5 years.

Lactulose treatment (**choice C**) is for hepatic encephalopathy. It decreases the flora of ammonia-forming bacteria in the colon. Lactulose treatment has no influence on TIPS or liver transplantation success.

Low-protein diet (**choice D**) is used to decrease the amount of ammonia formed by colonic bacterial flora in the treatment of hepatic encephalopathy.

Severity of ascites (**choice E**) is related to the severity of portal hypertension and the degree of hypoalbuminemia, both of which are associated with cirrhosis. TIPS is also used for patients with ascites refractory to diuretics or sodium restriction.

32. **The correct answer is C.** Severe pain that is significantly better when the patient lies quietly should specifically suggest peritonitis to the examining physician. Other features of peritonitis include abdominal guarding, localized or diffuse tenderness, and, in severe cases, absent peristalsis. Acute peritonitis may have a wide variety of etiologies, including ruptured or infarcted viscera (intra-abdominal esophagus, stomach, duodenum, bowel, appendix, gallbladder or biliary tree, urinary bladder), trauma, foreign bodies, pelvic inflammatory disease, infected blood in peritoneum, and pancreatitis. Emergency exploratory laparotomy is often required for diagnosis and therapy, with exceptions including acute pancreatitis and pelvic inflammatory disease.

The pain of cholelithiasis (**choice A**) may be relieved by walking and may be referred to the right scapula.

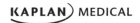

Peptic ulcer disease (**choice B**) may be relieved by antacids and tends to produce burning pain.

Pyelonephritis (**choice D**) may cause dull, aching pain over the kidneys or may be referred to the pubis or vagina.

A rupturing aortic aneurysm (**choice E**) causes severe, knifelike, tearing pain in the mid-back that may move downward as the tear evolves.

33. **The correct answer is C.** The most common cause (>80%) of amenorrhea is pregnancy. Once this option has been excluded, a thorough physical exam is performed, and a well-established ACOG (American College of Obstetrics and Gynecology) algorithm is used. This patient gives a history suggestive of an intracranial process (headache and specific visual deficits). The one diagnosis that could explain both these symptoms and her lack of menses is a prolactin-secreting adenoma of the pituitary.

A 17-beta-estradiol level (**choice A**) is not indicated in the evaluation of amenorrhea.

Serum LH and FSH (**choice B**) is indicated only if PRL levels are normal and polycystic ovarian disease or gonadal dysgenesis of some variety (e.g., early menopause or premature ovarian failure) is being considered.

MRI of the brain (**choice D**) is indicated only if prolactin is elevated, since brain masses are an uncommon cause of headache and the reason for her amenorrhea will typically lay elsewhere.

A visual evoked potential study (**choice E**) is not indicated in the evaluation of a patient with amenorrhea. This study is used in patients with suspected multiple sclerosis or retinal nerve damage.

34. **The correct answer is B.** This question relates to infectious diseases, their manifestations, and their geographic distribution. *Coccidioides immitis*, a fungus that exists as a spherule in the tissue, is endemic to the southwestern U.S., and infection is caused by inhalation. Some people develop an influenza-like illness that often resolves spontaneously.

Candida albicans (**choice A**) causes cutaneous infections and mucosal infections. It appears as pseudohyphae.

Cryptococcus neoformans (**choice C**) typically causes meningitis or pneumonia in immunocompromised patients. India ink preparation shows budding yeast forms.

Histoplasma capsulatum (**choice D**) is endemic in the central and eastern U.S. Spores are engulfed by macrophages. Diagnosis is made by tissue examination showing oval budding yeasts inside macrophages.

35. **The correct answer is D.** Normal pressure hydrocephalus (NPH) must be considered in any elderly patient with a subacute onset of mild dementia, urinary incontinence, and gait disturbance ("wacky, wobbly, and wet"). NPH is a communicating hydrocephalus presumed to be due to defective reabsorption of CSF by subarachnoid villi. The etiology is unknown, but some have suggested that obstruction of the normal flow of CSF over the cerebral convexity and delayed absorption into the venous system may be causative. Intracranial pressure is generally normal or high normal. Ventriculoperitoneal shunting is sometimes beneficial.

Alzheimer disease (**choice A**) is characterized by a slowly progressive decrease in cognitive functioning and memory over time in elderly patients.

Huntington disease (**choice B**) causes dementia, but is also associated with a choreoathetotic movement disorder that was not observed in this patient. In addition, Huntington disease generally presents around age 45-50.

Multi-infarct dementia (**choice C**) is characterized by a step-wise decrease in cognitive function associated with hypertension, atrial fibrillation, smoking, and transient ischemic events (TIAs) or strokes.

Pick disease (**choice E**) is rare and characterized by progressive dementia (similar to Alzheimer disease) associated with circumscribed cerebral atrophy (lobar sclerosis).

36. **The correct answer is B.** Atrial fibrillation may be the first sign of *hyperthyroidism*, especially in the absence of any cardiac anomalies or coronary artery disease. In such cases, thyroid hormone levels should be evaluated. The TSH level is a more sensitive parameter for the evaluation of thyroid dysfunction, as long as a sensitive (second- or third-generation) assay is used.

Maintaining the patient on the same medication (**choice A**) would be inappropriate without clarifying the underlying etiology.

The dexamethasone suppression test (**choice C**) is used to confirm a clinical suspicion of hypercortisolism. The patient is given 1 mg of dexamethasone at 11 P.M. At 8 A.M. the next morning, after overnight fasting, the cortisol level is measured in a serum sample. Failure to suppress cortisol secretion is evidence of Cushing syndrome/disease. This patient does not have clinical evidence of hypercortisolism (i.e., truncal obesity, dermal striae, and "moon face").

Anticoagulation with warfarin (**choice D**) would be appropriate if electrical or pharmacologic cardioversion were planned. This measure is necessary to prevent the formation of clots within the atria, with subsequent embolization when the heart resumes its normal rhythm.

Coronary arteriography (**choice E**) is useless since there is no clinical evidence of coronary artery disease, namely a history of anginal pain. On the other hand, hyperthyroidism can itself cause anginal pain, as well as atrial fibrillation.

37. **The correct answer is C.** The clinical presentation is consistent with *osteogenesis imperfecta*, which is due to mutations in one of the two genes that encode procollagen I. Type I collagen is the most abundant form in the body. Different mutations associated with osteogenesis imperfecta have been identified, some causing structurally abnormal collagen, others leading to decreased expression of procollagen I gene. There are two main clinical variants. The *fetal* type leads to *in utero* fractures and congenital deformities. The *adult* type results in extreme bone brittleness and frequent fractures and is also associated with a characteristic constellation of signs including bluish sclerae, brown or bluish misshapen teeth, and conductive hearing loss. Family history is usually positive since the disorder is usually transmitted as autosomal dominant.

Mutations resulting in defects in fibrillin (**choice A**) cause *Marfan syndrome*. Fibrillin protein forms the scaffold for the deposition of elastin in tissues of the heart valves, aorta, and lens suspensory ligaments. Major clinical manifestations include mitral valve prolapse, aortic dissection, aortic insufficiency, and dislocation of the lens. Body habitus is characteristic, with long arms and legs, long fingers (arachnodactyly), pectus excavatum, and bossing of frontal eminence.

A point mutation in the gene coding for FGF-receptor 3 (**choice B**) is the molecular defect causing *achondroplasia*, one of the most common causes of dwarfism. This mutation results in abnormal cell signaling that impairs proliferation of chondrocytes in the growth plate. Activation of FGFR3 inhibits normal proliferation of chondrocytes. Mutations associated with achondroplasia cause this receptor to be in constant activation.

Mutations affecting procollagen III (**choice D**) account for the majority of *Ehlers-Danlos syndrome*, characterized by hyperextensible skin and hypermobile joints.

Accumulation of mucopolysaccharides (**choice E**), as occurs in *mucopolysaccharidoses*, is often associated with short stature, chest wall deformities, and various bone malformations. Chondrocytes are among the cells most severely affected by these disorders.

38. **The correct answer is A.** Cryptococcal meningoencephalitis is one of the most frequent opportunistic infections in patients with AIDS. Cryptococcal organisms invade the subarachnoid space and extend into the perivascular (Virchow-Robin) spaces in the brain parenchyma, often without eliciting a significant inflammatory reaction. Cryptococcal meningitis presents with fever and headache, but nuchal rigidity may be minimal. Cranial nerve palsy may be present. Very high CSF cryptococcal antigen titers are characteristic of this condition. IV

administration of amphotericin B is necessary, followed by oral fluconazole.

The clarithromycin-rifabutin combination (**choice B**) is currently recommended to treat infections caused by *Mycobacterium avium-intracellulare* (MAI). MAI infections are exceptionally rare in immunocompetent hosts but occur frequently in AIDS patients.

Oral fluconazole (**choice C**) alone can be used to treat cryptococcal CNS infections in the absence of significant neurologic compromise.

Sulfadiazine-pyrimethamine (**choice D**) is an effective combination for treatment of cerebral toxoplasmosis, one of the most common opportunistic infections in AIDS.

Trimethoprim-sulfamethoxazole (**choice E**) is currently the treatment of choice for *Pneumocystis carinii* pneumonia, the most common opportunistic infection in AIDS.

39. **The correct answer is C.** Marfan syndrome is characterized by long limbs and fingers (arachnodactyly), ectopia lentis (dislocation of the lens), and proximal aortic dilatation resulting in aortic insufficiency, mitral valve prolapse (hence, the midsystolic click), and laxity of joints. Patients with Marfan syndrome are usually very tall: most of the height is due to the long lower extremities. Pectus excavatum and pectus carinatum (pigeon breast), and protuberant forehead are frequent associated skeletal anomalies. A mutation in the *fibrillin* gene is the underlying molecular defect. Cardiovascular complications, particularly aortic dissection, represent the most common cause of death in Marfan patients.

Ehlers-Danlos syndrome (**choice A**) is a heterogeneous group of disorders related to mutations in the genes encoding one of several types of collagen, most commonly collagen III. Clinically, it is characterized by laxity of joints and ligaments. The skin can be abnormally stretched.

Klinefelter syndrome (**choice B**) is a chromosomal disorder due to a 47,XXY karyotype. Patients are phenotypically males, but show hypogonadism and a characteristic *eunuchoid* habitus, with gynecomastia and long legs. Klinefelter syndrome is one the most frequent causes of male infertility.

McCune-Albright syndrome (**choice D**) or Albright syndrome is a rare hereditary condition caused by somatic mutations in the c-*fox* gene. It leads to multiple endocrinopathies, unilateral skin hyperpigmentation, multifocal fibrous dysplasia (on the side of the body with hyperpigmented skin), and precocious puberty.

Osteogenesis imperfecta (**choice E**) is an inherited condition, usually autosomal dominant, due to mutations in the gene for collagen type I. The resulting clinical picture is characterized by bone fragility, leading to multiple fractures *in utero* (fetal form) or adult life (adult form).

40. **The correct answer is E.** Virtually all patients with adult respiratory distress syndrome (ARDS) have reduced lung compliance. ARDS begins with compromise of capillary integrity, which causes extravasation of fluid, fibrin, and protein into the alveoli. Thus, the lungs become wet and stiff, causing reduced lung compliance. Clinical features include progressive tachypnea. Specific physical features are usually absent, except for bilateral diffuse rales. ARDS can be initiated by many different events and conditions, including shock, aspiration of fluid, disseminated intravascular coagulation (DIC), sepsis, trauma, blood transfusion, pancreatitis, smoke inhalation, and heroin overdose. The ultimate goal of treatment is to provide adequate tissue perfusion and oxygenation while addressing the precipitating event.

ARDS leads to tachypnea and increased ventilation. Thus, arterial P_{CO_2} is reduced (compare with **choice A**).

Chest x-ray films typically show patchy, diffuse, bilateral fluffy infiltrates, rather than a localized mass (**choice B**).

ARDS is characterized by severe hypoxia caused by extreme ventilation-perfusion ($\dot{V}/\dot{Q}$) imbalance and shunting of blood in the fluid-filled areas of the lung. Oxygenation is severely reduced, not normal (compare with **choice C**).

A pulmonary embolism (**choice D**) may result from prolonged immobilization, but is not necessarily a direct sequelae of ARDS.

41. **The correct answer is C.** Treatment with steroids is standard for polymyositis. Prednisone is used daily in single doses of 1 to 2 mg/kg. In responsive patients, muscle strength usually improves in 1 or 2 months, and the creatine phosphokinase (CPK) level normalizes in 3 months. Daily high-dose steroids are continued until the CPK has remained normal for a period of 3 to 6 weeks. Once the patient is in remission, the steroids should be tapered off slowly.

Intravenous fluid replacement (**choice A**) and plasma exchange (**choice B**) play no role in the management of polymyositis.

Neostigmine (**choice D**) is used in the treatment of myasthenia gravis.

Azathioprine (**choice E**) is used in patients whose condition is refractory or in those who continue to require high doses of steroids. It is not used as an initial therapy.

42. **The correct answer is A.** Hemolytic disease is associated with the production of black pigment gallbladder stones.

Brown pigment stones (**choice B**) form in the common duct, in the presence of infected bile.

Calcium stones (**choice C**) are found in the urinary tract rather than the biliary tract. Pigment stones in the biliary tract often have enough calcium to be radiopaque, but they are not pure calcium stones.

Mixed stones (**choice D**) are the usual gallbladder stones, seen in obese females who have had multiple pregnancies. They are not associated with hemolysis.

Pure cholesterol stone (**choice E**) is occasionally seen as a single large stone filling the entire gallbladder.

43. **The correct answer is D.** Urinary 5-hydroxyindoleacetic acid (5-HIAA), a serotonin metabolite, is increased in patients with carcinoid syndrome.

Calcitonin levels (**choice A**) would be elevated in patients with medullary thyroid carcinoma.

Serum gastrin levels (**choice B**) are elevated in patients with gastrinoma. Levels greater than 1,000 pg/mL in patients with typical clinical features of gastrinoma are sufficient to establish the diagnosis.

Upper gastrointestinal tract endoscopy (**choice C**) might reveal multiple peptic ulcers, implying Zollinger-Ellison syndrome. However, this is not the most appropriate diagnostic test.

Urine vanillylmandelic acid (**choice E**), a catecholamine metabolite, would be elevated in pheochromocytoma.

44. **The correct answer is A.** The young woman has a brain tumor. MRI will provide the best diagnostic images.

Skull x-rays (**choice B**) rarely are used nowadays. When patients sustain head trauma, CT scan is much more valuable. When we suspect brain tumor, x-rays are completely worthless. They cannot penetrate past the bone to show the brain.

Spinal tap (**choice C**) is absolutely contraindicated. The patient has increased intracranial pressure. A tap might produce herniation and death.

Pheochromocytomas produce headaches, but they do so as part of a pattern of pounding headache, palpitations, perspiration, pallor, and blood pressure elevation. In that case, measuring catecholamines (**choice D**) is indicated. In this vignette, it is not.

Visual fields (**choice E**) might help establish if the chiasma or the optic nerves or tracts are involved, but they would be completely normal if the tumor is elsewhere. This is obviously not the correct answer.

45. **The correct answer is D.** The patient is in diabetic ketoacidosis (DKA). The precipitant is probably the recent infection. The patient has become hyperglycemic, leading to an osmotic diuresis. The low insulin levels have induced a fasting state, leading to catabolism of fatty acids into ketones. She needs continuous short-acting

insulin to reverse this process. Regular insulin is short-acting and can be administered via continuous intravenous infusion, with monitoring of the patient's blood glucose response. This patient is also dehydrated because of the osmotic diuresis; the dehydration is the cause of the observed orthostasis. Therefore, fluid replacement with regular insulin infusion is the ideal treatment.

Severe dehydration can produce lactic acidosis from decreased perfusion and ischemia. Thus, isotonic solution replacement (**choice A**) is a partial, but not complete, treatment for this patient. Her acidosis is significantly worsened by her diabetes, and the underlying problem will be corrected by insulin administration.

NPH insulin would be too erratic in maintaining euglycemia (**choice B**). Her dehydration needs to be corrected rapidly. NPH effects peak after 4 to 6 hours, which will not allow the adequate and immediate reversal of this patient's DKA.

Although administration of continuous IV regular insulin is part of the solution (**choice C**), it is not the complete solution, since the lost fluids must be replaced as well.

In the initial stages of DKA, this patient needs *continuous* insulin infusion. Administration of regular insulin every 4 hours (**choice E**) might not prove adequate, since her DKA control will be too episodic and erratic.

46. **The correct answer is C.** The diagnosis is obvious (bony metastasis from the recent breast cancer), but the question is to what extent the spinal cord is involved. MRI is the best study to evaluate the spinal cord.

Lumbar puncture (**choice A**) will not provide useful information unless it is done to provide access for contrast material for x-rays. One of the advantages of the MRI is that detailed information can be seen without resorting to invasive studies.

She may well have a second cancer in her other breast, but looking for it (**choice B**) is not going to influence what we do for the current problem that is affecting her back.

By the same token, she could have bony metastasis elsewhere, but a bone scan of the thoracic area (**choice D**) would be redundant. We already know from the x-ray that she has a metastasis in the thoracic spine. The MRI will show other metastasis in that region if they are present. Bone scan of the whole body might add information, but it would not be critical for the management of the current symptomatic lesion.

MRI is better than CT scan (**choice E**) when the target of our studies is the spinal cord.

47. **In the correct answer is B.** Most mucosa-associated lymphoid tissue lymphoma is related to *Helicobacter pylori* infection. Studies have shown that eradication of infec-tion of *H. pylori* results in regression of such infection. This treatment involves a prolonged course of antibiotic therapy aimed at eliminating the bacteria.

Combination chemotherapy has been used in the diffuse aggressive lymphoma that arises from mucosa-associated lymphoid tissue lymphoma (**choice A**).

Because MALT lymphomas can progress to diffuse, large, B cell lymphomas, observation is not appropriate (**choice C**).

Primary management for most lymphoma is combination chemotherapy, not radiation therapy (**choice D**).

Gastric mucosa-associated lymphoid tissue lymphomas can progress to diffuse, large, B cell lymphomas. Many forms of treatment produce responses, but until recently most therapies were considered palliative and had not been shown to extend survival. Combination chemotherapy regimens that include fludarabine have shown improvements in response rate and durability of response (**choice E**).

48. **The correct answer is B.** This patient has cold autoimmune hemolytic anemia, a disease primarily seen in the elderly although it is classically associated with mycoplasma (and other pulmonary pathogens) infection and lymphoproliferative disorders. IgM antibodies are created, which react with polysaccharide antigens on the erythrocyte surface only at temperatures below that of the core temperature of the body. In severe cases, acral cyanosis (often easily reproducible) and livedo reticularis are both present. Anemia is usually Coombs-positive, which reveals surface complement and antibody attached to the erythrocyte membrane. The indirect Coombs test (**choice D**) looks for circulating antibodies (such as in testing blood before transfusion) and is not commonly used in evaluating autoimmune hemolytic anemias. The usual treatment centers on staying warm.

A bone marrow biopsy (**choice A**) will show nonspecific erythroid hyperplasia and some lymphocytoplasmic aggregates. It is not necessary for the diagnosis, unless there is other evidence to suspect a lymphoproliferative disorder (lymphoma is associated with cold agglutinins).

This patient has a normocytic anemia with laboratory work consistent with hemolysis. LDH, an intracellular enzyme, is elevated, indicating cell lysis. Indirect bilirubin, also elevated, indicates increased heme catabolism, further suggesting hemolysis. The haptoglobin, which binds free hemoglobin, is low, suggesting that extracellular hemoglobin is present. Given these findings, it is not necessary to first rule out iron deficiency anemia by ordering a ferritin and iron binding capacity (**choice C**). If, in the course of this patient's treatment, there appears to be an iron deficiency component to his anemia, then these would be appropriate tests.

Mycoplasma is one of a handful of conditions that have well described associations with cold autoimmune hemolytic anemia. However, this patient's current condition exists independent of any obvious precipitating factor. As such, mycoplasma pneumonia titers (**choice E**) are unlikely to be helpful because the current condition exists independent of any precipitating cause.

49. **The correct answer is K.** This is the characteristic clinical presentation of schwannomas of the acoustic nerve (AKA acoustic neurinomas). Loss of speech discrimination is an early sign, often associated with tinnitus. In the Weber test, the tuning fork is applied to the forehead: the sound will appear louder in the deaf ear because of a conductive deficit. In this case, the sound appears louder in the good ear, which indicates sensorineural loss.

50. **The correct answer is D.** Guillain-Barré syndrome is an acute/subacute demyelinating inflammatory polyneuropathy manifesting with typical "ascending" paralysis. This condition may be fatal if respiratory muscles are involved. It is probably of autoimmune origin and is often triggered by an upper respiratory infection occurring a few weeks before the onset of the neurologic symptoms. Typical CSF findings include elevated protein with a normal cell count or mild lymphocytosis.

Botulism (**choice A**) manifests with sudden development of diplopia, dysphagia, and nasal speech, followed by paralysis of respiratory muscles and limbs.

Charcot-Marie-Tooth disease (**choice B**) is an autosomal dominant polyneuropathy that manifests in childhood with distal weakness and wasting of calf muscles.

The most common form of diabetic neuropathy (**choice C**) is a distal symmetric polyneuropathy, manifesting with depressed tendon reflexes, reduced sensation, paresthesias, and burning pain in the distal extremities (typically feet before hands).

Lead neuropathy (**choice E**) follows chronic lead poisoning, manifesting with learning disorders (in children) and motor deficits (wrist drop).

Ménière syndrome (**choice F**) consists of recurrent attacks of vertigo, tinnitus, and a characteristic sensation of pressure in the ear. Fluctuating sensorineural hearing loss is also present.

Neurofibromatosis (**choice G**) type 2 (the "central" type) is associated with intracranial tumors. Bilateral schwannomas are pathognomonic of this condition.

Otosclerosis (**choice H**) affects the footplate of the stapes, leading to increased rigidity of the ossicular chain and producing conductive hearing loss (usually bilateral and symmetric). Otosclerosis has a strong familial basis.

Polyarteritis nodosa (**choice I**) may involve the vasa nervorum and manifests with random involvement of single peripheral nerves (*mononeuritis multiplex*), with sensory-motor disturbances.

Presbyacusis (**choice J**) is the progressive hearing loss associated with aging. It is symmetric and preferentially affects high-frequency sounds. Impaired speech discrimination in a noisy environment is characteristic.

Traumatic neuroma (**choice L**) is a tumor-like nodule resulting from haphazard regeneration of the distal end of a peripheral nerve following transection. It manifests with acute pain.

Vertebrobasilar insufficiency (**choice M**) is a common cause of vertigo in old age. It may result from atherosclerosis of the posterior cerebral circulation or osteoarthritis of the cervical column.

Obstetrics/Gynecology: **Test One**

1. A 24-year-old woman presents to the emergency department complaining of right lower quadrant pain and vaginal spotting. Her last menstrual period was 5 weeks ago. Her temperature is 37.0° C (98.6° F), blood pressure is 112/70 mm Hg, pulse is 74/min, and respirations are 14/min. The abdomen is soft and nontender. Pelvic examination reveals scant blood in the vagina, a closed cervical os, no pelvic masses, and right pelvic tenderness. Her leukocyte count is 8,000/mm^3, hematocrit is 38%, and platelet count is 250,000/mm^3. Which of the following is the most appropriate step next in diagnosis?

    (A) Bedside hCG

    (B) Serum TSH

    (C) Abdominal x-ray

    (D) Abdominal/pelvic CT

    (E) Laparoscopy

2. A 35-year-old African American woman presents to a physician complaining of irregular menstrual periods. She had her first menses at age 15 and states that her periods come irregularly every 2 to 6 months. She has been in a monogamous relationship with her husband for 15 years; for 10 years they have been trying unsuccessfully to conceive. She gets yearly Pap smears, which have been normal. Her height is 5 feet 2 inches (157.5 cm), and her weight is 200 pounds (90.9 kg). Her temperature is 37.0° C (98.6° F), blood pressure is 118/78 mm Hg, pulse is 80/min, and respirations are 14/min. She has acne, as well as excess hair on her face and between her breasts. Her abdomen is obese. Examination is otherwise within normal limits. This patient is at greatest risk for developing which of the following diseases?

    (A) Cervical cancer

    (B) Endometrial cancer

    (C) Lung cancer

    (D) Osteoporosis

    (E) Ovarian cancer

3. A 32-year-old Hispanic woman presents to the emergency department complaining of heavy vaginal bleeding. Her temperature is 37.0° C (98.6° F), blood pressure is 80/50 mm Hg, pulse is 110/min, and respirations are 18/min. Her abdomen is soft, nontender, and nondistended. Her pelvic examination reveals approximately 200 mL of clotted blood in the vagina, an open cervical os with tissue protruding from it, and a 10-week-sized, nontender uterus. Leukocyte count is 9,000/mm^3, hematocrit is 22%, and platelet count is 275,000/mm^3. Quantitative hCG is 100,000 mIU/L (normal: 5-200,000 mIU/L). Pelvic ultrasound shows echogenic material within the uterine cavity consistent with blood or tissue, no adnexal masses, and no free fluid. No viable pregnancy is seen. Which of the following is the most appropriate next step in management?

    (A) Discharge to home

    (B) Culdocentesis

    (C) Dilation and evacuation

    (D) Laparoscopy

    (E) Laparotomy

4. A 25-year-old Caucasian woman, gravida 1, para 0, at 26 weeks' gestational age presents to her physician's office complaining of spotting from the vagina. She has no contractions and reports normal fetal movement. She denies any history of a bleeding disorder. Her temperature is 37.3° C (99.1° F), blood pressure is 100/60 mm Hg, pulse is 75/min, and respirations are 14/min. Her abdomen is gravid and benign, with a fundal height of 26 cm. A placenta previa is ruled out by ultrasound examination. Pelvic examination reveals some scant blood in the vagina, a closed os, and no uterine tenderness. Leukocyte count is 12,000/mm^3, hematocrit is 33%, and platelet count is 140,000/mm^3. Her blood type is A, Rh negative. Which of the following is the most appropriate pharmacotherapy?

    (A) Antibiotics

    (B) Blood transfusion

    (C) Magnesium sulfate

    (D) Platelet transfusion

    (E) RhoGAM™

5. A 29-year-old primigravid woman is admitted to the labor and delivery ward with strong contractions every 2 minutes and cervical change from 3 to 4 cm. Over the next 5 hours she progresses to full dilation. After 3 hours of pushing, the physician cuts a mediolateral episiotomy, and the woman delivers a 3770-g (8-lb, 4-oz) boy. Which of the following is the main advantage of a mediolateral episiotomy over a median (midline) episiotomy?

    (A) Easier surgical repair of the episiotomy

    (B) Improved healing of the episiotomy

    (C) Less blood loss

    (D) Less likely to cause a fourth-degree extension

    (E) Less pain

6. A 22-year-old woman presents with mouth sores, sore throat, vaginal discharge, fever, and myalgia. She has no other medical problems. She takes oral contraceptive pills. She is in a monogamous relationship and states that her partner occasionally uses barrier contraception. Physical examination reveals a temperature of 38.3° C (101.0° F), cervical and inguinal lymphadenopathy, exudative pharyngitis, and multiple ulcers on the oral mucosa, the labia, and cervix. The vaginal discharge is profuse, and Gram stain indicates many neutrophils. Which of the following is the most likely diagnosis?

    (A) Chancroid

    (B) Condyloma acuminatum

    (C) Herpes simplex virus

    (D) Lymphogranuloma venereum

    (E) Syphilis

7. A 34-year-old woman, gravida 3, para 2, at 38 weeks' gestation presents to the labor and delivery ward complaining of headache. She has no contractions. Her prenatal course was unremarkable until she noted the onset of swelling in her face, hands, and feet this week. Her obstetric history is significant for two normal spontaneous vaginal deliveries. She has no significant past medical or surgical history. Her temperature is 37.0° C (98.6° F), blood pressure is 160/92 mm Hg, pulse is 78/min, and respirations are 16/min. Examination reveals 3+ patellar reflexes bilaterally. A cervical examination reveals that her cervix is 3 cm dilated and 50% effaced and soft, and that the fetus is at 0 station and vertex. The fetal heart rate has a baseline of 140/min and is reactive. The results from a 24-hour urine collection show 5,200 mg of protein (normal <300 mg/24 hours). The patient is given magnesium sulfate intravenously for seizure prophylaxis. Which of the following is the most appropriate next step in the management of this patient?

    (A) Expectant management

    (B) Intramuscular glucocorticoids

    (C) IV oxytocin

    (D) Subcutaneous terbutaline

    (E) Cesarean section

8. A 64-year-old woman undergoes left radical mastectomy for breast cancer. A 4-cm infiltrating ductal carcinoma is found on pathologic examination. Four of 20 axillary lymph nodes are positive for malignancy. Neoplastic cells are immunoreactive for estrogen and progesterone receptors. No evidence of metastatic disease is found on bone scanning with ^{99m}Tc-labeled phosphate or chest x-ray films. The patient receives appropriate radiation therapy and multidrug chemotherapy. Which of the following is the most appropriate adjunctive therapy in this setting?

   (A) Danazol

   (B) Ethinyl estradiol

   (C) Megestrol acetate

   (D) Medroxyprogesterone acetate

   (E) Natural progesterone

   (F) Tamoxifen

9. A 23-year-old gravida 3, para 2 is admitted to the hospital at 31 weeks' gestation with painful uterine contractions. Her cervix is initially 3 cm dilated. Magnesium sulfate is started. Over the next 5 hours, she progresses to full dilation. After a 1-hour second stage, she delivers a 2013-g (4-lb, 7-oz) newborn. In the neonatal intensive care unit, the infant develops respiratory distress and pneumonia. Over the following days the infant develops septicemia. Preliminary blood cultures demonstrate gram-positive cocci in chains. Treatment with which of the following would most likely have prevented this neonatal outcome?

   (A) Folic acid

   (B) Gentamicin

   (C) Naloxone

   (D) Oxytocin

   (E) Penicillin

10. A 26-year-old nulligravid patient presents to her physician seeking preconceptional advice. She plans to conceive in about 1 year. Her past medical history is significant for chickenpox as a child. She had an appendectomy 2 years ago. She takes no medications and is allergic to penicillin. Her complete physical examination, including a pelvic examination, is unremarkable. Which of the following is the most appropriate next step in diagnosis to prevent morbidity in this patient's offspring?

   (A) Blood cultures

   (B) Group B *Streptococcus* culture

   (C) Pelvic ultrasound

   (D) Rubella titer

   (E) Urine culture

11. A 26-year-old black gravida 2, para 1, at 32 weeks' gestation presents to the physician for a prenatal visit. Her prenatal course has been remarkable for hyperemesis gravidarum in the first trimester. She also had a urine culture in the first trimester that grew out group B *Streptococcus*. She has had type 1 diabetes for the past 2 years and has had good control of her blood glucose levels during this pregnancy. Her first pregnancy resulted in a low transverse cesarean section for dystocia. Other than insulin, she takes no medicines and has no known drug allergies. After a routine prenatal visit, the physician sends her to the antepartum fetal testing unit to undergo a nonstress test (NST). Which of the following characteristics makes this patient a good candidate for antepartum fetal testing with an NST?

   (A) Black race

   (B) Diabetes mellitus

   (C) Group B *Streptococcus* urine culture

   (D) History of cesarean section

   (E) Hyperemesis gravidarum

12. A 19-year-old gravida 2, para 1 woman presents at her first prenatal visit complaining of a rash, hair loss, and spots on her tongue. Her temperature is 37.0° C (98.6° F), blood pressure is 112/74 mm Hg, pulse is 68/min, and respirations are 14/min. Physical examination is significant for a maculopapular rash on her trunk and extremities, including her palms and soles. She has "moth-eaten" alopecia and white patches on her tongue. Her uterus is 10-week size, which is consistent with her dating by last menstrual period. The rest of her examination is unremarkable. RPR and MHA-TP are positive. Which of the following is the most appropriate pharmacotherapy?

    (A) Clindamycin
    (B) Gentamicin
    (C) Nitrofurantoin
    (D) Penicillin
    (E) Tetracycline

13. A 34-year-old woman with breast cancer presents to her physician complaining of increased weakness, lower back pain, and urinary incontinence. She was diagnosed with breast cancer 2 years ago and is undergoing radiation and chemotherapy. Her back pain developed 2 days ago. Physical examination shows lower extremity weakness and hyporeflexia. Which of the following is the most appropriate next step in this patient's care?

    (A) Obtain a neurologic consultation
    (B) Obtain an emergency spinal MRI
    (C) Administer narcotics for pain relief
    (D) Administer high-dose steroids
    (E) Perform a lumbar puncture

14. An otherwise healthy, 65-year-old woman comes to the physician because of bloody discharge from the right nipple for 2 weeks. On examination, no retraction, erosion, or other abnormal change is present. Palpation reveals an ill-defined, 1-cm nodule located deep in the right areola. Which of the following is the most appropriate next step in diagnosis?

    (A) Cytologic examination of nipple discharge
    (B) Mammography alone
    (C) Ultrasonography
    (D) Biopsy under mammographic localization
    (E) Mammography followed by fine-needle cytology

15. A 34-year-old woman, gravida 3, para 2, at 16 weeks' gestation comes to the physician concerned that she may have been exposed to an infectious disease. Yesterday, she and her 5-year-old son spent a day at the beach with one of his classmates. This morning, the classmate was sent home from school with a fever and rash that the teacher thought were suspicious for chickenpox. The patient is unsure whether she had chickenpox as a child. Her temperature is 37° C (98.6° F), blood pressure is 100/70 mm Hg, pulse is 88/min, and respirations are 16/min. Her examination is unremarkable. An inquiry made by the physician confirms that the classmate has chickenpox. Which of the following is the most appropriate next step in management?

    (A) Check an IgG varicella serology
    (B) Wait to see whether a rash develops
    (C) Administer IV acyclovir
    (D) Administer oral acyclovir
    (E) Administer varicella vaccine

16. A 26-year-old primigravid woman at 10 weeks' gestation comes to the physician for a routine prenatal appointment. Her dating is based on a 6-week ultrasound. She has sickle-cell anemia. She has no past surgical history, takes prenatal vitamins, and has no known drug allergies. She tells the physician that she recently learned that the father of the baby has sickle-cell trait. On examination, her uterus is appropriate for a 10-week gestation, and fetal heart tones are heard. Her hematocrit is 37%. What is the most appropriate next step in the management of this patient?

    (A) Genetic counseling
    (B) Obstetric ultrasound
    (C) Hydroxyurea
    (D) IV hydration
    (E) Blood transfusion

17. A 23-year-old woman, gravida 1, para 0, at 25 weeks' gestation comes to the physician because of right upper quadrant pain, nausea and vomiting, and malaise for the past 2 days. Her temperature is 37.0° C (98.6° F), blood pressure is 104/72 mm Hg, pulse is 92/min, and respirations are 16/min. Physical examination reveals right upper quadrant tenderness to palpation. The cervix is long, closed, and posterior. There is generalized edema. Laboratory values are as follows:

Leukocyte count	10,500/mm³
Platelet count	62,000/mm³
Hematocrit	26%
Sodium	140 mEq/L
Chloride	100 mEq/L
Potassium	4.5 mEq/L
Bicarbonate	26 mEq/L

A peripheral blood smear reveals hemolysis. Which of the following laboratory findings would be most likely in this patient?

(A) Decreased fibrin split products

(B) Decreased lactate dehydrogenase

(C) Elevated AST

(D) Elevated fibrinogen

(E) Elevated glucose

18. A 17-year-old woman, gravida 1, para 0, at 38 weeks' gestation comes to the labor and delivery ward because of contractions. Her dating was determined by a 7-week ultrasound. Her prenatal course was complicated by gestational diabetes. Her past surgical history is significant for shoulder surgery. She takes insulin and prenatal vitamins. She has no known drug allergies. She smokes 3 to 4 cigarettes per day. She is initially found to be 4 cm dilated and is contracting every 2 to 3 minutes. She is admitted to the labor and delivery ward and, over the next 4 hours, progresses to full dilation. After pushing for 2 hours, she delivers the fetal head but has great difficulty delivering the fetal shoulders. Eventually, the fetus is delivered by the posterior arm. In the process of delivery the newborn's humerus is fractured. Which of the following factors contributed the most to the difficult delivery of the fetus?

(A) Cigarette smoking

(B) Gestational age

(C) Gestational diabetes

(D) Maternal age

(E) Maternal shoulder surgery

19. A 22-year-old woman comes to the physician seeking advice. Last night, while she was having sexual intercourse, the condom broke. She is very concerned that she may become pregnant and wants to know whether she can do anything at this point. She has no medical problems and has never had surgery. She takes ibuprofen for dysmenorrhea. She is allergic to sulfa drugs. On physical examination, she is anxious and intermittently sobbing. Her temperature is 37.0° C (98.6° F), blood pressure is 140/90 mm Hg, pulse is 98/min, and respirations are 24/min. The remainder of her physical examination is unremarkable. A urine pregnancy test is negative. Which of the following is the most appropriate pharmacotherapy?

(A) Clomiphene

(B) Gentamicin

(C) Labetalol

(D) Norgestrel/ethinyl estradiol (or levonorgestrel)

(E) Trimethoprim-sulfamethoxazole

20. A 42-year-old woman comes to the physician because of vaginal itch and discharge, dysuria, and dyspareunia. These symptoms have been steadily worsening over the past 3 days. Pelvic examination reveals an erythematous vagina and a thin, green, frothy vaginal discharge with a pH of 6. Microscopic examination of the discharge demonstrates the presence of a pear-shaped, motile organism. Which of the following is the most likely pathogen?

(A) *Candida albicans*

(B) *Gardnerella vaginalis*

(C) Herpes simplex virus

(D) *Treponema pallidum*

(E) *Trichomonas vaginalis*

21. A 34-year-old woman, gravida 4, para 3 at 38 weeks' gestation comes to the labor and delivery ward because of contractions. Her prenatal course was significant for low maternal weight gain. She had a normal 18-week ultrasound survey of the fetus and normal 36-week ultrasound to check fetal presentation. Her blood type is O positive, and she is rubella immune. Three years ago, she had a multiple myomectomy. She takes prenatal vitamins and has no known drug allergies. She smokes one pack of cigarettes per day. Which of the following complications is most likely to occur?

    (A) Amniotic fluid embolism

    (B) Anencephaly

    (C) Macrosomia

    (D) Rh isoimmunization

    (E) Uterine rupture

22. A 39-year-old woman, gravida 3, para 2 at 34 weeks' gestation, with a known history of chronic hypertension, is found to have a blood pressure of 180/115 mm Hg at a routine prenatal visit. Her prenatal course had been otherwise unremarkable. She is transferred to the labor and delivery ward for further management. IV antihypertensive medications should be given to this patient with a goal of which of the following blood pressures?

    (A) 90/60 mm Hg

    (B) 100/75 mm Hg

    (C) 120/80 mm Hg

    (D) 150/95 mm Hg

    (E) 180/110 mm Hg

23. A 33-year-old woman comes to the physician because she has not had a menstrual period for 6 months. Prior to this she had a normal period every 29 days that lasted for 4 days. She has noted some weight gain in the past few months. She has a history of hepatitis A infection 6 years ago and had an appendectomy at age 12. She takes no medications and has no allergies to medications. Her father died of acute pancreatitis 3 years ago. Her mother is alive and well with no medical problems. Which of the following is the most appropriate next step in diagnosis?

    (A) Lipase

    (B) FSH

    (C) Beta-hCG

    (D) Liver function tests

    (E) TSH

24. A 24-year-old woman, gravida 2, para 2, comes to the physician for a yearly physical and birth control counseling. She is currently using the rhythm method of birth control, but has heard that this method has a high failure rate and would like to try a different method. Several of her friends use the intrauterine device (IUD), and she is wondering whether she could also use this method. Past medical history is significant for eczema. Past surgical history is significant for a right ovarian cystectomy 2 years ago. Past gynecologic history is significant for multiple episodes of *Chlamydia* cervicitis and two episodes of pelvic inflammatory disease (PID), the most recent episode occurring 1 year ago. She takes acetaminophen for occasional tension headaches. She is allergic to penicillin. She smokes one-half pack of cigarettes per day. Physical examination is unremarkable. Which of the following would be the best recommendation for this patient regarding her birth control method?

    (A) "The IUD is absolutely contraindicated."

    (B) "The IUD is recommended."

    (C) "The IUD is recommended if cervical cultures are negative."

    (D) "The oral contraceptive pill is absolutely contraindicated."

    (E) "The rhythm method is recommended."

25. A 26-year-old woman, gravida 2, para 1 at 28 weeks' gestation, comes to the physician for a follow-up ultrasound after a previous ultrasound demonstrated a marginal placenta previa. The present ultrasound shows complete resolution of the marginal previa, but the fetus is noted to be in breech presentation. The patient has otherwise had an unremarkable prenatal course. She has no medical problems and has never had surgery. She takes prenatal vitamins and is allergic to sulfa drugs. Assuming that the fetus stays in breech presentation, when should an external cephalic version be attempted?

    (A) After 30 weeks

    (B) After 33 weeks

    (C) After 37 weeks

    (D) After 40 weeks

    (E) After 42 weeks

26. A 19-year-old woman, gravida 1, para 1, is immediately status post a normal spontaneous vaginal delivery and normal third stage when she develops brisk bright red bleeding from the vagina. Her prenatal course was unremarkable. She has asthma, which worsened during the pregnancy. Ten years ago, she had a tonsillectomy. She takes a steroid and albuterol inhaler. She has no known drug allergies. Her temperature is 37.0° C (98.6° F), blood pressure is 100/70 mm Hg, pulse is 115/min, and respirations are 16/min. Her abdomen is soft and nontender. Her uterus is soft and "boggy" to palpation. Pelvic examination reveals no evidence of a laceration. Which of the following treatments should be avoided in managing this patient's postpartum hemorrhage?

   (A) Acetaminophen

   (B) IV hydration

   (C) Methylergonovine

   (D) Oxytocin

   (E) 15-Methyl-prostaglandin $F_{2\alpha}$ ($PGF_{2\alpha}$)

27. A 36-year-old woman, gravida 3, para 3, is 2 days status post cesarean section for dystocia when she begins wandering the hallways of the hospital at 2 A.M. She is extremely confused and thinks that she is at the police station. She states that she cannot sleep, feels very anxious, and wants to hurt her baby. Her prenatal course was unremarkable. She has no medical problems and had never had surgery. She has been taking Tylenol with codeine postpartum for incisional pain. Which of the following is the most appropriate next step in the management?

   (A) Fluoxetine

   (B) Morphine

   (C) Naloxone

   (D) Psychiatric hospitalization

   (E) Supervised visit to the nursery

28. A 19-year-old gravida 1, para 0 woman at 38 weeks' gestation comes to her physician because she has passed bloody mucus discharge. Her prenatal course was unremarkable including a normal 19-week ultrasound. On speculum examination, there are no vaginal or cervical lesions. On vaginal examination, the cervix is 2 cm dilated and 100% effaced, and the fetus is at +1 station. The fetal heart rate has a baseline of 140 and is reactive. She has painful contractions every 2 minutes. One hour later the patient's cervix is 3 cm dilated, and a small amount of bloody mucus is noted on the examining glove. Which of the following is the most likely diagnosis?

   (A) Early labor

   (B) Placental abruption

   (C) Placenta previa

   (D) Urinary tract infection

   (E) Vasa previa

29. A 23-year-old woman, gravida 2, para 1 at 26 weeks' gestation, comes to the physician because of fevers and pain in the middle of the back on the right side. Her fevers started 2 days ago, and the back pain began yesterday. Her temperature is 38.3° C (101.0° F), blood pressure is 110/70 mm Hg, pulse is 110/min, and respirations are 16/min. She has left costovertebral angle tenderness. Her abdomen is benign and gravid. Her laboratory values show leukocytes of 18,000/mm³. Urinalysis reveals white blood cells that are too numerous to count per high-powered field. Which of the following is the most appropriate pharmacotherapy for this patient?

   (A) Acyclovir

   (B) Ceftriaxone

   (C) Levofloxacin

   (D) Metronidazole

   (E) Tetracycline

30. A 42-year-old woman, gravida 4, para 3, at 38 weeks' gestation, comes to the labor and delivery ward complaining of contractions. She has had type 1 diabetes since the age of 20. She has a history of syphilis that was adequately treated 4 years ago. She took insulin and prenatal vitamins throughout the pregnancy. Otherwise, her prenatal course was unremarkable, including normal screening. Her blood pressure is 140/90 mm Hg. Her cervix is 4 cm dilated and 100% effaced. She is admitted. Which of the following IV medications will this patient likely require during labor and delivery to prevent neonatal complications?

    (A) Hydralazine
    (B) Insulin
    (C) Labetalol
    (D) Meperidine
    (E) Penicillin

31. A 75-year-old woman comes to the physician complaining of vulvar itch that has been worsening for the past 2 years. She has had no bleeding from the vagina since she underwent menopause at the age of 52. She smokes five cigarettes per day. On physical examination she has a raised, pigmented lesion on the right labia majora. The rest of her physical examination is unremarkable. Which of the following is the most appropriate next step in the management of this patient?

    (A) Prescribe an antibiotic
    (B) Prescribe an antifungal
    (C) Prescribe steroid cream
    (D) Refer to psychiatry
    (E) Biopsy the lesion

32. A 33-year-old, white woman, gravida 3, para 2, at 37 weeks' gestation comes to the emergency department because of painful uterine contractions and heavy vaginal bleeding that started after she used intranasal cocaine. The patient's prenatal course was significant because she conceived while on the oral contraceptive pill, she occasionally used cocaine and heroin during the pregnancy, and she was found to be positive for group B *Streptococcus* colonization at 35 weeks. Fetal monitoring is not reassuring. The patient undergoes cesarean section, at which the uterus has a bluish hue. On inspection, the placenta is noted to have an adherent, retroplacental clot on 50% of its surface. Which of the following is the most likely initiating factor for this patient's presentation?

    (A) Cocaine
    (B) Gestational age
    (C) Group B *Streptococcus* colonization
    (D) Oral contraceptive pill use
    (E) White race

33. A 22-year-old primigravid woman at 32 weeks' gestation comes to the emergency department because of heavy vaginal bleeding and abdominal pain. Her prenatal course was unremarkable, including a normal 20-week ultrasound. Physical examination demonstrates a contracted uterus with hypertonus. A large "gush" of blood occurs during the cervical examination, which demonstrates a long and closed cervix. The fetal heart rate tracing shows severe late decelerations. Which of the following is the most appropriate next step in management?

    (A) Expectant management
    (B) Magnesium sulfate
    (C) Oxytocin
    (D) Terbutaline
    (E) Cesarean section

34. A premenopausal, 48-year-old woman undergoes a routine mammographic screening. Physical examination is normal. Mammography identifies a suspicious focus with clustered microcalcifications located deeply in the lateral upper quadrant of the right breast. No abnormality can be detected in this area on breast examination. Which of the following is the most appropriate next step in diagnosis?

    (A) Mammographic reexamination in 1 year

    (B) Ultrasonography

    (C) Biopsy guided by mammographic localization

    (D) Fine-needle aspiration cytology

    (E) Large needle (core needle) biopsy

35. A 64-year-old woman comes to the physician because she is "leaking" urine. She states that, over the past 3 years, she has had incontinence several times daily. She describes these episodes as small squirts of urine that come out whenever she laughs, coughs, sneezes, or engages in physical activity. Physical examination shows mild uterine prolapse and a moderate cystocele. Urine culture is negative. Postvoid residual is 25 mL (normal <50 mL) Cystometrogram is normal. Which of the following is the most likely diagnosis?

    (A) Detrusor instability (DI)

    (B) Genuine stress urinary incontinence (GSUI)

    (C) Neurogenic bladder

    (D) Pyelonephritis

    (E) Urinary tract infection

36. A 30-year-old woman with a genetic disorder characterized by a deficiency of phenylalanine hydroxylase is planning a first pregnancy. Her physician explains the increased risk of mental retardation, as well congenital heart disease, in the infant. Which of the following should also be recommended?

    (A) Low phenylalanine diet should be initiated before conception

    (B) Dietary supplementation with glycine is recommended

    (C) Dietary supplementation with L-carnitine is recommended

    (D) There is no need for diet control if phenylalanine levels are mildly elevated

    (E) Vitamin B_6 should be administered to the neonate on delivery

37. A 19-year-old woman comes to the physician because of irregular vaginal bleeding. She has asthma and has never had surgery. She takes albuterol for her asthma and has been taking the oral contraceptive pill for 2 years. She has no allergies to medications. On examination she is found to have a vaginal lesion, which is biopsied. The biopsy shows clear cell adenocarcinoma of the vagina. This patient's malignancy is most likely associated with which of the following types of exposure?

    (A) Current albuterol use

    (B) Current oral contraceptive pill use

    (C) In utero aspirin exposure

    (D) In utero warfarin exposure

    (E) In utero diethylstilbestrol (DES) exposure

38. A 22-year-old woman, gravida 2, para 1, comes to the physician for her first prenatal visit. She had a previous full-term, normal vaginal delivery 2 years ago. She has no medical problems and has never had surgery. She takes no medications and has no known drug allergies. Pelvic examination reveals a mucopurulent cervical discharge, no cervical motion tenderness, and an 8-week-sized, nontender uterus. A cervical swab is performed. Two days later, the laboratory calls to notify the physician that the patient is positive for *Chlamydia trachomatis*. Which of the following is the most appropriate pharmacotherapy?

    (A) Ceftriaxone

    (B) Erythromycin

    (C) Metronidazole

    (D) Penicillin

    (E) Tetracycline

39. A 39-year-old nulligravid woman comes to the physician because of a persistent vaginal itch, vaginal discharge, and dysuria. She has had these same symptoms several times over the past 2 years and each time has been diagnosed with *Candida* vulvovaginitis. On physical examination, she has a thick, white vaginal discharge and significant vulvar and vaginal erythema. A potassium hydroxide (KOH) smear shows pseudohyphae; the normal saline smear is negative. Which of the following is the most appropriate next step in management?

    (A) Refer to psychiatry

    (B) Screen for cocaine abuse

    (C) Screen for diabetes

    (D) Screen for thalassemia

    (E) Treat with metronidazole

40. A 59-year-old patient with a 2-year history of metastatic breast cancer presents with the acute onset of severe low back pain. She underwent a radical mastectomy and lymphadenectomy 3 years ago. Four of seven nodes were positive at the time of her original diagnosis. One year ago she developed an asymptomatic metastasis to her right femur. On physical examination, she is in severe discomfort and finds movement extremely difficult. She has exquisite tenderness in the lumbar vertebral area, and any motion of her legs or lower back produces extreme pain. An emergent MRI reveals large lytic lesions in L3 and L4. Which of the following is the most appropriate next step in management?

    (A) Discuss her wishes regarding cardiopulmonary resuscitation (CPR)

    (B) Refer her to a pain management consultant

    (C) Prescribe bed rest with high-dose nonsteroidal anti-inflammatory drugs (NSAIDs)

    (D) Schedule her for radiation therapy to the lumbar spine

    (E) Schedule her for an emergency nuclear bone scan

41. A 22-year-old woman comes to the physician with her husband because of vaginal irritation and a malodorous vaginal discharge. Her symptoms started 4 days ago. She also notes pain with intercourse and dysuria. Pelvic examination reveals vaginal and cervical erythema and a copious greenish, frothy discharge. The pH of this discharge is 6.0. A wet preparation is done with normal saline, which shows numerous flagellated organisms that are slightly larger than the surrounding white blood cells. Which of the following is the most appropriate management?

    (A) Do not treat the patient or her partner

    (B) Treat only the patient with metronidazole

    (C) Treat the patient and her partner with metronidazole

    (D) Treat only the patient with penicillin

    (E) Treat the patient and her partner with penicillin

42. A 24-year-old woman asks her physician about the possibility of genetic screening for BRCA1 mutations. Her mother died of breast carcinoma at age 44, and a sister had a diagnosis of in situ ductal carcinoma at age 38. Which of the following is the most appropriate advice to give this woman?

    (A) Explain that BRCA1 mutations are not associated with an increased risk of breast cancer

    (B) Recommend screening only if she is of Ashkenazi Jewish descent

    (C) Recommend counseling before genetic screening is undertaken

    (D) Suggest prophylactic bilateral mastectomy instead of screening

43. A 29-year-old woman presents with complaints of a vaginal discharge. She has had two sexual partners over the past 4 weeks, and she reports that she uses oral contraceptives and that her partners were not using condoms. Examination shows she is afebrile, with no lymphadenopathy. Pelvic examination shows no ulcers, but a thick white discharge is noted at the cervical os on speculum examination. A Gram stain of the discharge reveals gram-negative diplococci. A sample of the discharge is also sent out for culture. The patient is appropriately treated and returns unhappily 3 weeks later with identical symptoms. A Gram stain of the discharge is again done, and this time reveals no organisms. Which of the following is the most likely cause of her symptoms?

    (A) Noncompliance with antibiotic therapy

    (B) Reinfection due to an occult urethral source

    (C) Reinfection from an untreated sexual partner

    (D) A resistant strain of the original organisms

    (E) An undetected, underlying immunosuppression

44. A 21-year-old nulligravid woman comes to her physician to discuss birth control options. She became sexually active for the first time 2 weeks ago. She is currently using condoms for contraception. Her past medical history is significant for asthma, which has been inactive for 2 years. She takes no medications and has no allergies to medications. She has no family history of cancer. Her examination is within normal limits. After a discussion with the physician, she chooses to take the oral contraceptive pill (OCP). She stays on the pill for the next 6 years. She now has most significantly decreased her risk of developing which of the following malignancies?

    (A) Breast cancer

    (B) Cervical cancer

    (C) Liver cancer

    (D) Lung cancer

    (E) Ovarian cancer

45. A 33-year-old woman presents to the physician because of a malodorous vaginal discharge that has been present for the past 3 days. She has no vaginal or vulvar irritation, and has no urinary complaints. Pelvic examination demonstrates a copious, gray discharge with a pH of 5.0. When 1 drop of potassium hydroxide (KOH) is added to a sample of the discharge there is an intense amine odor. A normal saline wet preparation is performed that demonstrates epithelial cells whose borders and nuclei are obscured by the presence of bacteria. Which of the following is the most likely pathogen?

    (A) *Candida albicans*

    (B) *Chlamydia trachomatis*

    (C) *Gardnerella vaginalis*

    (D) *Lactobacillus species*

    (E) *Trichomonas vaginalis*

46. A 62-year-old woman comes to the physician because of vaginal itch and pain with intercourse. She had her last menstrual period at age 52. She has no medical problems, takes no medications, and is allergic to penicillin. Pelvic examination demonstrates pale vaginal mucosa with no rugae present. The vagina is dry with no discharge. A potassium hydroxide (KOH) and normal saline wet preparation is negative. Which of the following is the most appropriate initial step in management?

    (A) Clotrimazole vaginal cream

    (B) Estrogen vaginal cream

    (C) Metronidazole vaginal cream

    (D) Oral fluconazole

    (E) Oral metronidazole

47. A 32-year-old woman is brought to the operating room for diagnostic laparoscopy because of chronic pelvic pain and chronic right upper quadrant pain. She has had these pains for the past 2 years. Her bowel and bladder function are normal. Past medical history is significant for two episodes of gonorrhea. She drinks one beer per day. Laboratory studies show:

Urine hCG	negative
Hematocrit	39%
Leukocyte count	8,000/mm^3
Platelet count	200,000/mm^3
AST	12 U/L
ALT	14 U/L

Intraoperatively, the patient is noted to have dense adhesions involving her fallopian tubes, ovaries, and uterus. The fallopian tubes themselves appear clubbed and occluded. A survey of her upper abdomen is remarkable for perihepatic adhesions extending from the liver surface to the diaphragm. The liver otherwise appears unremarkable. Which of the following is the most likely diagnosis for her right upper quadrant pain?

(A) Alcoholic cirrhosis

(B) Fitz-Hugh-Curtis syndrome

(C) Hepatitis

(D) Hepatocellular carcinoma

(E) Wolff-Parkinson-White syndrome

48. A 29-year-old woman comes to the emergency department because of constant, severe lower abdominal pain. She also complains of fever and chills. Three weeks ago she had an intrauterine device (IUD) placed for contraception. Her temperature is 38.3° C (101.0° F), blood pressure is 110/76 mm Hg, pulse is 110/min, and respirations are 16/min. She has bilateral lower quadrant abdominal tenderness. On pelvic examination, she has cervical motion tenderness and bilateral adnexal tenderness. A urinalysis is negative. A pelvic ultrasound is negative, with normal uterus and adnexae and no free fluid. What is the most likely diagnosis?

(A) Appendicitis

(B) Hemorrhagic ovarian cyst

(C) Ovarian torsion

(D) Pelvic inflammatory disease (PID)

(E) Pyelonephritis

49. A 14-year-old girl comes to the physician because of lower abdominal cramping. This cramping starts a few hours before, and lasts through, her menses, and then resolves completely. The cramping is primarily in the lower abdomen but also radiates to the back and thighs. She first noted this cramping approximately 6 months after her first menstrual period at age 12. She is not sexually active. Physical examination is unremarkable, including a normal pelvic examination. A pregnancy test is negative. Which of the following is the most appropriate next step in management?

(A) Trial of nonsteroidal anti-inflammatory drugs (NSAIDs)

(B) Trial of antibiotics

(C) GnRH agonist therapy

(D) Laparoscopy

(E) Laparotomy

50. A 26-year-old woman presents to her physician because of pain in her breast. She gave birth 3 months ago and is breast-feeding. Soon after she began lactating she developed cracks in the nipples, and for the past 5 days her left breast has become progressively more tender. On physical examination, her affected breast is red, hot, swollen, and painful to palpation. Her temperature is 38.3° C (101.0° F), and her white cell count is 13,000/mm^3. Which of the following is the most likely diagnosis?

(A) Breast abscess

(B) Breast cancer

(C) Intraductal papilloma

(D) Mastalgia

(E) Traumatic hematoma

Obstetrics/Gynecology Test One:
Answers and Explanations

ANSWER KEY

1.	A	26.	E
2.	B	27.	D
3.	C	28.	A
4.	E	29.	B
5.	D	30.	B
6.	C	31.	E
7.	C	32.	A
8.	F	33.	E
9.	E	34.	C
10.	D	35.	B
11.	B	36.	A
12.	D	37.	E
13.	D	38.	B
14.	E	39.	C
15.	A	40.	D
16.	A	41.	C
17.	C	42.	C
18.	C	43.	C
19.	D	44.	E
20.	E	45.	C
21.	E	46.	B
22.	D	47.	B
23.	C	48.	D
24.	A	49.	A
25.	C	50.	A

KAPLAN MEDICAL

1. **The correct answer is A.** A woman of childbearing age who presents with pain or vaginal bleeding must have a pregnancy test (bedside hCG) checked as one of the initial steps in her evaluation. Ectopic pregnancy is a potentially fatal condition in which a pregnancy develops outside of the uterus, most commonly in the Fallopian tube. The three most common presenting complaints for women with ectopic pregnancy are amenorrhea, abdominal pain, and vaginal bleeding. A woman may have an ectopic pregnancy and appear in no apparent distress with stable vital signs and a benign examination. Early diagnosis, however, is essential in ectopic pregnancy to avoid the significant morbidity and mortality that can result from an ectopic pregnancy that enlarges or ruptures.

Serum TSH (**choice B**) is an appropriate test to send as part of an outpatient evaluation of a woman having menstrual irregularities, because hypo- or hyperthyroidism can cause irregular bleeding. In the case of a young woman with abdominal pain and irregular bleeding, however, it is essential to first determine whether she is pregnant.

Abdominal x-ray (**choice C**) is a useful modality for identifying intestinal obstruction or perforation and some abdominal masses. In this patient, however, the physician would want to know the result of the pregnancy test (hCG) prior to ordering a diagnostic study. If the hCG is positive in this woman with bleeding and abdominal pain, the appropriate diagnostic study would be pelvic ultrasound and not abdominal x-ray.

Abdominal/pelvic CT (**choice D**) is an effective study for identifying masses in the abdomen and pelvis. It tends to be used in cases in which the differential diagnosis includes appendicitis, abscess, or tumor. For this patient, however, the physician must determine whether she is pregnant prior to scheduling a diagnostic study.

Laparoscopy (**choice E**) would not be an appropriate next step in the diagnosis, as it is too invasive a procedure to perform without first checking a serum or urine hCG, and using a diagnostic study to attempt to identify the cause of this woman's pain.

2. **The correct answer is B.** This patient has the constellation of findings on history and physical that are most consistent with polycystic ovarian syndrome (PCOS). Patients with PCOS typically have infertility, oligomenorrhea, hirsutism, and obesity. These women characteristically have elevated serum androgen levels, high LH to FSH ratios, and bilaterally enlarged ovaries, often with multiple cysts (which appear as "strings of pearls" on ultrasound). The oligomenorrhea that characterizes this syndrome places these women at increased risk for developing endometrial cancer. In women who ovulate each month, the second half of the menstrual cycle is characterized by production of progesterone from the ovary. This progesterone has a protective effect on the endometrium, preventing the development of hyperplasia and carcinoma. Women with PCOS, however, do not ovulate regularly and therefore do not make this "protective" progesterone each cycle. The prolonged exposure to unopposed estrogen, that is, estrogen that is not opposed by progesterone, places these women at increased risk of developing endometrial cancer.

This patient would not be considered at increased risk for developing cervical cancer (**choice A**). The risk factors for cervical cancer are multiple sexual partners, early age at first intercourse, history of sexually transmitted diseases, HIV, genital warts, cigarette smoking, and a history of cervical dysplasia. This patient is in a monogamous relationship and has had normal Pap smears for many years.

There is no known association between PCOS and lung cancer (**choice C**). Women with PCOS are at increased risk of developing type 2 diabetes and dyslipidemia, however.

Osteoporosis (**choice D**) is a major health risk for many women. However, this patient has characteristics that make osteoporosis less of a risk for her. Osteoporosis is less common among black women than among whites or Asians. It is also less common among obese women than among thin or small framed women. Finally, osteoporosis is not considered to be a characteristic of PCOS.

Ovarian cancer (**choice E**) is decreased in oligoovulatory women such as PCOS patients. Endometrial cancer is the cancer that women with PCOS are at the greatest risk of developing.

3. **The correct answer is C.** This patient has an incomplete abortion at roughly 10 weeks. We know that this is the diagnosis from a number of clues. Her os is open and she has tissue protruding from it. She has an hCG value that is consistent with a 10-week gestation (100,000 mIU/L), and her uterus is 10-week sized on examination. In her case, this abortion is causing her to lose a significant amount of blood, as evidenced by her tachycardia, low blood pressure, the large amount of clot in the vagina, and the low hematocrit. The most appropriate management for an incomplete abortion at 10 weeks with bleeding causing hemodynamic compromise is to evacuate the contents of the uterus with a dilation and evacuation. This will help to stop the bleeding by allowing the uterus to contract fully.

Discharge to home (**choice A**) would not be appropriate in this case because the patient has active bleeding, is hemodynamically unstable, and has a low hematocrit (22%). Delaying treatment with observation in this case might lead to a further drop in the hematocrit, further hemodynamic instability, and the eventual need for a blood transfusion with its associated risks and complications.

Culdocentesis (**choice B**) is a procedure used in the diagnosis of ectopic pregnancy in which a needle is placed into the posterior cul-de-sac to determine whether there is nonclotting blood there. Ultrasound has almost completely replaced culdocentesis in the diagnosis of ectopic pregnancy.

Laparoscopy (**choice D**) would not be appropriate in this case. It is true that in a pregnant woman with unstable vital signs and evidence of blood loss, the physician must think about ectopic pregnancy first. In this case, however, the diagnosis of incomplete abortion is certain enough that the risks of laparoscopy would outweigh the benefits. Several things make the diagnosis of ectopic pregnancy very unlikely here. First, the hCG is 100,000 mIU/L; most ectopic pregnancies do not reach this level. Second, the uterus is 10-week-size; most ectopic pregnancies do not lead to uterine growth that is consistent with the dates of the pregnancy. Third, there is no evidence of ectopic pregnancy on the ultrasound. Ultrasonic evidence of ectopic pregnancy includes an adnexal mass, free fluid in the pelvis, and no intrauterine gestational sac.

Laparotomy (**choice E**) would not be appropriate in this case for the same reasons mentioned with regard to laparoscopy. When the bleeding is coming from the uterus itself from an incomplete abortion, entering the peritoneal cavity (for laparoscopy or laparotomy) will not provide a remedy for the hemorrhage.

4. **The correct answer is E.** A woman who is pregnant and bleeding should have her blood type checked. If her blood type is Rh negative, she should receive RhoGAM unless the father of the child is known with certainty to be Rh-negative. RhoGAM is anti-D immune globulin, which will bind to the D subtype of the Rh antigen. It is given to prevent Rh isoimmunization. The Rh, or Rhesus, antigen is found on the red blood cells of most people. However, a certain percentage of women will not have the Rh antigen on their red blood cells. Rh isoimmunization occurs when an Rh-negative mother gets sensitized by being exposed to the Rh antigen of her fetus' red blood cells. This exposure may occur whenever the woman has an episode of bleeding (with trauma, an amniocentesis, or delivery). She then may make antibodies against the Rh antigen. These antibodies typically do not affect the initial pregnancy of the exposure. However, in a subsequent pregnancy, if that fetus also is Rh positive and the Rh-negative mother has been previously sensitized by an Rh-positive fetus, the mother may mount an immune response against the red blood cells of her fetus. The antibodies that she makes may cross the placenta and destroy the fetal red blood cells. This process can lead to significant fetal morbidity and mortality. RhoGAM should be given to any Rh-negative pregnant woman who has an episode of bleeding. If there is no bleeding during the pregnancy, then it should be given routinely at about 28 weeks and again postpartum if the neonate is Rh positive.

Antibiotics (**choice A**) would not be indicated here. There is a normal leukocytosis of pregnancy, with white cell counts ranging from 5,000 to 12,000/mm^3. During labor and immediately postpartum, it may become even more elevated, averaging 14,000-16,000/mm^3. This patient has no evidence of infection on the basis of her vital signs, examination, or laboratory values; therefore, antibiotics would not be indicated.

Blood transfusion (**choice B**) would not be indicated here. On average, healthy pregnant women will have lower hematocrits than nonpregnant women. Some refer to this as the "physiologic anemia of pregnancy." Therefore, a hematocrit of 33% is a routine finding during normal pregnancy and would not be an indication for transfusion.

Magnesium sulfate (**choice C**) is a drug commonly used in obstetrics. It is used for the treatment of preterm labor and for the prevention of seizures in patients with preeclampsia. Although bleeding from the vagina can be a sign of preterm labor, this patient has a normal, closed cervical os and has had no contractions. She also has no symptoms or findings to suggest preeclampsia, which is diagnosed on the basis of hypertension, edema, and proteinuria. Therefore, magnesium sulfate would not be used in this patient.

Platelet transfusion (**choice D**) would not be indicated here. Many normal pregnancies are characterized by a drop in the platelet count to a low-normal or even below normal value. When it is below normal, it is termed gestational thrombocytopenia. No intervention is necessary in the case of gestational thrombocytopenia. Platelet transfusions are reserved for more severe cases of bleeding, in the presence of a bleeding disorder, or for a surgical procedure.

5. **The correct answer is D.** A mediolateral episiotomy is made from the introitus at a 45-degree angle from the midline. Its main advantage over the median episiotomy, which starts from the introitus and goes down the perineum in the midline, is that the mediolateral episiotomy is less likely to result in a fourth-degree extension, which is a tear of the tissues from the vaginal mucosa to and through the rectal mucosa.

Easier surgical repair of the episiotomy (**choice A**), improved healing of the episiotomy (**choice B**), less blood loss (**choice C**), and less pain (**choice E**) are all characteristics of the median episiotomy and they are all advantages that the median episiotomy has over the mediolateral episiotomy. Again, however, the main advantage of the mediolateral episiotomy is that it is less likely to result in a fourth-degree extension.

6. **The correct answer is C.** Primary herpes infection can cause systemic symptoms of fever and myalgia and can affect the pharynx, urethra, external genitalia, and cervix. Although no effective therapy is available, acyclovir is used to reduce morbidity of the disease and decrease the incidence of recurrences.

Chancroid (**choice A**) does not cause systemic symptoms and leads to a soft, nonindurated, painful ulcer. The etiologic agent is *Haemophilus ducreyi*, which requires growth on an enriched chocolate medium. Management consists of oral erythromycin.

Condyloma (**choice B**) causes characteristic large, soft, fleshy, cauliflower-like excrescences around the vulva, urethral orifice, anus, and perineum. The causative agent is the human papilloma virus (HPV). Most HPV lesions resolve spontaneously. Frequently used therapies include cryosurgery, application of caustic agents, electrodesiccation, surgical excision, and laser ablation. Topical podophyllin has also been used with some success.

Lymphogranuloma venereum (**choice D**) leads to fever, arthritis, pericarditis, painless papules, and erythema nodosum. This is a sexually transmitted infection caused by *Chlamydia trachomatis* strains. A frequent presenting symptom is painful inguinal lymphadenopathy. Azithromycin may be of utility in treatment.

Syphilis (**choice E**) usually causes a single ulcer and does not produce exudative pharyngitis. Clinical manifestations of syphilis include primary, secondary, and tertiary syphilis. The primary chancre usually begins as a single painless papule, which rapidly becomes eroded and usually, but not always, is indurated with a characteristic cartilaginous consistency on palpation of the edge and base of the ulcer. Penicillin G is the drug of choice for all stages of syphilis.

7. **The correct answer is C.** This patient has the symptoms, signs, and laboratory values consistent with severe preeclampsia. Preeclampsia is diagnosed on the basis of hypertension, edema, and proteinuria. A patient is considered to have severe preeclampsia when she has any of the following manifestations: 1) headache, visual changes, or grand-mal seizure (eclampsia); 2) blood pressure greater than 160-180 mm Hg systolic or 110 mm Hg diastolic; 3) pulmonary edema; 4) right upper quadrant pain or elevated liver function tests; 5) oliguria (<500 mL/24 hours), elevated serum creatinine, or severe proteinuria (>5 g/24 hours); 6) microangiopathic hemolytic

anemia or thrombocytopenia; and 7) oligohydramnios or fetal intrauterine growth restriction. This patient meets the criteria of severe preeclampsia on the basis of her headache and her 24-hour urine with greater than 5 g of protein in 24 hours. The only cure for preeclampsia is delivery of the fetus. With a favorable cervix and a history of two prior normal spontaneous vaginal deliveries, this patient would be an excellent candidate for labor induction with IV oxytocin.

There is no role for expectant management (**choice A**) in the treatment of severe preeclampsia after 32 weeks. Some physicians choose to follow expectant management with women with severe preeclampsia prior to 32 weeks to allow for the administration of glucocorticoids and maturation of the fetus. This patient, however, is at 38 weeks' gestation; therefore, expectant management would not be appropriate.

Glucocorticoids (**choice B**) given to the mother have been shown to be effective in preventing certain sequelae of prematurity in the neonate. Maternal steroids have been shown to reduce the incidence of respiratory distress syndrome (RDS), intraventricular hemorrhage (IVH), and necrotizing enterocolitis (NEC). They have also been shown to reduce perinatal mortality. This patient, however, is at 38 weeks' gestation and therefore not having a premature delivery. Thus, administration of glucocorticoids would not be appropriate.

Subcutaneous terbutaline (**choice D**) is used as a uterine relaxant in cases of preterm labor or uterine tetany (prolonged contraction of the uterus). It would have no role in this patient.

Cesarean section (**choice E**) would not be considered the mode of choice for the delivery of a patient with severe preeclampsia with two prior vaginal deliveries and a favorable cervix. Severe preeclampsia at 38 weeks' gestation is certainly an indication for delivery, but vaginal delivery would be preferred over cesarean section in this patient.

8. **The correct answer is F.** After surgery and radiation therapy, chemotherapy and other forms of adjunctive treatments are recommended for most cases of potentially curable breast cancer. Chemotherapeutic regimens vary in relation to whether patients are pre- or postmenopausal, but hormonal adjunctive treatment has proven beneficial in both groups. Tamoxifen is an antiestrogen used for treatment of breast cancer, and tumors that express estrogen/progesterone receptors respond better to it. In addition, tamoxifen results in better survival regardless of tumor staging or grading. Therefore, receptor status is evaluated routinely in breast cancer by immunohistochemical staining with antibodies to estrogen/progesterone receptors. However, the physician

must be on the alert for paradoxical tamoxifen-induced endometrial hyperplasia.

Danazol (**choice A**) and medroxyprogesterone acetate (**choice D**) are used to treat a variety of gynecologic conditions, including endometriosis and abnormal uterine bleeding, but certainly not breast cancer. Danazol has also been used for symptomatic mammary dysplasia (fibrocystic changes).

Ethinyl estradiol (**choice B**) is used for treatment of abnormal uterine bleeding, estrogen replacement therapy, and adjunctive hormonal treatment for prostatic carcinoma.

Megestrol acetate (**choice C**) has been used for treatment of prostatic hyperplasia and endometrial cancer. This compound is also used for postmenopausal women with breast cancer in whom tamoxifen is not effective. In the latter situation, megestrol acetate is thus used as a second-line hormonal agent.

Natural progesterone (**choice E**) may benefit women with premenstrual syndrome.

9. **The correct answer is E.** This infant most likely has sepsis due to group B streptococci (GBS). GBS are a part of the normal flora of many women. During pregnancy, as many as 20% to 40% of women will be colonized with GBS. Most neonates born to colonized mothers will not develop infection with GBS; however, approximately 1% to 4% will. The likelihood of infection is increased if the mother has preterm labor and delivery (<37 weeks), prolonged rupture of the membranes (>18 hours), or intrapartum temperature greater than 100.4° F. Two primary methods are used to determine which women should receive antibiotics during labor. The first method is based on five risk factors: 1) history of a GBS-affected neonate; 2) urine culture with GBS; 3) preterm labor (<37 weeks); 4) membranes ruptured for more than 18 hours in labor; and 5) temperature greater than 100.4° F in labor. A woman with any one of these five risk factors should receive antibiotics. The second method is based on screening, with pregnant women being screened for GBS at 35-37 weeks with a culture of the vagina, perineum, and anus. In this patient, however, labor and delivery occurred at 31 weeks' gestation. Treatment with penicillin may have prevented the neonate from developing GBS sepsis.

Folic acid (**choice A**) is a supplement that women should take preconceptionally and during pregnancy to help prevent neural tube defects. This neonate does not have a neural tube defect.

Gentamicin (**choice B**) is an antibiotic that is effective in the treatment of gram-negative bacteria. As this infection was caused by a gram-positive coccus, gentamicin would not be the drug of choice.

Naloxone (**choice C**) is an opioid antagonist. It is given to neonates who demonstrate signs of depression after the laboring mother has been treated with narcotics. This infant has no signs of narcotic depression; therefore, naloxone would not be indicated.

Oxytocin (**choice D**) is given to women to induce or to augment labor. It can also be given postpartum to assist in uterine contractions in the case of atony and postpartum hemorrhage. This patient is preterm and has no indication for early delivery; therefore, oxytocin would not be indicated.

10. **The correct answer is D.** Preconceptional counseling is an essential part of the care of any young woman who plans to become pregnant. A detailed history and physical should be performed, including past obstetric history and any family history of congenital anomalies. Laboratory tests should include a rubella titer and a varicella-zoster titer. If the patient has a negative rubella titer, she should be given the MMR (measles-mumps-rubella) vaccine. Being vaccinated against rubella will prevent her from acquiring rubella during pregnancy. Rubella infection during pregnancy can lead to congenital rubella syndrome, a potentially devastating disorder that can lead to ear, eye, brain, and heart anomalies in the fetus. The patient should be counseled to avoid becoming pregnant for 3 months after the immunization since this is a live attenuated vaccine.

Blood cultures (**choice A**) are performed on patients when there is concern for bacteremia (bacteria present in the blood). This patient has no evidence of infection, and routine preconceptional blood cultures are not indicated.

Group B *Streptococcus* (GBS) culture (**choice B**) is performed on pregnant women in the third trimester to determine whether they have been colonized with this bacterium. If a woman is colonized, she should be given antibiotics in labor to prevent GBS disease in the newborn. This culture is performed in the third trimester and would not be indicated preconceptionally.

Pelvic ultrasound (**choice C**) is an excellent diagnostic tool for imaging the pelvis. It is useful in the diagnosis of ectopic pregnancy, ovarian torsion, tubo-ovarian abscess, ovarian masses, and other pelvic processes. It would not be indicated in an asymptomatic 26-year-old with a normal pelvic examination.

Urine culture (**choice E**) is used to diagnose a urinary tract infection (UTI). This patient has nothing in her history or physical that suggests active UTI or susceptibility to UTI. Therefore, urine culture would not be indicated in this patient.

11. **The correct answer is B.** Women with diabetes mellitus are at increased risk for sudden intrauterine death. In

the past, antepartum fetal death occurred in as many as 20% to 30% of patients with type 1 (insulin requiring) diabetes. Now, with improved maternal care and fetal surveillance, sudden intrauterine death is rare. Fetal surveillance usually begins at 28-32 weeks' gestation and consists of twice weekly nonstress tests (NST) until the mother delivers. An NST is reactive if there are two accelerations of the fetal heart rate (an increase of 15/min for 15 seconds) in 20 minutes. If the NST is not reactive, uteroacoustic stimulation should be performed, followed by a contraction stress test or biophysical profile. Management would then be based on the outcome of those tests.

Many obstetric outcomes vary according to race. However, black race (**choice A**) would not be an indication for antepartum fetal testing. In this patient, her diabetes mellitus makes her a candidate for such testing, not her race.

A urine culture positive for group B *Streptococcus* (GBS) (**choice C**) is an indication for antibiotic prophylaxis during labor and delivery to prevent GBS invasive disease in the newborn. A positive GBS urine culture is not an indication for antepartum fetal testing.

History of cesarean section (**choice D**) is an important aspect of the patient's past obstetric history. However, in the absence of diabetes mellitus, a prior c-section is not an indication for antepartum fetal testing.

Hyperemesis gravidarum (**choice E**) is a condition of pregnancy characterized by persistent nausea and vomiting. It is most often limited to the first trimester and usually resolves by 16 weeks' gestation. Although hyperemesis gravidarum can be a difficult condition for the patient, it is not an indication for antepartum fetal testing.

12. **The correct answer is D.** This patient has syphilis, a disease caused by *Treponema pallidum*, a spirochete, as evidenced by the positive rapid plasma reagin (RPR) test and microhemagglutination assay for antibodies to *T. pallidum* (MHA-TP). Primary syphilis is characterized by a painless ulcer, called a chancre, typically found on the vagina or cervix. Untreated primary syphilis can progress to secondary syphilis, which is characterized by "moth-eaten" alopecia, a maculopapular skin rash involving the palms and soles, and white patches on the tongue. Tertiary syphilis is characterized by gumma formation, cardiac lesions, and CNS abnormalities. Syphilis in pregnancy is associated with increased rates of preterm delivery, intrauterine growth retardation, and fetal demise. However, the most devastating complication of syphilis in pregnancy is congenital infection of the fetus, which can lead to severe effects on fetal morbidity and mortality. The key to preventing congenital infection is

adequate treatment of the mother. The drug of choice for syphilis is penicillin.

Clindamycin (**choice A**) is effective for some gram-positive and anaerobic infections. It does not treat syphilis and would not be indicated for this patient.

Gentamicin (**choice B**) is mostly used for gram-negative infections. It does not treat syphilis and would not be indicated.

Nitrofurantoin (**choice C**) is often used in pregnancy to treat urinary tract infections. However, it does not treat syphilis and therefore would not be indicated for this patient.

Tetracycline (**choice E**) should not be used in pregnancy, as it is known to cause discoloration of deciduous teeth and it can be deposited into fetal long bones. It is considered a second-line treatment of syphilis in the nonpregnant patient.

13. **The correct answer is D.** This patient probably has breast cancer metastases to the spine and is in danger of spinal cord compression, which is an emergency. It is essential to administer steroids immediately to help decrease the swelling and relieve some compression. She might ultimately need surgical intervention or radiation.

A neurologic consultation (**choice A**) will help localize the lesion; however, this is an emergency and must be treated immediately.

An MRI (**choice B**) will localize the lesion but should not delay emergent intervention.

Narcotics (**choice C**) would provide only symptomatic relief.

A lumbar puncture (**choice E**) might reveal malignant cells on cytologic evaluation but would not contribute to her immediate management.

14. **The correct answer is E.** Nipple discharge in the nonlactating breast may be the presenting sign of a number of diseases, the most common of which are intraductal papilloma, carcinoma, and fibrocystic changes. Carcinoma is more likely in women older than 50. Regardless of whether this sign is present, a clinically malignant palpable mass in a postmenopausal woman should be investigated with mammography followed by fine-needle cytology (or excisional biopsy). The features suspicious for malignancy in this case include ill-defined margins of the mass and the hemorrhagic nature of the discharge.

Cytologic examination of nipple discharge (**choice A**) may reveal malignant cells but is associated too frequently with false negative results to be reliable.

Mammography alone (**choice B**) is adequate if the breast mass appears benign on clinical grounds. Biopsy or fine-needle aspiration may then be carried out depending on the mammographic findings.

Ultrasonography (**choice C**) is mainly used to differentiate between solid and cystic masses. However, it does not allow any inference on the malignant versus benign nature of a lesion. If a lesion is cystic, the fluid should be aspirated and examined cytologically.

Biopsy under mammographic localization (**choice D**) (i.e., a "stereotactic" biopsy) is not necessary in this case because the lesion is palpable and can be easily sampled by fine-needle aspiration or conventional biopsy.

15. **The correct answer is A.** The varicella-zoster virus, the virus that causes the clinical manifestations that are commonly referred to as "chickenpox," can have severe consequences for a mother and her fetus during pregnancy. Fortunately, most pregnant women have already been exposed. And, of those pregnant women who are not sure whether they had chickenpox, the overwhelming majority will also have already been exposed and be immune to infection. The ideal time to screen for immunity to varicella is preconceptionally. If a pregnant women thinks she has been exposed, then the first step is to verify that the infected person truly has varicella. The next step is to check the mother's IgG serology. If her serology is positive, then she has immunity and there is no risk to her or her fetus. If the serology is negative, she should be given varicella-zoster immune globulin (VZIG), which is about 75% effective in preventing an infection if given within 96 hours of exposure.

Waiting to see whether a rash develops (**choice B**) would not be appropriate. The incubation period for the virus is 10-14 days. VZIG is most effective if given within 96 hours of exposure. Therefore, this patient may not develop a rash for 10 or more days, and by that time it would be too late for VZIG.

Administration of IV acyclovir (**choice C**) would be inappropriate. First, the mother most likely has already had varicella infection and is therefore immune. Second, the mother has no evidence of being infected. Finally, even in the case of a confirmed maternal infection, IV acyclovir is used only when serious complications of varicella infection (e.g., pneumonia or encephalitis) develop.

Administration of oral acyclovir (**choice D**) would be inappropriate for the above listed reasons.

Administration of the varicella vaccine (**choice E**) would be contraindicated because it is an attenuated live-virus vaccine. These vaccines are not recommended for pregnant women.

16. **The correct answer is A.** Sickle-cell anemia results from a single A–T substitution that leads to valine being substituted for glutamic acid on the beta-chain of the hemoglobin molecule. This change in the configuration of the hemoglobin molecule makes the erythrocyte sickle when it becomes deoxygenated. Patients with sickle-cell anemia have a number of maladies, including severe pain crises, pulmonary infarction, bony abnormalities, cerebrovascular accidents, and an increased likelihood of infection with gram-positive organisms. This patient has sickle-cell anemia (SS), and the father of the baby has sickle-cell trait (AS). This gives the fetus a 50% likelihood of having sickle-cell disease and a 50% likelihood of having sickle-cell trait. Amniocentesis and chorionic villus sampling can be used to determine the genotype of the fetus. This patient should at least be offered the option of having genetic counseling to better understand the inheritance of the disease and the fetus' likelihood of having each outcome.

Obstetric ultrasound (**choice B**) is a very useful diagnostic modality to examine the fetus, umbilical cord, placenta, amniotic fluid, and maternal pelvic structures. This patient, however, does not have an indication for an ultrasound at this time. This patient already had a 6-week ultrasound, which is especially useful for dating the pregnancy. The best time to do a "screening" ultrasound to look for fetal anomalies is during the second trimester. This patient, at 10-weeks' gestation with an ultrasound done 4 weeks ago, would have no indication for another ultrasound at this time.

Hydroxyurea (**choice C**) is a drug used to increase the production of hemoglobin F in patients with sickle-cell anemia who are not pregnant. It is considered a class D drug, and its use in pregnancy is limited.

IV hydration (**choice D**) is frequently used in patients with sickle-cell anemia during pain crises. This patient has no evidence of having a pain crisis; therefore, IV hydration would not be indicated during a prenatal visit.

Blood transfusion (**choice E**) during pregnancy for the patient with sickle-cell anemia is an area of controversy. Some argue for routine transfusion to maintain the hematocrit above 25% and the level of hemoglobin A above 40%. This patient is asymptomatic, with a hematocrit of 37% at 10 weeks' gestation. Therefore, blood transfusion would not be indicated as the next step in management.

17. **The correct answer is C.** This patient has the findings consistent with HELLP syndrome. HELLP stands for Hemolysis, Elevated Liver enzymes, and Low Platelets, and is related to preeclampsia. A patient with HELLP typically presents with complaints of abdominal pain, nausea, and vomiting, as well as a history of malaise or flu-like symptoms. The patients are usually afebrile and often have normal vital signs. Although HELLP

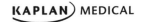

is related to preeclampsia, hypertension and protein-uria may be absent or minimal. Examination usually reveals right upper quadrant or epigastric tenderness. Laboratory values show evidence of hemolysis (e.g., abnormal peripheral blood smear, elevated lactate dehydrogenase, and increased bilirubin), elevated liver enzymes (e.g., elevated AST and ALT), and low platelets ($<100,000/mm^3$). The treatment is essentially the same as for severe preeclampsia.

Decreased fibrin split products (**choice A**) would not be consistent with HELLP syndrome. Up to 40% of patients with HELLP syndrome will develop disseminated intra-vascular coagulation (DIC). In DIC, fibrin split products are elevated.

Decreased lactate dehydrogenase (**choice B**) would also not be consistent with HELLP syndrome. As noted above, lactate dehydrogenase rises as hemolysis takes place and the liver is damaged.

Elevated fibrinogen (**choice D**) would also not usually be seen in HELLP syndrome. In the up to 40% of patients with HELLP who develop DIC, the fibrinogen level would be decreased.

Elevated glucose (**choice E**) would not usually be seen in HELLP syndrome.

18. **The correct answer is C.** Gestational diabetes is defined as glucose intolerance that develops or is first recognized during pregnancy. To diagnose gestational diabetes, a 50-g oral glucose tolerance test (OGTT) is given between 24 and 28 weeks. Any woman with a plasma glucose value above 140 mg/dL on the 50-g OGTT is then sent for a 100-g, 3-hour OGTT, in which a 100-g glucose load is given and plasma glucose levels are checked at 1, 2, and 3 hours. Any woman with two or more abnormal values is considered to have gestational diabetes. A class A1 gestational diabetic does not have fasting hyperglycemia (glucose >105 mg/dL) and can usually be treated with diet alone. A class A2 gestational diabetic has fasting hyperglycemia and needs insulin treatment. Gestational diabetics are at increased risk for fetal macrosomia. Fetal macrosomia is a risk factor for shoulder dystocia, a condition in which the fetus' anterior shoulder becomes impacted against the mother's pubic symphysis. This fetus had a shoulder dystocia that was relieved only with delivery of the posterior arm. In the process, the humerus was fractured. The shoulder dystocia was likely the result of the fetal macrosomia, which was most likely caused by the mother's gestational diabetes.

Cigarette smoking (**choice A**) has not been shown to be related to shoulder dystocia.

Gestational age (**choice B**) is related to shoulder dystocia when the patient is post-dates (>40 weeks). This patient, however, is at 38 weeks' gestation.

There is some evidence that advanced maternal age (**choice D**) may be related to shoulder dystocia. This patient is 17; therefore, advanced maternal age is not a factor.

Maternal shoulder surgery (**choice E**) is not related to the occurrence of shoulder dystocia.

19. **The correct answer is D.** Postcoital contraception is a safe and highly effective method of preventing preg-nancy. It is useful to check a pregnancy test prior to giving any treatment to ensure that the patient is not already pregnant. One of the most common methods of postcoital contraception is to administer norgestrel/ethinyl estradiol (Ovral). Ovral is given as 2 tablets stat and then 2 more tablets 12 hours later. This regimen is close to 99% effective in preventing pregnancy when given within 72 hours. Ovral would be the most effec-tive pharmacotherapy for this patient. There is a high incidence of nausea and vomiting with this regimen; antiemetics may be required. Levonorgestrel is available over the counter.

Clomiphene (**choice A**) works as an anti-estrogen. It is used to increase FSH levels and induce ovulation in infertile patients. It is not used for postcoital contraception.

Gentamicin (**choice B**) is an IV antibiotic most commonly used against gram-negative organisms. This patient may be at risk for sexually transmitted disease (STD) given that the condom broke. It is important to discuss the issue of STD with the patient and to decide whether prophylactic antibiotics will be given. However, IV gentamicin is not used for antibiotic prophylaxis.

Labetalol (**choice C**) is an alpha-1 and nonselective beta blocker. It is used commonly in pregnancy to treat hyper-tension. This patient has no history of hypertension. Her blood pressure is only mildly elevated and it is probably elevated during this visit because of anxiety. She should have follow-up blood pressure checks, but labetalol would not be indicated at this point.

Trimethoprim-sulfamethoxazole (**choice E**), also known as Bactrim, is used to treat infections. Among its most common uses is to treat urinary tract infections. As discussed above, this patient may require antibiotic prophylaxis because of her exposure. However, Bactrim is not typically used for STD prophylaxis. Furthermore, this patient has an allergy to sulfa drugs, which would make trimethoprim-sulfamethoxazole contraindicated.

20. **The correct answer is E.** This patient has the symptoms and signs most consistent with a *Trichomonas vaginalis* infection. Patients with *T. vaginalis* typically experi-

ence vaginal itch and discharge, dysuria, frequency and urgency of urination, and dyspareunia. However, a significant minority (around 20%) of patients infected with *T. vaginalis* will be asymptomatic. The key finding to diagnose the infection is the presence of motile, pear-shaped, flagellated organisms on the normal saline, wet-mount smear preparation. These organisms will be smaller than the surrounding vaginal epithelial cells but larger than white blood cells. The treatment for *T. vaginalis* is metronidazole.

Candida albicans (**choice A**) is a common cause of vaginitis. We know from the findings, however, that this patient does not have a *Candida* infection. Her discharge is not consistent with *Candida* infection. *Candida* typically causes a thick, white ("cottage-cheese") discharge with a pH of 4 to 5. Also, microscopic examination demonstrates the organism *T. vaginalis* and not the pseudohyphae seen with a *Candida* infection.

Gardnerella vaginalis (**choice B**) is a common organism in bacterial vaginosis, in association with increased levels of anaerobic bacteria. The discharge in bacterial vaginosis can appear similar to that caused by *T. vaginalis*. However, bacterial vaginosis is usually characterized by a strong odor, and irritation of the vaginal epithelium is usually not seen. Furthermore, this patient has an identifiable organism on wet-mount.

Herpes simplex virus (**choice C**) infection is characterized by vesicles and ulcers and an extremely tender vulva and vaginal area. This patient has no vesicles or ulcers and has an obvious organism on wet-mount.

Treponema pallidum (**choice D**) is the organism that causes syphilis. Primary infection with *T. pallidum* is characterized by a painless chancre on the vulva, vagina, or cervix. The organism is identified on dark-field microscopy and not wet-mount preparation.

21. **The correct answer is E.** This patient, with a prior multiple myomectomy, would be at increased risk for uterine rupture. Uterine rupture is a rare, potentially catastrophic outcome in which there is complete separation of all layers of the uterine musculature. The most commonly cited risk factor is prior surgery involving the myometrium (e.g., prior c-section or myomectomy). However, uterine rupture may also be associated with blunt abdominal trauma, incorrect use of oxytocin, perforation with an intrauterine pressure catheter, grand multiparity, fetal malpresentation, or difficult delivery with forceps or breech extraction. The classic symptoms are severe abdominal pain with vaginal bleeding, although the presentation can vary. Fetal distress will often be found on electronic fetal monitoring. Management involves immediate laparotomy in cases where the suspicion for uterine rupture is high.

Amniotic fluid embolism (**choice A**) is a very rare but potentially fatal occurrence in obstetrics. It is believed to occur when a significant amount of amniotic fluid enters the maternal circulation. The classic presentation is with maternal respiratory distress, followed by cardiovascular collapse, hemorrhage, and coma. It is not clear what risk factors exist for the development of this syndrome, although some investigators have shown that many women with amniotic fluid embolism had allergy or atopy. This patient's history would not place her at particular risk for this rare outcome.

Anencephaly (**choice B**) is a neural tube defect in which there is an absence of development of the cranium and cerebral hemispheres. The defect can be diagnosed by ultrasound. The fetus appeared normal at the 18- and 36-week ultrasounds and therefore would not be considered at risk for anencephaly.

Fetal macrosomia (**choice C**) is associated with maternal diabetes and obesity. This patient's cigarette smoking puts her at greater risk for having a low birth weight infant.

This mother is not considered to be at risk for Rh isoimmunization (**choice D**), as she is Rh positive.

22. **The correct answer is D.** The management of an acute hypertensive episode during pregnancy presents a challenge. On the one hand, it is important to lower the blood pressure of the mother to prevent the development of a hypertensive emergency (e.g., hypertensive encephalopathy, cardiac decompensation, or damage to other organs). Extreme hypertension is also a risk for placental abruption. On the other hand, lowering the blood pressure too much may lead to underperfusion of the placenta and fetal distress. The goal of antihypertensive therapy during an acute episode of severe hypertension is not to lower the blood pressure to normotensive levels but rather to a mild-moderate hypertensive level, with a diastolic blood pressure of 90-100 mm Hg. In this patient, 150/95 mm Hg is a good target blood pressure.

Blood pressures of 90/60 mm Hg (**choice A**) or 100/75 mm Hg (**choice B**) are too low. Lowering the maternal blood pressure to this level could lead to hypoperfusion of the placenta and fetal distress.

A blood pressure of 120/80 mm Hg (**choice C**) is normal for nonpregnant patients. However, acutely lowering this patient's blood pressure from 180/115 mm Hg to 120/80 mm Hg could lead to fetal distress.

A blood pressure of 180/110 mm Hg (**choice E**) is too high to use as a goal for antihypertensive therapy. A level of 150/95 mm Hg represents the best compromise between too high versus too low in a chronically hypertensive pregnant patient.

23. **The correct answer is C.** The first step in the diagnosis of secondary amenorrhea is a pregnancy test. Secondary amenorrhea is defined as the cessation of menses for 3 months in a woman with previously regular periods or 6 months in a woman with a history of oligomenorrhea. This patient had normal periods up until the last 6 months. The most common cause of secondary amenorrhea in a 33-year-old with previously normal cycles is pregnancy. Therefore, beta-hCG would be indicated as the first step.

Lipase (**choice A**) is a useful laboratory value to check in cases in which pancreatitis is on the differential diagnosis. The fact that this patient's father died of pancreatitis almost certainly has no relationship to her current amenorrhea.

FSH (**choice B**) is a useful test in women with secondary amenorrhea after a pregnancy test, TSH, and prolactin have been checked, and after the patient's estrogen status is assessed with a progesterone withdrawal test. If the patient is found to be amenorrheic from estrogen deficiency, assessment of the FSH level allows one to distinguish between a centrally mediated deficiency (FSH low) and an ovarian deficiency (FSH high).

Liver function tests (**choice D**) would not be indicated in this patient as part of her workup for secondary amenorrhea. Hepatitis A is a virus that affects hepatocytes and can cause abnormal liver function tests. However, it does not cause chronic infection and almost certainly is not causing this patient's secondary amenorrhea.

TSH (**choice E**) is an excellent test in the workup of secondary amenorrhea after pregnancy has been ruled out. Women with abnormal thyroid function can have menstrual irregularities, so a TSH is a good test for any woman with abnormal menses. However, a pregnancy test should still be done first in the evaluation of secondary amenorrhea.

24. **The correct answer is A.** Active, recent, or recurrent sexually transmitted diseases (STDs) are considered an absolute contraindication to intrauterine device (IUD) use. This patient has a gynecologic history that is significant for multiple episodes of chlamydia cervicitis and two episodes of pelvic inflammatory disease (PID). In a patient with an IUD in place, these infections have an increased likelihood of causing significant morbidity and mortality. Many physicians consider even the risk for STDs (i.e., multiple sexual partners or sexual relations with someone with multiple sexual partners) to be a contraindication to IUD use. The presence of such numerous and recent episodes of STDs would certainly make the IUD absolutely contraindicated for this patient.

The IUD is contraindicated, not recommended (**choice B**), for the reasons given above.

The IUD would not be recommended if cervical cultures were negative (**choice C**) for two reasons. First, cervical cultures have a high false negative rate. Therefore, even if the cultures are negative, it does not completely rule out an infection. Second, even if the cultures are truly negative this time, her recent history of multiple STDs places her at far too great a risk to be a candidate for the IUD.

The oral contraceptive pill is not absolutely contraindicated (**choice D**). The pill is absolutely contraindicated in women older than 35 who smoke; however, this patient is 24 years old. She should certainly be encouraged to stop smoking, and smoking cessation advice and counseling should be offered to her.

The rhythm method would not be a correct recommendation for this patient (**choice E**). Even with perfect use, the rhythm method has a failure rate of greater than 10%. Furthermore, because of the nature of the technique, the actual failure rate is significantly higher, probably greater than 30%. The rhythm method is not recommended as a first-line birth control option.

25. **The correct answer is C.** External cephalic version is a procedure in which the physician manually rotates the fetus from a breech to a vertex presentation with pressure applied on the maternal abdomen. It is usually performed after 37 weeks' gestation because of some of the risks of the procedure. One risk is that the successfully verted fetus will revert back to its breech position. This is more likely if the procedure is performed prior to 37 weeks. Also, there is a risk that fetal distress from cord compression or placental abruption will occur during the procedure, necessitating cesarean delivery. If the procedure is attempted prior to 37 weeks, there is a risk of delivering a premature fetus. Finally, about 5% of women will have a fetal to maternal transfusion during the procedure; therefore, Rh-negative women should be given RhoGAM™.

Performing the procedure after 30 (**choice A**) or 33 (**choice B**) weeks could lead to iatrogenic prematurity or a spontaneous reversion to the breech position as discussed above.

Waiting until after 40 (**choice D**) or 42 (**choice E**) weeks would not be correct management. The later in gestation that version is attempted, the more likely it is to fail, as the breech becomes more deeply engaged with advancing gestation. Furthermore, by 40 or 42 weeks many of the patients with breech fetuses will have already gone into labor.

26. **The correct answer is E.** Postpartum hemorrhage is an important cause of maternal morbidity and mortality in obstetrics. Postpartum hemorrhage is defined as blood loss in excess of 500 mL at vaginal delivery or 1,000 mL

at cesarean section. The main causes of postpartum hemorrhage are uterine atony and laceration. Other possible causes include retained placenta, coagulopathy, and uterine inversion. This patient has uterine atony, as indicated by the soft, "boggy" uterus on physical examination. The postpartum uterus should be firm and at the level of the umbilicus. The treatments for atony include oxytocin, methylergonovine, and PGF$_{2\alpha}$. However, PGF$_{2\alpha}$ is contraindicated in patients who have asthma, as it may increase airway resistance and exacerbate the condition.

Acetaminophen (**choice A**) is not considered a treatment for postpartum hemorrhage. However, it should not necessarily be avoided either. This patient has no contraindication to the use of acetaminophen.

IV hydration (**choice B**) should be given in the case of a postpartum hemorrhage. Any patient experiencing significant blood loss should have IV access. IV hydration will allow this patient to maintain her intravascular volume and organ perfusion.

Methylergonovine (**choice C**) should be given in the case of postpartum hemorrhage caused by uterine atony. It is a medication from the ergot family. Ergot drugs can cause vasoconstriction and should therefore be used with caution or avoided altogether in patients with hypertension.

Oxytocin (**choice D**) should be given for postpartum hemorrhage caused by uterine atony. Forty units oxytocin in 1 L crystalloid may be given as a rapid infusion (500 mL over 10 minutes). Oxytocin will help the uterus to contract and thus resolve the atony.

27.   **The correct answer is D.** This patient has postpartum psychosis. Postpartum psychosis typically occurs hours to days postpartum and is characterized by anxiety, agitation, insomnia, confusion, and ideation of hurting oneself, the baby, or others. Postpartum psychosis, especially when there are concerns regarding suicide or homicide, must be managed with psychiatric hospitalization for the patient.

Fluoxetine (**choice A**) is an effective antidepressant. However, this patient has a full-blown postpartum psychosis including homicidal ideation. Management with fluoxetine would not be the most appropriate next step.

Morphine (**choice B**) is an opioid used for pain control. This patient has no complaints of pain. As such, morphine would not be an appropriate next step.

Naloxone (**choice C**) is an opioid antagonist used in cases of opioid overdose, especially when there is a concern for respiratory depression. Although this patient is taking codeine (an opioid), she has no evidence of opioid overdose. Thus, naloxone would not be recommended.

A visit to the nursery (**choice E**) would not be recommended for this patient as the next step in her management. She is voicing homicidal thoughts regarding her infant; therefore, a visit to the nursery would not be appropriate at this time.

28.   **The correct answer is A.** Bleeding in the third trimester can be caused by a number of processes and must be taken very seriously by the physician. The differential diagnosis for third-trimester bleeding includes placenta previa; placental abruption; vasa previa (when fetal vessels course over the internal cervical os); cervical, vaginal, or vulvar lesions; hematuria; and hematochezia. Also on the differential is "bloody show," the bloody mucus that a woman in labor passes as she undergoes cervical dilation. This patient has regular, painful contractions, is passing bloody mucus, and is changing her cervix. These findings are most consistent with early labor.

Placental abruption (**choice B**) is characterized by vaginal bleeding, abdominal pain, and uterine contractions (or increased uterine tone). Fetal distress is seen in more than 50% of cases. The bleeding of an abruption is not bloody mucus but rather frank blood that is often dark red. This patient had bloody mucus, not frank blood, and consistent contractions with cervical change. Her signs and symptoms make labor, and not abruption, the most likely diagnosis.

Placenta previa (**choice C**) can also cause third-trimester bleeding. Whereas abruption is typically characterized by painful vaginal bleeding, previa is classically characterized as painless vaginal bleeding. Diagnosis of a placenta previa is made by ultrasound. This patient had a normal ultrasound at 19 weeks' gestation, with no evidence of previa; therefore, placenta previa would not be the most likely diagnosis.

Urinary tract infection (**choice D**) can present with hematuria. Typically it is a microscopic hematuria, not bloody mucus. Although this patient could have a urinary tract infection, given her signs and symptoms this is not the most likely diagnosis.

Vasa previa (**choice E**) occurs when the fetal vessels pass over the internal cervical os. Bleeding from vasa previa will lead to fetal distress evidenced by changes in the fetal heart tracing. Fetal tachycardia or bradycardia may be seen. When fetal anemia results, a sinusoidal heart rate is often seen. This patient has a reactive fetal heart tracing and a more likely cause for her bleeding (labor).

29.   **The correct answer is B.** This patient has pyelonephritis. The incidence of pyelonephritis in pregnancy is approximately 1% to 2%. The usual symptoms are fever, chills, back pain, dysuria, frequency, and urgency. On examination, these patients will often have a fever and

costovertebral angle tenderness. Urinalysis will typically show white and red blood cells. The causative organism is often *Escherichia coli*. Other organisms commonly isolated are *Klebsiella* and *Proteus*. If the patient is otherwise completely stable, outpatient treatment with cephalexin or amoxicillin may be tried, although many suggest that a pregnant woman with pyelonephritis should be hospitalized. Inpatient management includes IV cefazolin, with or without gentamicin. The major complications of pyelonephritis in pregnancy are sepsis, adult respiratory distress syndrome (ARDS), and preterm labor.

Acyclovir (**choice A**) is an antiviral therapy used for the treatment of severe cases of varicella-zoster virus infection in pregnancy or herpes virus infections. Pyelonephritis is a bacterial infection. Thus, acyclovir would not be appropriate.

Levofloxacin (**choice C**) is a DNA gyrase inhibitor that is contraindicated in pregnancy because it is associated with musculoskeletal anomalies.

Metronidazole (**choice D**) is an antibiotic most often used to treat anaerobic organisms. During pregnancy it is used in the treatment of bacterial vaginosis and *Trichomonas vaginalis*. This patient has pyelonephritis; therefore, metronidazole would not be indicated.

Tetracycline (**choice E**) is contraindicated in pregnancy. Its use during pregnancy has been associated with brown discoloration of the deciduous teeth and hypoplasia of the enamel. It can also be deposited into fetal long bones and cause inhibition of bone growth.

30. **The correct answer is B.** Patients with type 1 diabetes mellitus often require insulin during labor and delivery. The insulin is given to prevent the mother from developing hyperglycemia. Maternal hyperglycemia during labor and delivery can lead to fetal hyperglycemia, which can lead to neonatal hypoglycemia. The goal during labor and delivery is a plasma glucose of 100 mg/dL. This is best accomplished using a continuous infusion of regular insulin.

Hydralazine (**choice A**) and labetalol (**choice C**) are antihypertensives that can be given intravenously antepartum when the diastolic blood pressure exceeds 110 mm Hg. This patient has a diastolic blood pressure of 90 mm Hg; therefore, neither drug would be indicated.

Meperidine (**choice D**) is a narcotic that can be given intravenously for pain control during labor. IV narcotic use, however, is becoming less common with the more widespread use of epidural anesthesia during labor and delivery.

Penicillin (**choice E**) is an antibiotic that is given to women during labor and delivery to prevent group B streptococcal disease of the newborn. On the basis of this patient's unremarkable prenatal course and normal screening she would

not need penicillin during labor and delivery. Syphilis is also treated with penicillin. However, this patient was already adequately treated for syphilis and would not need penicillin for this indication.

31. **The correct answer is E.** A history of chronic vulvar itching is a common presentation in women with squamous cell carcinoma of the vulva. Other features include bleeding, pain, and a discharge. The lesions can appear ulcerated, pigmented, or raised, although infrequently there is no lesion at all. Any postmenopausal woman with chronic vulvar itch should undergo biopsy to rule out malignancy.

Prescribing an antibiotic (**choice A**) or an antifungal (**choice B**) would be inappropriate management. This patient does not have an obvious infection for which either of these agents would be effective. Furthermore, trying antibiotics or antifungals could lead to further delay of the biopsy being performed.

Prescribing a steroid cream (**choice C**) would also be inappropriate management. In postmenopausal women, certain vulvar lesions (e.g., lichen sclerosis) would respond to steroid cream. In this case, however, it is most important to first establish a diagnosis with a biopsy prior to instituting treatment.

Attempting to ascribe this patient's itching to a possible psychiatric process (**choice D**) without first trying to establish a diagnosis by biopsying the lesion is inappropriate.

32. **The correct answer is A.** This patient has the classic presentation for placental abruption, which occurs when there is premature separation of a normally implanted placenta from its attachment to the uterus. The classic triad of presentation is third-trimester vaginal bleeding, painful uterine contractions or hypertonus, and fetal distress. Definitive diagnosis can be made when there is a retroplacental clot. The most common causes of abruption are maternal hypertension and trauma (e.g., motor vehicle accidents or domestic violence). The relationship between cocaine use and abruption is well established. It is believed that the vasoconstrictive and hypertensive effects of cocaine lead to abruption.

In this case, the gestational age (**choice B**) is not the most likely initiating factor for the placental abruption, as 37 weeks is considered a term pregnancy. It is most likely that the cocaine use, rather than the gestational age, precipitated this course.

Group B *Streptococcus* colonization (**choice C**) is not known to be associated with placental abruption.

Oral contraceptive pill use (**choice D**) around the time of conception is a frequent concern for patients. It has never been proven to cause increased rates of anomalies and is not known to be associated with placental abruption.

White race (**choice E**) is not considered a risk factor for placental abruption. Rates of placental abruption are higher in African American women.

33. **The correct answer is E.** This patient presents with the classic triad of placental abruption: third-trimester bleeding, uterine contractions or hypertonus, and fetal distress. Placental abruption occurs when a normally implanted placenta separates prematurely from its attachment to the uterus. Management of a placental abruption depends on its severity and the status of the maternal cervix. This patient has a severe abruption with fetal distress and a closed cervix. Cesarean section is indicated both for fetal and maternal indications. To not perform cesarean section in this case places the fetus at risk of death and the mother at risk of significant morbidity and mortality from hemorrhage.

Expectant management (**choice A**) would not be appropriate with this presentation of abruption. Sometimes small abruptions occur with only a limited amount of placental separation, a small amount of bleeding, and no fetal distress. These abruptions, particularly when the fetus is premature, may be managed expectantly.

Magnesium sulfate (**choice B**) and terbutaline (**choice D**) are tocolytic drugs used to stop contractions. In general tocolytics are contraindicated in the setting of placental abruption. In select patients with minor abruptions and no fetal distress who are remote from term, tocolytics may be used. In general, however, they are contraindicated for use during a placental abruption.

Oxytocin (**choice C**) is used to induce labor. It may be used in certain cases of placental abruption. This patient, however, has a severe abruption and fetal distress requiring cesarean section.

34. **The correct answer is C.** With widespread use of mammographic screening for breast cancer, radiologic detection of breast lesions that cannot be identified by palpation is increasingly common. The next steps in the diagnostic tree depend on whether the lesion is considered "suspicious" on radiologic grounds. Clustered microcalcifications, spiculated densities, and parenchymal distortions are suspicious for malignancy. A stereotactic biopsy is probably the most appropriate approach to nonpalpable lesions with high index of suspicion. With this procedure, a biopsy needle is inserted into the lesion under mammographic guidance, and a core of tissue can be removed for pathologic examination.

Mammographic reexamination in 1 year (**choice A**) is not appropriate for nonpalpable breast lesions with either a high or low index of suspicion. Mammographic

reevaluation within 3-6 months is acceptable for nonpalpable lesions that appear benign on mammograms.

Ultrasonography (**choice B**) is principally used to determine whether a breast lesion is solid or cystic. In this example, the presence of microcalcifications makes the lesion highly suspicious, which warrants pathologic examination (i.e., biopsy).

Fine-needle aspiration cytology (**choice D**) is a practical technique with excellent diagnostic accuracy if used by an experienced pathologist. Cells are aspirated by inserting a small (22-gauge) needle into the lesion. The cells are then smeared onto glass slides and examined microscopically after appropriate staining. This technique cannot be used, however, if the lesion is nonpalpable.

Large-needle (core needle) biopsy (**choice E**) extracts a core of tissue by using a large-bore needle inserted into the lesion. As with the fine-needle aspiration technique, it may not be applied to nonpalpable breast lesions.

35. **The correct answer is B.** Genuine stress urinary incontinence (GSUI) is caused by a change in the normal angle between the bladder and urethra such that urine is lost when there is an increase in intra-abdominal pressure (such as with physical activity, sneezing, and coughing). Physical examination often reveals pelvic organ prolapse, although it may be normal. The postvoid residual (the amount of urine left in the bladder after voiding) and cystometrogram are normal. Noninvasive treatments include Kegel exercises, behavior modification, and, for postmenopausal women, estrogen cream. Invasive therapy includes several surgical options.

Detrusor instability (DI; **choice A**) is characterized by sudden urgency followed by a medium-to-large loss of urine. It is caused by uninhibited bladder contraction. A cystometrogram will often demonstrate bladder contractions.

Neurogenic bladder (**choice C**) is characterized by a high postvoid residual, as the patient is unable to fully empty the bladder. This patient has a normal postvoid residual.

Pyelonephritis (**choice D**) is characterized by fevers, chills, back or flank pain, and costovertebral angle tenderness on examination. This patient has none of these findings.

Urinary tract infection (**choice E**) is characterized by frequency, urgency, and dysuria. This patient has none of these findings and a negative urine culture.

36. **The correct answer is A.** The adverse effects of maternal phenylketonuria (PKU) correlate with the degree of hyperphenylalaninemia. Lowering the maternal phenylalanine level into the normal range by dietary means before conception affords optimal protection to the infant.

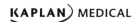

Glycine supplementation (**choice B**) is used as a treatment option in patients with isovaleric acidemia. This is an organic acid disorder resulting from deficiency of isovaleryl CoA dehydrogenase, which is an enzyme involved in the oxidative decarboxylation of leucine. Severe neonatal ketoacidosis may occur.

Isovaleric acidemia may also occur because of a secondary depletion of L-carnitine, preventing conjugation of isovaleric acid and elimination of the water-soluble isovaleryl carnitine in the urine. Dietary supplementation with L-carnitine is recommended (**choice C**).

Choice D is incorrect because even mildly elevated levels of phenylalanine can induce adverse fetal outcomes.

Vitamin B_6 (**choice E**) is used in the partial treatment of homocystinuria. This occurs because of an autosomal recessive inherited deficiency of the enzyme cystathionine beta-synthase leading to the accumulation of homocystine. Vitamin B_6 is a cofactor of this enzyme.

37. **The correct answer is E.** Clear cell adenocarcinoma is a rare malignancy that is associated with in utero exposure to diethylstilbestrol (DES). For approximately 25 years, up until the early 1970s, pregnant women were treated with DES to prevent abortion, preeclampsia, diabetes, and preterm labor. However, it was discovered that in utero exposure to this drug leads to an increased risk of clear cell adenocarcinoma of the vagina and cervix, as well as genital tract anomalies, in the daughters of DES-ingesting mothers.

Albuterol use (**choice A**) has no known association with clear cell adenocarcinoma of the vagina.

Oral contraceptive pill (OCP) use (**choice B**) has no known association with clear cell adenocarcinoma of the vagina. OCP use is known to decrease a woman's risk of ovarian and endometrial cancer. There is conflicting evidence regarding the effect of OCP use on breast and cervical cancer.

In utero aspirin exposure (**choice C**) can cause constriction of the ductus arteriosus in the fetus. Pregnant women who take aspirin also may have delayed onset of labor, prolonged labor, and an increased risk of a prolonged pregnancy. However, there is no known association between aspirin and clear cell adenocarcinoma.

In utero warfarin exposure (**choice D**) is associated with chondrodysplasia punctata in about 5% to 10% of exposed pregnancies. Chondrodysplasia punctata is a syndrome characterized by nasal hypoplasia, bone and eye abnormalities, and mental retardation. In utero warfarin exposure is not associated with clear cell adenocarcinoma.

38. **The correct answer is B.** *Chlamydia trachomatis* is the most common sexually transmitted bacterial pathogen in the U.S. Infection during pregnancy has been associated with preterm delivery and preterm premature rupture of the membranes. Several clinical syndromes are associated with chlamydial infection, including urethritis, cervicitis, and salpingitis. The drug of choice to treat chlamydial infection in pregnancy is erythromycin. Azithromycin is also an accepted option. (Erythromycin base or erythromycin ethylsuccinate should be used because erythromycin estolate may cause hepatotoxicity.)

Ceftriaxone (**choice A**) is the drug of choice for infection with *Neisseria gonorrhoeae*. This patient has *Chlamydia*, not gonorrhea; therefore, ceftriaxone would not be the drug of choice.

Metronidazole (**choice C**) is the drug of choice for infection with *Trichomonas vaginalis* and bacterial vaginosis, not chlamydia.

Penicillin (**choice D**) is the drug of choice for infection with *Treponema pallidum*, the organism that causes syphilis. Penicillin is also used in labor to prevent group B streptococcal infection of the newborn.

Tetracycline (**choice E**) should not be used in pregnancy, as it has been associated with brown discoloration of the deciduous teeth and hypoplasia of the enamel. It can also be deposited into fetal long bones and cause inhibition of bone growth.

39. **The correct answer is C.** There is a well-established association between recurrent *Candida* infections and diabetes mellitus. Diabetes mellitus is known to alter the metabolic and nutritional milieu of the vulva and vagina, which makes infections with *Candida* more likely. A patient who has recurrent *Candida* infections should therefore be screened for diabetes mellitus. Screening for HIV would also be appropriate, as immunosuppression can certainly lead to recurrent infections.

Referral to a psychiatrist (**choice A**) would not be proper management. This patient comes to the physician several times a year with vulvar complaints because of her recurrent infections with *Candida*. On this visit she also has a *Candida* infection that is diagnosed on the basis of the symptoms (vulvovaginal itch and discharge and dysuria), her examination (erythema and a thick, white discharge), and KOH smear findings (pseudohyphae). She needs treatment and screening for diabetes and HIV and not referral to psychiatry for this issue.

To screen for cocaine abuse (**choice B**) or thalassemia (**choice D**) would not be proper management. There is no proven association between either of these conditions and recurrent *Candida* infections.

To treat with metronidazole (**choice E**) would not be proper management. Metronidazole is used to treat infection with *Trichomonas vaginalis* or bacterial vaginosis. This patient has no evidence of either of these infections.

40. **The correct answer is D.** The presence of a large lytic lesion in the lumbar spine in a patient with metastatic breast cancer is an indication for emergency radiotherapy.

    Although it would be appropriate to have a pain management consultant involved in this patient's care (**choice B**) and to discuss her wishes regarding CPR (**choice A**), the patient should first undergo radiation therapy while narcotic analgesics are being administered.

    Prescribing bed rest with high-dose NSAIDs (**choice C**) would not be appropriate management for progressive metastatic disease.

    An emergency nuclear bone scan (**choice E**) is unnecessary since an emergency MRI revealed large lytic lesions at L3 and L4.

41. **The correct answer is C.** Trichomoniasis, a sexually transmitted disease, is a common cause of vulvovaginitis. It is caused by the organism *Trichomonas vaginalis*. The most common symptoms are a profuse, malodorous, frothy vaginal discharge and vaginal itch and pain. Occasionally patients will have dysuria, dyspareunia, and pelvic pain. Examination will demonstrate the copious, frothy discharge. The pH of this discharge will usually be equal to or greater than 6.0. On a normal saline smear, motile trichomonads will be seen in most symptomatic patients. The drug of choice to treat trichomoniasis is metronidazole, and it is imperative that both the patient and her partner be treated. They should refrain from intercourse until they have completed the treatment and are asymptomatic.

    Failing to treat the patient or her partner (**choice A**) would not be an appropriate course of action. The patient has obvious trichomoniasis and therefore needs to be treated. Her partner also must be treated so that he does not continue to reinfect the patient if he is infected as well.

    Treating only the patient with metronidazole (**choice B**) would leave her partner untreated. If he is infected and does not receive treatment, he may continue to infect her. This is important as men are frequently asymptomatic.

    Treating only the patient (**choice D**) or the patient and her partner (**choice E**) with penicillin would not be appropriate. Penicillin is not a drug of choice for trichomoniasis. The first-line treatment is metronidazole. If the patient cannot tolerate metronidazole, topical clotrimazole or boric acid may be tried.

42. **The correct answer is C.** The identification of BRCA1 in 1990 was followed by the finding that mutations of this gene were frequent in a high proportion of women with familial predisposition for breast and ovarian cancer. This discovery suggested the possibility of genetic screening for breast cancer susceptibility genes. A commercially available genetic test was then developed. However, how this test should be applied and what to do when disease-related mutations are detected are still highly controversial issues. Suffice it to say that the most current studies discourage the widespread use of this form of genetic screening, unless there is a strong family history of breast cancer, especially if associated with ovarian cancer and arising at young ages. It is recommended that this screening be performed only along with genetic counseling to assess the individual psychological response to a positive result. However, it can be comforting for a woman to know that she does not carry BRCA1 mutations.

    To say that BRCA1 mutations are not associated with increased risk of breast cancer (**choice A**) would certainly be a highly inaccurate statement. The lifetime risk of breast and ovarian cancer associated with BRCA1 mutations is, respectively, 85% and 50%. Mutations are inherited as autosomal dominant traits.

    Mutations of the BRCA1 gene may occur throughout the length of this gene. At this time, more than 130 germline mutations have been identified in the general population, and 1 in 500 individuals carry one of such mutations. In contrast, 1 in 100 Ashkenazi Jewish individuals (**choice B**) carry a BRCA1 mutation in a specific location of the gene.

    A recommendation of prophylactic bilateral mastectomy (**choice D**) would be highly problematic in a young woman, although in theory it is the only definitive measure to reduce the risk of developing breast cancer. The problem is what to do with individuals with BRCA1 mutations. Is increased surveillance sufficient, or should they undergo bilateral mastectomy? In the latter case, as some authors have written, "the prevention is worse than the disease."

43. **The correct answer is C.** This patient has vaginal discharge and multiple sexual partners and does not use condoms, all of which suggests the presence of a sexually transmitted disease such as gonorrhea. Although Gram stain of cervical cultures is positive only 60% of the time, the presence of gram-negative diplococci is specific for the disease. It is extremely important to treat both patients and their partners for gonorrhea, because reinfection is usually caused by sexual exposure to an untreated partner. The standard treatment is a single intramuscular injection of ceftriaxone followed by a 7-day course of doxycycline to cover for the commonly co-occurring *Chlamydia* (note that in pregnant women, erythromycin is used instead of doxycycline to avoid tooth-mottling in the fetus).

    The remaining choices answer choices are possible sources of recurrence, but are not the most likely cause of this patient's presentation.

44. **The correct answer is E.** Numerous studies demonstrate that use of the oral contraceptive pill (OCP) significantly decreases a woman's likelihood of developing ovarian cancer. Some studies show a protective effect with as little as 6 months of use, and others show an even greater effect with longer use. One theory to explain the decreased ovarian cancer risk is that the OCP provides hormones that feedback inhibit the pituitary, which then decreases the amount of gonadotropins that are produced and helps to suppress monthly ovarian germinal capsule disruptions caused by ovulation.

The relationship between breast cancer (**choice A**) and the OCP remains unclear at this time. There is some evidence that current users and those who have recently stopped may be at some increased risk of breast cancer. However, there is also evidence that when breast cancer is diagnosed in an OCP user, it tends to be more localized than in a nonuser.

The relationship between cervical cancer (**choice B**) and the OCP also remains unclear at this time. Overall the results have been inconclusive. All sexually active patients should have regular screening for cervical dysplasia with a pap smear.

The OCP does not protect against liver cancer (**choice C**); it is believed to increase the risk of certain benign liver tumors.

There is no known association between lung cancer (**choice D**) and the OCP.

45. **The correct answer is C.** There is still an incomplete understanding of the exact pathophysiology underlying bacterial vaginosis (BV). However, it is believed that an increase in the levels of anaerobic bacteria coupled with overabundance of *Gardnerella vaginalis* are involved. The symptoms of BV include vaginal odor and an increased vaginal discharge. Local discomfort is uncommon. Physical examination will often demonstrate a copious vaginal discharge that has a pH greater than 4.7. There will be an intense, amine (fishy) odor when potassium hydroxide (KOH) is added to the discharge (a positive "whiff test"). Finally, the normal saline wet preparation is characterized by "clue cells" (epithelial cells whose borders and nuclei are obscured by the presence of bacteria). The treatment is with metronidazole.

Candida albicans (**choice A**) is the causative organism of yeast infections. These infections are characterized by a thick, "cottage cheese" vaginal discharge. Physical examination reveals the vaginal discharge, as well as evidence of local inflammation. The KOH preparation shows pseudohyphae. This patient has findings consistent with BV and not yeast infection.

Chlamydia trachomatis (**choice B**) is the causal organism for chlamydial cervicitis. *Chlamydia* infection is characterized by a vaginal discharge with local irritation. Physical examination will often demonstrate a mucopurulent cervical discharge and an erythematous and friable cervix. The normal saline wet preparation usually shows the presence of numerous white blood cells.

Lactobacillus species (**choice D**) are considered normal inhabitants of the vaginal flora. It is believed that the replacement of *Lactobacillus* species by *Gardnerella vaginalis* and other bacteria leads to BV.

Trichomonas vaginalis (**choice E**) causes trichomoniasis, which is characterized by vaginal and vulvar irritation. On normal saline wet preparation, *Trichomonas vaginalis* will be seen as a motile, flagellated organism, somewhat larger than a white blood cell.

46. **The correct answer is B.** This patient has the signs and symptoms that are consistent with atrophic vaginitis, which affects women who are estrogen deficient. Most often it occurs after menopause. Estrogen helps to keep the vaginal mucosa moist and well supported; without estrogen, the mucosa becomes thin and pale and the rugae diminish. Patients with atrophic vaginitis tend to have pruritus, vaginal dryness, and dyspareunia. The most appropriate course of action for this patient would be to treat with estrogen vaginal cream. Systemic hormone replacement therapy could also be used, as it would also affect the vaginal mucosa.

Treatment with clotrimazole vaginal cream (**choice A**) or oral fluconazole (**choice D**) would not be appropriate. Although this patient does have pruritus, she does not have the physical examination findings that are consistent with *Candida* infections: thick, white vaginal discharge, erythema of the vulvovaginal area, and pseudohyphae on KOH preparation. Thus, atrophic vaginitis, not *Candida* infection, is this patient's diagnosis, and the treatment is estrogen.

Treatment with metronidazole vaginal cream (**choice C**) or oral metronidazole (**choice E**) would not be appropriate. Metronidazole is used to treat bacterial vaginosis or trichomoniasis. This patient does not have the symptoms (e.g., vaginal discharge) or physical examination findings (e.g., vaginal pH >4.5, malodorous vaginal discharge, or clue cells or trichomonads on wet preparation) that would support the diagnosis of bacterial vaginosis or trichomoniasis.

47. **The correct answer is B.** Fitz-Hugh-Curtis syndrome occurs when patients with pelvic inflammatory disease (PID) develop perihepatic inflammation and adhesions extending from the liver surface to the diaphragm. This syndrome is believed to occur in 1% to 10%

of patients with acute PID. Symptoms may include right upper quadrant pain and pleuritic pain, though many cases are asymptomatic. It is believed to be caused by hematogenous dissemination or transperitoneal dissemination of *Chlamydia trachomatis* or *Neisseria gonorrhoeae*, though other organisms may be involved.

Alcoholic cirrhosis (**choice A**) is not the most likely diagnosis given that this patient's liver appears unremarkable except for the perihepatic adhesions. A cirrhotic liver usually appears fibrotic, scarred, and shrunken, although alcoholics may have an enlarged liver because of fatty infiltration. Furthermore, one beer per day is unlikely to lead to cirrhosis in an otherwise healthy 32-year-old woman.

Hepatitis (**choice C**) will often present as a systemic illness. Usually there are alterations in the liver function tests (ALT and AST). This patient has pelvic pain and right upper quadrant pain only, normal liver function tests, and laparoscopic findings most consistent with prior PID and Fitz-Hugh-Curtis syndrome.

Hepatocellular carcinoma (**choice D**) is one of the most common cancers in the world. Often patients who develop these tumors will have cirrhosis and significant weight loss and ascites. This patient has the perihepatic adhesions only.

In Wolff-Parkinson-White syndrome (**choice E**), patients may develop paroxysmal supraventricular tachycardia because of the presence of an accessory muscle bundle that bypasses the AV node of the heart and produces a reentry loop. This patient has no complaints of cardiac arrhythmia.

48. **The correct answer is D.** Pelvic inflammatory disease (PID) is an infection of the upper genital tract. It most often starts as a vaginal or cervical infection that then extends along the endometrium and eventually involves the fallopian tubes, adnexae, and parametrial tissues. In some cases it may involve the liver and diaphragm by causing perihepatic inflammation and adhesions (Fitz-Hugh-Curtis syndrome). Patients often present with systemic illness, complaining of fever, chills, and myalgias, as well as with lower abdominal pain. To make the diagnosis, the patient should have the triad of abdominal tenderness, cervical motion tenderness, and adnexal tenderness. Along with this triad, the patient should also have a fever (>38° C), leukocytosis (>11,000/mm³), or an adnexal mass. This patient clearly meets these diagnostic criteria. Also, this patient had an IUD placed recently, which is a well-established risk factor for PID.

Appendicitis (**choice A**) is a possible diagnosis here. However, it is not the most likely diagnosis given the patient's history and physical. Appendicitis often starts with periumbilical pain that becomes severe at

McBurney's point. It is usually characterized by nausea, vomiting, and decreased appetite. On examination, the patient with appendicitis may have an elevated temperature, tenderness at McBurney's point, and cervical motion tenderness. Laboratory studies will often demonstrate an elevated white blood cell count. This patient, with her bilateral pain and tenderness, as well as her recent history of IUD placement, is more likely to have PID.

A hemorrhagic ovarian cyst (**choice B**) can often present with abdominal pain and peritoneal signs. However, the pain is often of sudden onset as the cyst ruptures. Furthermore, ultrasound will reveal a cyst or free fluid in the pelvis, if the cyst has completely ruptured and drained.

Ovarian torsion (**choice C**) presents with severe abdominal pain, often along with nausea, vomiting, diaphoresis, and an acute abdomen. Torsion occurs when an adnexal mass causes the adnexa to twist on its pedicle, compromising the blood supply. In an adult, ovarian torsion is extremely unlikely when there is no adnexal mass present.

Pyelonephritis (**choice E**) usually presents with urinary complaints and back or flank pain, along with fever and chills. This patient has no urinary complaints, no costovertebral angle tenderness on examination, and a negative urinalysis.

49. **The correct answer is A.** This patient's presentation is most consistent with primary dysmenorrhea. Primary dysmenorrhea typically has its onset 6-12 months after menarche. Cramping occurs before menses and last 48-72 hours. Uterine ischemia and prostaglandins are believed to be responsible for the pain of primary dysmenorrhea. Pelvic examination is normal. Treatment of primary dysmenorrhea is with a trial of either nonsteroidal anti-inflammatory drugs (NSAIDs) or oral contraceptive pills (OCPs). If these therapies fail to provide relief, further evaluation with ultrasound or laparoscopy may be warranted.

A trial of antibiotics (**choice B**) would not be appropriate. Although infection can cause lower abdominal pain, this patient's history and physical are much more consistent with primary dysmenorrhea. A woman who presents with crampy lower abdominal pain should certainly be evaluated for an infection, but a trial of antibiotics would not be appropriate.

GnRH agonist therapy (**choice C**) is used for patients with secondary dysmenorrhea caused by endometriosis. This patient's presentation is more consistent with primary dysmenorrhea than with endometriosis. Even if this patient were to have endometriosis, she would benefit from a trial of OCPs prior to instituting GnRH agonist therapy.

Laparoscopy (**choice D**) and especially laparotomy (**choice E**) are too invasive to be the most appropriate next step in management. This patient may have a case of primary dysmenorrhea that responds well to NSAIDs. In that case, surgical evaluation would be completely unnecessary and not worth the risks. As noted before, if the trial of NSAIDs or OCPs fails, then the patient may be a candidate for a diagnostic laparoscopy.

50. **The correct answer is A.** Virtually the only time in life when a woman can get a breast abscess is during lactation; therefore, a red, hot, tender breast at that time is most likely to represent an abscess. The fever and leukocytosis provide further confirmation of the diagnosis.

    Breast cancer (**choice B**) should be the number one choice if an identical vignette were given for a nonlactating woman. Breast infections are extremely rare outside of the postpartum period (unless precipitated by trauma); thus, what appears to be breast abscess in a nonlactating woman is breast cancer until proven otherwise. Because this patient is breast-feeding, a breast abscess is more likely.

    Intraductal papilloma (**choice C**) manifests itself with bloody discharge from the breast.

    Mastalgia (**choice D**) is part of the "fibrocystic disease" complex; as such, it is the most common benign breast disorder. It indeed produces pain, but the pain is related to the menstrual cycle and comes with "lumpiness" of the breast, rather than redness, warmth, fever, and leukocytosis.

    Hematoma (**choice E**) is also painful, but it would come after a traumatic injury and would probably produce a mass rather than a red, hot, swollen breast with fever and leukocytosis.

Obstetrics/Gynecology: **Test Two**

1. A 25-year-old nulligravid woman comes to the physician for her annual visit. She has no complaints. She has a history of hepatitis A but denies prior surgeries. She has been taking the oral contraceptive pill for 2 years. She has no known drug allergies. She is sexually active and occasionally uses condoms. A Pap smear shows perinuclear cytoplasmic vacuolization and nuclear enlargement, irregularity, and hyperchromasia. The report states that she has a low-grade squamous intraepithelial lesion (LGSIL). Which of the following organisms is most likely responsible for these cellular changes?

   (A) *Donovania granulomatis*

   (B) *Haemophilus ducreyi*

   (C) Hepatitis A

   (D) Hepatitis B

   (E) Human papillomavirus

2. A 41-year-old woman comes to the physician complaining of depression. She states that her depression started about 4 months ago and she cannot recall any precipitating event that led to it. She also notes insomnia and decreased appetite over the past 4 months. Her feelings grow worse at the time of menses but are always there. She states that she has had no thoughts of hurting herself or others. She is taking no medications. Physical examination is normal. Which of the following is the most appropriate next step in management?

   (A) Reassure the patient that these symptoms are normal

   (B) Perform or refer for a thorough psychological evaluation

   (C) Admit the patient to inpatient psychiatry

   (D) Prescribe fluoxetine for premenstrual syndrome (PMS)

   (E) Prescribe vitamin B_6 for premenstrual syndrome (PMS)

3. A 42-year-old woman comes to the physician because of irregular vaginal bleeding. She has a normal menstrual period every 29 days that lasts 3-4 days. Then, a few days after the cessation of her normal menses, she has a "second period" that lasts 1-2 days. Physical examination is unremarkable, including a normal pelvic examination. Urine hCG is negative. Endometrial biopsy suggests the presence of an endometrial polyp. Pap smear is within normal limits. Office hysteroscopy reveals a 2-3 cm endometrial polyp at the fundus. Which of the following is the most appropriate next step in management?

   (A) GnRH agonist therapy

   (B) Medroxyprogesterone acetate therapy

   (C) Hysteroscopic polypectomy

   (D) Total vaginal hysterectomy

   (E) Total abdominal hysterectomy

4. A 19-year-old woman is brought to the emergency department because of severe lower abdominal pain. Over the past 24 hours, she has had several episodes of severe abdominal pain lasting for 15 to 20 minutes and then resolving. With the episodes of pain, she has nausea, vomiting, and diaphoresis. Her temperature is 37.7° C (100.0° F), blood pressure is 114/78 mm Hg, pulse is 110/min, and respirations are 14/min. Her lower abdomen is bilaterally tender, more on the left than the right. Pelvic examination is somewhat limited because of the patient's inability to tolerate it, but there is the suggestion of a left adnexal mass. Urine hCG and urinalysis are negative. Which of the following is the most appropriate next step in diagnosis?

   (A) Pelvic ultrasound

   (B) Abdominal x-ray

   (C) CT scan

   (D) MRI

   (E) Culdocentesis

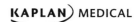

5. A 20-year-old nulligravid woman comes to the physician because of abnormal menstrual periods. She states that menarche occurred at age 12. Since then, her menstrual period has occurred every 45 to 60 days, and has lasted for 5 days. A rough estimate of blood loss with each period is about 60 mL. She was on depot medroxyprogesterone acetate (DMPA or Depo Provera) for 2 years, from age 17 to 19; during the second year, she had no menstrual periods. Which of the following makes this patient's menstrual history abnormal?

(A) Her cycle lasts 45 to 60 days

(B) Her menses lasts 5 days

(C) Her menstrual blood loss is 60 mL

(D) Menarche was at age 12

(E) She had no menses for 1 year on DMPA

6. A 25-year-old woman comes to her physician on the same date each year for her examination and Pap smear. One week later, the Pap smear result is returned as atypical squamous cells of undetermined significance (ASCUS). Which of the following is the most appropriate next step in management?

(A) Repeat Pap smear in 1 week

(B) Repeat Pap smear in 3 months

(C) Repeat Pap smear in 1 year

(D) Repeat Pap smear in 2 years

(E) Perform cervical cone biopsy

7. A 28-year-old, HIV-positive woman comes to the physician complaining of "pimples" on the vulva and perineal skin. The lesions do not bother her except for occasional mild itching. Examination shows multiple small (2-5 mm), dome-shaped, flesh-colored papules with a smooth surface. Several of the lesions have a central dimple. Which of the following is the most likely causal organism?

(A) *Epidermophyton floccosum*

(B) Human papillomavirus

(C) Molluscum contagiosum virus

(D) *Phthirus pubis*

(E) *Sarcoptes scabiei*

8. A 27-year-old woman at 12 weeks' gestation presents to the physician for her first prenatal visit. She has had nausea, but no other complaints. Pelvic examination shows a bulky cervix with a mass involving the cervix and the upper vagina. A biopsy of the mass reveals squamous cell carcinoma of the cervix. Which of the following is the most appropriate management?

(A) Expectant management

(B) Pap smear in 3 to 6 months

(C) Colposcopy in 4 to 6 weeks

(D) Cone biopsy

(E) Radical hysterectomy

9. A 32-year old woman presents to her physician for advice about attempting to conceive. She has no complaints currently. Her past medical history is significant for a urinary tract infection 4 years ago. She has never had surgery. She takes no medications and has no known drug allergies. Physical examination is unremarkable, including a normal pelvic examination. Which of the following should this patient be taking daily?

(A) Ampicillin

(B) Caffeine

(C) Folic acid

(D) Nitrofurantoin

(E) Vitamin A

10. A 26-year-old nulligravid woman comes to the physician for her first prenatal visit. She has no complaints. She is unsure of the date of her last menstrual period. Examination is unremarkable. Given her uncertainty regarding her last menstrual period, ultrasound is performed. It shows a 7-week intrauterine pregnancy and a 5 by 4 cm right simple cyst. Which of the following is the most appropriate next step in the management of this cyst?

(A) Repeat ultrasound in second trimester

(B) Oral contraceptive pills

(C) Laparoscopy

(D) Laparotomy

(E) Termination of the pregnancy

11. An 85-year-old woman comes to the physician because of pelvic pressure and the feeling that something is coming out of her vagina. She has a history of coronary artery disease and is status post a three-vessel coronary artery bypass graft 10 years ago. She had a cerebrovascular accident 2 years ago that left her with decreased right-sided sensory and motor function. She takes multiple cardiac medications. Examination shows morbid obesity. Her uterus is noted to have mild to moderate prolapse. Which of the following is the most appropriate next step in management?

    (A) Oral contraceptive pill

    (B) Hormone replacement therapy

    (C) Trial of pessary

    (D) Vaginal hysterectomy

    (E) Abdominal hysterectomy

12. A 34-year-old black woman comes to the physician complaining of pelvic pain. Past medical history is significant for gonorrhea. She has had four spontaneous vaginal deliveries. She smokes 1 to 2 packs of cigarettes per day. She is 170 cm (5 feet 7 inches) tall and weighs 54.5 kg (120 pounds). Examination shows a 12-week sized uterus. Pelvic ultrasound reveals an enlarged uterus containing what appear to be several fibroids. Which of the following factors places this patient at greatest risk of having fibroids?

    (A) Black race

    (B) Cigarette smoking

    (C) History of gonorrhea

    (D) Low body mass index

    (E) Multiparity

13. A 29-year-old woman comes to the physician because of "warts" on her external genitalia. She first noted their appearance approximately 9 months ago. Since that time she states that they have become numerous. She has no medical problems. Examination shows multiple, small, raised lesions and a few larger cauliflower-like lesions on her vulva and the posterior fourchette. Rapid plasma reagin (RPR) is negative. Which of the following is the most likely diagnosis?

    (A) Condylomata acuminata

    (B) Condylomata lata

    (C) Herpes genitalis

    (D) Molluscum contagiosum

    (E) Syphilis

14. A 34-year-old primigravid woman at 9 weeks' gestation comes to the physician for her first prenatal visit. She has had some mild nausea but is otherwise doing well. She has no medical problems and has never had surgery. She occasionally takes acetaminophen for headaches. She has no known drug allergies. She wants to know what level of alcohol consumption is considered safe during early pregnancy. Which of the following is the most appropriate response?

    (A) The level is unknown

    (B) 2 drinks/day

    (C) 2 ounces/day

    (D) 4 drinks/day

    (E) 4 ounces/day

15. A 21-year-old woman comes to the physician because of painful menstrual periods. Menarche was at age 13. During her first several cycles, her cramping was bearable, but since then it has grown increasingly worse. Her episodes are now characterized by lower abdominal pain that starts several hours prior to the onset of menses, lasts about 2 days, and then resolves completely. She has diarrhea and fatigue during this time. A year ago, a physician had her try ibuprofen, which helped significantly. Physical examination is unremarkable, and pelvic examination is normal. This patient's painful menstrual periods are related to which of the following substances?

    (A) Endotoxin

    (B) Nonsteroidal anti-inflammatory drugs (NSAIDs)

    (C) Prolactin

    (D) Prostaglandins

    (E) Thyroid stimulating hormone (TSH)

16. A 21-year-old primigravid woman at term presents to the physician because of lightheadedness. She states that she has noticed this feeling for the past 2 days. The lightheadedness comes on only when she is lying on her back. She notices it a short time after lying down. The episode resolves completely when she sits up or is standing. She does not notice the symptoms when she is lying on her side. Which of the following is the most likely cause of this patient's lightheadedness?

    (A) Atrial fibrillation

    (B) Fetal movement

    (C) Inferior vena cava compression

    (D) Pulmonary embolus

    (E) Ventricular tachycardia

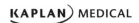
KAPLAN) MEDICAL

17. A 31-year-old primigravid woman at 35 weeks' gestation comes to the physician complaining of pain and tingling in the first three fingers of her right hand. She has had these symptoms on and off for the past 2 weeks. She has no history of trauma to the arm, wrist, or hand. She has had an otherwise uncomplicated prenatal course. Examination, including complete neurologic examination, is unremarkable. Which of the following is the most likely diagnosis?

    (A) Carpal tunnel syndrome

    (B) Cerebrovascular accident

    (C) Malingering

    (D) Seizure disorder

    (E) Wrist fracture

18. A 37-year-old primigravid woman comes to the physician for her first prenatal visit. She is at 8 weeks' gestation based on a firm last menstrual period. She has migraine headaches, for which she takes acetaminophen and occasional butalbital. She has never had surgery. She has no allergies to medications. Which of the following would be proper counseling to this patient?

    (A) Acetaminophen cannot be used in pregnancy

    (B) Ergot-derived medications should be used in pregnancy

    (C) Migraine symptoms usually improve with pregnancy

    (D) Narcotics cannot be used in pregnancy

19. A 31-year-old woman comes to the obstetrician at 12 weeks' gestation for a prenatal examination. She has no complaints, takes no medications, and has no known drug allergies. She does not smoke or use illegal drugs but states that she drinks daily. Which of the following questions is most likely to create confrontation with this patient?

    (A) Have you ever been annoyed by criticism of your drinking?

    (B) Have you ever felt guilty about your drinking?

    (C) Have you ever felt the need to cut down on your drinking?

    (D) Have you ever had a morning drink to get started?

    (E) Have you ever tried to stop this harmful behavior that is hurting your baby?

20. A 32-year-old woman comes to the physician seeking advice regarding contraception. She has no medical problems and takes no medications. She was fitted for a diaphragm earlier in the day. She asks the physician when the diaphragm should be removed from the vagina after intercourse. Which of the following is the correct response?

    (A) Immediately after intercourse

    (B) 1 hour after intercourse

    (C) 6 hours after intercourse

    (D) 12 hours after intercourse

    (E) 24 hours after intercourse

21. A 34-year-old primigravid woman at 39 weeks' gestation comes to the labor and delivery ward because of contractions. Her prenatal course was significant for anemia in the third trimester. Examination shows the cervix to be 6 cm dilated and the fetus in footling breech position. External fetal monitoring shows the fetal heart rate to be in the 140s and reactive. A cesarean section is performed. Which of the following risk factors places this patient at greatest risk for developing postpartum endometritis?

    (A) Anemia

    (B) Cesarean section

    (C) External fetal monitoring

    (D) Intact membranes

    (E) Socioeconomic status

22. A 24-year-old woman comes to the physician 2 weeks after experiencing a spontaneous abortion at 6 weeks' gestation. She has no vaginal bleeding, abdominal pain, fevers, or chills. Examination is unremarkable, including a normal pelvic examination. She states that this was her first pregnancy and she wants to know whether she and her husband need testing to determine why the miscarriage occurred. After comforting the patient, which of the following is the most appropriate response?

    (A) Investigation is initiated after the first, first-trimester miscarriage

    (B) Investigation is initiated after two consecutive first-trimester miscarriages

    (C) Investigation is initiated after three consecutive first-trimester miscarriages

    (D) Investigation is initiated after four consecutive first-trimester miscarriages

    (E) There is no need to investigate recurrent miscarriages

23. A 33-year-old woman, gravida 3, para 3, comes to the physician for advice regarding birth control methods. She has no medical problems and takes no medications. She has been in a monogamous relationship with her husband for 9 years. She thinks that she does not want any more children, but does not want a tubal ligation. Her physician recommends the intrauterine device (IUD). Which of the following is more likely to occur with this method of contraception compared with other methods of contraception?

    (A) Amenorrhea

    (B) Ectopic pregnancy

    (C) Intrauterine pregnancy

    (D) Venous thromboembolism

    (E) Weight gain

24. A 37-year-old woman, gravida 3, para 3, comes to the physician complaining of worsening depression and irritability over the past several years. She states that these symptoms have been worsening since she was about 28 years old. She notes that the depression and irritability come on about 1 to 2 weeks prior to her menses and resolve completely a few days after the start of the menses. She also states that she feels swollen and develops breast tenderness, headaches, and insomnia during these times of depression. Those symptoms disrupt her day-to-day activities. She has no medical problems and takes no medications. Examination is unremarkable. Which of the following is the most likely diagnosis?

    (A) Endometriosis

    (B) Manic-depressive disorder

    (C) Premenstrual dysmorphic disorder

    (D) Recurrent situational anxiety of pregnancy

    (E) Schizophrenia

25. A 29-year-old woman comes to the physician for birth control counseling. She is sexually active and has been using condoms, but would like to switch to a different method. She has no medical problems. She had a left ovarian cystectomy 4 years ago. She takes no medications and has no allergies to medications. Physical examination, including pelvic examination, is normal. After a thorough discussion of the birth control options, the patient wishes to start on depot medroxy-progesterone acetate (DMPA). Which of the following is this patient most likely to experience while on this form of contraception?

    (A) Elevated circulating estrogen levels

    (B) Increased bone density

    (C) Increased HDL cholesterol

    (D) Menstrual abnormalities

    (E) Pregnancy

26. A 48-year-old Caucasian woman comes to the physician because of uterine prolapse. She feels as if her uterus is "falling out" and complains of a constant sensation of pressure. She has asthma and has never had surgery. She uses an albuterol inhaler and has no allergies to medications. Examination shows a significant uterine prolapse, with the uterus in descent to the level of the introitus. After a full preoperative evaluation, the decision is made to perform a vaginal hysterectomy. On the day of the operation, which of the following is the most appropriate pharmacotherapy regimen?

(A) No medications are needed

(B) Antibiotics 30 minutes prior to surgery

(C) Beta blocker 30 minutes prior to surgery

(D) Antibiotics prior to closing

(E) Antibiotics 6 hours after the surgery

27. An 18-year-old woman has a 2-cm, firm, rubbery mass in the upper outer quadrant of her left breast. It has been present for at least 3 or 4 months. The mass is easily movable, not tender, and otherwise asymptomatic. Which of the following is the most appropriate initial step in management?

(A) Clinical observation

(B) Sonogram

(C) Mammogram

(D) Incisional biopsy

(E) Excisional biopsy

28. A 39-year-old woman comes to the emergency department because of right lower quadrant abdominal pain and vaginal spotting. Examination is remarkable for a diffusely tender abdomen with rebound and guarding. Halfway through the examination, the patient begins to complain of shoulder pain. Urine hCG is positive. Serum hCG is 5,500 mIU/dL. Transvaginal ultrasound shows nothing in the uterus and significant free fluid in the abdomen and pelvis. Which of the following is the most likely cause of this patient's shoulder pain?

(A) Diaphragmatic ectopic pregnancy

(B) Diaphragmatic irritation

(C) Malingering

(D) Rotator cuff tear

29. A 29-year-old woman comes to the physician complaining of persistent dysmenorrhea and dyspareunia. Both began approximately 4 years ago. The patient has tried nonsteroidal anti-inflammatory drugs (NSAIDs) and has been on the oral contraceptive pill (OCP) for a few years without relief. The patient is brought to the operating room for laparoscopy, during which multiple lesions along her anterior and posterior cul-de-sac are noted. Many of these lesions appear like "gun-powder burns," whereas others are reddish or bluish. The patient also has thickening of her uterosacral ligaments with nodularity. In addition to dysmenorrhea and dyspareunia, which of the following conditions does this patient most likely have?

(A) Basal cell carcinoma

(B) Infertility

(C) Lengthy menstrual cycles

(D) Lung cancer

(E) Menorrhagia

30. A 24-year-old primigravid patient comes to the physician because of vaginal bleeding. Her last menstrual period was 8 weeks ago. Since then, she has had no problems with the early pregnancy except for some nausea and vomiting. She is afebrile, and her vital signs are stable. Pelvic examination shows a small amount of brown blood in the vagina. The cervical os is closed. The uterus is 8-week size and nontender. There are no adnexal masses or tenderness. Pelvic ultrasound shows an 8-week fetus with a heart rate of 158/min and no abnormalities. The patient wants to know what the prognosis is for her pregnancy. Which of the following is the correct response?

(A) There is no risk of miscarriage

(B) There is approximately a 10% risk of miscarriage

(C) There is an approximately 50% risk of miscarriage

(D) There is an approximately 75% risk of miscarriage

(E) Miscarriage is almost certain

31. A 22-year-old primigravid African American woman comes to the physician for her first prenatal visit. She has no complaints. Her last menstrual period was 7 weeks ago. Past medical history is significant for sickle cell trait. Her partner is also known to have sickle cell trait. She takes no medications and has no allergies to medications. Physical examination is unremarkable except for a mildly enlarged uterus consistent with early pregnancy. Which of the following represents this couple's risk of having a child with sickle cell anemia?

    (A) 0%

    (B) 25%

    (C) 50%

    (D) 75%

    (E) 100%

32. A 39-year-old woman, gravida 3, para 2, at 20 weeks' gestation comes to the physician because of fevers, chills, and a cough for the past week. Her prenatal course had been otherwise unremarkable. Her temperature is 38.0° C (100.4° F), blood pressure is 100/60 mm Hg, pulse is 98/min, and respirations are 14/min. Examination demonstrates crackles and harsh breath sounds at the right lung base. The physician recommends a chest x-ray, but the patient is concerned about radiation exposure during pregnancy. Which of the following is the most appropriate response?

    (A) Exposure from a chest x-ray does not cause harmful fetal effects

    (B) Exposure from a chest x-ray leads to birth defects

    (C) Exposure from a chest x-ray leads to spontaneous abortion

    (D) When a chest x-ray has occurred, fetal pneumonia is more common

    (E) When a chest x-ray has occurred, termination should be considered

33. A 43-year-old woman, gravida 2, para 1, at 34 weeks' gestation comes to the physician because of shortness of breath, which began yesterday while she was lying down. Today, she notices pain when she takes a deep breath. Her temperature is 37.0° C (98.6° F), blood pressure is 110/70 mm Hg, pulse is 110/min, and respirations are 25/min. Oxygen saturation is 93% on room air. Examination is unremarkable. ECG shows sinus tachycardia. A chest x-ray film is negative. Which of the following is the most appropriate initial step in management?

    (A) Antibiotic therapy

    (B) Warfarin therapy

    (C) Heparin therapy

    (D) Pulmonary ultrasonography

    (E) Ventilation-perfusion scan

34. A 29-year-old woman, gravida 2, para 1, comes to the physician for a prenatal visit at 36 weeks' gestation. At 28 weeks, she was diagnosed with gestational diabetes on the basis of an abnormal glucose tolerance test. Since then, she has been able to control her blood sugar levels with an improved diet regimen. She has no medical problems and has taken only prenatal vitamins during the pregnancy. Which of the following is the most appropriate postpartum management of this patient?

    (A) No postpartum follow-up is necessary

    (B) Perform 2-hour, 75-g glucose tolerance test at 6-week postpartum visit

    (C) Start oral hypoglycemics at 6-week postpartum visit

    (D) Start subcutaneous insulin at 6-week postpartum visit

    (E) Refer for pancreatic transplantation after 6-week postpartum visit

35. A 14-year-old girl comes to the physician complaining of pelvic pain each month. She states that approximately every 30 days she develops crampy lower abdominal pain that resolves after a day or two. She has never had a menstrual period. Examination shows normal development of the breasts and the presence of axillary and pubic hair. Pelvic examination demonstrates a vaginal bulge. Rectal examination reveals a mass anterior to the rectum. Urine hCG is negative. Which of the following is the most likely diagnosis?

    (A) Colon cancer

    (B) Ectopic pregnancy

    (C) Endometriosis

    (D) Imperforate hymen

    (E) Vaginal cancer

36. A 44-year-old woman comes to the physician because of heavy periods. She states that her periods have gotten increasingly heavy over the past year. She now has a 6-day menstrual flow and needs to change pads far more frequently than before. She also complains of constant lower abdominal pressure. She has four children and does not wish to have any more. Examination shows a 16-week-sized uterus. Hematocrit is 29%. Endometrial biopsy demonstrates benign endometrial tissue. Pelvic ultrasound shows an enlarged fibroid uterus with multiple fibroids. What is the most appropriate next step in management?

    (A) Hormone replacement therapy

    (B) Diagnostic laparoscopy

    (C) Myomectomy

    (D) Tubal ligation

    (E) Hysterectomy

37. A 23-year-old woman comes to the physician because of vaginal bleeding. Her last menstrual period was 8 weeks ago, and a home pregnancy test 2 weeks ago was positive. She has had mild uterine cramping but is otherwise asymptomatic. Pelvic examination reveals a 10- to 12-week, nontender uterus. The remainder of the physical examination is unremarkable. Urine hCG is positive. Pelvic ultrasound reveals multiple echogenic areas in a "snowstorm" pattern with no evidence of a fetus. Which of the following is the most appropriate next step in management?

    (A) Expectant management

    (B) Folic acid supplementation

    (C) Methotrexate therapy

    (D) Dilation and evacuation

    (E) Laparotomy

38. A 14-year-old girl comes to the emergency department because of heavy vaginal bleeding. She states that she has been soaking 1 to 2 pads per hour for the past 24 hours. She has no medical problems and no history of easy bleeding or bruising. Her temperature is 37.0° C (98.6° F), blood pressure is 118/76 mm Hg, pulse is 92/min, and respirations are 14/min. Pelvic examination reveals some blood in the vagina and oozing from the cervical os; it is otherwise unremarkable. Pelvic ultrasound is unremarkable. Urine hCG is negative. Hematocrit is 31%. Platelet count is 275,000/mm^3. PT and PTT are within normal limits. Six hours later the hematocrit is 30%. Which of the following is the most appropriate next step in management?

    (A) Blood transfusion

    (B) Fresh frozen plasma

    (C) IV conjugated estrogens

    (D) Oral contraceptive pill

    (E) Platelet transfusion

39. A 22-year-old primigravid woman at 35 weeks' gestation comes to the physician complaining of a severe frontal headache that has not improved with acetaminophen. She also notes changes in her vision over the past 12 hours. Within the past 6 hours, she has developed constant epigastric pain. Her temperature is 37.0° C (98.6° F), blood pressure is 150/90 mm Hg, pulse is 88/min, and respirations are 12/min. Examination shows moderate to severe edema in the face, hands, and feet. Urinalysis shows 3+ proteinuria. Which of the following is the most likely diagnosis?

    (A) Eclampsia

    (B) Hepatitis

    (C) Migraine

    (D) Myocardial infarction

    (E) Systemic lupus erythematosus

40. A 29-year-old woman comes the physician for an annual examination. She has no complaints but is interested in becoming pregnant. She has had type 1 diabetes mellitus for the past 9 years, for which she takes insulin daily. She does not smoke or drink alcohol. Examination is unremarkable, including a normal pelvic examination. Urine hCG is negative. When should management and counseling regarding fetal anomalies take place with this patient?

    (A) Prior to conception

    (B) In the first trimester

    (C) Prior to an 18-week ultrasound

    (D) After an 18-week ultrasound

    (E) In the third trimester

41. A 27-year-old woman, gravida 4, para 0, at 6 weeks' gestation comes the physician for her first prenatal visit. Her past obstetric history is significant for three second-trimester losses. She states that each time she presented to the hospital and was found to have a widely dilated cervix. She does not recall having painful contractions prior to the diagnosis of dilation in any of the previous pregnancies. She has no medical problems and has never had surgery. Physical examination is unremarkable, including a pelvic examination that shows her cervix to be long and closed. After a lengthy discussion with the patient, she chooses to have a cerclage placed during this pregnancy. Which of the following is the most appropriate time to place the cerclage?

    (A) Immediately

    (B) 10 to 14 weeks

    (C) 20 to 24 weeks

    (D) 24 to 28 weeks

    (E) 32 to 36 weeks

42. A wealthy, 32-year-old primigravid woman at 39 weeks' gestation comes to the labor and delivery ward because of ruptured membranes. She states that 10 minutes ago, as she was walking by the hospital, she felt a large gush of fluid and has continued to leak fluid. Her prenatal course was unremarkable, except for her obesity (300 pounds) and inactive asthma, for which she has not taken medications for many years. On initial examination, she is found to have a fetus in breech position and she is quickly brought to the operating room for primary cesarean section. The cesarean delivery is performed rapidly and without complication. Which of the following characteristics is a risk factor for this patient developing a wound infection?

    (A) Asthma

    (B) High socioeconomic status

    (C) Obesity

    (D) Short duration of ruptured membranes

    (E) Short operative time

43. A 25-year-old nulligravid patient calls the physician complaining of right leg pain. She states that the pain started 1 day ago and has been growing worse throughout the day. She also feels that her right leg is "bigger" than her left leg. She has no medical problems and has never had surgery. She takes the oral contraceptive pill for birth control. She is allergic to aspirin. She does not smoke. Her family history is significant for ulcer disease but is otherwise unremarkable. Which of the following is the most appropriate next step in management?

(A) Have the patient come in for evaluation

(B) Prescribe acetaminophen

(C) Recommend warm soaks and evaluation in 1 week

(D) Schedule a pelvic ultrasound

(E) Prescribe anticoagulants

44. A 22-year-old woman, gravida 2, para 1, at 8 weeks' gestation, comes to the physician for her first prenatal visit. Past obstetric history is significant for induction at 28 weeks for severe preeclampsia, with delivery via classic cesarean section for nonreassuring fetal heart rate tracing. Past medical and surgical histories are otherwise unremarkable. She takes prenatal vitamins and has no known drug allergies. The patient wants to know which mode of delivery will be used this pregnancy. Which of the following is the correct response?

(A) Cesarean delivery is contraindicated

(B) Forceps-assisted vaginal delivery is recommended

(C) Vacuum-assisted vaginal delivery is recommended

(D) Vaginal birth is contraindicated

(E) Vaginal birth is not contraindicated

45. A 34-year-old woman, gravida 3, para 2, at 39 weeks' gestation comes to the hospital for elective repeat cesarean delivery. She had a cesarean delivery 5 years ago for arrest of dilation, followed by an elective repeat cesarean delivery 2 years ago. She had nausea and vomiting in the first and early second trimester, but otherwise had an unremarkable prenatal course. Other than her two cesarean deliveries, she has no past medical or past surgical history. She took prenatal vitamins throughout the pregnancy and is allergic to penicillin. Which of the following outcomes is most likely given this mode of delivery?

(A) Fracture of the fetal clavicle

(B) Fracture of the fetal femur

(C) Maternal perineal trauma

(D) Shoulder dystocia

(E) Transient tachypnea of the newborn

46. A 23-year-old woman comes to the physician seeking advice regarding birth control options. She has multiple sexual partners. She has migraine headaches for which she occasionally takes acetaminophen or sumatriptan. She was hospitalized for pelvic inflammatory disease when she was 19. Physical examination is unremarkable. Urine hCG is negative. Which of the following is the most appropriate contraception option for this patient?

(A) Condoms

(B) Intrauterine device

(C) Oral contraceptive pill

(D) Rhythm method

(E) Withdrawal method (coitus interruptus)

47. A 33-year-old primigravid patient comes to the physician for her first prenatal visit. Her last menstrual period was 5 weeks ago, and a urine pregnancy test was positive. She has no complaints. She had an appendectomy at age 15. She has occasional migraine headaches, for which she takes acetaminophen. She is allergic to penicillin. Examination shows that her height is 163 cm (64 in) and her weight is 54.5 kg (120 lb). Her vital signs are stable, and her physical examination is normal. Which of the following is the recommended amount of total weight gain for this patient during her pregnancy?

    (A) 5 to 15 lb
    (B) 15 to 25 lb
    (C) 25 to 35 lb
    (D) 35 to 45 lb
    (E) 45 to 55 lb

48. A 32-year-old woman comes to the emergency department because of abdominal pain and vaginal spotting. Her temperature is 37.0° C (98.6° F), blood pressure is 110/70 mm Hg, pulse is 90/min, and respirations are 14/min. Examination shows scant blood in the vagina and right adnexal tenderness. Hematocrit is 40%. Platelet count is 200,000/mm^3. Serum human chorionic gonadotropin is 4,000 mIU/dL. Aspartate aminotransferase is 110 U/L. Creatinine is 0.7 mg/dL. Pelvic ultrasound shows no evidence of an intrauterine pregnancy but does reveal a right adnexal mass with features consistent with ectopic pregnancy. Which of the following makes this patient ineligible for methotrexate treatment of her ectopic pregnancy?

    (A) Aspartate aminotransferase of 110 U/L
    (B) Blood pressure 110/70 mm Hg
    (C) Creatinine of 0.7 mg/dL
    (D) Hematocrit 40%
    (E) Platelet count of 200,000/mm^3

49. A schoolteacher calls her physician to request information about a recent outbreak of the varicella zoster virus (chickenpox) at her school. She teaches the third grade, and several of her students have been affected in the past week. She has no symptoms but cannot remember having varicella as a child. She is most concerned because she is 16 weeks pregnant with her first child. She is advised to come to the office in the morning for some laboratory tests. These are available within a few hours and show that she has tested positive for IgG to the varicella virus and negative for IgM. Which of the following is the most appropriate management?

    (A) She can go back to school without worrying
    (B) She should remain out of school until the outbreak is over to prevent infection
    (C) She should be retested because she is still in the incubation stage of the illness
    (D) She should have an abortion because her fetus is affected and, at this gestation, the effects are severe
    (E) She should have an ultrasound to see if her fetus is affected by the infection

50. A 42-year-old woman, gravida 4, para 3, at 31 weeks' gestation comes to the labor and delivery ward because of contractions. The contractions started 3 hours ago and are now coming every 5 minutes. The patient has had no leakage of fluid. Examination reveals that her cervix is 2 cm dilated and 75% effaced. A previous cervical examination done 2 days ago during a prenatal visit showed her cervix to be long and closed. The fetal heart rate is in the 150s and reactive. The patient is started on IV magnesium sulfate and penicillin. Which of the following is the most appropriate additional pharmacotherapy for this patient?

    (A) Ampicillin
    (B) Dexamethasone
    (C) Gentamicin
    (D) Terbutaline
    (E) Tetracycline

Obstetrics/Gynecology Test Two:
Answers and Explanations

ANSWER KEY

1.	E	26.	B
2.	B	27.	B
3.	C	28.	B
4.	A	29.	B
5.	A	30.	B
6.	B	31.	B
7.	C	32.	A
8.	E	33.	E
9.	C	34.	B
10.	A	35.	D
11.	C	36.	E
12.	A	37.	D
13.	A	38.	D
14.	A	39.	A
15.	D	40.	A
16.	C	41.	B
17.	A	42.	C
18.	C	43.	A
19.	E	44.	D
20.	C	45.	E
21.	B	46.	A
22.	B	47.	C
23.	B	48.	A
24.	C	49.	A
25.	D	50.	B

1. **The correct answer is E.** It is now generally accepted that the human papillomavirus (HPV) is the most likely etiologic agent for cervical dysplasia. Overwhelming epidemiologic evidence supports the association between cervical dysplasia and HPV. Infection with HPV leads to cellular changes: perinuclear cytoplasmic vacuolization and nuclear enlargement, irregularity, and hyperchromasia. Under the Bethesda system of Papanicolaou smear grading, these HPV-associated changes are considered to be a low-grade squamous intraepithelial lesion (LGSIL).

    Donovania granulomatis (**choice A**) is the bacterium that causes granuloma inguinale. This condition is characterized by papules and ulcers of the external genitalia. Diagnosis is made by the presence of Donovan bodies (encapsulated bacteria found in mononuclear cells) in tissue samples specially stained. Treatment is with tetracycline.

    Haemophilus ducreyi (**choice B**) is the bacterium that causes chancroid. This condition is characterized by papules and painful ulcers of the external genitalia, as well as by local lymphadenopathy. The diagnosis is made by Gram stain, culture, and biopsy. The treatment is with erythromycin.

    Hepatitis A (**choice C**) and hepatitis B (**choice D**) are viruses that infect the liver. They do not cause the cellular changes on Pap smear that are described in this patient and they are not known to cause cervical dysplasia.

2. **The correct answer is B.** Premenstrual syndrome (PMS) is very common, occurring in approximately 10% to 30% of women. However, when a patient presents with psychologic symptoms, it should not be assumed she just has PMS. This patient with insomnia, depression, and decreased appetite most likely does not have PMS. For PMS to be diagnosed, symptoms should remit shortly after menses. This patient states that even though her feelings grow worse at the time of menses, her symptoms are always there. She is more likely to have depression than PMS. Thus, when a patient presents with worrisome psychologic symptoms, a thorough psychologic evaluation should be performed. If the physician does not feel capable of doing this, then referral should be made to an appropriate provider of care.

    To reassure the patient that these symptoms are normal (**choice A**) would not be appropriate. Having insomnia, depression, and decreased appetite over the course of 4 months cannot be considered normal.

    Admitting the patient to inpatient psychiatry (**choice C**) would not be appropriate. Although this patient does have insomnia, depression, and decreased appetite, she does not have any thoughts of hurting herself or others. She can therefore be evaluated in the outpatient setting.

    To prescribe fluoxetine (**choice D**) or vitamin B$_6$ (**choice E**) for PMS would be inappropriate. As explained above, one cannot simply assume that psychologic complaints in a woman equal PMS. She first deserves a complete psychologic evaluation.

3. **The correct answer is C.** This patient has an endometrial polyp. Endometrial polyps are localized, hyperplastic overgrowths of glands and stroma that project out from the endometrial surface. The most common symptoms are irregular bleeding and postmenopausal spotting, although many are asymptomatic. Polyps may be diagnosed on the basis of an endometrial biopsy. Office hysteroscopy or sonohysterogram (an ultrasound performed while the endometrial cavity is distended with saline) may also be used to diagnose polyps. This patient has a symptomatic polyp (i.e., the polyp is causing irregular bleeding). The management of a symptomatic polyp involves removal with a hysteroscopic polypectomy (polypectomy performed with hysteroscopic guidance). If a dilation and curettage is performed without a hysteroscopy, the polyp could be missed.

    GnRH agonist therapy (**choice A**) is used to treat several gynecologic conditions, including adenomyosis, endometriosis, and leiomyomas. To understand the mechanism of action of the GnRH agonists, one must understand that the hypothalamus normally produces GnRH in a pulsatile fashion. These pulses of GnRH stimulate the pituitary to produce FSH and LH, which then act on the ovary. When GnRH is given in a continuous fashion, as it is in GnRH agonist therapy, FSH and LH production by the pituitary decreases. Although GnRH agonists are useful in the treatment of the aforementioned conditions, they are not appropriate in the management of an endometrial polyp.

    Medroxyprogesterone acetate therapy (**choice B**) is commonly used as a birth control method and as a method to reverse endometrial hyperplasia. The depot form of medroxyprogesterone acetate (DMPA) is given to women as an intramuscular injection. It inhibits ovulation through its effect on the hypothalamus. Medroxyprogesterone acetate is also given to women with neoplastic or proliferative disorders of the endometrium. It is not used in the treatment of endometrial polyps.

    Total vaginal hysterectomy (**choice D**) or total abdominal hysterectomy (**choice E**) would not be the most appropriate next step in the management of this patient. These procedures are too drastic for this patient's problem. This patient has irregular bleeding with an obvious source (i.e., the polyp). To take out this patient's entire uterus with a hysterectomy is not indicated at this point. The correct next step is the hysteroscopic polypectomy.

4. **The correct answer is A.** This patient's presentation is classic for ovarian torsion, which occurs when an adnexal mass (e.g., an ovarian cyst or paraovarian cyst) twists on its pedicle. When this happens, blood supply to the ovary may be compromised, causing infarction. The symptoms are lower abdominal pain, which may wax and wane as the torsion and detorsion occur, nausea, vomiting, and diaphoresis. On examination, the patient will have abdominal tenderness, often with peritoneal signs if infarction has occurred. Pelvic examination will demonstrate an adnexal mass with adnexal tenderness. Pelvic ultrasound is the diagnostic modality of choice in the emergency department, as it rapidly allows for evaluation and characterization of adnexal masses. If the pelvic ultrasound shows an adnexal mass, the patient should be brought to the operating room for laparoscopy for presumed ovarian torsion.

Abdominal x-ray (**choice B**) is not the most effective method for evaluating the uterus and adnexae. It is a good study for intestinal obstruction or perforation and some abdominal masses. However, this patient's presentation is much more consistent with ovarian torsion.

CT scan (**choice C**) is useful for evaluating the abdomen and pelvis, particularly for identifying masses in these regions. It is often used in situations in which the differential diagnosis includes appendicitis, abscess, or tumor. For this patient, however, the diagnosis of ovarian torsion is significantly more likely than any of these conditions.

MRI (**choice D**) can provide an excellent evaluation of the pelvic organs. However, in the emergency department setting, and with a patient who has a classic presentation for ovarian torsion, pelvic ultrasound will more rapidly establish the presence of an adnexal mass. This will allow the patient to be brought to the operating room for laparoscopy and attempted detorsion or adnexectomy.

Culdocentesis (**choice E**) is a procedure in which a spinal needle is introduced through the vagina into the posterior cul-de-sac and any fluid is aspirated. Prior to the widespread availability and use of ultrasound, culdocentesis played an important role in the diagnosis of ectopic pregnancy. This patient has no indication for culdocentesis.

5. **The correct answer is A.** A normal menstrual cycle lasts 28 +/- 7 days. This patient has a cycle that lasts from 45 to 60 days, which is considered oligomenorrhea. Several processes can cause oligomenorrhea, including polycystic ovarian syndrome (PCOS), thyroid abnormalities, diabetes, and medications. Furthermore, a woman can be pregnant and think she has oligomenorrhea because of intermittent first or second trimester bleed-

ing. Therefore, a pregnancy test should be checked in a woman of reproductive age with irregular bleeding.

Menses lasting 5 days (**choice B**) is normal. The average duration of the menstrual flow is from 3 to 7 days.

A menstrual blood loss of 60 mL (**choice C**) is normal. The average amount of blood lost during a normal menstrual period is from 40 to 80 mL.

Menarche, or the onset of first menses, is dependent on a number of factors, including geographic location, body weight, and psychological issues. In the U.S., the mean age of menarche is approximately 12 (**choice D**) to 13 years.

Approximately 50% of women on depot medroxyprogesterone acetate (DMPA) for more than 1 year will report amenorrhea (**choice E**). This likely is the result of the atrophy of the endometrial lining that occurs with this drug.

6. **The correct answer is B.** ASCUS is a cytologic diagnosis used to describe abnormal cells that do not fit the criteria for low- or high-grade squamous intraepithelial lesion (LGSIL or HGSIL). Although most patients with ASCUS will have normal follow-up Pap smears, a significant proportion (approximately 25%) will have dysplasia. Thus, a patient with ASCUS should have a repeat Pap smear in 3-6 months. If the patient is not reliable and may be lost to follow-up, then colposcopy should be performed immediately. This patient is reliable and can therefore be followed with a repeat Pap smear in 3 months.

A repeat Pap smear in 1 week (**choice A**) would not be appropriate. This is not a sufficient time interval to correctly determine resolution or persistence of the ASCUS. Three months, however, is adequate. If the ASCUS persists after 3 months, then it is truly a persistent finding.

A repeat Pap smear in 1 year (**choice C**) or 2 years (**choice D**) is not appropriate because the time interval is too long. Some Pap smears that are read as ASCUS will be discovered to be from an HGSIL or worse. Therefore, waiting longer than 3 to 6 months to repeat the Pap smear is not appropriate.

A cervical cone biopsy (**choice E**) is not appropriate. Cone biopsy is indicated in certain circumstances when premalignant or malignant lesions are found. ASCUS represents cells of *undetermined significance* and not premalignant or malignant cells. Therefore, jumping to cone biopsy in this patient would not be appropriate.

7. **The correct answer is C.** Molluscum contagiosum is a poxvirus. Infection can occur with or without sexual contact. It is a rare infection that tends to occur in patients who are immunosuppressed, such as those with HIV or on immunosuppressive agents. It is largely asymptomatic, although it can cause mild pruritus. The lesions have a

typical appearance in that they are small, dome-shaped, flesh-colored papules with a smooth surface. Many of the lesions will be umbilicated, that is, they will have a central dimple. Diagnosis is made by biopsying the lesion or expressing the contents of the lesion onto a slide for histologic evaluation. Treatment is with destruction of the lesions with laser, liquid nitrogen, or trichloroacetic acid.

Epidermophyton floccosum (**choice A**) causes tinea cruris (jock itch). This lesion appears pink to red and has well-defined scaly borders.

Human papillomavirus (**choice B**) causes condyloma acuminata. These lesions are often grouped together on the vulva and perineum and may involve the vagina and cervix. They have the appearance of warts that are small or large and cauliflower-like.

Phthirus pubis (**choice D**) is the pubic louse that causes severe pruritus and erythema. This patient has only mild pruritus, no erythema, and lesions classic for molluscum contagiosum.

Sarcoptes scabiei (**choice E**) is the female itch mite that causes scabies. Scabies is characterized by severe pruritus (often at night) and papular lesions on the hands, wrists, other joints, and pubis.

8. **The correct answer is E.** Gynecologic cancer is the most common form of cancer occurring during pregnancy. Of the gynecologic cancers, endometrial cancer is the most common, followed by ovarian, cervical, and vulvar cancer. This patient has cervical cancer in the first trimester of pregnancy. Prompt therapy is required to treat invasive cervical cancer during pregnancy. Depending on the stage, cervical cancer may be treated with surgery or radiation. An advanced stage cervical cancer in early pregnancy (as suggested by the findings in this case) would require radical hysterectomy or radiation, which would lead to termination of the pregnancy. If cervical cancer is diagnosed late in pregnancy, one can wait for fetal maturity prior to delivery and treatment.

Expectant management (**choice A**) would not be appropriate. This patient has an invasive cancer. Waiting 28 or more weeks for the patient to deliver could allow progression of the cancer.

A Pap smear in 3-6 months (**choice B**) would be appropriate management for a nonpregnant patient with atypical squamous cells of undetermined significance (ASCUS). This patient has invasive cancer. Therefore, cytologic screening with Pap smear is not necessary; what is needed is treatment.

The diagnosis of invasive cervical cancer has already been made. Therefore, a diagnostic modality like colposcopy (**choice C**) is not needed.

Cone biopsy (**choice D**) can be used in pregnancy to exclude invasive cancer if a biopsy shows microinvasion. This patient does not require a cone biopsy for diagnosis, as she has tumor involving the upper portion of the vagina, which makes her at least stage II. Cone biopsy would therefore play no role in the management of this patient.

9. **The correct answer is C.** Numerous studies have established that periconceptional folic acid supplementation can significantly decrease a mother's risk of having a fetus with a neural tube defect, such as anencephaly or spina bifida. The U.S. Public Health Service recommendation is that all women of childbearing age should take 0.4 mg of folic acid per day periconceptionally. Women who have previously given birth to an infant with a neural tube defect should take 4.0 mg/day periconceptionally, according to the Centers for Disease Control and Prevention.

Ampicillin (**choice A**) would not be recommended for this patient. Some women with chronic urinary tract infections (UTIs) do require antibiotic prophylaxis. This patient, however, had only one isolated UTI 4 years ago. Therefore, she would not be a candidate for antibiotic prophylaxis.

The relationship between caffeine (**choice B**) intake and pregnancy difficulties is controversial. Most obstetricians believe that moderate caffeine intake prior to and during pregnancy is acceptable. However, the fact that moderate intake may be acceptable does not make it recommended in the same way that folic acid is recommended periconceptionally for women.

Nitrofurantoin (**choice D**) is sometimes used as antibiotic prophylaxis in patients who are susceptible to developing a UTI or pyelonephritis, e.g., those with chronic UTIs or pyelonephritis and those with Foley catheters in place. This patient had one UTI and therefore would not require daily nitrofurantoin.

Vitamin A (**choice E**) supplementation prior to pregnancy is probably unnecessary and possibly harmful. Some studies have shown a relationship between high amounts of daily vitamin A intake and birth defects, particularly neural crest malformations.

10. **The correct answer is A.** It is quite common to find cysts in the first trimester of pregnancy. These cysts are most often corpus luteum cysts. The corpus luteum is the name of the structure that is formed from the ovarian follicle after ovulation occurs. Its role is to produce progesterone to support the pregnancy until the placenta can take over that function. Sometimes corpus luteum cysts can form. These cysts can cause complications if they undergo torsion or if they hemorrhage. However, not all cysts in early

pregnancy are corpus luteum cysts; some represent malignancies. Therefore, the correct management of a cyst in early pregnancy is with follow-up ultrasound to look for resolution of the cyst. If, on the second trimester ultrasound, the cyst is not resolving or is growing larger, or if there are other worrisome characteristics, then operative intervention is indicated.

Oral contraceptive pills (**choice B**) are often given to nonpregnant women to prevent cyst formation. They would be contraindicated in pregnancy.

Laparoscopy (**choice C**) and laparotomy (**choice D**) are too invasive to be used for a relatively small, simple cyst that is likely a corpus luteum cyst in an asymptomatic patient in the first trimester. If the patient were having significant symptoms or there were evidence of torsion, hemorrhage, or malignancy, then operative intervention might be warranted.

Termination of the pregnancy (**choice E**) would not be an appropriate next step in management. This is a desired pregnancy in a patient with a simple cyst in the first trimester. The cyst is most likely benign and will not cause significant complications during the pregnancy.

11. **The correct answer is C.** This patient has uterine prolapse, which is believed to result from damage to pelvic fascia, muscles, and ligaments during childbirth. Prolapse is more common among Caucasian woman than among other ethnic groups. Patients with uterine prolapse will often complain of a bulge from the vagina or of pelvic pain or pressure. Some patients also may have urinary or sexual complaints. On examination, the uterus will be found to be prolapsing toward or through the introitus. The management is either with a pessary (a Lucite or rubber structure used to support pelvic organs) or with surgery (hysterectomy). This patient, with her numerous medical problems, represents a significant surgical and anesthesia risk. Therefore, a nonsurgical approach (the pessary) should be attempted first.

The oral contraceptive pill (OCP; **choice A**) or hormone replacement therapy (HRT; **choice B**) would not be appropriate treatment. Uterine prolapse is essentially a mechanical problem that requires a mechanical solution (i.e., pessary or surgery). The OCP or HRT would not address this problem. Also, there is accumulating evidence that shows that hormones increase the risk of thrombosis. This patient, with her history of coronary artery disease and recent stroke, would not represent a good candidate for hormone therapy.

Vaginal hysterectomy (**choice D**) or abdominal hysterectomy (**choice E**) would not be the most appropriate next step in the management of this patient. Uterine prolapse can be treated with a pessary or with surgery. This patient has numerous medical problems, placing her at increased surgical risk; therefore, the pessary should be attempted first.

12. **The correct answer is A.** There is a well-established association between black race and the presence of fibroids. Numerous studies quote a relative risk between 1.5 and 3.5. The exact mechanism underlying this increased risk has not been proven.

Cigarette smoking (**choice B**) is associated with a decreased incidence of leiomyomas. One possible explanation for this is that cigarette smoking increases the concentrations of sex-hormone-binding globulin, thereby lowering levels of bioavailable estrogen. Elevated estrogen concentrations, as are seen in pregnancy, obesity, and certain tumors, are known to increase the incidence of fibroids.

A history of gonorrhea (**choice C**) does not place this patient at greater risk for having fibroids. *Neisseria gonorrhoeae* is known to cause cervicitis and contribute to pelvic inflammatory disease, but it is not implicated in the pathophysiology of fibroids.

Low body mass index (**choice D**) is associated with a decreased risk of fibroids. Again, obese women are more likely to have fibroids, and the likely mechanism for this is an increase in bioavailable estrogens.

Multiparity (**choice E**) is associated with a decreased risk of fibroids. The exact mechanism underlying this association is unknown.

13. **The correct answer is A.** Condyloma acuminata is caused by the human papillomavirus. It is believed to be a sexually transmitted disease that is transmitted when viral particles come into contact with the female genitalia or surrounding skin. The lesions tend to occur at the sites most affected by coitus, namely the posterior fourchette and lateral vulva. The smaller lesions appear to be warts, whereas the larger lesions are verrucous or cauliflower-like. Diagnosis is based on the appearance of the lesion or by biopsy. Treatment is through local destruction with laser, cryotherapy, trichloroacetic acid, podophyllin, excision, or immunomodulators, such as imiquimod.

Condylomata lata (**choice B**) is a manifestation of secondary syphilis. These lesions are elevated areas and moist grayish patches that occasionally cause ulceration. This patient has a negative RPR; therefore, her lesions do not represent condylomata lata.

Herpes genitalis (**choice C**) is characterized by painful vesicles and ulcers. This patient has raised warts and verrucous lesions.

Molluscum contagiosum (**choice D**) is characterized by numerous, small, dome-shaped papules with a smooth surface and, sometimes, an umbilicated center. These lesions are occasionally pruritic. Molluscum contagiosum usually occurs in patients who are immunosuppressed secondary to HIV or to immunosuppressive medications.

Syphilis (**choice E**) can present with many different manifestations. Primary syphilis is characterized by a chancre, which is a painless ulcer. Secondary syphilis may be characterized by condylomata lata as described above. However, this patient has a negative RPR, which makes syphilis very unlikely.

14. **The correct answer is A.** Alcohol consumption during pregnancy is a major cause of significant fetal birth defects. Alcohol is known to cause fetal alcohol syndrome (FAS). FAS is characterized by growth retardation both before and after birth, facial anomalies, and CNS dysfunction. FAS is the most commonly recognized cause of mental retardation. It is usually seen in the children of women who drink more than 3 ounces of alcohol per day during pregnancy. Lesser amounts of alcohol are associated with fetal alcohol effects. These effects include minor anomalies, growth deficiency, mental defects, and behavior abnormalities. Alcohol is also associated with an increased risk of perinatal death and low intelligence quotient scores. Although most studies have focused on daily or consistent alcohol intake, occasional binge drinking also likely represents a significant threat to the fetus. There is no safe level for maternal drinking during pregnancy.

Two drinks per day (**choice B**), 2 ounces per day (**choice C**), 4 drinks per day (**choice D**), and 4 ounces per day (**choice E**) are not considered to be safe levels of alcohol consumption. The occasional drink during pregnancy has not been proven to be unsafe, but no degree of alcohol intake has been proven to be safe. Alcohol intake of 2-4 drinks/day or 2-4 ounces/day would certainly be considered unsafe in pregnancy.

15. **The correct answer is D.** This patient most likely has primary dysmenorrhea, which is painful menstruation without any demonstrable pelvic disease. The relationship between prostaglandins and primary dysmenorrhea is now reasonably well established. Prostaglandin $F_{2\alpha}$ and prostaglandin E_2 are released from endometrial cells, as these cells undergo lysis at the time of menstruation. These prostaglandins then induce uterine smooth muscle contractions that are the cause of the cramping pain of primary dysmenorrhea. Prostaglandins can cause smooth muscle contraction in other tissues as well, such as bowel—which is how dysmenorrhea can be associated with diarrhea. The treatment for primary dysmenorrhea is with nonsteroidal anti-inflammatory drugs (NSAIDs) or oral contraceptive pills (OCPs).

Endotoxin (**choice A**) is a lipopolysaccharide that is released when the cell wall of gram-negative bacteria is lysed. It is implicated in the pathophysiology of septic shock. There is no known association between endotoxin and primary dysmenorrhea.

Nonsteroidal anti-inflammatory drugs (NSAIDs) (**choice B**) are a first-line treatment for primary dysmenorrhea. As described above, prostaglandins are believed to play a central role in the pathophysiology of primary dysmenorrhea. NSAIDs block the formation of prostaglandins and therefore help to relieve the pain.

Prolactin (**choice C**) is a protein hormone that is synthesized and secreted by lactotrophs of the anterior pituitary. Initiating and maintaining lactation is the primary function of prolactin, but there is a significant amount of evidence showing that prolactin plays a role in numerous processes of the reproductive system and other systems. There is no proven link between prolactin and the pathophysiology of primary dysmenorrhea.

Thyroid stimulating hormone (TSH; **choice E**) is produced by thyrotrophs of the anterior pituitary. TSH acts on the thyroid gland itself, regulating thyroid iodine metabolism and the release of thyroid hormones. There has been no demonstrated link between TSH and primary dysmenorrhea.

16. **The correct answer is C.** This patient has a presentation that is most consistent with the supine hypotensive syndrome of pregnancy. In late gestation, if a woman lies flat on her back, the gravid uterus can compress the inferior vena cava. This decreases cardiac return to the heart and thus decreases cardiac output. The most common symptom is lightheadedness. A small minority of patients may even experience fainting. The gravid uterus can also compress the aorta, resulting in hypotension in the arteries distal to the compression. The management of this supine hypotensive syndrome is to make sure that the patient does not have underlying cardiac, pulmonary, or neurologic disease and then to recommend that she stay on her side, in the left lateral position, when lying down.

Atrial fibrillation (**choice A**) can also cause a feeling of lightheadedness. However, this patient experiences these symptoms only when lying down, and they promptly resolve when sitting or standing. Also, she has no complaints of heart palpitations, which patients with atrial fibrillation will often have.

Fetal movement (**choice B**) can cause the mother to experience a variety of symptoms. Women sometimes perceive fetal movement as contractions or abdominal pain. Fetal movement does not usually cause lightheadedness, and this patient has a presentation classic for supine hypotension syndrome.

Pulmonary embolus (**choice D**) is a concern during pregnancy because of the relative "hypercoagulability" of pregnancy. Pulmonary embolus often presents with chest pain, palpitations, tachycardia, tachypnea, and cough or chest pressure. This patient has none of these complaints and has symptoms that promptly resolve with a change in position.

Ventricular tachycardia (**choice E**) is not very common in otherwise healthy young pregnant women with no history of heart disease. It may present with lightheadedness, but again, this patient's history is much more consistent with supine hypotension syndrome.

17. **The correct answer is A.** This patient presents with a history that is most consistent with carpal tunnel syndrome. The carpal tunnel runs along the underside of the wrist. Through this "tunnel" run the median nerve and flexor tendons. In pregnancy, the size of the carpal tunnel is reduced secondary to weight gain and edema. With this reduction in size, there is an increased likelihood of compression of the median nerve, resulting in pain, numbness, or tingling in the distribution of the nerve. This distribution includes the thumb, index, and middle fingers and the palmar surface of the radial side of the ring finger. Treatment is with a wrist splint to keep the wrist in neutral position. In severe cases, surgical decompression may be necessary.

Cerebrovascular accident (**choice B**) usually does not present with symptoms along only one nerve and with a normal neurologic examination. This condition is also very unlikely in a young, pregnant patient.

Malingering (**choice C**) should never be assumed as a principal diagnosis. This patient has findings consistent with carpal tunnel syndrome.

Seizure disorders (**choice D**) are highly unlikely to present with pain and tingling along the distribution of the median nerve.

A wrist fracture (**choice E**) could cause pain and tingling in the hand. However, this patient has no history of trauma to the wrist, and a more likely diagnosis is carpal tunnel syndrome.

18. **The correct answer is C.** Migraine headache describes a severe headache that is often unilateral and can cause nausea, vomiting, and visual scotomata, among other neurologic findings. Migraine headache is a common problem in women of childbearing age. Therefore, issues surrounding migraine headache and its management come up often during the care of pregnant women. Approximately two-thirds of migraine sufferers will report improvement of their symptoms during pregnancy.

To state that acetaminophen cannot be used in pregnancy (**choice A**) is incorrect. Acetaminophen is widely used in pregnancy and believed to be safe.

Ergot-derived medications (**choice B**) cause vasoconstriction, and there is concern that these medications are harmful to the fetus.

As with most medications during pregnancy, it is better to limit the use of narcotics or not use them at all, if possible. However, in cases where pain relief is needed, such as for migraine headache or nephrolithiasis, narcotics can and should be used (compare with **choice D**).

19. **The correct answer is E.** When asking screening questions for alcohol and drug dependence, it is important not to ask judgmental questions. "Have you ever tried to stop this harmful behavior that is hurting your baby?" is clearly a judgmental question that places the patient on the defensive. This type of question is most likely to create confrontation. Drinking is described as "harmful behavior" and the woman is told that she is "hurting" her baby. The implication in the question is that the mother is a "bad mother" for doing something injurious to her baby.

The CAGE questionnaire is a four-question screening test to detect problem drinking. The questions are as follows: Have you ever felt the need to cut down on your drinking? (**choice C**); have you ever been annoyed by criticism of your drinking? (**choice A**); have you ever felt guilty about your drinking? (**choice B**); and have you ever had a morning drink to get started? (**choice D**). One positive response to these questions is a cause for concern. Two positive responses indicate that a problem is likely. Any patient who needs an drink to get started in the morning is much more likely to have alcohol dependence. This screening test allows the physician to determine which patients will need alcohol counseling and other interventions to prevent or stop problem drinking.

20. **The correct answer is C.** The diaphragm is a barrier form of contraception. It is a dome made of rubber or latex that covers the cervix when placed correctly. Correct placement means that the most posterior portion is placed into the posterior vaginal fornix and the most anterior portion lies immediately below the urethra in close proximity to the pubic symphysis. It should be used in conjunction with a spermicidal lubricant. The lubricant should be placed along the surface of the diaphragm that is closest to the cervix. The diaphragm should be placed prior to the first episode of intercourse. If a second coital episode takes place, then additional spermicide should be used. After intercourse, the diaphragm should be left in for 6 hours to allow for complete immobilization of sperm. The diaphragm should be taken out in 6 hours or, at most, the next morning so as to avoid the risk of toxic shock syndrome, which has been described following the use of the diaphragm. The diaphragm is a form of contraception that requires a highly motivated patient. With

correct use, it is roughly 98% effective at preventing pregnancy. In addition, the diaphragm must be fitted correctly to work properly. Sizes range from 60 to 105 mm, but most woman fall into the 70 to 80 mm range. The main side effect is bladder irritation with the risk of developing cystitis.

The diaphragm should not be removed immediately after intercourse (**choice A**) or 1 hour after intercourse (**choice B**). It should be left in for 6 hours to ensure that the sperm are completely immobilized. Removing the diaphragm too soon after intercourse runs the risk of allowing still viable sperm to reach the cervix, continue up the female reproductive tract, and fertilize the ovum.

The diaphragm should not be removed 12 hours (**choice D**) or 24 hours (**choice E**) after intercourse. Leaving the diaphragm in this long increases the risk of infection, particularly bladder infections and possibly toxic shock syndrome. Toxic shock syndrome is typically associated with tampon use and toxins produced by *Staphylococcus aureus*; however, there have been reports associating toxic shock syndrome with extended placement of the diaphragm.

21. **The correct answer is B.** Cesarean section is by far the most significant risk factor for the development of postpartum endometritis. Patients undergoing cesarean section have several times the risk for developing endometritis compared with patients having a vaginal delivery. Other patients who have an increased risk are those with prolonged rupture of membranes, long labors, multiple vaginal examinations, internal fetal monitoring, and low socioeconomic status. The use of prophylactic antibiotics (cefazolin, clindamycin-gentamicin, or metronidazole) at the time of cord clamping significantly decreases the risk of developing endometritis.

Anemia (**choice A**), although often cited as a risk factor for the development of endometritis, has not been proven to be associated with it. If there is any increased risk, it is significantly less than that posed by cesarean section.

External fetal monitoring (**choice C**) does not place the patient at risk for developing endometritis. Internal fetal monitoring with a scalp electrode does increase the risk.

Intact membranes (**choice D**) do not place the patient at risk for developing endometritis. Having ruptured membranes for an extended period of time is what places the patient at risk for endometritis, especially when cesarean section is the eventual mode of delivery.

Socioeconomic status (**choice E**) has been shown to be associated with the development of endometritis. Patients of low socioeconomic status are more likely to develop postpartum endometritis compared with their counterparts of higher socioeconomic status. However, cesarean section would be the factor that places this patient at greatest risk compared with socioeconomic status.

22. **The correct answer is B.** Spontaneous abortion (what is commonly called miscarriage by the lay population) is a common event. Approximately 10% to 20% of all clinically recognized pregnancies end in spontaneous abortion. If one includes chemical pregnancies (i.e., pregnancies in which a fertilization event takes place and there is an increase in the serum hCG level in the woman), the spontaneous loss rate is probably greater than 50%. However, although it may be a common event, it can still be an emotionally difficult time for a woman and a couple. Therefore, comfort and reassurance must be the first steps in dealing with the patient. In terms of investigating the reasons behind the spontaneous abortion, the current recommendation is that investigation be performed on couples after two consecutive first-trimester miscarriages. This investigation includes an evaluation of the parental chromosomes and the uterine cavity, and screening for diabetes, lupus, thyroid disease, autoimmune antibodies, and infection.

Because the background spontaneous abortion rate is so high, to investigate every couple after their first first-trimester miscarriage (**choice A**) would lead to a costly and invasive evaluation being done on a large number of couples who do not have a problem.

Investigation initiated after three consecutive first-trimester miscarriages (**choice C**) had formerly been the accepted practice, but is no longer the case.

To state that investigation is initiated after four consecutive first-trimester miscarriages (**choice D**) is incorrect.

To state that there is no need to investigate recurrent miscarriages (**choice E**) is incorrect. The investigation of recurrent spontaneous abortions can lead to the discovery of a treatable condition in the patient. For example, an infection can be treated, as can certain uterine anomalies.

23. **The correct answer is B.** In the correctly selected patient, the intrauterine device (IUD) is an excellent method of birth control. One of the major positive characteristics of the IUD is that it is easy for the patient to use. There is no pill to take daily, as with the oral contraceptive pill. There are no regular injections, as with intramuscular depot medroxyprogesterone acetate. And, there is no need to remember the method with each act of sexual intercourse, as with condoms, spermicides, and the diaphragm. One of the disadvantages often cited is that there is a higher rate of ectopic pregnancy associated with the use of the IUD compared with other birth

control methods. However, the risk of ectopic pregnancy in IUD users is significantly less than in patients using no birth control. This is because the overall number of pregnancies is so much lower in patients using the IUD.

Amenorrhea (**choice A**) is not considered to be a side effect of the IUD. Amenorrhea is commonly seen in patients on depot medroxyprogesterone acetate after 1 year of use. Amenorrhea also occurs in patients on the oral contraceptive pill for extended periods of time. Menorrhagia is more common with the IUD.

Intrauterine pregnancy (**choice C**) is less likely with the IUD than with several other types of birth control. One reason is that the rates of pregnancy with perfect use of the IUD are equivalent to the rates with actual use. This is not the case with many other methods. For example, patients often forget to take their birth control pills every day or they do not use condoms every time they have sexual intercourse.

Venous thromboembolism (**choice D**) is a complication of the oral contraceptive pill, not the IUD.

Weight gain (**choice E**) is a side effect of depot medroxyprogesterone acetate, not the IUD.

24. **The correct answer is C.** This patient has symptoms that are most consistent with premenstrual dysmorphic disorder (PMDD). PMDD is characterized by psychological and somatic symptoms that develop in the luteal phase of the menstrual cycle and resolve with menses. These symptoms must be separate from a preexisting psychiatric disorder, and a thorough assessment should be made to identify any underlying psychiatric disorders prior to diagnosing PMDD. The psychological symptoms may include depression, hopelessness, anxiety, mood lability, anger, irritability, lethargy, difficulty concentrating, and appetite and sleep changes. The physical symptoms may include breast tenderness and swelling, headaches, joint and muscle pain, and weight gain. Treatment can involve lifestyle changes or psychotherapy, although fluoxetine and other serotonin-specific reuptake inhibitors (SSRIs) are considered more effective.

Endometriosis (**choice A**) can present with symptoms around the menses. However, these symptoms are typically pelvic pain, dyspareunia, and dyschezia. This patient has psychological and somatic complaints that are much more consistent with PMDD.

Manic-depressive disorder (**choice B**) is characterized by episodes of intense mood elevation with grandiosity, pressured speech, and reckless behavior and depression. This patient's symptoms are confined to the luteal phase and not characterized by mood elevations.

Recurrent situational anxiety of pregnancy (**choice D**) is the diagnosis given to some women who desire permanent sterilization. This patient has no complaints regarding pregnancy.

Schizophrenia (**choice E**) is characterized by psychotic behavior, which this patient does not exhibit.

25. **The correct answer is D.** Depot medroxyprogesterone acetate (DMPA) is an injectable contraceptive given intramuscularly every 3 months. It is a synthetic progestin that provides contraception by inhibiting ovulation and creating an inhospitable environment in the female genital tract for conception (e.g., thickened cervical mucus). The most common side effects are menstrual abnormalities. Irregular bleeding patterns, including spotting, occur frequently in the first few months of use. Amenorrhea is also frequent and increases in incidence as the duration of therapy increases. Another major side effect of DMPA is weight gain, with the average user experiencing gains of approximately 3-5 pounds. Other adverse effects may include headache, decreased libido, tiredness, depression, and hair loss. Women should be counseled regarding these effects prior to starting this contraception.

DMPA does not cause an elevation of circulating estrogen levels (**choice A**). On the contrary, DMPA has been shown to cause decreased circulating estrogen levels. These decreased levels are believed to result from the central hypothalamic suppression that DMPA causes, which decreases ovarian activation and estrogen production.

DMPA does not cause increased bone density (**choice B**). In fact, DMPA has been shown to lead to decreased bone density over time, likely secondary to the decreased estrogen levels. However, this decreased bone density on DMPA has not yet been proven to lead to an increased rate of fractures.

DMPA does not cause increased HDL cholesterol (**choice C**), but rather has been shown to decrease HDL (or "healthy") cholesterol levels.

DMPA is less likely to lead to pregnancy (**choice E**) compared with many other forms of contraception. Administration of 150 mg every 3 months has been shown to prevent pregnancy very effectively, with pregnancy rates approximately 0.3 per 100 women per year.

26. **The correct answer is B.** Antibiotic prophylaxis is important for certain operations in obstetrics and gynecology. Vaginal hysterectomy is one gynecologic procedure for which prophylactic antibiotics have been proven to be of benefit in the prevention of infection. The goal of antibiotic prophylaxis in a vaginal hysterectomy is to have the antibiotics present in the tissue prior to the opening of the vaginal cuff, because vaginal organisms can gain entrance to the peritoneal cavity at that point. When

antibiotics are administered 30 minutes prior to surgery, there is sufficient time for the antibiotics to reach the appropriate tissues and provide prophylaxis.

No medications are needed (**choice A**) during many procedures. However, during vaginal hysterectomy, the risk of infection is increased compared with certain other procedures because there are numerous bacteria within the vagina that are not completely eradicated, even with an aggressive vaginal preparation prior to surgery.

A beta blocker 30 minutes prior to surgery (**choice C**) would not be indicated in this patient. First, she has no cardiac history. Second, she has asthma; therefore, beta blockers would not be recommended.

Antibiotics prior to closing (**choice D**) are not routinely indicated. In certain cases (e.g., a long operative time), a second dose of antibiotics should be given. Typically, however, one preoperative dose of antibiotics is sufficient.

Antibiotics 6 hours after the surgery (**choice E**) would not be indicated. A postoperative antibiotic dose is sometimes needed for endocarditis prophylaxis in patients with valvular disease. This patient has no cardiac disease.

27. **The correct answer is B.** The clinical diagnosis is fibroadenoma, which is seen in this age group with exactly the findings described. Fibroadenomas can be diagnosed with fine needle aspiration, which was not offered as a choice, or with ultrasonography. On confirmation of the diagnosis, the woman has the option for excision or continued clinical observation. Most women elect to have the mass removed, but it should be their choice.

Clinical observation (**choice A**) is fine, once we know the lesion is a fibroadenoma. Otherwise, when the rare case of cancer comes along in this age group (yes, it can happen), diagnostic and therapeutic delays would be inexcusable.

If a mammogram (**choice C**) were ordered, the physicians in the radiology department would have a good laugh. They do not perform mammograms in women younger than 20. The breast tissue is too dense in this population, and the study is not useful. Ultrasonography is a better option.

Incisional biopsy (**choice D**) would be too aggressive to make the diagnosis and not complete enough to actually serve as treatment. If one elects a surgical approach for a 2-cm mass, one should take it all out.

Excisional biopsy (**choice E**) would be better than incisional biopsy, but it would be an even more aggressive way to confirm the clinical diagnosis and would not allow the patient the choice of therapy.

28. **The correct answer is B.** When an ectopic pregnancy ruptures, there is often a significant amount of bleeding into the peritoneum. When a hemoperitoneum occurs, the blood can track upward and irritate the diaphragm. This diaphragmatic irritation is perceived by the patient as shoulder pain because of the phenomenon of referred pain. Referred pain describes the process by which pain in one area of the body is perceived as pain somewhere else (or referred to somewhere else) because of the nerve pathways that innervate the body. The same phenomenon is seen in myocardial infarction; patients often complain of jaw or arm pain. Thus, in a patient who is at risk for ectopic pregnancy, the complaint of shoulder pain may signal that the ectopic pregnancy has already ruptured and there is enough of a hemoperitoneum to cause diaphragmatic irritation. This patient has an hCG of 5,500 mIU/dL, nothing in the uterus on ultrasound (a pregnancy should be seen at an hCG of approximately 1,500 mIU/dL), and significant free fluid (likely blood). She therefore almost certainly has an ectopic pregnancy, and the shoulder pain is caused from diaphragmatic irritation.

A diaphragmatic ectopic pregnancy (**choice A**) is extraordinarily rare, if not impossible. Irritation from blood along the diaphragm causes referred pain to the shoulder—the presence of the ectopic on the diaphragm is not necessary.

Malingering (**choice C**) should never be assumed until all other possibilities have been explored. The complaint of shoulder pain may, at first glance, seem odd. However, when one understands the phenomenon of referred pain it makes sense, and the patient is not incorrectly labeled a malingerer.

A rotator cuff tear (**choice D**) can certainly cause shoulder pain. However, it is unlikely that this patient suddenly tore her rotator cuff halfway through the examination. Much more likely is that diaphragmatic irritation is causing her shoulder pain.

29. **The correct answer is B.** This patient has a presentation that is classic for endometriosis. Endometriosis is a condition in which implants of endometrial glands and stroma are found outside of their normal location within the endometrial lining of the uterine cavity. In endometriosis, these implants are often found along several sites in the pelvis, including the anterior and posterior cul-de-sac, the tubes and ovaries, and the pelvic sidewalls bilaterally. Endometriotic implants have also been found in the lung and kidney. The classic triad of findings in endometriosis is dysmenorrhea, dyspareunia, and dyschezia (painful defecation). Definitive diagnosis is made with laparoscopy and biopsy of the lesions. At laparoscopy, the lesions can have a number of appearances, including powder-burn lesions, red and blue lesions, fibrotic lesions, or cystic lesions. There is a strong association between endometriosis and infertility.

There is no proven association between endometriosis and basal cell carcinoma (**choice A**).

Patients with endometriosis do not tend to have lengthy menstrual cycles (**choice C**). In fact, many patients with endometriosis have short menstrual cycles (<28 days).

There is no proven association between endometriosis and lung cancer (**choice D**).

Patients with endometriosis typically do not have menorrhagia (**choice E**). In fact, patients with endometriosis tend to have a lighter menstrual flow than do women without the condition.

30. **The correct answer is B.** Approximately 20% to 25% of women will have first-trimester bleeding, and the chief concern is with ectopic pregnancy and spontaneous abortion. Of those women, about 50% will go on to have a spontaneous abortion (miscarriage). However, once fetal cardiac activity is seen, the risk of spontaneous abortion is around 10%. This patient has fetal cardiac activity and a normal exam and ultrasound. Therefore, she should be counseled that her risk of miscarriage is approximately 10%.

To state that there is no risk of miscarriage (**choice A**) would not be correct. This is never appropriate counseling because in any pregnancy there is a risk of miscarriage, no matter how normal or healthy the pregnancy may seem.

To state that there is an approximately 50% (**choice C**) or 75% (**choice D**) risk of miscarriage would be incorrect. As stated above, the risk of miscarriage with vaginal bleeding in the first trimester when fetal cardiac activity is present is approximately 10%.

To state that miscarriage is almost certain (**choice E**) would not be correct.

31. **The correct answer is B.** Sickle cell anemia results when a person has two copies of the sickle gene. This gene is on chromosome 11 and represents a mutation of the normal beta hemoglobin gene. The gene that codes for sickle hemoglobin has a single base pair substitution that results in coding for the amino acid valine rather than the glutamic acid, which is present in the normal beta globin chain. This amino acid substitution results in a hemoglobin that is susceptible to sickling at times of stress, infection, or decreased oxygen tension. These patients have sickle crises, which are acute, painful episodes believed to be associated with sickling in the microcirculation. They also may have increased susceptibility to infection, leg ulcers, autosplenectomy, thromboses, and cerebrovascular accidents. The disease is transmitted in an autosomal recessive fashion and is most common among persons of African descent. This patient has the sickle trait and so does her partner. Therefore, the child has a 25% chance

of being born with sickle cell anemia. This disease will not affect the fetus in utero; fetal hemoglobin, which does not have a beta globin chain, is the primary hemoglobin type in the fetus. However, because of the risk of sickle cell anemia, some patients wish to have genetic testing performed.

Chance of 0% (**choice A**) is incorrect. With a disease that is transmitted in an autosomal recessive fashion, when both parents have the trait, they have a 25% chance of having offspring affected with the disease. If one parent does not have the trait, then the chance of having offspring with the disease would be 0%.

Chance of 50% (**choice C**) is incorrect. This couple has a 50% chance of having a fetus with sickle trait—that is, one normal copy of the beta-hemoglobin gene and one copy for sickle hemoglobin—but only a 25% chance of having a child with sickle disease.

Chance of 75% (**choice D**) is incorrect for the above-given reasons.

Chance of 100% (**choice E**) is incorrect. With an autosomal recessive disease, only if both partners have the disease is the likelihood 100% that the offspring will have the disease.

32. **The correct answer is A.** Exposure to radiation, particularly in the form of an x-ray, is a major cause of anxiety for pregnant patients. There is a generally held belief that exposure to any radiation during pregnancy will lead to miscarriage or birth defects. There is no evidence, however, of any increase in spontaneous abortion or fetal anomalies at doses of radiation less than 5 rad. This dose is above the level of radiation exposure of diagnostic procedures. The fetal exposure from a chest x-ray with 2 views is approximately 0.05 mrad. This amount is several orders of magnitude below the 5 rad limit. Therefore, it is currently believed that x-ray exposure from any single diagnostic procedure will not cause harm to the fetus. This patient has signs and symptoms consistent with pneumonia and could therefore benefit from a chest x-ray. She should be reassured that the exposure to the fetus from a chest x-ray is minimal and has not been shown to cause birth defects or fetal loss.

A chest x-ray exposes the fetus to minute amount of radiation compared with the amount needed to cause birth defects (**choice B**).

There is no evidence that the exposure of 0.02 to 0.07 mrad of radiation caused by a chest x-ray leads to spontaneous abortion (**choice C**).

To state that when a chest x-ray has occurred, fetal pneumonia is more common (**choice D**) is incorrect. The presence or absence of a fetal infection is not dependent on a chest x-ray being performed to evaluate for maternal pneumonia.

To state that when a chest x-ray has occurred, termination should be considered (**choice E**) is incorrect. Exposure to x-ray during pregnancy is not an indication for therapeutic abortion.

33. **The correct answer is E.** This patient has signs and symptoms that are suggestive of pulmonary embolism (PE). The most common presenting symptom for PE is shortness of breath, followed by pleuritic chest pain, apprehension, and cough. This patient has shortness of breath and pleuritic chest pain. On physical examination, tachypnea and tachycardia are the most common findings. This patient has tachycardia on the ECG, but has no tachypnea. Given her complaints, her tachycardia, the increased likelihood of PE in pregnancy, and the catastrophic outcome that can result from an undiagnosed PE, doing a ventilation-perfusion ($\dot{V}/\dot{Q}$) scan makes sense in this patient. Many patients are reluctant to undergo a $\dot{V}/\dot{Q}$ scan during pregnancy because they are concerned about radiation exposure of the fetus. These patients should be reassured that a $\dot{V}/\dot{Q}$ scan leads to approximately 50 mrad of radiation exposure to the fetus. Exposure to less than 5,000 mrad total during pregnancy is not associated with spontaneous abortion or fetal anomalies. Since the radionucleotides used during the scan collect in the urine, the patient should empty her bladder immediately after the scan or consider having a Foley catheter inserted to facilitate rapid evacuation of the bladder. It should be noted that the sensitivity and specificity of $\dot{V}/\dot{Q}$ scans drop considerably if the patient's x-ray is abnormal.

CT angiography of the chest is also used to diagnose pulmonary embolus. Although this test also subjects both mother and fetus to radiation, CT allows greater diagnostic accuracy and can result in discovery of other unsuspected causes of pain (aortic dissection, pulmonary infiltrate, etc). The use of CT angiography in pregnant patients is still evolving.

Antibiotic therapy (**choice A**) is not indicated in this patient. Although she does have dyspnea and tachycardia, she has no fever or chest x-ray findings consistent with pneumonia.

Warfarin therapy (**choice B**) is contraindicated during pregnancy. In the first trimester, warfarin can lead to chondrodysplasia punctata, which includes nasal hypoplasia, bony abnormalities, and mental retardation. In the second and third trimesters, it can also lead to fetal structural abnormalities and clotting difficulties.

Heparin therapy (**choice C**) can be used during pregnancy. In this case, however, it is important to first diagnose PE prior to instituting heparin therapy.

Pulmonary ultrasonography (**choice D**) is not used to evaluate for PE.

34. **The correct answer is B.** Patients who are diagnosed with gestational diabetes are known to be at increased risk for the eventual development of overt diabetes. In fact, there is an approximately 50% likelihood that a woman with gestational diabetes will develop overt diabetes within the next 20 years. Therefore, women with gestational diabetes should be screened postpartum to determine whether they have diabetes so that prompt intervention can be initiated.

To state that no postpartum follow-up is necessary (**choice A**) is incorrect. One of the benefits of screening for gestational diabetes in pregnancy is to identify women who may eventually develop overt diabetes.

To start either oral hypoglycemics (**choice C**) or subcutaneous insulin (**choice D**) at the 6-week postpartum visit would be incorrect. This patient may not have diabetes and may never develop diabetes. To start her on oral hypoglycemics or subcutaneous insulin on the basis of her gestational diabetes would therefore not be proper. She should, however, be screened for diabetes at the 6-week postpartum visit.

To refer the patient for pancreatic transplantation after her 6-week postpartum visit (**choice E**) would not be correct management.

35. **The correct answer is D.** This patient presents with signs and symptoms most consistent with imperforate hymen. With an imperforate hymen, there is no egress for the monthly menstrual flow. Therefore, the patient will often complain of monthly cramping. Because there is no hormonal abnormality, the patient will have normal breast development as well as axillary and pubic hair. Pelvic examination will sometimes show a bulge as the monthly menstrual flow accumulates in the vagina. Rectal examination may reveal an anterior bulge, as the accumulation in the vagina can be palpated through the rectum. Management is with hymenectomy to allow for the egress of the monthly menstrual flow.

Colon cancer (**choice A**) is unlikely in an otherwise healthy 14-year-old, and this patient's signs and symptoms are more consistent with imperforate hymen.

Ectopic pregnancy (**choice B**) is extremely unlikely with a negative hCG. Ectopic pregnancies almost never present as a bulge in the vagina, as they are usually located in the fallopian tube.

Endometriosis (**choice C**) can present with monthly dysmenorrhea. However, this patient also has a bulge in the vagina, which is more consistent with imperforate hymen.

Vaginal cancer (**choice E**) is unlikely in an otherwise healthy 14-year-old. This patient has monthly dysmenorrhea and a bulge in the vagina, both of which are most consistent with imperforate hymen.

36. **The correct answer is E.** This patient has fibroids (leiomyomata). Fibroids are believed to be monoclonal tumors arising from uterine smooth muscle cells. Most often they are asymptomatic. When they are symptomatic, the symptoms include pain, pressure, urinary symptoms, or irregular uterine bleeding. This patient has significant menorrhagia causing her to have anemia to a hematocrit of 29%. She does not wish to have any more children; therefore, hysterectomy would be the most appropriate next step in management.

Hormone replacement therapy (HRT) (**choice A**) would not be appropriate for this patient. This patient is neither postmenopausal nor estrogen deficient, so HRT would not be indicated.

Diagnostic laparoscopy (**choice B**) would not be appropriate for this patient. This procedure is used for diagnosis in cases of acute or chronic pelvic pain or ectopic pregnancy. In this patient, the diagnosis is clear, given her findings on physical examination and ultrasound.

Myomectomy (**choice C**) can be used in the treatment of fibroids, but it is usually reserved for patients who wish to preserve their childbearing potential. Myomectomy is usually quite effective in removing the fibroids; however, 25% to 50% of patients will have a recurrence, and as many as 10% of patients will require a second operation. This patient does not wish to preserve her uterus; therefore, hysterectomy would be preferred over myomectomy.

Tubal ligation (**choice D**) would effectively address this patient's desire not to have any more children; however, it would not address her pelvic pressure and menorrhagia.

37. **The correct answer is D.** This patient has the signs and symptoms most consistent with a complete hydatidiform mole, which is one type of gestational trophoblastic disease. Other types include partial mole and choriocarcinoma. Patients with a complete mole often present with complaints of bleeding. Physical examination is typically significant for a uterus that is larger than the dates of the pregnancy would predict. Diagnosis is most often made by ultrasound, with the appearance of multiple echogenic areas. This pattern is usually described as a "snowstorm." Management of a complete mole is with dilation and evacuation. This effectively removes the molar tissue from the patient. These patients then need close follow-up, with the serum hCG level being followed to ensure that there is no persistent or metastatic molar tissue.

Expectant management (**choice A**) is not appropriate for a patient with a complete mole. These patients need therapy to prevent spread of the disease and/or

the development of preeclampsia, hyperthyroidism, or other metabolic abnormalities.

Folic acid supplementation (**choice B**) is not the next most appropriate step in management for someone with a complete mole. There is some evidence of a link between folic acid deficiency and complete mole. However, once a mole has been diagnosed, treatment is with dilation and evacuation.

Methotrexate therapy (**choice C**) can be used to treat a persistent or metastatic complete mole. However, the first step in management is with dilation and evacuation.

Laparotomy (**choice E**) is usually not necessary for the treatment of complete mole. Occasionally, some patients will elect or require hysterectomy for definitive treatment, but most cases can be treated with dilation and evacuation.

38. **The correct answer is D.** In an adolescent, many of the initial menstrual cycles will be anovulatory. Anovulatory cycles put the woman at greater risk for menorrhagia, as there is often an excess build-up and loss of synchronicity of the endometrium when compared with an ovulatory cycle. As long as the episode of bleeding is not too excessive or causing any hemodynamic compromise, the oral contraceptive pill (OCP) is appropriate treatment. However, one should not immediately assume that acute vaginal bleeding in an adolescent is due to an anovulatory cycle. It is most important to check an hCG to establish the patient's pregnancy status. History should focus on any bleeding disorder, history of trauma, or medications taken. This patient most likely has excessive bleeding from an anovulatory cycle. Her hematocrit is low (30%), and she still has some oozing; therefore, treatment is warranted. Treatment with the OCP should help to stabilize her endometrium and stop her bleeding.

Blood transfusion (**choice A**) would not be indicated in this patient. Blood transfusions should be reserved for patients with very low hematocrits and signs of hemodynamic compromise. This patient has a hematocrit of 30% and stable vital signs. The risks of blood transfusion (e.g., infection and transfusion reaction) outweigh any benefit to be gained in this case.

Fresh frozen plasma (**choice B**) is indicated in situations in which clotting factors are needed. This patient has a normal PT and PTT and no history of a bleeding disorder; therefore, fresh frozen plasma would not be indicated.

IV conjugated estrogens (**choice C**) is the correct management in cases of acute bleeding caused by anovulation when the hematocrit is very low or when there are signs of hemodynamic compromise. IV conjugated estrogens work at both the capillary level and the level of the endometrium to stop bleeding. This patient, with her stable vital signs and stable hematocrit, would not need IV conjugated estrogens.

Platelet transfusion (**choice E**) would not be the most appropriate next step in management, as this patient has a normal platelet count. She also has no history of a bleeding disorder to suggest that her platelets are functionally ineffective.

39. **The correct answer is A.** This patient has the constellation of signs and symptoms consistent with severe preeclampsia: hypertension, edema, and proteinuria. Her headache, visual changes, and epigastric pain indicate that her condition is severe and troublesome, because these symptoms often precede the development of convulsions (eclampsia). The management of severe preeclampsia is delivery of the fetus, as this is the only way the disease process will resolve. Magnesium sulfate should be started immediately and continued for 24 hours postpartum to prevent eclampsia.

Hepatitis (**choice B**) can present with epigastric or right upper quadrant pain. However, this patient has a variety of other signs and symptoms that make severe preeclampsia the diagnosis, and eclampsia the most immediate concern.

Migraine (**choice C**) can present with headache and visual changes. Again, however, this patient also has elevated blood pressure, edema, proteinuria, and epigastric pain. This constellation of symptoms is more consistent with preeclampsia than with migraine.

Myocardial infarction (**choice D**) occurs during pregnancy at a rate of less than 1 in 10,000. This would not be of most immediate concern in this patient.

Systemic lupus erythematosus (**choice E**) can present with hypertension and proteinuria. However, this patient has these findings as well as other signs and symptoms that make eclampsia a more immediate concern.

40. **The correct answer is A.** Women with type 1 diabetes mellitus are at increased risk of having offspring with congenital malformations. Various studies have shown that these fetuses are at a two- to sixfold increased risk compared with normal pregnancies. Anomalies commonly found in infants of diabetic mothers (IDM) include those of the cardiac, renal, and central nervous systems. Sacral agenesis, the most characteristic anomaly of diabetic embryopathy, is found 200-400 times more commonly in IDM. Most of these anomalies arise during the first 7 weeks of gestation as the fetal organs are forming. Women at this stage of pregnancy often do not yet know that they are pregnant. Therefore, it is essential that women with type 1 diabetes be counseled regarding fetal anomalies prior to conception. Good glycemic control prior to conception decreases the risk of spontaneous

abortions and congenital malformations and increases the likelihood of good pregnancy outcomes. Folic acid (4 mg/day) may help prevent neural tube defects in overt diabetics.

If women with type 1 diabetes are given management and counseling in the first trimester (**choice B**) regarding fetal anomalies, then it is likely that the window of opportunity to attain good glycemic control during organogenesis will be missed. Again, organ formation and development occur during the first 7 weeks of pregnancy. Many patients do not realize they are pregnant until after 7 weeks' gestation. Also, those who do present prior to 7 weeks may have difficulty in achieving good glycemic control in a short time span.

A woman with type 1 diabetes should have an ultrasound at around 18 weeks to evaluate for anomalies. However, waiting until just prior to (**choice C**) or after (**choice D**) an 18-week ultrasound or until the third trimester (**choice E**) is too late to counsel the patient regarding fetal anomalies.

41. **The correct answer is B.** This patient has a history that is most consistent with cervical incompetence, which is defined as painless cervical dilation in the second trimester. This definition is meant to distinguish cervical incompetence from preterm labor, in which there is progressive cervical dilation with painful contractions. In actual practice, many women present with a history of cervical dilation and some "cramping." In these cases, it can be difficult to determine whether the process was cervical incompetence or preterm labor. When a patient has a history of cervical incompetence, a cerclage may be placed. This cerclage is a suture that is placed at the level of the internal os (a Shirodkar cerclage) or a purse string suture that is placed as high as possible (a McDonald cerclage). The idea is that the suture will support the cervix and maintain its "competence." Timing of cerclage placement is important. There are two kinds of cerclages to consider when discussing timing. One is a prophylactic cerclage that is placed based on the woman's history. The second is an emergency cerclage that is placed based on findings of cervical dilation with bulging membranes. This patient would qualify for a prophylactic cerclage, as she is at 6 weeks' gestation. To place a cerclage immediately (**choice A**) runs the risk of performing a procedure on a patient who may have a spontaneous abortion. It is better to wait until the pregnancy is well established (e.g., late first or early second trimester, or 10-14 weeks) so that there is less likelihood of performing a cerclage on a woman who was going to miscarry anyway.

To wait until 20-24 weeks (**choice C**) would not be correct because this may be too late. The process of incompetence may be under way at this point in the pregnancy.

To wait until 24-28 weeks (**choice D**) or 32-36 weeks (**choice E**) would also be incorrect. Again, the process of incompetence may have already started. Also, performing a cerclage this late in the pregnancy runs the risk of iatrogenic prematurity by stimulating preterm labor or rupturing the membranes. A woman, regardless of her history, who makes it to 24 or 32 weeks has a good chance of not delivering prematurely. Cerclage placement carries the risks of ruptured membranes, infection, or preterm labor.

42. **The correct answer is C.** This patient is at increased risk for developing a postcesarean wound infection because of her obesity. The main risk factors are poor surgical technique, low socioeconomic status, extended duration of labor and ruptured membranes, chorioamnionitis, obesity, type 1 diabetes mellitus, immunodeficiency, corticosteroid therapy, and immunosuppressive therapy. Postcesarean wound infections are usually caused by staphylococci or streptococci. Treatment should be directed against gram-positive organisms, with nafcillin or vancomycin if the patient is allergic to penicillins.

This patient has a distant history of asthma (**choice A**) and she has taken no medications for many years. Thus, her asthma does not increase her risk for postcesarean wound infection. However, if she were to have more active asthma and had been taking steroids, this immunosuppression would place her at greater risk of wound infection.

Low socioeconomic status, not high socioeconomic status (**choice B**), is a risk factor for postcesarean wound infection.

Short duration of ruptured membranes (**choice D**) is not a risk factor for wound infection. When the membranes are ruptured for a long time, there is a greater risk for the development of both endometritis and wound infection.

Short operative time (**choice E**) is not a risk factor for wound infection. Certain studies have shown that long operative times make the patient more likely to develop postoperative infections.

43. **The correct answer is A.** One of the most serious complications of the oral contraceptive pill (OCP) is deep venous thrombosis (DVT). OCPs, particularly the estrogen component, are known to make some patients hypercoagulable. Patients who are especially at risk are those with an inherited resistance to activated protein C and those with the factor V Leiden mutation. However, even in patients without these traits, the OCP can lead to an increased risk of DVT, pulmonary embolus, and cerebral thrombosis. All patients who are started on an OCP should be warned and educated regarding the symptoms of a blood clot. If leg pain and swelling develop, the main concern is DVT, and that patient must be evaluated (e.g., with duplex Doppler studies).

To prescribe acetaminophen (**choice B**) over the phone without first evaluating the patient would not be appropriate. As noted above, DVT is a major concern in women taking the OCP with leg pain and swelling. Delay could lead to propagation of a thrombus, embolism, and even death.

To recommend warm soaks and evaluation in 1 week (**choice C**) would not be appropriate. Again, this patient may have a DVT, and delay in diagnosis and treatment could result in significant morbidity or mortality.

To schedule a pelvic ultrasound (**choice D**) would be improper management. Although this patient is a woman, her complaint is leg pain and swelling. The appropriate study would be ultrasound of the leg, or another study, to evaluate for the presence of a thrombus in the lower extremities.

Prescribing warfarin (**choice E**) would not be appropriate. The patient must be evaluated first to determine whether she has a DVT. If a thrombus is discovered, then anticoagulation would be appropriate.

44. **The correct answer is D.** A patient with a prior cesarean delivery is at increased risk of uterine rupture. When the prior uterine scar is from a classic cesarean delivery (i.e., a vertical uterine incision involving the upper, contractile portion of the uterus), the risk of uterine rupture with labor is approximately 12%. With such a high risk of uterine rupture, patients who have had a previous classic cesarean delivery are not allowed to have a VBAC (vaginal birth after cesarean). Vaginal birth is contraindicated. In contrast, patients with a prior low transverse uterine incision or low vertical uterine incision have a much lower rate of uterine rupture (around 1% to 2%); these patients are allowed a trial of labor.

To state that cesarean delivery is contraindicated (**choice A**) is incorrect. Cesarean delivery is, in fact, mandated in patients with a prior classic cesarean delivery, and it is vaginal delivery that is contraindicated.

To state that forceps-assisted vaginal delivery is recommended (**choice B**) or that vacuum-assisted vaginal delivery is recommended (**choice C**) is not correct. Vaginal delivery of any type is contraindicated in a woman with a prior classic cesarean delivery.

To state that vaginal birth is not contraindicated (**choice E**) is incorrect. As explained above, vaginal birth is contraindicated after a prior classic cesarean delivery.

45. **The correct answer is E.** Newborns delivered by cesarean have a higher rate of transient tachypnea compared with newborns delivered via vaginal delivery. One hypothesis for this finding is that vaginal delivery leads to compres-

sion of the fetal thorax and removal of pulmonary fluid, which can cause transient tachypnea of the newborn. Also, some would argue that other factors in the process of vaginal delivery better prepare the newborn for extra-uterine life from a pulmonary standpoint. Most of these cases resolve without serious sequelae.

Fracture of the fetal clavicle (**choice A**) and fracture of the fetal femur (**choice B**) can occur during a cesarean delivery but are more common with a vaginal delivery. However, when obtaining consent from a patient for cesarean delivery, it is important to inform her that there is a risk of injury to the baby. Many patients are under the mistaken assumption that cesarean delivery implies no risk whatsoever of injury.

Maternal perineal trauma (**choice C**) is far more likely to occur with a vaginal than with a cesarean delivery. An uncomplicated cesarean delivery should lead to no perineal trauma at all. Some physicians argue that because the perineal trauma that women experience with a vaginal delivery can lead to incontinence and pelvic organ prolapse in the future, women should be allowed to choose cesarean delivery as an elective procedure. However, this is not the standard of care for most practitioners or institutions.

Shoulder dystocia (**choice D**) is far more likely to occur with a vaginal delivery than with a cesarean delivery. However, there is still some risk of shoulder dystocia and fetal injury during a cesarean delivery.

46. **The correct answer is A.** This patient has two issues that must be addressed when considering a birth control option. The first is birth control. All of the options would address birth control, although the rhythm and withdrawal methods are not recommended because of their high failure rates. The second is prevention of sexually transmitted diseases (STDs). Of these options, only condoms can prevent the transmission of STDs. Along with the emphasis on condoms, this patient needs to be advised that her sexual behavior places her at risk for a number of STDs, including HIV, hepatitis B and C, herpes, *Chlamydia*, gonorrhea, syphilis, and trichomoniasis.

The intrauterine device (IUD; **choice B**) would be absolutely contraindicated in this patient. Her prior history of pelvic inflammatory disease (PID) and current sexual behavior place her at increased risk for contracting an STD. STDs (most notably *Chlamydia* and gonorrhea) in the setting of an IUD can lead to severe PID, sepsis, and even death.

The oral contraceptive pill (OCP; **choice C**) is an option for this patient. However, although use of the OCP will prevent pregnancy, it will do nothing to prevent STDs. Therefore, even if this patient does use the OCP, she must also use condoms.

The rhythm (**choice D**) and withdrawal (**choice E**) methods are both associated with high failure rates. The rhythm method relies on timing intercourse during the period of the woman's cycle in which ovulation is unlikely. The withdrawal method relies on the male partner withdrawing from the vagina prior to ejaculation. Both have prohibitively high failure rates and do not provide good protection from STDs.

47. **The correct answer is C.** This patient is considered to have an appropriate weight, with a BMI of 20.6. BMI is calculated by dividing the prepregnant weight in kilograms by the height in meters squared. Thus, with a BMI of 20.6, she is neither overweight nor underweight. In a patient of normal weight, pregnancy should be associated with a weight gain of 25-35 lb. This weight gain is composed of fetal weight, amniotic fluid, uterine growth, placenta, breast enlargement, volume expansion, and increased fat stores. Patients usually gain about 5-10 pounds in the first 20 weeks of pregnancy and then roughly 1 pound per week for the final 20 weeks, although a wide range of weight changes in pregnancy are still compatible with good maternal and fetal outcomes. Several studies, however, do show increased complications with weight gains that are at the extreme high or low ends.

A weight gain of 5-15 pounds (**choice A**) or 15-25 pounds (**choice B**) is considered less than recommended for a woman of normal body weight. Certain studies have shown that too low a weight gain is associated with low birthweight infants and preterm labor. However, for women who enter the pregnancy overweight (BMI of 26-29), the recommended gain is 15-25 pounds. For obese women (BMI greater than 29), the recommended gain is 15 pounds.

A weight gain of 35-45 pounds (**choice D**) or 45-55 pounds (**choice E**) is considered more than recommended for a woman of normal body weight. Excessive weight gain has been linked to large-for-gestational age infants and increased risk of cesarean delivery. However, for patients who enter the pregnancy underweight (BMI less than 19.8), the recommended gain is 28-40 pounds.

48. **The correct answer is A.** Methotrexate, an inhibitor of the enzyme dihydrofolate reductase, can be used in certain cases to treat ectopic pregnancy. This enzyme is essential for the eventual production of purine and pyrimidine subunits of nucleic acid. By blocking this enzyme, methotrexate destroys the rapidly dividing cells of the ectopic pregnancy. However, certain patients are not considered eligible for methotrexate treatment. Many physicians consider this therapy contraindicated if the ectopic pregnancy has a certain size (e.g., greater than 3.5 cm), has an elevated hCG value (e.g., greater

than 15,000 mIU/dL), or has cardiac activity. However, these criteria do vary depending on the institution and physician. Also, methotrexate can cause bone marrow depression as well as hepatotoxicity and nephrotoxicity. Therefore, patients with anemia, leukopenia, thrombocytopenia, elevated liver function tests, or elevated creatinine levels are also considered ineligible for methotrexate treatment. This patient has an elevated liver function test: her aspartate aminotransferase level is 110 U/L.

A blood pressure of 110/70 mm Hg (**choice B**), a creatinine of 0.7 mg/dL (**choice C**), a hematocrit of 40% (**choice D**), and a platelet count of 200,000/mm^3 (**choice E**) are all normal and would not constitute a contraindication to methotrexate treatment in this patient.

49. **The correct answer is A.** This patient, although she cannot remember having varicella, has evidence of prior infection and natural immunity. Most women who have no known history of varicella infection will have detectable antibodies. This patient's immunity will protect her fetus from infection, and no further treatment is needed.

Avoidance of possible infection (**choice B**) is a strategy for women without natural immunity. However, this patient has been shown to have immunity. In addition, this patient has a documented exposure. If she were without immunity, she would need to be treated with varicella zoster immunoglobulin in an effort to prevent infection or severe manifestations of infection.

The incubation of varicella ranges from 10 to 20 days, with a mean of 14 days. This patient's exposure does fall in the incubation stage, but she has documented immunity. Further immunologic testing (**choice C**) is not indicated.

Fetal infection is usually very severe and may lead to fetal death. Elective termination should be offered to those who have evidence of fetal infection. Fortunately, fetal infection is very rare, occurring in less than 5% of infected mothers. Fetal infection is likely to have the worst outcome in those affected earlier than 20 weeks' gestation. Ultrasound is used to look for signs of fetal infection, such as hydrops, microcephaly, limb anomalies, cardiac malformations, and intrauterine growth restriction. However, this mother has signs of immunity as discussed previously, and there is no risk of fetal infection. Termination of pregnancy (**choice D**) or an ultrasound (**choice E**) is not needed.

50. **The correct answer is B.** This patient has preterm labor. This diagnosis can be made on the basis of her regular contractions and cervical change. The magnesium sulfate is a tocolytic designed to quiet the uterus and halt the preterm labor. The penicillin is given to prevent group B streptococcal (GBS) disease of the newborn should the patient deliver. Dexamethasone should also be given to reduce the risk of respiratory distress syndrome (RDS), intraventricular hemorrhage (IVH), and perinatal mortality. A large amount of data have accumulated over the past 3 decades, demonstrating that antenatal corticosteroids are effective in the prevention of RDS, IVH, and neonatal mortality. The two corticosteroids used are betamethasone and dexamethasone. They are similar in structure, have a half-life of approximately 72 hours, and cross the placenta in an active form.

It is not necessary to add ampicillin (**choice A**) to this patient's pharmacologic regimen. This patient is already on penicillin for GBS prophylaxis and further treatment with ampicillin is therefore not needed.

Gentamicin (**choice C**) should not be added to this patient's regimen. There is no evidence that this patient has chorioamnionitis, but if she did, she should be treated with gentamicin. However, in that case the fetus should also be delivered and tocolysis should not be given.

Terbutaline (**choice D**) should not be added to this patient's regimen. This patient is already on magnesium sulfate for tocolysis. The addition of another tocolytic would only place this patient at greater risk of complications.

Tetracycline (**choice E**) is not used during pregnancy because of its effects on fetal teeth and bone.

Pediatrics: **Test One**

1. An 8-year-old boy is brought to his physician by his mother, who is worried by the child's frequent episodes of daydreaming, which have apparently resulted in a decline in school performance. The child's psychomotor development appears normal. EEG recording reveals bilateral and symmetric 3-Hz spike-and-wave discharges, which begin and end abruptly on a normal background. Which of the following is the most likely diagnosis?

   (A) Absence seizures (petit mal)

   (B) Complex partial seizures

   (C) Pseudoseizures

   (D) Simple partial seizures

   (E) Tonic-clonic seizures (grand mal)

2. A pregnant woman has premature rupture of membranes. Her baby is born 3 days later, at 37 weeks' gestation. The 5-minute APGAR score is 4. Lung sounds are reduced, and the infant appears to be in respiratory distress. Peripheral blood smear with differential counts demonstrates a neutrophil count of 30,000/mL, with toxic granules evident in many neutrophils. Gram stain of buffy coat demonstrates small gram-positive cocci in chains. Which of the following is the most likely causative organism?

   (A) Group A *Streptococcus*

   (B) Group B *Streptococcus*

   (C) Methicillin-resistant *Staphylococcus aureus*

   (D) Methicillin-sensitive *Staphylococcus aureus*

   (E) *Neisseria meningitidis*

3. A 6-year-old boy has multiple, honey-colored, crusted lesions on his face, periungual areas, and forearms. The first lesion appeared 2 weeks ago on his philtrum. Since then the lesions have spread to his hands and arms. Each began as a small pustule on an erythematous base and eventually ruptured to form the crusted lesions now present. His temperature is 38.1° C (100.6° F), pulse is 100/min, and respirations are 14/min. The remainder of the physical examination is unremarkable. Which of the following is the most appropriate treatment?

   (A) Clarithromycin

   (B) Dicloxacillin

   (C) Penicillin G

   (D) Penicillin V

   (E) Vancomycin

4. A 15-year-old girl has a round, 1-cm cystic mass in the midline of her neck, at the level of the hyoid bone. The mass is deep to the skin and moves slightly when the patient swallows. When the mass is palpated at the same time that the tongue is pulled, there seems to be a connection between the two. The mass has been present for at least 10 years, but only recently bothered the patient because it became infected. Which of the following is the most likely diagnosis?

   (A) Branchial cleft cyst

   (B) Cystic hygroma

   (C) Epidermal inclusion cyst

   (D) Metastatic thyroid cancer

   (E) Thyroglossal duct cyst

KAPLAN MEDICAL

5. A 2-year-old boy who emigrated from Eastern Europe 1 year ago is brought to the physician because of fever, cough, and night sweats for 3 weeks. The child's grandmother, who lives with him, has similar symptoms. The child's temperature is 39.2° C (102.6° F), blood pressure is 110/65 mm Hg, pulse is 90/min, and respirations are 28/min. A Mantoux test is reactive, and a chest x-ray film shows a right middle lobe infiltrate and hilar lymphadenopathy. Which of the following is the most appropriate next step in diagnosis?

(A) Cervical lymph node biopsy

(B) Gastric aspiration

(C) Pleurocentesis

(D) Sputum induction

6. A mother brings her 6-year-old daughter for evaluation because she has never been able to toilet train her. The child states that she perceives the sensation of having to void, and empties her bladder normally at normal intervals, but is nonetheless wet with urine all the time. Which of the following is the most likely diagnosis?

(A) Low implantation of one ureter

(B) Meatal stenosis

(C) Ureteropelvic junction obstruction

(D) Ureterovesical reflux

(E) Urethral valves

7. A neonate is noted to have an abnormally shaped face with a very small jaw. Several hours after birth, the baby develops convulsions and tetany. Serum chemistries show the following:

Sodium	140 mEq/L
Potassium	4 mEq/L
Chloride	100 mEq/L
Bicarbonate	24 mEq/L
Magnesium	2 mEq/L
Calcium	5 mg/dL
Glucose	100 mg/dL

This child's disorder is associated with aplasia or hypoplasia of which of the following organs?

(A) Ovaries

(B) Pancreas

(C) Pituitary

(D) Thymus

(E) Thyroid

8. A 10-year-old girl is brought to the physician because of throat pain, anorexia, and fever for 2 days. Her temperature is 38.9° C (102.0° F). The patient's history is negative for allergic diseases. She has had two episodes of pharyngotonsillitis over the past several years. Examination reveals a purulent exudate in the posterior oropharynx and enlarged tonsils. There is bilateral tender enlargement of anterior cervical lymph nodes. Cardiac and chest auscultation is normal. A rapid strep test is positive. Which of the following is the most appropriate next step in management?

(A) Confirmatory throat cultures before treatment

(B) Symptomatic treatment with nonsteroidal anti-inflammatory drugs

(C) Symptomatic treatment and oral penicillin V

(D) Symptomatic treatment and a broad-spectrum cephalosporin

(E) Surgical referral for tonsillectomy

9. A 12-year-old girl is seen by a pediatrician for a mild case of pneumonia. She is treated with an intramuscular injection of penicillin. About 15 minutes later, she develops extreme itchiness, accompanied by the development of wheals scattered over her chest and extremities. She also begins to wheeze and complain of difficulty breathing. The color of her lips and face remains rosy. Which of the following is the most appropriate first step in management?

(A) Epinephrine injection

(B) IV corticosteroids

(C) Intubation

(D) Oral corticosteroids

(E) No specific therapy is needed

10. An 11-month-old boy is brought to the emergency department by his parents. The child has a fracture of the right femur. The father reports this was sustained as a result of falling out of the crib. The child is also noted to have bruises on his shoulders and back. The rest of his examination is unremarkable. Which of the following is the most appropriate next step in diagnosis?

(A) Social services consult

(B) Chest x-ray

(C) CT of the head

(D) Funduscopic exam

(E) Lumbar puncture

11. A 4-month-old infant is evaluated by a dermatologist because of thick, erythematous skin with fine scaling, principally involving his face. The mother reports that the infant is "always scratching his face." An older brother and a maternal uncle had a similar condition. Screening hematologic studies show the following:

Erythrocyte count	5.1 million/mm^3
Leukocyte count	12,000/mm^3
Segmented neutrophils	80%
Bands	5%
Eosinophils	3%
Basophils	1%
Lymphocytes	5%
Monocytes	6%
Platelet count	35,000/mm^3, with the comment that the platelets are smaller than normal

Serum immunoglobulin studies demonstrate the following:

IgA	120 mg/dL
IgE	2,300 IU/mL
IgG	900 mg/dL
IgM	15 mg/dL

Patients with this condition have a significantly increased incidence of which of the following?

(A) Basal cell carcinoma

(B) Hodgkin lymphoma

(C) Melanoma

(D) Non-Hodgkin lymphoma

(E) Squamous cell carcinoma of the skin

12. A 7-month-old boy is brought to his physician because of increased agitation and restlessness. Lung examination reveals crackles and decreased breath sounds bilaterally. Chest x-ray films are notable for bilateral pneumonia. Arterial blood gas analysis reveals an oxygen tension of 45 mm Hg and a carbon dioxide tension of 60 mm Hg. Which of the following is the most appropriate next step in management?

(A) Obtain blood cultures

(B) Perform a rapid test for RSV and influenza

(C) Administer bronchodilators

(D) Administer antibiotics

(E) Insert endotracheal tube

13. A 4-year-old boy from India presents with weakness. His parents note that he has been looking increasingly pale. Hemoglobin electrophoresis demonstrates an abnormal hemoglobin species. Genetic analysis indicates that the patient has the substitution of a valine for a glutamine in the sixth position of the beta-hemoglobin chain. Which of the following will most likely be seen on his blood smear?

(A) Hypochromic, sickled red blood cells

(B) Hypochromic, spherical red blood cells

(C) Macrocytic, hypochromic red blood cells

(D) Normocytic, hypochromic red blood cells

(E) Normocytic, normochromic red blood cells

14. A 2-week-old boy in the neonatal intensive care unit had a birth weight of 1,200 g. Ultrasound of the head reveals grade II intraventricular hemorrhage and periventricular leukomalacia. An ophthalmologic examination reveals retinopathy of prematurity of both eyes. In addition, a hearing screen demonstrates bilateral hearing deficits. Which of the following is the most important determinant of this child's neurodevelopmental outcome?

(A) Length of gestation

(B) Maternal education

(C) Outcome of the mother's previous pregnancies

(D) Quality of prenatal care

(E) Socioeconomic status of the family

15. A 2-year-old girl is brought to her pediatrician by her parents because of increasing lethargy and irritability. She has just started walking, is teething, and likes to chew on the woodwork around the windows. Physical examination reveals a tender abdomen. Laboratory studies indicate high iron and ferritin levels. The peripheral blood smear shows basophilic stippling. Which of the following laboratory anomalies will be seen in this patient?

(A) Increased free erythrocyte protoporphyrin levels

(B) Increased homocysteine and methylmalonic acid levels

(C) Increased hemoglobin A$_2$ on electrophoresis

(D) Increased urinary aminolevulinic acid (ALA) porphobilinogen (PBG)

(E) Low serum ferritin and elevated total iron binding capacity (TIBC)

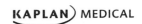

16. A 12-year-old boy with cystic fibrosis presents to the emergency department with a 3-day history of severe coughing, which is productive of a yellow-greenish purulent sputum. He had fever and chills at home. He also complains of chest congestion and chest pain that is worse with coughing. On physical examination, his temperature is 39.6° C (103.2° F), blood pressure is 98/68 mm Hg, pulse is 102/min, and respirations are 24/min. He is noted to be lethargic. He has rales on the left lower lung field on auscultation, and chest radiography shows an infiltrate in the left lower lobe. Which of the following is the most appropriate initial antimicrobial therapy for this patient?

    (A) Amoxicillin-clavulanate and gentamicin

    (B) Azithromycin and ceftriaxone

    (C) Ceftazidime and tobramycin

    (D) Levofloxacin and metronidazole

    (E) Trimethoprim-sulfamethoxazole and vancomycin

17. A 12-year-old boy is brought to the physician because of pain in his right leg for the past 3 weeks. The pain frequently occurs at night and is localized to the tibia, a few centimeters below the knee. The mother reports that the pain is promptly relieved by aspirin and that the child has had no fever. Examination reveals no tissue swelling or redness about the site of pain. X-ray films show a 1-cm radiolucent focus in the tibial cortex surrounded by marked bone sclerosis. Which of the following is the most likely diagnosis?

    (A) Aneurysmal bone cyst

    (B) Enchondroma

    (C) Ewing sarcoma

    (D) Osteoid osteoma

    (E) Osteosarcoma

18. A 15-year old girl presents with a 5-day history of sore throat, low-grade fever, and easy fatigability. Physical examination shows bilateral tonsillar enlargement with exudate. Her spleen is palpable 3 cm below the left costal margin. Her throat culture is negative for group A *Streptococcus*. Monospot test is positive. Which of the following is the most appropriate management for this patient?

    (A) Abdominal ultrasound

    (B) Avoidance of all contact sports

    (C) Complete blood count

    (D) Oral penicillin

    (E) Splenectomy

19. A 3-year-old child is taken to a pediatrician because he develops burning pain, erythema, and swelling minutes after being exposed to the sun. Physical examination demonstrates erythema with swelling of the hands and arms. The skin is thickened on the backs of the hands but does not show blistering or scarring. Which of the following is the most likely diagnosis?

    (A) Acute intermittent porphyria

    (B) Erythropoietic protoporphyria

    (C) Hepatoerythropoietic porphyria

    (D) Porphyria cutanea tarda

    (E) Variegate porphyria

20. A 16-year-old girl has had a fever, vomiting, and watery diarrhea for the past 24 hours. She also complains of intermittent abdominal pain and generalized myalgia. On examination, she is slightly lethargic. Her temperature is 39.4° C (103.0° F), blood pressure is 75/50 mm Hg, and pulse is 150/min. Her conjunctivae and pharynx are hyperemic. She has a generalized erythematous maculopapular rash that spares the wrists. Which of the following will be the most appropriate treatment?

    (A) Amantadine

    (B) Gentamicin

    (C) Ketoconazole

    (D) Nafcillin

    (E) Prednisone

21. A 7-year-old girl was found in a routine health supervision visit to have bilateral breast tissue development. She also had long, pigmented hair over the labia majora. Her height and weight are both at the 80th percentile for her age. Which of the following is the most appropriate management?

    (A) CT of the head and abdomen

    (B) Pelvic ultrasonography

    (C) Radiography of the head and wrist

    (D) Reassurance to the parents that it is normal

    (E) Thyroid stimulating hormone (TSH) level

22. The mother of a 2-year-old boy comes to the physician because her child awakens at night, with a blank gaze, screaming in bed without recognizing his parents. These episodes have occurred three times in the past 2 weeks, always in the first few hours of the night. The child goes back to sleep and seems to retain no memory of the episode the next morning. Which of the following is the most appropriate next step in management?

    (A) Reassurance of parents about the nature of these manifestations

    (B) Avoidance of TV before going to bed

    (C) Behavioral therapy

    (D) Therapy with chloral hydrate

    (E) Therapy with a tricyclic antidepressant

23. A 12-year-old girl is taken to a pediatrician complaining of a sore mouth. On questioning, the child states that she has been feeling poorly, with fatigue and weakness. She began menstruating briefly and then stopped. Physical examination is notable for focal white crusting of the oral cavity; biopsy of one of these areas later shows candidiasis. Laboratory studies show the following:

Sodium	127 mEq/L
Potassium	5.3 mEq/L
Bicarbonate	24 mEq/L
Calcium	7.5 mEq/dL
Phosphorus	5.5 mg/dL
Glucose	87 mg/dL

    Which of the following is the most likely diagnosis?

    (A) Multiple endocrine neoplasia, type I

    (B) Multiple endocrine neoplasia, type IIA

    (C) Polyglandular deficiency syndrome, type I

    (D) Polyglandular deficiency syndrome, type II

    (E) Polyglandular deficiency syndrome, type III

24. An 8-year-old boy is brought to the pediatrician with a rash on his abdomen. The mother first noticed the rash about 3 weeks ago. The boy has no fever or other symptoms. On examination, there is a well-circumscribed, circular, erythematous, scaly annular patch on his abdomen. The border of the skin lesion is raised and well defined. Which of the following is the most likely diagnosis?

    (A) Erythema multiforme

    (B) Erythema nodosum

    (C) Impetigo

    (D) Nummular eczema

    (E) Tinea corporis

25. A 10-year-old boy is brought to the clinic because of increasing weakness and dyspnea over the past 6 months. He had been healthy and is taking no medications. There is no significant family history of illness. On examination, he appears pale. His hematocrit is 20% and mean corpuscular volume (MCV) is $60/\mu m^3$. Ferritin and total iron binding capacity (TIBC) are within normal levels. Peripheral blood smear reveals basophilic stippling, and capillary lead level is less than 10 $\mu g/dL$. Hemoglobin electrophoresis shows an elevation of hemoglobin A_2 and an absence of one beta-globin gene. Which of the following is the most likely diagnosis?

    (A) Elliptocytosis

    (B) Hemoglobin S-C disease

    (C) Iron deficiency anemia

    (D) Lead poisoning

    (E) Sickle cell anemia

    (F) Thalassemia

26. A 16-month-old girl is brought to medical attention because of irritability, poor feeding, and temperatures up to 39.4° C (103.0° F). Careful history and physical examination fail to disclose any identifiable cause of her fever. There is some degree of abdominal tenderness on palpation. Which of the following is the most appropriate next step in diagnosis?

    (A) Abdominal radiographs

    (B) Culture of urine obtained by transurethral catheterization

    (C) Microscopic examination and culture of stool

    (D) Renal ultrasound

    (E) Voiding cystourethrogram

27. A premature neonate with respiratory distress syndrome is maintained on mechanical ventilation in a neonatal intensive care unit. Two weeks after delivery, the nurses in the intensive care unit notice that higher ventilation settings are needed and that more secretions are being suctioned from the endotracheal tube. A chest x-ray film shows questionable new infiltrates. Which of the following is the most likely pathogen?

    (A) Coagulase-negative oxacillin-resistant *Staphylococcus*

    (B) Coagulase-negative oxacillin-sensitive *Staphylococcus*

    (C) Group B *Streptococcus*

    (D) Methicillin-resistant *Staphylococcus aureus*

    (E) Methicillin-sensitive *Staphylococcus aureus*

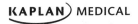

28. During a diaper change, a 3-day-old infant in the nursery is noted to have uneven gluteal folds. The infant was born via cesarean section due to failure of progression but otherwise has been well since birth. The infant's temperature is 37.2° C (99.0° F), pulse rate is 125/min, and respiratory rate is 50/min. The infant weighs 3,250 g. Physical examination of the infant reveals that the left hip is more easily dislocated posteriorly with a jerk and a "click" and returns to its normal position with a snapping sound. The mother is concerned because she has a history of tetracycline use before she was known to be pregnant. Which of the following is most likely to confirm the diagnosis?

    (A) Bone scan

    (B) CT scan

    (C) Frog-leg lateral radiographs

    (D) Joint fluid aspiration

    (E) Serum tetracycline levels

    (F) Ultrasound

29. A 3-year-old boy is brought to the emergency department because of a worsening cough over the past week. His temperature is 38.9° C (102.0° F), and inspiratory stridor is noted. A plain film of the neck reveals subglottic swelling. He is noted to have copious thick secretions and a barking cough. He has not had such events previously, and his parents deny recent contact with sick children. The patient is in respiratory distress and is noted to be retracting his subcostal muscles to breathe. Which of the following is the next most appropriate step in management?

    (A) Administer albuterol

    (B) Administer racemic epinephrine

    (C) Administer corticosteroids

    (D) Administer IV penicillin

    (E) Endotracheal intubation

30. A 7-year-old girl is brought to the physician because of an exanthematous rash associated with malaise and headache for 2 days. On examination, the child shows a fiery red facial rash with a characteristic "slapped cheek" pattern and pallor around the mouth. There is no fever. In immunocompromised patients, the pathogen that causes this condition may result in which of the following manifestations?

    (A) Aplastic anemia

    (B) Encephalitis

    (C) Non-Hodgkin lymphoma

    (D) Progressive multifocal leukoencephalopath (PML)

    (E) Symmetric polyarthritis

31. A 2-year-old girl is brought to the physician because of protracted irritability, crying, and loss of appetite. She recently had a sore throat. Her temperature is 38.5° C (101.3° F). Physical examination is unremarkable, except for abnormalities of the tympanic membrane detected on otoscopic examination. Which of the following signs or symptoms correlates best with a diagnosis of acute otitis media?

    (A) Color change of tympanic membrane

    (B) Fever

    (C) Opacification of tympanic membrane

    (D) Otalgia

    (E) Otorrhea

    (F) Reduced tympanic membrane mobility

32. A woman comes to an emergency department because she is in labor. She has had no prenatal care. Her baby is delivered and appears to be of about 32 weeks' gestation. The newborn is very pale and shows severe, generalized edema. Cord-blood hematocrit is 22%, and cord-blood bilirubin is 7 mg/dL. Ultrasound examination demonstrates pleural effusions, ascites, cardiomegaly, and hepatomegaly. Which of the following is the most likely diagnosis?

    (A) ABO incompatibility

    (B) Beta thalassemia

    (C) Congenital spherocytosis

    (D) Sickle cell anemia

    (E) Rh incompatibility

33. A term neonate is examined following a protracted breech delivery. A complete neurologic examination reveals an asymmetrical Moro reflex, with the left arm being nonreactive. The left arm falls limply and close to the side of the body when drawn upward, and the resting position is adducted and internally rotated with pronation of the forearm. The neonate's fingers show a normal response to the hand grasp reflex bilaterally. Vital signs are within normal limits, and no other abnormalities are noted on examination. Which of the following is the most likely diagnosis?

    (A) Bell's palsy

    (B) Erb's palsy

    (C) Klumpke paralysis

    (D) Pseudobulbar palsy

    (E) Spinal cord injury

    (F) Supranuclear palsy

34. A 3-month-old infant is taken to the emergency department with constipation and behavioral changes. Physical examination demonstrates ptosis and an absence of facial expression. The child appears conscious but has trouble following a toy with her gaze. The crying is very weak, and saliva is pooling in her mouth. She is also developing a generalized hypotonia, and breathing is becoming more shallow. A lumbar puncture is performed, and analysis of the cerebrospinal fluid is within normal limits. Early treatment with which of the following would most likely have prevented morbidity in this infant?

    (A) Antibiotics

    (B) Antitoxin

    (C) Antiviral medications

    (D) Corticosteroids

    (E) Intravenous gammaglobulin

    (F) Plasmapheresis

35. A 3-year-old-boy ingests 40 of his older sister's chewable vitamin tablets, as well as 3 tablets of 250 mg of acetaminophen. The ingredients in the multivitamin tablets are as follows:

Vitamin A	3,000 IU
Thiamine	1 mg
Vitamin C	75 mg
Vitamin B$_6$	1 mg
Vitamin D	400 IU
Iron	12 mg
Fluoride	1 mg

    The child is brought to the emergency department in no acute distress. Which of the following complications may occur if appropriate therapy is not undertaken?

    (A) Acute renal failure from vitamin D toxicity

    (B) Hepatic failure from acetaminophen toxicity

    (C) Hepatic failure from iron toxicity

    (D) Increased intracranial pressure from vitamin A toxicity

    (E) Intestinal ischemia from fluoride toxicity

36. A 7-year-old boy presents with tenderness and erythema of one knee joint. He has had troubles with infections since about 3 months of age. A brother and a maternal uncle both died of infectious disease at an early age. A detailed immunologic evaluation performed at 2 years of age demonstrated plasma IgG less than 50 mg/100 mL. Normal numbers of circulating T cells and normal cellular immunity were found. The boy had been treated monthly since then with IV immunoglobulin. This therapy had markedly reduced, but not eliminated, the boy's infection rate. Which of the following is the most likely pathogen to cause infectious arthritis in this patient?

    (A) *Aspergillus*

    (B) Herpes

    (C) *Mycobacterium*

    (D) *Mycoplasma*

    (E) *Toxoplasma*

KAPLAN) MEDICAL

37. A 6-month-old infant is taken to the emergency department because he had a seizure. Physical examination demonstrates premature closure of cranial sutures and markedly bowed legs. Laboratory studies demonstrate low serum phosphate levels, with normal vitamin D and parathyroid hormone levels. Urinalysis shows high phosphate levels, but no increased excretion of glucose, amino acids, or protein. The child's maternal grandfather had crippling bone disease, and his mother has mild bowing of the legs. Which of the following is most likely diagnosis?

(A) Fanconi syndrome

(B) Hypophosphatemic rickets

(C) Osteogenesis imperfecta

(D) Osteomalacia

(E) Paget disease of bone

38. A 2-year-old girl is brought to the emergency department with a fever, chills, poor appetite, and vomiting. On examination, she is irritable and diaphoretic. Her temperature is 39.2° C (102.5° F), blood pressure is 80/48 mm Hg, pulse is 88/min, and respirations are 17/min. She is tender at the left costovertebral angle. Initial laboratory tests show the following:

Leukocyte count	16,300/mm^3
Hemoglobin	12.5 g/dL
Platelet count	245,000/mm^3
Blood urea nitrogen	6 mg/dL
Creatinine	0.5 mg/dL

Urinalysis is positive for leukocyte esterase and nitrite, with 150 white blood cells/hpf. After IV antibiotic administration and stabilization, what is the most appropriate diagnostic study?

(A) CT of the abdomen and pelvis

(B) IV pyelography

(C) Plain abdominal radiography

(D) Radionuclide imaging of the kidneys

(E) Voiding cystourethrography

39. A 12-year-old girl complains of intermittent palpitations. She had previously been in excellent health and has met all development milestones. There is no family history of heart disease. She is on no medications and takes no drugs. She states that the palpitations begin and end suddenly and usually last a couple of hours. She is otherwise asymptomatic between episodes. The physical examination is normal. An ECG reveals a shortened PR interval and a slow upstroke of the QRS wave in lead III. Which of the following is the most likely diagnosis?

(A) Anxiety attack

(B) Lown-Ganong-Levine syndrome

(C) Nodal reentrant tachycardia

(D) Sinus tachycardia

(E) Wolff-Parkinson-White syndrome

40. A term neonate is delivered via normal spontaneous delivery without complication. Within the first 2 hours of life, he becomes tachypneic, with occasional apneas and two seizure episodes. The infant is large for gestational age, and his weight is in the 95th percentile for his age. There are no evident dysmorphic features, and the rest of the physical examination is unremarkable. Serum studies demonstrate a blood glucose level of 30 mg/dL. Which of the following conditions is most likely present in the mother?

(A) Diabetes mellitus

(B) Graves disease

(C) Hepatic cirrhosis

(D) Rheumatoid arthritis

(E) Seizure disorder

(F) Systemic lupus erythematosus (SLE)

41. A 4-month-old infant is brought to the clinic by his mother because of 3 days of diarrhea and mild fever. The stools are nonbloody, watery, and voluminous and continue even when the infant is fasting. The infant's only significant history is premature birth at 34 weeks' gestation. He is in the 60th percentile in weight and length for his age, and he has met his developmental milestones. A stool examination is negative for leukocytes, ova, and parasites. Which of the following is the most likely cause of this infant's diarrhea?

    (A) *Campylobacter jejuni*

    (B) *Cryptosporidium*

    (C) Enteroinvasive *Escherichia coli*

    (D) Pancreatic insufficiency

    (E) *Giardia lamblia*

    (F) Lactose intolerance

    (G) Rotavirus

    (H) *Salmonella* species

    (I) *Shigella* species

42. A 2-year-old child has had red, weeping, crusted lesions of the face, scalp, diaper area, and extremities since about age 2 months, with multiple periods of exacerbation and improvement. Attempts to remove potentially irritating substances have not modified the course of the rashes. The child is noted to be constantly scratching and rubbing involved areas. There is a strong family history of hay fever and asthma. Which of the following is the most likely diagnosis?

    (A) Atopic dermatitis

    (B) Cellulitis

    (C) Contact dermatitis

    (D) Lichen simplex chronicus

    (E) Seborrheic dermatitis

43. A 5-year-old boy is brought to clinic with increasing right lower foot pain. He stepped on a nail several days ago. At that time, the family had sought medical attention. The child was given a tetanus shot, and the wound was extensively irrigated. On examination, the foot is tender, swollen, warm, and erythematous. Osteomyelitis is suspected. Which of the following is the most appropriate next step in diagnosis?

    (A) White cell count

    (B) CT scan of the foot

    (C) Gallium scan

    (D) Technetium bone scan

    (E) X-ray of the foot

44. A 3-day-old girl has trouble feeding and pulmonary congestion. The mother says that the infant is so busy breathing, that she literally has no time to suckle. The girl was born at home, with the delivery attended by a midwife. Physical examination confirms that she is in respiratory distress and shows bounding peripheral pulses with a loud continuous precordial machinery-like murmur. X-ray films show increased pulmonary vascular markings. Shortly thereafter, the infant goes into overt heart failure. Which of the following would most likely be required to correct this problem?

    (A) Indomethacin

    (B) Digitalis and diuretics

    (C) Emergency surgical closure of atrial septal defect

    (D) Emergency surgical closure of ventricular septal defect

    (E) Emergency surgical division of patent ductus arteriosus

45. A 12-year-old girl presents with a 2-month history of vaginal discharge. She describes it as clear and states that it stains her underwear. She says that she hates boys, and that "no way" has she ever had sex or even kissed a boy. She reports having had developing breasts for 2 years and thinks that her growth spurt was about a year ago. Genital findings include a pubic hair stage of Tanner III with no evidence of redness or irritation of the vulvovaginal area. A slight amount of odorless, clear mucus is seen. Microscopic examination of the mucus reveals epithelial cells and a few bacteria, but no white cells. The pH is between 3.5 and 4. Which of the following is the most appropriate next step in management?

    (A) No treatment, but the girl should be reassessed in a few months

    (B) Advise the girl to discontinue all bubble baths and wipe herself front to back after voiding

    (C) Pelvic examination to obtain cultures for gonorrhea and *Chlamydia*

    (D) Clotrimazole cream to be applied once a day for 10 days

    (E) Sitz baths one or two times a day and 1% hydrocortisone cream applications once a day for a week

46. A 10-year-old girl is involved in a motor vehicle accident, sustaining multiple injuries to her head, arms, and abdomen. Her blood pressure is 90/60 mm Hg, and her pulse is 120/min. Her forearm is disfigured, and bone can be seen through the wound. She is breathing periodically and has cyanotic lips. Her abdomen is rigid, and there is flank discoloration. Which of the following is the most appropriate next step in management?

    (A) Splint the arm and cover wound with sterile gauze

    (B) Administer crystalloid solution

    (C) Administer vasopressors immediately

    (D) Administer packed red blood cells

    (E) Perform exploratory laparotomy

47. A 15-year-old Caucasian boy is injured during a football game. He is taken to the emergency department for x-ray films of his leg to rule out a possible fracture. The radiologist reports that the boy has evidence of an aggressive bone tumor with both bone destruction and a soft tissue mass. Later, the pathologist reports that the bone biopsy reveals a bone cancer, with some of the tumor tissue displaying neural differentiation. Which of the following is the most appropriate next step in management?

    (A) Chemotherapy

    (B) Radiation therapy

    (C) Surgery

    (D) Surgery and chemotherapy

    (E) Surgery, chemotherapy, and radiation therapy

48. A 7-year-old boy has a history of repeated urinary tract infections that have been treated with the empiric use of antibiotics. The parents are not satisfied with the care the child is receiving, and they take him to a pediatric urologist. Evaluation by voiding cystourethrogram shows that the patient has vesicoureteral reflux without ureteral or upper tract dilatation (grade one reflux). Which of the following is the appropriate management for this child?

    (A) Alpha blockers

    (B) Long-term, low-dose antibacterial therapy

    (C) Nephrectomy on the affected site

    (D) Reassurance and observation

    (E) Surgical reimplantation of the ureter

The response options for items 49-50 are the same. You will be required to select one answer for each item in the set.

(A) Acute lymphocytic leukemia

(B) Chondromalacia patella

(C) Ewing sarcoma

(D) "Growing pains"

(E) Juvenile rheumatoid arthritis

(F) Legg-Calvé-Perthes disease

(G) Osgood-Schlatter disease

(H) Osteoid osteoma

(I) Septic arthritis

(J) Slipped capital femoral epiphysis

For each patient with leg pain, select the most likely diagnosis.

49. A 14-year-old girl is brought to the pediatrician with a 4-day history of pain and swelling in her left knee. She plays soccer on her school team regularly, and her knee has become too painful for her to participate. There is no history of trauma and no previous episodes of pain. On physical examination, there is marked swelling and tenderness over her left anterior tibial tuberosity. A radiograph of her left knee reveals irregularities of the tubercle contour and haziness of the adjacent metaphyseal border.

50. A 4-year-old, previously well boy has moderate pains in both of his legs for the past 3 weeks. On physical examination, his temperature is 37.7° C (99.8° F), blood pressure is 108/68 mm Hg, pulse is 96/min, and respirations are 17/min. On examination, he is noted to have marked pallor on his lips and palpebral conjunctiva. Numerous purpura and petechiae are noted on his skin, and his spleen is palpable 3 cm below his left costal margin. Both legs show normal range of motion without tenderness or swelling of the joints. A complete blood count reveals a white blood cell count of 1,600/mm^3, hemoglobin of 6.9 g/dL, and platelet count of 36,000/mm^3.

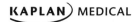

Pediatrics Test One:
Answers and Explanations

ANSWER KEY

1.	A	26.	B
2.	B	27.	A
3.	B	28.	F
4.	E	29.	B
5.	B	30.	A
6.	A	31.	F
7.	D	32.	E
8.	C	33.	B
9.	A	34.	B
10.	D	35.	C
11.	D	36.	D
12.	E	37.	B
13.	A	38.	E
14.	A	39.	E
15.	A	40.	A
16.	C	41.	G
17.	D	42.	A
18.	B	43.	D
19.	B	44.	E
20.	D	45.	A
21.	C	46.	B
22.	A	47.	E
23.	C	48.	B
24.	E	49.	F
25.	F	50.	A

1. **The correct answer is A.** Children with absence seizures manifest periodic and sudden episodes of impaired consciousness, which are often interpreted by the unaware parent as "daydreaming." These episodes may recur frequently during the day (even hundreds of times) and disturb play and school activities. EEG evidence of 3 Hz spike-and-wave activity during attacks is diagnostic of petit mal. The onset of this type of seizures is between the ages of 4 and 12 years; the seizures often resolve before the age of 20 years.

   Epilepsy can be divided into *partial* seizures, if the abnormal activity is localized to a specific part of the brain, or *generalized* seizures, if the entire brain is involved. In complex partial seizures (**choice B**), there is loss of consciousness associated with focal motor (e.g., convulsions and jerking movements) and/or sensory (e.g., visual, auditory, olfactory, and tactile) symptoms that affect different parts of the body depending on the cortical localization. It may be difficult to differentiate complex partial seizures from absence seizures on clinical grounds alone without EEG studies. Simple partial seizures (**choice D**) manifest with motor or somatosensory symptoms but with preservation of consciousness.

   Pseudoseizures (**choice C**) refer to attacks that are superficially similar to tonic-clonic seizures but are related to hysterical conversion or malingering. The differential diagnosis with true seizures is usually easy with the aid of EEG studies and serum prolactin measurement. Serum prolactin increases after true tonic-clonic convulsions but is unchanged following pseudoseizures.

   Tonic-clonic seizures (**choice E**) are generalized seizures characterized by a sudden loss of consciousness accompanied by a tonic phase (the patient becomes rigid and falls to the ground) and followed by a clonic phase (convulsive manifestations). Each attack usually lasts 2-3 minutes, after which the patient may regain consciousness or fall asleep. Tongue biting and loss of sphincter control are common during the attack.

2. **The correct answer is B.** This is neonatal sepsis, which in the first few days of life is most likely to be due to group B *Streptococcus* or gram-negative enteric organisms. Physicians should maintain a high index of suspicion, since neonatal sepsis may be subtle or nonspecific in its symptoms ("not doing well," respiratory distress, apnea, bradycardia, seizures, jaundice). Gram stain of the buffy coat from a blood sample may be particularly helpful in establishing the diagnosis. Predisposing conditions include obstetric complications, toxemia, and maternal infection.

   Group A *Streptococcus* (**choice A**) does not commonly infect infants; it causes sore throats, pneumonia, and meningitis in older children.

   Staphylococcus aureus, in either its methicillin-sensitive (**choice D**) or methicillin-resistant (**choice C**) forms, can cause skin pustules, sepsis, pneumonia, and meningitis in infants, but would be described as gram-positive cocci in clusters rather than chains.

   Neisseria meningitidis (**choice E**) is a gram-negative diplococcus that can cause meningitis and respiratory infections in children but is not common in neonates.

3. **The correct answer is B.** This is a case of impetigo, a common superficial infection caused by group A beta hemolytic streptococci or *Staphylococcus aureus*. Dicloxacillin is an oral preparation that is effective for infections caused by staphylococci and some streptococci. The drug is not deactivated by penicillinase, which is often present in staphylococci.

   Clarithromycin (**choice A**) is a macrolide antibiotic that is used for mild to moderate respiratory tract infections, uncomplicated skin infections, and prophylaxis for *Mycobacterium avium* complex.

   Penicillin G (**choice C**) is available for oral, intramuscular, or intravenous use and is active against streptococci. However, most staphylococci produce beta-lactamases, which break down penicillin.

   Penicillin V (**choice D**) is an oral preparation of penicillin and has a similar coverage as penicillin G.

   Vancomycin (**choice E**) is active against gram-positive species and is reserved for those bacteria that are resistant to beta-lactamase-resistant antibiotics. It is used intravenously and orally for treatment of *Clostridium difficile* colitis.

4. **The correct answer is E.** The age, description, location, and "connection with the tongue" are classic for a thyroglossal duct cyst. The thyroid gland initially develops in close proximity to the tongue, then descends into the neck via the thyroglossal duct, which is normally obliterated but occasionally persists as thyroglossal duct cysts or nodules.

   Branchial cleft cysts (**choice A**) are seen in the lateral aspect of the neck, along the anterior edge of the sternocleidomastoid muscle, anywhere from in front of the tragus to near the base of the neck.

   Cystic hygroma (**choice B**) is seen at the base of the neck, as a soft, fluid-filled mass that goes deep into the mediastinum.

   Epidermal inclusion cysts (**choice C**) are attached to the skin, not connected to the tongue. If this cyst had been present for 10 years, it would have caused problems long ago. Furthermore, its location at the midline and level of the hyoid would have been an incredible coincidence.

   Thyroid cancer (**choice D**), if primary, would have been lower in the neck, where the thyroid is located. If it were metastatic, it would have been in the lateral side of the neck at the jugular nodes. Also, although thyroid cancers are notorious for slow growth, a cancer would be larger than 1 cm in size after 10 years.

5. **The correct answer is B.** This child has primary pulmonary tuberculosis. The infection was most likely acquired from his grandmother, who is sick with similar symptoms. The initial pneumonic area may be anywhere in the lung, especially in the middle and lower lobes. This age group of patients rarely has a positive Mantoux test in the absence of recent infection. Early-morning gastric aspiration is the best method for identifying acid-fast bacilli, which are swallowed during the night. Gastric aspiration is optimal in the early morning before the gastric acid destroys the bacilli.

    This patient does not have miliary tuberculosis, and so a cervical lymph node biopsy (**choice A**) would not be of diagnostic value.

    This patient has does not have evidence of a pleural effusion; therefore, pleurocentesis (**choice C**) is not indicated.

    It would be difficult for a 2-year-old to comply with sputum induction (**choice D**). In addition, sputum induction may be negative in more than 50% of cases of pulmonary tuberculosis.

6. **The correct answer is A.** One ureter is normally implanted into the bladder, and that one is responsible for the filling that leads to the normal voiding pattern. The other ureter has a low implantation, beyond the sphincter, into the vagina or the perineum. Having no sphincter, that ureter constantly leaks urine. Incidentally, this is a congenital anomaly that is symptomatic only in little girls. Boys have a longer sphincteric segment; even if a ureter has low implantation it does not leak.

    Meatal stenosis (**choice B**) is a very common source of obstruction in little boys in the newborn period. It would not occur in little girls.

    Ureteropelvic junction obstruction (**choice C**) is another common problem, but the clinical presentation is flank pain when urinary flow is much larger than usual. Typically this happens to adolescents when they drink a lot of beer for the first time in their lives.

    Ureterovesical reflux (**choice D**) is also a common congenital anomaly, but the presentation is that of recurrent urinary tract infections.

    Urethral valves (**choice E**) are seen in newborn boys who fail to void during the first day of life.

7. **The correct answer is D.** The only abnormal finding in the serum chemistries is the low calcium level. The disease is DiGeorge syndrome, in which fetal malformations of the third and fourth branchial arches cause failure of development of both the parathyroid glands and the thymus. An abnormal face with a small jaw may be noted at birth. The absence of the parathyroid glands causes hypocalcemic convulsions and tetany in infancy. Aplasia or near aplasia of the thymus predisposes for infections; circulating T cells may be very low to absent. The presence of even a small amount of functioning thymic tissue may allow these children to "outgrow" their immunodeficiency over a period of 4 or 5 years; children with severe disease often die. These children are also likely to have cardiac malformations, which may cause death.

    Abnormal ovaries (**choice A**) are associated with Turner syndrome.

    The pancreas (**choice B**) is vulnerable to congenital anomalies either as an isolated finding or in association with other congenital anomalies, but the description is most suggestive of DiGeorge syndrome.

    Developmental abnormalities of the pituitary gland (**choice C**) are unusual, possibly because significant in utero damage to this important endocrine organ leads to fetal death.

    Developmental abnormalities of the thyroid gland (**choice E**) can cause cretinism (infantile hypothyroidism).

8. **The correct answer is C.** This child has an acute pharyngotonsillitis (sore throat). Most cases are caused by viruses, of which rhinovirus, coronavirus, and parainfluenza virus are the most frequent agents. Bacteria, and specifically *group A beta-hemolytic Streptococcus* cause approximately 15% to 30% of cases. It is clinically important to determine whether pharyngitis is due to viruses or *Streptococcus* because of the different treatment involved. The classic symptomatology of "strep throat" is fever, anorexia, throat pain, tender and swollen lymph nodes, and purulent exudate on the oropharyngeal mucosa. Occasionally, there is an associated scarlatiniform rash. Clinical observation alone is not entirely reliable in differentiating between viral and streptococcal pharyngitis. Throat cultures or rapid strep test (the latter based on an enzyme immunoassay method that detects streptococcal antigens) help the clinician confirm or rule out streptococcal infection. Available rapid strep tests are highly sensitive (95%) but not very specific. Thus, a positive test confirms streptococcal infection and does not need confirmatory throat cultures before treatment (**choice A**). If the rapid strep test is negative, on the other hand, cultures are necessary to rule out streptococcal infection. The treatment of choice is a full course of oral penicillin, combined with acetaminophen or anti-inflammatory drugs for symptomatic relief.

    Symptomatic treatment alone with nonsteroidal anti-inflammatory drugs (**choice B**) would not be adequate

KAPLAN) MEDICAL

in this case because a rapid strep test has confirmed the streptococcal etiology. Antistreptococcal antibiotic therapy is mandatory to prevent complications (i.e., rheumatic fever).

Symptomatic treatment and a broad-spectrum cephalosporin (**choice D**) should be discouraged, since the indiscriminate use of broad-spectrum antibiotics facilitates the emergence of antibiotic resistance. Antistreptococcal treatment should be based on agents with narrow activity against group A *Streptococcus* (penicillin V or, in penicillin-allergic patients, erythromycin).

Surgical referral for tonsillectomy (**choice E**) is unnecessary in this case. Indications for tonsillectomy are rather limited, namely tonsillar enlargement causing persistent respiratory problems, swallowing difficulties, or obstructive sleep apnea.

9. **The correct answer is A.** The girl is having a systemic anaphylactic reaction to the penicillin. The itchiness and wheals (swollen, erythematous patches of skin) are the result of changes in small cutaneous vessels that favor shift of fluid out of the vascular space. The shortness of breath and wheezing are due to edema and bronchoconstriction of the upper airways. Epinephrine injection (either intramuscularly or subcutaneously) is the most appropriate first step in management, as this will usually quickly reverse the anaphylactic reaction if given promptly.

IV corticosteroids (**choice B**) and histamine blockers are sometimes given after epinephrine in severe cases of anaphylaxis, especially when the stimulating antigen cannot be immediately removed.

Intubation (**choice C**) is not initially indicated, since epinephrine usually reverses the airway edema within a few minutes. If her blood begins to desaturate significantly, as evidenced by pulse oximetry, or if respiratory distress or arrest occurs, intubation would be performed.

Oral corticosteroids (**choice D**) are used either as prophylaxis in situations where anaphylaxis may occur, or sometimes after milder cases of anaphylaxis in which the antigen may not have been completely removed.

No specific therapy (**choice E**) is incorrect, since untreated anaphylactic reactions to penicillin can be fatal.

10. **The correct answer is D.** This child is presenting with multiple atypical injuries, and child abuse must be suspected. Injuries from being shaken and subtle head trauma are common findings in abused children. Retinal hemorrhage may be noted. Funduscopic examination is imperative before other measures are undertaken.

A social services consult will probably be needed if there is suspicion of child neglect and abuse (**choice A**). In such situations, the child may be placed in a foster home.

Chest x-ray (**choice B**) may be needed to assess for rib fractures. Although this ultimately may be required to complete the child's evaluation, it is not needed initially. Nondisplaced fractures should heal without intervention.

A head CT (**choice C**) may be needed to assess for brain injury, including intracranial hemorrhage. Cranial fractures may be seen, and coup/contra-coup contusions may be noted as well.

Lumbar puncture (**choice E**) may be needed if there is strong suspicion of head trauma and the child is exhibiting neurologic deficits. Even if the head CT is negative, the lumbar puncture may indicate the presence of a hemorrhage. This should be done with caution, since the intracranial pressure may be elevated and there is risk of herniation.

11. **The correct answer is D.** The disease is Wiskott-Aldrich syndrome. This X-linked condition is characterized by thrombocytopenia (with characteristically small platelets) and lymphopenia with depressed cellular immunity. The lymphocytes have a reduced level of the adhesion molecule sialophorin (CD43) on their surfaces, which forms the basis of a helpful diagnostic test in this condition. Atopic eczema, as seen this child, is very common and may be the presenting complaint in these patients. It is typically accompanied by high serum IgE, often with low serum IgM. If the thrombocytopenia is very severe, splenectomy may be helpful in controlling the bleeding tendency. For reasons that are not yet biochemically clear, but have to do with their already abnormal lymphoid cells, these patients are very prone to develop non-Hodgkin lymphomas. They do not have a significantly increased tendency to develop skin malignancies, such as melanomas, squamous cell carcinomas, and basal cell carcinomas.

Associate basal cell carcinoma (**choice A**) with xeroderma pigmentosa and basal cell nevus syndrome.

Hodgkin disease (**choice B**) does not have any noteworthy associations with genetic diseases.

Associate melanoma (**choice C**) with xeroderma pigmentosa and very large congenital nevi.

Associate squamous cell carcinoma of the skin (**choice E**) with xeroderma pigmentosa.

12. **The correct answer is E.** The child is in respiratory failure and needs emergent care. Alveolar ventilation must be restored to lower the carbon dioxide level. The child's restlessness is a clue to the extent of respiratory insufficiency. Intubation will improve ventilation while delivering oxygen.

Blood cultures (**choice A**) will be crucial in guiding antibiotic selection, but these can be obtained after the child is intubated.

RSV and influenza test (**choice B**) is incorrect.

The patient is not wheezing and bronchodilators (**choice C**) will not obviate the need for mechanical ventilation.

Antibiotics (**choice D**) should be administered after the patient is stabilized. Intubation should not be delayed.

13. **The correct answer is A.** Sickle cell anemia is very common in the Mediterranean, Africa, and the Indian subcontinent. The valine to glutamine substitution in hemoglobin is the most common genetic defect underlying this illness. This amino acid substitution leads to polymerization of hemoglobin in low oxygen states, causing sickling, and hemolysis in small vessels. The increased use of iron leads to anemia, and the peripheral blood smear shows characteristic sickling of red cells. The cells will also be hypochromic secondary to the low iron content.

Hereditary spherocytosis (**choice B**) is caused by a genetic defect in the cell wall of the erythrocytes. This leads to spontaneous loss of cell wall material, which causes the red cell to assume a spherical shape. Splenic sequestration and destruction follow.

Macrocytic and hypochromic red cells (**choice C**) can be seen in megaloblastic anemia caused by folate and B_{12} deficiency.

Most forms of anemia will lead to some decrease in the iron content of the red cells (**choice D**). Thus, normochromic cells would not likely be seen in the smear.

This patient has sickle cell anemia and, depending on the severity of his illness, some abnormality should be seen on the smear (**choice E**).

14. **The correct answer is A.** The length of gestation is the single most important determinant of the neuro-developmental outcome of any very low birth weight (<1,500 g) infant. Infants born before 23 weeks' gestation have an 85% perinatal mortality rate. Mortality decreases to about 25% at 25 weeks.

The quality of prenatal care (**choice D**) also plays a significant role in the neurodevelopmental outcome of the infant. Improved obstetric care has reduced the rate of perinatal asphyxia. Antenatal administration of corticosteroids to mothers who might have preterm labor has decreased the incidence and severity of respiratory distress syndrome (hyaline membrane disease). However, the impact of prenatal care impact is not as great as that of the length of gestation.

Maternal education (**choice B**) and socioeconomic status (**choice E**) are also found to have some impact on the long-term neurodevelopmental outcome of infants. Limited financial and educational resources, as well as suboptimal home environment, may have contributed to this finding.

The outcome of the mother's previous pregnancies (**choice C**) has not been shown to have significant impact on the long-term neurodevelopmental outcome of a very low birth weight infant. Nonetheless, a previous preterm delivery is a risk factor for a future preterm pregnancy.

15. **The correct answer is A.** This child has developed lead poisoning, which can occur when toddlers eat chips of old lead paint. Lead inhibits ferrochelatase, leading to the accumulation of erythrocyte protoporphyrin. Ferrochelatase catalyzes the insertion of iron into protoporphyrin, thus inhibiting the production of hemoglobin (the high iron levels reflect the inhibition of ferrochelatase). In the presence of elevated lead levels (55 µg/dL and higher), erythrocyte protoporphyrin is an adjunct for the diagnosis. At lead levels below 55 µg/dL, erythrocyte protoporphyrin is not a very sensitive measure and its positivity declines. Therefore, erythrocyte protoporphyrin is not used as a primary screening tool. Note that basophilic stippling can be seen in both thalassemia and lead poisoning.

Cobalamin deficiency is characterized by increased levels of homocysteine and methylmalonic acid (**choice B**). It can occur in pernicious anemia, leading to megaloblastic anemia. Cobalamin deficiency can result in neurologic symptoms, paresthesia in the hands and feet, early loss of vibration and position sense, and progressive weakness.

Increased hemoglobin A_2 (**choice C**) on electrophoresis confirms the diagnosis of beta-thalassemia trait (minor). Thalassemia is an inherited defect in hemoglobin chain synthesis, resulting in red blood cell hemolysis. However, beta-thalassemia minor is asymptomatic and doesn't require treatment.

The desire to eat mud, paint, and ice is indicative of a condition called pica, which is suggestive of iron deficiency. Laboratory abnormalities characteristically show low serum ferritin and an elevated total iron binding capacity (TIBC; **choice E**).

In porphyria, heme synthesis is affected because of a defect in one of several enzymes involved in the formation of hemoglobin molecule. The characteristic laboratory abnormality is elevated levels of urinary aminolevulinic acid (ALA) and porphobilinogen (PBG; **choice D**). Children with porphyria often present with abdominal pain and sensitivity to light.

16. **The correct answer is C.** Cystic fibrosis (CF) is one of the most common genetic diseases in the white population, with an incidence of about 1:3,300. It is an autosomal-recessive disease caused by an genetic defect in the long arm of chromosome 7. CF affects mainly the pulmonary and the gastrointestinal systems. It causes recurrent, severe, lower respiratory tract infections leading to

progressive pulmonary obstructive disease. Pneumonia is one of the major causes of morbidity and mortality in these patients. Pulmonary exacerbation of CF often manifests as fever, coughing productive of purulent sputum, retraction, tachypnea, shortness of breath, and chest congestion. The primary pathogen in children is *Pseudomonas aeruginosa*. Other pathogens include *Staphylococcus aureus*, *Haemophilus influenzae*, and gram-negative bacilli, such as *Escherichia coli*. The choice of initial antibiotic therapy is based on the above possible organisms. In addition, these patients have to be treated aggressively and promptly, because recurrent untreated episodes will result in bronchiectasis and significant decreases in pulmonary function. As a general rule, gram-negative organisms need to be covered with two antibiotics. In the case of *P. aeruginosa* infections, two different IV antibiotics that have antipseudomonal activity should be used. The most common choices are ceftazidime and tobramycin; an alternative combination is ticarcillin and tobramycin. Adjunctive therapies, such as chest physical therapy and bronchodilators, are also important.

Amoxicillin-clavulanate (**choice A**) is ineffective because resistance of *P. aeruginosa* is not secondary to the production of beta-lactamase.

Azithromycin (**choice B**) is a macrolide that is not commonly used for *P. aeruginosa*, and ceftriaxone is not effective against *P. aeruginosa*.

Levofloxacin, metronidazole (**choice D**), trimethoprim-sulfamethoxazole, and vancomycin (**choice E**) are not used to treat *P. aeruginosa*, but vancomycin can be useful if methicillin-resistant *S. aureus* is recovered from the sputum culture.

17. **The correct answer is D.** Nocturnal bouts of bone pain in a child that are promptly relieved by aspirin should raise the suspicion of osteoid osteoma. The diagnosis is supported by the radiographic finding of a radiolucent nidus surrounded by a wide rim of osteosclerosis in a typical location. Typically, this benign tumor is located in the metaphyseal cortex of long bones, especially the femur and tibia, and bones of the hands and feet. Osteoid osteoma consists of haphazardly arranged bone trabeculae separated by fibrovascular tissue. It is treated with surgical resection.

Aneurysmal bone cyst (**choice A**) most commonly affects the metaphysis of the tibia and femur close to the knee in children and young adults. It is a spongy hemorrhagic multilocular cyst that expands the bone, eroding the cortex. X-ray films show an eccentric area of osteolysis, which is well demarcated and surrounded by thinned cortex. It manifests with pain and functional impairment of the adjacent joint.

Enchondroma (**choice B**), or chondroma, is a benign cartilaginous tumor that most frequently develops in the medullary cavity of phalangeal, metacarpal, and metatarsal bones. X-ray films show an osteolytic area in the diaphysis surrounded by thinned cortex. Frequently asymptomatic, it may manifest with pain.

Ewing sarcoma (**choice C**) is a malignant tumor occurring most frequently in long bones, especially the femur and humerus. Radiographically, the tumor gives rise to a moth-eaten area of osteolysis associated with a periosteal reaction and an onion-skinning pattern. It manifests with pain and systemic symptoms (e.g., fever, leukocytosis, and elevated erythrocyte sedimentation rate).

Osteosarcoma (**choice E**) is the most common primary malignant tumor of the bone. It most frequently affects males between 10 and 20 years of age. Preferential locations include the metaphysis of the tibia and femur around the knee and the upper metaphysis of the humerus. Intense local pain, swelling, and pathologic fractures are clinical manifestations. X-ray films show destruction of the cortical bone with a periosteal reaction manifesting with the *Codman triangle*.

18. **The correct answer is B.** This girl has infectious mononucleosis (IM), a common infection in adolescents caused by the Epstein-Barr virus (EBV). IM is characterized by fatigue, sore throat, fever, exudative tonsillitis, abdominal symptoms, and splenomegaly. It occurs commonly in high school and college students. Patients may have a positive Monospot test (up to 50% of patients under 4-5 years of age may have a false negative result). EBV is usually spread in saliva and is very contagious, as suggested by the name of the disease. One of the feared complications of IM is splenic enlargement and subsequent splenic rupture, an emergency that can result in death from hemorrhagic shock. In this case, the patient has a palpable spleen 3 cm below the left costal margin, which suggests marked splenomegaly. Contact sports should be absolutely forbidden in this patient. In fact, strict bed rest, or even hospitalization, may need to be considered until the splenomegaly resolves.

Abdominal ultrasound (**choice A**) is usually not necessary when the diagnosis of IM is apparent and the spleen is palpable.

A complete blood count (**choice C**) may not help to diagnose IM. EBV infection may induce some atypical lymphocytes (which along with clinical symptoms may allow a diagnosis of IM to be made). Definitive diagnosis is made with serology.

The sore throat and tonsillitis of this patient are caused by a virus (EBV), not group A *Streptococcus*; therefore, penicillin (**choice D**) is not the appropriate treatment.

The splenic enlargement in IM is only temporary and usually resolves on its own. Splenectomy (**choice E**) is inappropriate at this point.

19. **The correct answer is B.** Erythropoietic protoporphyria is the most common form of erythropoietic porphyria. The clinical presentation illustrated is typical. Patients may also present with liver function test abnormalities. Protoporphyrin concentrations in plasma and red cells are markedly increased in these cases, whereas urine porphyrins are not. Lead poisoning can also raise red cell protoporphyrin concentrations, so this may need to be excluded in a young child. Beta carotene is particularly effective in treating this type of porphyria, but it must be taken in amounts large enough to cause slight yellowing of the skin.

Acute intermittent porphyria (**choice A**) usually presents with severe abdominal pain.

Hepatoerythropoietic porphyria (**choice C**) is a very rare condition that can have a presentation similar to that in the question stem.

Porphyria cutanea tarda (**choice D**) causes chronic skin blistering.

Variegate porphyria (**choice E**) can present with either abdominal pain or chronic skin blistering.

20. **The correct answer is D.** The clinical presentation is consistent with toxic shock syndrome, which is caused by *Staphylococcus aureus* and usually occurs in women using highly absorbent tampons. Toxic shock syndrome is caused by the release of a toxin from a *S. aureus* infection, and the condition is potentially fatal. The rash spares the wrists. Treatment includes controlling the symptoms of shock, removing any device from the vagina, and administering IV antibiotics. A beta-lactamase resistant antistaphylococcal antibiotic (e.g., nafcillin, oxacillin, methicillin) should be used. Appropriate cultures should be obtained to verify the identity of the pathogen.

Amantadine (**choice A**) would be used for a viral infection such as influenza.

Gentamicin (**choice B**) provides good coverage for gram-negative rods. However, this patient has infection by a gram-positive coccus.

Ketoconazole (**choice C**) is an antifungal agent that would be used in the treatment of candidal infections.

Prednisone (**choice E**) is a steroid and would be considered if the patient was going into anaphylaxis. In that case, epinephrine should be considered as well. If the patient is believed to be in shock from adrenal insufficiency, then stress dose steroids must be given.

21. **The correct answer is C.** The girl in this clinical vignette has precocious puberty, which is defined as the appearance of pubertal signs before age 8 in girls and age 9 in boys. In young girls, it involves early development of both breasts and pubic hair. Somatic development also increases to yield a higher-than-average height and weight.

A detailed history should be obtained, including the chronology of secondary sexual development, growth patterns, intercurrent illness, and medication. Physical examination should document the child's Tanner stage of breasts and pubic hair, and growth parameters, and should include neurologic and ophthalmologic examinations. Evaluation of precocious puberty should begin with radiography of the hand and wrist to determine the bone age. If the patient has a normal bone age, she has an incomplete form of sexual precocity. Outpatient follow-up of the patient for 6 to 12 months is indicated to determine whether complete precocious puberty or another condition is developing. A delayed bone age suggests hypothyroidism. An advanced bone age requires further evaluation.

CT scans of the head and abdomen (**choice A**) and pelvic ultrasonography (**choice B**) are indicated if the bone age is advanced. Ten percent of girls with true precocious puberty have a brain tumor. CT scan of the abdomen and pelvic ultrasonography are helpful in identifying an abdominal mass such as ovarian tumor or adrenal tumor.

Reassurance to the parents (**choice D**) that the early development of both breasts and pubic hair is normal is absolutely inappropriate. Seven years of age is too young for such advanced secondary sexual development.

A thyroid stimulating hormone (TSH) level (**choice E**) should be obtained if the bone age is delayed and precocious puberty secondary to hypothyroidism is suspected. Prolonged hypothyroidism causes growth retardation and delayed bone age. Since TSH and gonadotropins have a similar structure, increased TSH levels in hypothyroidism cause subsequent stimulation of ovaries and testes.

22. **The correct answer is A.** The most common disorders of sleep in childhood include difficulty falling and staying asleep, night terrors, nightmares, and sleepwalking. The clinical presentation in this case is consistent with *night terrors*. These usually begin after 18 months of age and affect as many as 6% of children. The frequency of episodes is highly variable. Night terrors occur in the first few hours after falling asleep in concomitance with the transition from non-REM to REM sleep. Night terrors will usually disappear in late childhood. There is evidence that this is a genetic disorder, since it is frequently associated with a family history of sleep disturbances, including night terrors, sleepwalking, and

sleep-talking. Management of this condition should simply be based on explaining the benign nature of this disorder to the parents. No other measure is necessary besides preventing physical injury during the episodes if the child is very agitated.

Avoidance of TV before going to bed (**choice B**) has no benefit in preventing night terrors. Nightmares, on the other hand, may be triggered by frightening TV shows. Nightmares occur in the last part of sleep, during the REM phase. The child appears frightened during nightmares, but recognizes his caretakers and is easily consoled. After nightmares, children may not fall back asleep easily, as happens after night terrors.

Behavioral therapy (**choice C**) and pharmacologic therapy with chloral hydrate (**choice D**) have no value in either night terrors or nightmares. Short-term treatment (1-2 weeks) with chloral hydrate may be tried in children with problems falling asleep.

Benzodiazepines or tricyclic antidepressants (**choice E**) have been used occasionally for night terrors and nightmares, based on their suppression of stage 3 and 4 sleep, but studies confirming the efficacy of these agents is lacking.

23. **The correct answer is C.** The polyglandular deficiency syndromes are autoimmune and are characterized by concurrent subnormal function of several endocrine glands. This child has the type I form, which can occur in children or younger adults, with peak incidence at 12 years. Polyglandular deficiency syndrome, type I, frequently has chronic mucocutaneous candidiasis, hypoparathyroidism (as evidenced by hypocalcemia and hyperphosphatemia), and Addison disease (adrenocortical failure, as indicated by hyponatremia and low bicarbonate). Other features encountered with some frequency in this condition are gonadal failure, alopecia, malabsorption, and, much less commonly, thyroid disease, pernicious anemia, diabetes mellitus, vitiligo, and chronic active hepatitis.

Multiple endocrine neoplasia, type I (**choice A**), is characterized by parathyroid adenomas with hypercalcemia, pancreatic islet cell tumors, and pituitary adenomas.

Multiple endocrine neoplasia, type IIA (**choice B**), is characterized by medullary carcinoma of the thyroid (which might produce hypocalcemia), pheochromocytomas (which would produce hypertension), and sometimes parathyroid adenomas (which might produce hypercalcemia).

Polyglandular deficiency syndrome, type II (**choice D**), occurs in adults and is commonly characterized by adrenocortical insufficiency, thyroid disease, and diabetes mellitus.

Polyglandular deficiency syndrome, type III (**choice E**), occurs in adults. It is similar to type II but specifically lacks adrenocortical insufficiency.

24. **The correct answer is E.** The description of this skin lesion is consistent with tinea corporis, a very common cutaneous infection in children. It is one of the dermatophytoses (ringworm), which is caused by a group of related fungi including *Microsporum* and *Trichophyton* species. These fungi can invade the stratum corneum, nails, and hairs. The lesions are annular, gyrate, scaling, and discrete. Secondary bacterial infection commonly occurs. Topical antifungal agents are the initial treatment of choice. Tinea pedis represents the same infection in the lower extremities, whereas tinea manuum affects the hands.

Erythema multiforme (**choice A**) is a skin eruption caused by a hypersensitivity reaction to drugs, infections, or toxins. Skin lesions usually appear as macules, papules, wheals, and vesicobullous lesions. There is often central clearing of those skin lesions, which are therefore termed "target lesions."

Erythema nodosum (**choice B**) is characterized by tender erythematous nodules, usually in the pretibial surfaces. It is caused by hypersensitivity reactions to a spectrum of infections, drugs, and disease states.

Impetigo (**choice C**) is a superficial bacterial infection of the skin usually caused by group A streptococci. Infection is usually induced by minor trauma or abrasion to the surface of the skin with prior colonization of the bacteria.

Nummular eczema (**choice D**) is a highly pruritic idiopathic skin disorder that commonly occurs in association with asthma or allergic rhinitis.

25. **The correct answer is F.** Thalassemia refers to any genetic defect in the production of the globin chains of hemoglobin. Patients may have deficient production of the globin beta chain (beta-thalassemia) or the alpha chain (alpha-thalassemia). In the homozygous state, beta-thalassemia (i.e., thalassemia major) causes severe, transfusion-dependent anemia. In the heterozygous state, the beta-thalassemia trait (i.e., thalassemia minor) causes mild to moderate microcytic anemia. Thalassemia minor usually presents as an asymptomatic, mild microcytic anemia, and it is detected through routine blood tests. Usually, the diagnosis of beta-thalassemia minor is suggested by the presence of an isolated, mild microcytic anemia, target cells on the peripheral blood smear, and a normal red blood cell count. An elevation of hemoglobin A_2, demonstrated by electrophoresis, confirms the diagnosis of the beta-thalassemia trait. Although basophilic stippling may also be seen in lead poisoning and severe vitamin B_{12} deficiency, the basophilic stippling

in thalassemia results from the retention of ribonucleo-protein particles and mitochondrial remnants in the red blood cells.

Elliptocytosis (**choice A**) is similar to spherocytosis in that it is caused by a defect in a cell wall structural protein and will lead to elliptical red cells on the peripheral blood smear.

Hemoglobin S-C disease (**choice B**) is a variant of sickle disease in which the cells carry two abnormal beta-alleles, those for hemoglobin S and those for hemoglobin C. Patients are sometimes severely affected, but generally less so than those with HbSS disease.

The normal iron study results (ferritin and total iron binding capacity) exclude iron deficiency anemia (**choice C**) and chronic disorders as the causes of this patient's microcytic anemia. Patients with thalassemia minor will not experience improvement of their anemia with iron supplementation, and transfusion-related iron overload is a major obstacle of therapy in thalassemia major.

Lead poisoning (**choice D**) results from the ingestion or inhalation of lead-containing substances. Chronic exposure results in hypochromic microcytic anemia and basophilic stippling of the erythrocytes. Screening capillary lead levels suggest lead poisoning when they are greater than 10 µg/dL. This prompts further testing for venous lead levels.

Sickle cell anemia (**choice E**) is due to a structural defect in hemoglobin that leads to sickling of red cells in conditions of low oxygen tension, low flow, and decreased blood vessel diameter, leading to hemolysis.

26. **The correct answer is B.** Urinary tract infections (UTIs) are extremely common in children, especially girls. Failure to diagnose and properly treat UTIs may lead to serious complications, including renal scarring, hypertension, and chronic renal failure. Renal scarring due to UTIs is one of the most common causes of renal failure in children and young adults. UTIs in children younger than 2 years usually present with nonspecific signs and symptoms. Irritability, poor feeding, diarrhea, and fever are the most common manifestations. Occasionally, abdominal tenderness and malodorous urine are present. A diagnosis of UTI becomes more likely in a child with fever (especially if the temperature is higher than 39.0° C) but no identifiable sources of infection. In such cases, urinalysis and urine culture are absolutely necessary to diagnose UTI. Bagged urine specimens are frequently associated with false positive results because of bacterial contamination. Transurethral catheterization is the most widely recommended method of urine collection for UTI screening. Urinalysis and culture are the most important diagnostic investigations in children younger than 2 years who present with unexplained fever.

Microscopic examination and culture of stool (**choice C**) or abdominal radiographs (**choice A**) should not be the first diagnostic investigations in cases of fever without an obvious source. Of course, careful history and physical examination are crucial to ruling out causes of fever other than UTIs.

Renal ultrasound (**choice D**) is now considered the method of choice to identify obstructive lesions that may predispose to UTIs. Renal ultrasound is performed after a diagnosis of UTI is established.

Voiding cystourethrogram (**choice E**) is the most sensitive technique to identify vesicoureteral reflux in children who have had an episode of pyelonephritis.

27. **The correct answer is A.** This infant has "late-onset" infant pneumonia, since it occurred more than 1 week after delivery. The most common cause in this setting is coagulase-negative *Staphylococcus*, which in this setting is usually resistant to oxacillin. Cultures of blood and tracheal aspirates can usually demonstrate the organism. Vancomycin is the initial drug of choice and may sometimes be replaced by a less toxic drug after culture sensitivities become available.

Most strains of coagulase-negative *Staphylococcus* isolated in this setting are resistant, rather than sensitive, to oxacillin (**choice B**).

Group B *Streptococcus* (**choice C**) is an important cause of early onset neonatal sepsis and pneumonia.

Methicillin-sensitive (**choice E**) and methicillin-resistant (**choice D**) *Staphylococcus aureus* tend to cause skin pustules of the periumbilical and diaper areas.

28. **The correct answer is F.** Developmental dysplasia of the hip (DDH) must be diagnosed and treated early in all infants because failure to diagnose it can result in significant morbidity. Physical examination maneuvers, such as the Barlow and Ortolani maneuvers performed in this case, suggest the diagnosis, but further evaluation is undertaken with the use of ultrasound. Ultrasonography is the preferred modality for evaluating the hip and diagnosing DDH in infants younger than 6 months because it directly images the cartilaginous portions of the hip that cannot be seen on plain radiographs. Furthermore, ultrasound examination enables dynamic study of the hip with stress maneuvering.

Bone scan (**choice A**) is useful in evaluating early osteomyelitis and bone tumors. Both conditions are unlikely due to the physical examination findings in this patient.

CT scan (**choice B**) is often not the first test performed to evaluate infants for DDH. Typically, the diagnosis is confirmed with ultrasound. However, CT scan is very useful for complicated hip dislocations and postoperative hip evaluations.

Frog-leg lateral radiographs (**choice C**) describe the hip that is in flexion and externally rotated. They are performed to look for reduction if the hips are displaced or dysplastic. Plain frontal radiographs are performed more commonly, but they have no diagnostic value for DDH in infants younger than 6 months.

Joint fluid aspiration (**choice D**) has no place in the evaluation of joint laxity in this infant. It may be performed in cases where a septic joint is suspected. There are, however, no clinical findings to suggest a septic joint in this otherwise healthy infant.

Although the patient's mother has a history of tetracycline ingestion during pregnancy, tetracycline is not a known cause of DDH. Furthermore, serum tetracycline levels (**choice E**) have no diagnostic value in evaluating cartilaginous damage from the exposure.

29. **The correct answer is B.** The patient has infectious laryngotracheitis (viral croup), which is caused by the parainfluenza virus. Symptoms are often worse at night and include a characteristic barking cough. Fever is usually low grade, but temperatures as high as 104.0° F have been noted. Epiglottitis is in the differential but is rapidly progressive and is marked by the abrupt onset of high fever. Racemic epinephrine by aerosol has been shown to provide symptomatic relief by vasoconstriction and reduction of local edema. This drug should be used in the moderately ill patient since it may eliminate the need for intubation.

Albuterol (**choice A**) would help in treating the bronchospasm but will be of little use in treating croup. In mild illness, humidification may help.

Some data support the use of corticosteroids (**choice C**) in severely ill patients, although this remains controversial. Patients given dexamethasone with a repeat dose in 2 hours have had a shorter course of illness than those not given steroids.

This is a viral illness, and antibiotics (**choice D**) will be of little utility. However, acute epiglottitis is caused by *Haemophilus influenzae* type B, and more recently, group A beta-hemolytic streptococci. A third-generation cephalosporin would be appropriate therapy until culture results are known.

Intubation (**choice E**) may be needed if the respiratory distress worsens and epinephrine and steroids fail.

30. **The correct answer is A.** *Parvovirus B19* is the etiologic agent of this benign exanthem of childhood, which manifests with a "slapped cheeks" facial rash and little or no fever. This exanthema is referred to as *fifth disease* or *erythema infectiosum*. B19 parvovirus may cause red cell aplasia (aplastic anemia) in patients with AIDS or with sickle cell disease. Older people develop

symmetric polyarthritis (**choice E**), which is not seen in children.

Encephalitis (**choice B**) in immunocompromised patients may have different etiologies. Herpes simplex 1 and 2, herpes zoster, measles, and cytomegalovirus may cause encephalitis in immunocompromised patients. HIV itself frequently affects the CNS, producing subacute encephalitis in AIDS patients.

Non-Hodgkin lymphoma (**choice C**) in immunocompromised patients, especially those with AIDS, is most commonly a high-grade B-cell lymphoma. Epstein-Barr virus has been implicated in its pathogenesis.

Progressive multifocal leukoencephalopathy (PML) (**choice D**) is a complication of *JC virus*, a papovavirus that causes no disease in immunocompetent individuals. PML affects patients with AIDS or lymphomas. It is a progressive demyelinating disease in which oligodendroglial cells are destroyed by the virus.

31. **The correct answer is F.** Acute otitis media (AOM) is one of the most frequent conditions affecting infants and young children. Accumulation of exudative fluid within the middle ear results in distention of the tympanic membrane and pain. By the age of 3 years, approximately 50% of children will have had at least one episode. Therefore, all primary care physicians should become skilled in the diagnosis of AOM, which entails a careful otoscopic examination. Physical signs of AOM include bulging and fullness of the tympanic membrane with reduced tympanic membrane mobility appreciated under positive pressure.

Color change of tympanic membrane (**choice A**) is neither sensitive nor specific of AOM.

Fever (**choice B**) is a nonspecific sign that has little correlation with AOM. Children with AOM often have a concomitant upper respiratory infection that justifies temperature elevation.

Opacification of tympanic membrane (**choice C**) is no longer considered a useful diagnostic criterion for AOM. Opacification of the tympanic membrane, with resultant absent light reflex, may be also observed in normal ears.

Otalgia, or pain localized to the ear (**choice D**), is absent in a substantial number of cases, especially in infants.

Otorrhea (**choice E**) becomes apparent in only 2% of cases, following spontaneous rupture of the tympanic membrane. One should not await this sign to make a diagnosis of AOM.

32. **The correct answer is E.** The infant has hydrops fetalis (erythroblastosis fetalis), which is due to severe hemolytic anemia in the fetus or newborn. Some of these infants die in utero of anemia or during delivery of

asphyxiation, since they are so anemic that they cannot tolerate hypoxia. Survivors have many problems, including kernicterus (bilirubin levels high enough to damage the brain), congestive heart failure (high output failure secondary to anemia), hepatosplenomegaly (mostly secondary to extramedullary hematopoiesis), and generalized edema. Although, in theory, hydrops fetalis can occur with any severe intrauterine hemolytic anemia, Rh incompatibility (Rh positive fetus in an Rh negative mother) is the most common cause.

ABO incompatibility (**choice A**) can cause fetal anemia, but is usually not sufficiently severe to cause the full-blown picture of hydrops fetalis.

Beta thalassemia (**choice B**) and sickle cell anemia (**choice D**) do not usually become clinically evident until about the sixth month of life, when the infant completes the switch from making fetal type hemoglobin to adult type hemoglobin.

Congenital spherocytosis (**choice C**) can cause anemia at birth, but is usually not sufficiently severe to cause hydrops fetalis.

33. **The correct answer is B.** Brachial plexus injuries can occur in neonates who have difficult deliveries with shoulder dystocia, breech extraction, or hyperabduction of the neck. This infant has Erb's palsy, which occurs when the upper part of the brachial plexus is injured and causes the signs illustrated in the question stem. Ipsilateral paralysis of the diaphragm may also be present. Sensory changes are usually not present and, if seen, suggest a much more serious tear or avulsion of the brachial plexus. Fortunately, most cases of Erb's palsy resolve within 3 months, and the only treatment needed is a protection of the shoulder from excessive motion by immobilizing the arm across the upper abdomen and daily passive range-of-motion exercises performed gently on involved joints starting at 1 week of age. Cases persisting longer than 3 months may require MRI to evaluate both the extent of the injury and the possibility of surgical repair.

Bell's palsy (**choice A**) causes unilateral facial paralysis, typically in adults.

Klumpke paralysis (**choice C**) is due to injury to the lower part of the brachial plexus and causes paralysis of the hand and wrist, often accompanied by ipsilateral Horner syndrome (miosis and ptosis). Like Erb's palsy, it can occur during delivery and usually resolves spontaneously in less than 3 months. Passive range-of-motion exercises are the only treatment required.

Pseudobulbar palsy (**choice D**) is a degenerative disorder of the nervous system that, over a period of years (often starting in adulthood), causes muscle stiffness and weakness in muscles innervated by the lower cranial nerves and thus produces difficulty swallowing.

Spinal cord injury (**choice E**) can result from excessive traction or rotation. It presents with stillbirth or neonatal death due to respiratory failure, especially when the upper cervical cord or lower brain stem is involved. The infant may survive, with weakness, hypotonia, and, later, spasticity, all of which can be mistaken for cerebral palsy.

Supranuclear palsy (**choice F**) is a rare disorder of adults with loss of eye movements, muscular rigidity, and difficulty swallowing.

34. **The correct answer is B.** This child has infant botulism. Typically, the infant ingests *Clostridium* spores that germinate and colonize the large intestine, producing a toxin *in vivo*. This differs from adult botulism, in which preformed toxin in canned foods is ingested. All forms of botulism can be fatal and are considered medical emergencies. Honey is a notorious source of *Clostridium* spores and is not recommended for children younger than 2 years. Botulism should be suspected in previously healthy infants aged ≤12 months who are constipated and exhibit weakness in sucking, swallowing, or crying, as well as hypotonia, progressive bulbar, and extremity muscle weakness. The major risk is respiratory failure, and approximately 50% of patients require mechanical ventilation during hospitalization. Lumbar puncture and brain imaging generally yield normal results but can help differentiate among other causes of flaccid weakness. The diagnosis is confirmed by finding *C. botulinum* toxin or organisms in the feces. Antitoxin should be given as promptly as possible because early antitoxin treatment dramatically alters the course of the disease, especially if it is administered within the first 24 hours.

In general, therapy with antibiotics (**choice A**) to clear the large bowel of *Clostridium* in infant botulism is contraindicated because the treatment increases toxin release and worsens the condition. Furthermore, aminoglycosides, such as gentamicin or tobramycin, may potentiate neuromuscular blockade and are contraindicated.

Antiviral medications (**choice C**) have no role in the management of infant botulism.

The lumbar puncture performed excluded Guillain-Barré syndrome, which typically shows a high level of protein in the cerebrospinal fluid (especially later in the course of the disease) compared with the reference levels seen in botulism. Corticosteroids (**choice D**), intravenous gammaglobulin (**choice E**), and plasmapharesis (**choice F**) are all appropriate choices in the management of Guillain-Barré but are ineffective therapies in the management of infant botulism.

35. **The correct answer is C.** Vitamin A, iron, and fluoride can cause acute toxic reactions. Iron is an important ingredient in chewable vitamins. Toxic effects occur after ingestion of 30 mg/kg of body weight and include acute corrosive necrosis of the stomach and acute hepatic necrosis. Deferoxamine, an iron chelator, may be used in treatment.

Vitamin D has no significant acute toxicity in the amounts available in chewable tablets, but chronic overuse may cause renal failure (**choice A**).

The most serious toxicity of acetaminophen toxicity (**choice B**) is irreversible hepatotoxicity, which may lead to death. If the presumed ingested dose is less than 100 mg/kg of body weight, the ingestion is mild and need not be treated.

Hypervitaminosis A occurs in amounts greater than 300,000 IU, which requires ingestion of 120 chewable tablets. Toxicity leads to an acute elevation of intracranial pressure (**choice D**).

An entire bottle of 100 tablets will need to be ingested to produce fluoride toxicity (**choice E**). Fluoride should not be administered to infants younger than 6 months. From age 6 months to 3 years, a daily supplement of 0.25 mg of fluoride is recommended if the water has less than 0.3 parts per million concentration.

36. **The correct answer is D.** The immunodeficiency disease described is Bruton (X-linked) hypogammaglobulinemia. This condition is due to a defective B cell specific tyrosine kinase, coded for by the XLA gene, which facilitates proliferation of pre-B cells in the marrow. The immunologic studies detailed in the question stem are typical of this condition. Affected children are vulnerable to recurrent infections that typically begin at about 3 months of age, when the maternal IgG that crosses the placenta is exhausted. Organisms that are likely to be a particular problem in these antibody-deficient children include *Haemophilus*, pneumococcus, *Mycoplasma*, *Ureaplasma*, *Campylobacter*, *Giardia*, and enteroviruses. Septic arthritis is a common problem because there are no antibodies coating and protecting the joint surfaces; common causative organisms include *Mycoplasma*, *Haemophilus*, and pneumococcus.

The other organisms listed are important pathogens in patients with depressed cell-mediated immunity.

The fungus *Aspergillus* (**choice A**) can cause lung infections.

Herpes viruses (**choice B**) can cause severe encephalitis.

Mycobacterium (**choice C**) can cause lung infections (tuberculosis, atypical mycobacterial infections).

Toxoplasma (**choice E**) is a protozoan associated with multisystem infections.

37. **The correct answer is B.** This is hypophosphatemic rickets, also known as vitamin D-resistant rickets. This is a usually familial (often with X-linked dominant genetics) and rarely acquired abnormality of phosphate metabolism with impaired renal tubular resorption of phosphate accompanied by decreased intestinal absorption of calcium and phosphate. Vitamin D and parathyroid hormone levels are normal in these cases. The underlying biochemistry can be either impaired renal synthesis of 1,25-dihydroxy-vitamin D_3, or impaired cellular response to this substance. Some patients may have only the hypophosphatemia (particularly heterozygous females), whereas others also show severe bone disease. Some patients, as the one in the question, present with craniostenosis (premature suture fusion with resulting abnormal head shape) and seizures before 1 year of age. Other patients present in childhood with bony abnormalities that can include bowed legs, other bone deformities, pseudofractures, short stature, bone pain, and bony outgrowths at muscle attachments that may limit joint motion. This condition can now be treated with combined oral phosphate and 1,25-dihydroxy-vitamin D_3.

Fanconi syndrome (**choice A**) can have hypophosphatemia as a component, but will show a generalized impairment of renal tubular absorption that also involves glucose, amino acids, and protein.

Osteogenesis imperfecta (**choice C**) causes brittle bones that fracture easily.

Osteomalacia (**choice D**) is the term used for abnormalities of calcium and phosphate metabolism. It is similar to rickets and affects adults who have reached full stature.

Paget disease of bone (**choice E**) is a bony remodeling disease of adults.

38. **The correct answer is E.** This girl has pyelonephritis, which is an upper urinary tract infection (UTI) that involves one or both of the kidneys. Children with pyelonephritis present with high fever, dysuria, vomiting, abdominal pain, back pain, and irritability. They often have costovertebral tenderness on examination. The laboratory evaluation often shows leukocytosis. Urinalysis shows the presence of leukocyte esterase, nitrite, and increased white blood cells (>5/hpf). It is also important to note the number of squamous epithelial cells. The urine specimen is considered contaminated and is a poor specimen if there are more than 5 squamous epithelial cells per hpf. Obtaining a urine culture is also important to identify the pathogen and its susceptibility to different antibiotics. In very young children, a clean catch may not be the best method to obtain a good urine sample; straight bladder catheterization may be necessary. The most common organisms are *Escherichia coli*, *Proteus*, *Klebsiella*, and *Enterobacter* sp. Voiding cystourethrog-

raphy (VCUG) is indicated in all girls younger than 5 years with the first episode of UTI, because 25% to 30% of such patients have vesicoureteral reflux. Older girls should be evaluated by VCUG after the second episode of UTI. VCUG is also indicated in all boys who have an episode of UTI regardless of age.

CT of the abdomen and pelvis (**choice A**) is indicated when there is a suspicion of structural abnormalities of the kidneys, but not for routine evaluation of UTI.

IV pyelography (**choice B**) is used to visualize the renal calyces, ureteral anatomy, urinary diversions, and ectopic ureteroceles. It is not routinely recommended after UTI.

Plain abdominal radiography (**choice C**) has no role in the evaluation of a known UTI.

Radionuclide imaging of the kidneys (**choice D**) involves the administration of a radioactive material, usually ^{99}Tc-DTPA, to assess the blood flow and excretory function of the kidney. Areas of differential function or obstruction can be detected.

39. **The correct answer is E.** The shortened PR interval and delta waves with the slow QRS upstroke are classic ECG manifestations of Wolff-Parkinson-White (WPW) syndrome. WPW syndrome is caused by the presence of a tract bypassing the AV node, causing preexcitation and leading to paroxysmal tachycardia. Ablation of the bypass tract is the treatment of choice.

An anxiety attack (**choice A**) would present with symptoms of agitation, clamminess, and chest tightness.

Lown-Ganong-Levine syndrome (**choice B**) is similar to WPW syndrome, but the PR interval is not shortened.

Nodal reentrant tachycardia (**choice C**) would present with P waves following QRS waves.

Sinus tachycardia (**choice D**) would not present with the shortened PR interval and QRS waves.

40. **The correct answer is A.** Maternal diabetes, particularly poorly controlled type 1 diabetes mellitus, predisposes for large-for-gestational-age (LGA) infants and hypoglycemia in the neonatal period. The latter occurs because the infant's endocrine system has learned, in utero, to secrete excessively large amounts of insulin in an attempt to regulate its own blood glucose (which is set by the maternal blood). Once the infant is born, serum glucose levels fall rapidly because the mother is no longer supplying the high levels of serum glucose. Some infants are asymptomatic, whereas others may have listlessness, poor feeding, hypotonia, jitters, apneic spells, tachypnea, or seizures. Treatment is with glucose-containing intravenous fluids, which are eventually tapered as enteric feeding progresses.

Infants of mothers with hyperthyroidism, such as Graves disease (**choice B**), may also develop a form of Graves disease secondary to the maternal antibodies to thyroid hormone receptor.

Hepatic cirrhosis (**choice C**) is associated with decreased maternal fertility and high rates of spontaneous abortion.

Rheumatoid arthritis (**choice D**) may begin in pregnancy and make delivery difficult, but it does not directly affect the infant.

Seizure disorder (**choice E**) in the mother may be complicated to manage during pregnancy because of the teratogenic effects of many of the anticonvulsive drugs. However, it is not the cause of the child's seizures, which are due to the metabolic disturbance secondary to relative hyperinsulinism.

Systemic lupus erythematosus (SLE; **choice F**) in the mother rarely causes neonatal lupus due to circulating maternal autoantibodies. SLE can cause congenital heart block or cutaneous symptoms in symptomatic infants.

41. **The correct answer is G.** Serious diarrhea in infants can take two forms: bloody, mucous stools or watery, voluminous stools, which this infant has. The latter is often called secretory diarrhea and, in infants, is most commonly caused by rotavirus and enterotoxigenic *Escherichia coli*. Severe dehydration and electrolyte imbalances are very dangerous in infants because they may lead to shock, arrhythmias, intracranial hemorrhage, and renal vein thrombosis. Consequently, fluid and electrolyte therapy is the primary and most urgent step. This can be done orally in less ill infants, but it may require peripheral or central intravenous therapy (or even intraosseous administration if a line cannot be started) in those who are more ill.

Campylobacter jejuni (**choice A**), enteroinvasive *Escherichia coli* (**choice C**), *Salmonella* species (**choice H**), and *Shigella* species (**choice I**) are all invasive bacteria that infect the large bowel and cause bloody, mucus-laden diarrhea. Examination of the stool in enteroinvasive infections of the large bowel reveals leukocytes, predominantly neutrophils, which in this case were absent. Stool leukocyte count is usually not elevated in viral-mediated and toxin-mediated diarrhea.

Cryptosporidium (**choice B**) is a parasite that can cause severe diarrhea in immunocompromised and immunosuppressed individuals. There is no significant history to suggest that this child is immunosuppressed, and other more common causes of infant diarrhea should be suspected first.

Pancreatic insufficiency (**choice D**), seen in cystic fibrosis, may be a cause of chronic diarrhea when children present with frequent passage of bulky, foul-smelling, oily stools and poor growth pattern. This infant's growth is normal for his age despite his premature birth, and there is nothing to suggest a chronic cause of his acute presentation of diarrhea.

Giardia lamblia (**choice E**) would be an unlikely cause of diarrhea in this child because of the absence of protozoa in the examined stool. *Giardia* typically causes flatus-associated, foul-smelling stools that float, suggesting fat malabsorption.

Lactose intolerance (**choice F**) can cause diarrhea in children after the ingestion of milk. These children often will not gain weight and may even present with failure to thrive. Characteristically, the diarrhea associated with lactose intolerance resolves with fasting. Infants may have temporary lactase deficiency following enteric infections or abdominal surgery, but this deficiency is unlikely to be the primary cause of this child's diarrhea.

42. **The correct answer is A.** This is atopic dermatitis. The presentation illustrated is typical for young children. Secondary bacterial infections and regional lymphadenitis may complicate the clinical picture. The dermatitis often improves by age 3 or 4 years, but periodic exacerbations may continue to occur into adulthood. Older children and adults tend to have more localized lesions, typically with erythema and lichenification. Common sites of involvement in older children and adults include the antecubital and popliteal fossas, eyelids, neck, and wrists. Once the diagnosis is made, the physician must remember not to make the mistake of automatically attributing all subsequent skin lesions the children develop to the atopic dermatitis, since they remain vulnerable to all other dermatologic diseases as well.

Cellulitis (**choice B**) is a streptococcal, or less commonly staphylococcal, infection causing acute inflammation of subcutaneous tissues associated with local erythema, tenderness, frequently lymphangitis, and regional lymphadenopathy. The skin is usually warm, edematous, and erythematous, and may exhibit a "peau d'orange" (orange peel) appearance.

Contact dermatitis (**choice C**) can resemble atopic dermatitis, but the long history illustrated in the question stem would not be typical of this condition.

Lichen simplex chronicus (**choice D**) is characterized by itchy, dry skin that may progress to well-demarcated, hyperpigmented, lichenified plaques of oval, irregular, or angular shape.

Seborrheic dermatitis (**choice E**) is an inflammatory scaling disease, usually of the scalp and face, that may initially resemble atopic dermatitis in infants. Unlike atopic dermatitis, however, it tends to remain confined to the head and scalp. (The diaper area may be initially involved, but this usually clears with time.)

43. **The correct answer is D.** A technetium bone scan is very effective in diagnosing osteomyelitis in its earliest stages. Technetium uptake reflects osteoblastic activity and skeletal vascularity, so this method is quite sensitive. However, it will give false positive results for fractures, tumors, infarction, or neuropathic osteopathy, and will give false negative results if the vascular supply is impeded in some way.

Blood count monitoring (**choice A**) is helpful in monitoring the progress and response to treatment but does not aid in the absolute diagnosis of osteomyelitis.

CT scan (**choice B**) would not be as sensitive as an MRI scan, and a technetium scan would be better than either.

Gallium scans (**choice C**) are effective in demonstrating response to treatment, but not in the initial diagnosis of osteomyelitis.

An x-ray of the foot (**choice E**) will not show osteomyelitis for approximately 1 week.

44. **The correct answer is E.** The diagnosis should be easy to make, since the "machinery-like murmur" is classic for patent ductus arteriosus. In premature infants who are not in failure, closure can be achieved medically with the use of indomethacin. Nonpremature infants are less likely to respond, and infants in overt heart failure cannot wait at all and need immediate surgical correction.

Indomethacin (**choice A**), as noted above, is ideal for the premature infant who is not in failure.

Digitalis and diuretics (**choice B**) will indeed be used as the infant is rushed to surgery, but, as the question is framed, they alone cannot correct the problem.

The infant does not have either an atrial septal defect (**choice C**) or a ventricular septal defect (**choice D**). Neither of those gives a continuous machinery-like murmur or produces bounding peripheral pulses.

45. **The correct answer is A.** Physiologic leukorrhea is the most likely diagnosis. It frequently occurs a few months prior to menarche. Menarche may occur at Tanner stage III, usually about 1 year following the peak height velocity. The onset of menarche seems imminent in this girl. The pH of vaginal fluid falls below 4 with the onset of puberty. Certain vaginal infections alter the pH. For example, both trichomoniasis and bacterial vaginosis are characterized by a pH of greater than 5. There is no evidence of abnormal vaginal discharge, either by amount, color, or odor. No inflammation of the perineum is evident.

Discussion of hygiene and possible irritants (**choice B**) is particularly appropriate for prepubertal girls who have symptoms of dysuria or perineal irritation from bubble baths. This does not describe this patient.

There are no indications at this time to perform a pelvic examination (**choice C**). The girl does not have the signs or symptoms of abnormal discharge or vulvovaginitis. A history of sexual contact was not obtained and seems unlikely in this case.

Clotrimazole (**choice D**), miconazole, terconazole, and butoconazole are all commonly used to treat candidal infections. *Candida* or monilial vaginitis is characterized by clumpy white discharge, described as cottage cheese in appearance. Microscopically, pseudohyphae are seen. None of these are present in this patient.

Sitz baths and a mild strength hydrocortisone cream (**choice E**) may be helpful in soothing an irritated or mildly inflamed vulva. These are sometimes recommended as treatment for types of dermatitis, such as contact dermatitis, that involve the perineum. This is not necessary in this patient.

46. **The correct answer is B.** The patient is losing blood, most likely in the retroperitoneum, as a result of traumatic injury. Her blood pressure is decreased, and she is compensating with an increased pulse. The immediate response is repletion of fluids to counter the hypovolemic shock the patient is experiencing. Perfusion to the brain and heart is of utmost importance.

The broken arm will need to corrected after she has been surgically stabilized. The emergency option is to splint the arm (**choice A**). However, an orthopedic surgeon should evaluate for nerve and vessel damage as well.

Although administration of vasopressors may correct the blood pressure, it is not addressing the underlying problem (**choice C**). The patient has lost blood volume, and pressors will simply clamp down blood supply to the viscera and limbs, leading to ischemic damage. Fluid should be given first, with pressors as an adjunct.

The patient is probably losing large quantities of blood and will need replenishment soon (**choice D**). However, the blood should not be replenished too quickly, as this may lead to worsening shock. Thus, the patient should first be stabilized with fluids; then, blood should be replenished.

The underlying problem is a retroperitoneal bleed, and exploratory laparotomy (**choice E**) will be needed to correct the problem. This is a surgical treatment, however, and it is ideal to stabilize the patient's hemodynamics before the surgical correction.

47. **The correct answer is E.** Ewing sarcoma (ES) is the second most common bone cancer in childhood and adolescence. It has a peak age incidence during adolescent years. It rarely occurs in blacks and is more prevalent in boys than girls. ES may have histopathologic features characteristic of neural differentiation; ES is thought to be a tumor of neural origin, whereas most bone tumors are thought to be of mesodermal origin. The tumor category of ES has recently been expanded to include more neural tumors, such as peripheral primitive neuroectodermal tumor. Like other bone tumors, ES is associated with a consistent chromosomal translocation, t(11;22)(q24;q12), which occurs in about 90% to 95% of cases.

ES is treated with a multimodal approach, including surgery, chemotherapy, and radiation therapy. ES is a highly radiosensitive tumor. In addition, most patients usually undergo surgery following induction chemotherapy. Chemotherapy is used because most patients who receive local therapy alone will do poorly. Osteosarcoma is treated with chemotherapy and surgery but not radiation. Unlike ES, osteosarcoma is radioresistant.

48. **The correct answer is B.** Low-grade reflux can be expected to resolve as the child grows, and the ureteral implantation into the bladder becomes more oblique. While waiting for that to happen, however, the kidney must be protected against infection. Long-term, low-dose antibacterial therapy is thus recommended.

The problem is caused by an abnormally short intramural ureteral tunnel rather than bladder neck obstruction. The use of alpha blockers (**choice A**) is thus not indicated.

The goal of therapy is to protect and preserve renal function. To do a nephrectomy (**choice C**) would do the opposite.

Spontaneous resolution is expected, but simple reassurance and observation (**choice D**) would leave the kidney unprotected.

Surgical correction (**choice E**) is needed in more severe cases in which spontaneous resolution is not likely to occur.

49. **The correct answer is F.** Osgood-Schlatter disease is an example of an overuse syndrome associated with physical exertion. It usually occurs around the pubertal growth spurt (ages 10 to 15) before skeletal maturity, when the quadriceps has enlarged but the apophysis has not yet fused with the tibia. The disease results in partial avulsion fracture through the ossification center. Patients complain of pain, tenderness, and a lump over the tibial tubercle. Pain is worsened with contraction of the quadriceps against resistance, and it may be bilateral in some patients. It is a benign, self-limiting condition with rest, immobilization, and gradual return to activity.

50. **The correct answer is A.** Acute lymphocytic leukemia (ALL), or lymphoblastic leukemia, is a primary neoplasm of the bone marrow. The malignant cells

are immature lymphoblastic cells. Children with ALL generally present with signs and symptoms of bone marrow infiltration and extramedullary disease. Major features are symptoms of bone marrow failure, including anemia, thrombocytopenia, and neutropenia, all of which manifest as fatigue, pallor, petechiae, bleeding, and fever. Additionally, lymphadenopathy and hepatosplenomegaly can reflect leukemic spread. Other signs and symptoms of leukemia include weight loss, bone pain, and dyspnea. The physical examination of children with ALL reflects bone marrow infiltration and extramedullary disease. Patients present with pallor as a result of anemia, petechiae, and bruising secondary to thrombocytopenia, as well as signs of infection because of neutropenia. In addition, leukemic spread may be seen as lymphadenopathy and hepatosplenomegaly.

Chondromalacia patellae (**choice B**) is the softening of the articular cartilage of the patella. The usual cause is overuse. Chondromalacia patellae is a significant cause of anterior knee pain in teenage girls. Symptoms include retropatellar pain that is worse upon rising from prolonged sitting or when climbing stairs. There may be some degree of patella misalignment, and there is a grating sensation on knee extension. Treatment involves rest and nonsteroidal anti-inflammatory drugs (NSAIDs).

Ewing sarcoma (**choice C**) is a malignant small cell tumor of long bones that is more common in males less than 20 years of age. It most often occurs around the knee joint, diaphysis of the femur, humerus, tibia, pelvis, and ribs. Ewing sarcoma may mimic an infection, with localized swelling, redness, heat, and fever. There may be both elevated white blood cell count and erythrocyte sedimentation rate.

Pediatrics: **Test Two**

1. A 13-year-old girl returns to her physician for follow-up of a strep throat, for which she had been treated 3 weeks previously. After performing a throat culture, the physician asks how school is going. There is dead silence. Her mother says that her daughter has missed the last 4 weeks of school. Which of the following is the most appropriate initial step in management?

   (A) Contract with the girl to go back to school as you explore the problem

   (B) Write a medical excuse for her until the throat culture results come back

   (C) Tell them you must report her to the school authorities for truancy

   (D) Send the mother for supportive counseling

   (E) Send the girl for psychotherapy

2. A 1-year old child is brought in for a well baby checkup. His parents report that he has been of good health and began walking a few weeks earlier. They are concerned that he tends to bump into things and falls more than his older sister did. Family history is significant for retinoblastoma. On examination, the pediatrician notes leukocoria of the left eye. No significant lymphadenopathy is present, and there is no enlargement of the liver or spleen. The child's height and weight are normal for his age. A complete ophthalmologic examination reveals retinoblastoma in the child's left eye, and enucleation is performed. This patient has the highest lifetime risk for which of the following conditions?

   (A) Glaucoma

   (B) Glioblastoma

   (C) Malignant melanoma

   (D) Osteosarcoma

   (E) Squamous cell carcinoma

3. A 4-day-old female infant presents to the emergency department with vomiting and abdominal distention. The mother states that the vomitus was green. The infant also has had difficulty feeding and has been hard to console. The mother had an uncomplicated pregnancy. The infant passed meconium within 12 hours after birth. She also had several small, seedy, yellowish stools each day since birth. On physical examination, she is very irritable. Her anterior fontanelle is slightly depressed. Her abdomen is distended. Which of the following is the most likely diagnosis?

   (A) Allergic reaction to formula

   (B) Gastroesophageal reflux disease

   (C) Hirschsprung disease

   (D) Meconium ileus

   (E) Midgut volvulus

4. An 8-year-old boy presents to the pediatrician's office with a headache for the past 3 weeks. His mother also states that he has been more tired and has had frequent nose bleeding for the past month. On physical examination, his height and weight are both below the fifth percentile for his age. His blood pressure is 152/86 mm Hg in all four extremities. His pulse is 74/min, and respirations are 16/min. His heart examination is normal with no murmur. His peripheral pulses are strong and symmetric. Urinalysis and serum electrolytes are ordered. Which of the following is the most appropriate next step in diagnosis?

   (A) 24-hour urine creatinine and protein

   (B) Blood urea nitrogen and creatinine concentration

   (C) Plasma and urine catecholamine levels

   (D) Serum aldosterone level

   (E) Serum cortisol level

KAPLAN) MEDICAL

5. An infant is brought to the office for health maintenance visit. On examination, the infant turns when her name is called. She is able to say "mama." Her mother mentions that she also says "dada" at home. She is able to look for her mother when she gets frightened. She also waves bye-bye to the doctor when the doctor steps out of the examination room. What age of this child is most consistent with these developmental milestones?

(A) 3 months

(B) 5 months

(C) 7 months

(D) 9 months

(E) 11 months

6. A 2-week-old infant is noted to be jaundiced. The baby's stools are pale, and his urine is darkly colored. Physical examination demonstrates hepatomegaly. Serum studies show elevations of AST, ALT, conjugated bilirubin, and unconjugated bilirubin. By 2 months of age, the baby is notably irritated by pruritus, has retarded growth, and has visible dilated veins in the periumbilical area. Ultrasound fails to demonstrate a gallbladder. Which of the following is the most likely diagnosis?

(A) Alpha-1-antitrypsin deficiency

(B) Biliary atresia

(C) Cystic fibrosis

(D) Hepatitis B

(E) Hepatitis C

(F) Toxoplasmosis

7. A 3-year-old girl with a ventricular septal defect (VSD) presents to the emergency department after a 15-minute focal seizure of her left arm and leg. A brief history reveals that the child has no known seizure disorder and has been having a low-grade fever at home for about 4 days. She also has been less active and has had poor appetite. On physical examination, her temperature is 40.2° C (104.3° F), and her pulse is 82/min. She is not responsive to her name, but she is responsive to painful stimuli with withdrawal of her extremities. Cardiac examination is significant for a grade 3 systolic murmur best heard at the left lower sternal border. Neurologic examination reveals anisocoria with a dilated right pupil. After stabilization, which of the following is the most appropriate next step in diagnosis?

(A) CT of the brain

(B) ECG

(C) Electroencephalography

(D) MRI of the brain

(E) Complete blood count and blood culture

(F) Lumbar puncture

8. A mother brings her 7-year-old son to the clinic because, over the past several days, his urine has become pink and his eyes have looked puffy. About 2 weeks ago, he missed school because of fever and a sore throat. On examination, the boy's blood pressure is 130/85 mm Hg, his eyelids and scrotum appear puffy, and he has 1+ tibial edema. No rashes are noted. Which of the following is the most likely diagnosis?

(A) Acute poststreptococcal glomerulonephritis

(B) Hemolytic-uremic syndrome

(C) Henoch-Schönlein purpura

(D) Nephrotic syndrome

(E) Vesicoureteral reflux

9. A 3-month-old infant is brought to the emergency department for severe vomiting over the past 6 hours. The mother tells the physician that she has vomited at least four times during this period. She also noticed the infant was having difficulty feeding for 2 days. On examination, she is very fussy, and there is a swelling over the left side of the head. CT of the head shows a skull fracture of the left parietal bone with no evidence of intracranial damage. The mother explains that the baby rolled off the sofa onto the floor yesterday. Which of the following is the most appropriate next step in management?

(A) Discharge the patient home with instructions concerning post-concussion symptoms

(B) Monitor the infant for 12 hours for signs of increased intracranial pressure, discharge the patient home if asymptomatic thereafter

(C) Obtain a neurosurgical consultation for the skull fracture

(D) Obtain a skeletal survey

(E) Repeat the CT scan of the head in 24 hours

10. A 9-month-old, chubby, healthy-appearing boy is brought to the pediatrician because of episodes of colicky abdominal pain and blood-tinged stools. The pain lasts from 1 to 10 minutes and causes the infant to double up; he then appears normal until his next bout of colic. During the examination, the infant has another episode, at which time a vague mass can be felt on the right side of the abdomen, and the right lower quadrant has an "empty" feeling to deep palpation. Which of the following is the most appropriate initial step in management?

(A) Barium/air contrast enema

(B) Colonoscopy

(C) Reassure the parents and arrange 24-hour follow-up

(D) Upper gastrointestinal endoscopy

(E) Exploratory surgery

11. A 12-year-old boy presents with an intensely pruritic rash for 3 days. He just went on a camping trip, during which he wore only short-sleeve shirts and short pants. His temperature is 37.6° C (99.7° F), blood pressure is 96/62 mm Hg, pulse is 65/min, and respirations are 12/min. There are numerous erythematous papules and vesicles on both arms and legs. Most of them are in a linear array. Which of the following is the most appropriate pharmacotherapy?

(A) Oral cephalexin

(B) Oral prednisone

(C) Topical diphenhydramine

(D) Topical mupirocin

(E) Topical 1% hydrocortisone

12. A premature infant has a difficult delivery with episodes of arrhythmia and suspected hypoxia-ischemia. After the delivery, the infant is lethargic and has periods of apnea. Intracranial hemorrhage is suspected. No obvious head trauma is noted. Cranial ultrasound identifies blood within the ventricles. Which of the following structures is the most likely source of the hemorrhage?

(A) Bridging veins of the skull

(B) Cerebral cortex

(C) Germinal matrix

(D) Middle meningeal artery

(E) Thalamus

(F) Vessels of the circle of Willis

13. A 6-year-old boy has had a fever for 8 days. He just finished a 5-day course of amoxicillin for otitis media. On examination, his temperature is 38.6° C (101.4° F). He has meningismus and palsy of the left sixth cranial nerve. Cerebrospinal fluid (CSF) analysis reveals 200 white cells per mL with 80% lymphocytes and 20% polymorphonuclear leukocytes, glucose of 18 mg/dL, protein of 260 mg/dL, and a negative Gram stain. There is basilar enhancement without focal lesions on CT. Which of the following CSF tests will most likely identify the cause of meningitis?

   (A) Antigen test for *Cryptococcus*

   (B) Bacterial culture

   (C) Culture for mycobacteria

   (D) Latex agglutination test for pneumococcus

   (E) Test for *Treponema pallidum*

14. A previously healthy 5-month-old boy has been irritable and has had a decreased oral intake for 2 days. His rectal temperature is 37.4° C (99.3° F), pulse is 220/min, and respirations are 50/min. The radial and posterior tibial pulses are diminished with good brachial and femoral pulses. ECG shows tachycardia; QRS complexes are narrow without preceding P waves. Which of the following is the most appropriate initial step in management?

   (A) Administer adenosine intravenously

   (B) Administer verapamil intravenously

   (C) Apply an ice-filled plastic bag to the entire face for 5 to 10 seconds

   (D) Cardiac pacing

   (E) Perform synchronized direct current cardioversion

15. A 3-month-old boy is brought to the pediatrician because of a red growth on his arm. The pregnancy had been uncomplicated, and the infant has been meeting all development milestones. He has been healthy so far and has received all scheduled immunizations. He is currently being breast-fed. His skin was clear at birth, but when he was 2 months old, his mother noted a light red growth on his arm. Within the past month, it has increased in size and has turned bright red. Which of the following is the most appropriate treatment for this disorder?

   (A) Observation

   (B) Topical corticosteroids

   (C) Argon laser therapy

   (D) Radiation therapy

   (E) Surgery

16. A 5-year-old girl is being evaluated for generalized swelling. Her blood pressure is 98/60 mm Hg. Her laboratory results show:

Creatinine	0.7 mg/dL
Albumin	1.6 g/dL
Cholesterol	360 mg/dL
Triglycerides	400 mg/dL
C3 complement	120 mg/dL (normal, >80 mg/dL)
Antinuclear antibody	Negative
Urinalysis	1 RBC/hpf protein 400 mg/dL

Which of the following is the most likely diagnosis?

   (A) Membranoproliferative glomerulonephritis

   (B) Membranous glomerulopathy

   (C) Minimal change disease

   (D) Postinfectious acute glomerulonephritis

   (E) Systemic lupus erythematosus

17. A 13-year-old girl presents with a 1-week history of a sore throat and a nonproductive cough. She has been previously healthy and has not been exposed to any other sick person. She has not been taking any medications. On examination, she has normal oxygen saturation and a low-grade fever. X-ray shows perihilar infiltrates. The remainder of the examination is unremarkable. Which of the following is the most appropriate pharmacotherapy?

    (A) Amoxicillin

    (B) Cefazolin

    (C) Erythromycin/azithromycin

    (D) Metronidazole

    (E) Trimethoprim-sulfamethoxazole

18. A 10-year-old girl is evaluated by a pediatrician. She is already 5′8″ tall and is taller than other members of her family were at this age. Her arms are disproportionately long compared with her trunk, and her sternum is outwardly displaced. Her joints are hyperextensible, particularly at the knees. Ocular examination demonstrates dislocation of one lens. Based on the most likely diagnosis, which of the following conditions is the most appropriate screening method to prevent morbidity?

    (A) Bone density

    (B) CT scan of the pituitary stalk

    (C) Dexamethasone suppression test

    (D) Echocardiography

    (E) Electrocardiogram

    (F) Glucose tolerance test

19. A 7-year-old boy is brought to the physician because of recurrent headaches. The child feels nauseated before and during each attack, and derives some relief from lying down in a dark room. Noises, bright light, and fatigue seem to trigger the episodes. The child frequently complains of headaches at school, and his mother has been occasionally compelled to take him home. The mother is worried about the possibility of a serious illness. She reports that the child's father has similar headaches. The child's growth is normal, and a neurologic examination fails to reveal any abnormality. Which of the following is the most likely diagnosis?

    (A) Brain tumor

    (B) Cluster headache

    (C) Conduct disorder

    (D) Migraine

    (E) Tension headache

20. A 12-year-old boy is brought to the emergency department with a temperature of 39.1° C (102.4° F) at home, difficulty speaking, and odynophagia for 2 days. Physical examination reveals marked erythema of the right tonsil pillar and edema of the uvula with deviation to the left. In addition to anaerobic bacteria, which of the following organisms is most likely to be isolated from a tonsillar pillar aspirate?

    (A) Beta-hemolytic *Streptococcus*

    (B) *Enterococcus*

    (C) *Haemophilus influenzae* type b

    (D) *Staphylococcus aureus*

    (E) *Streptococcus pneumoniae*

21. A term neonate is noted at birth to have multiple structural defects, many of which are midline in location. He has a bilateral cleft lip and palate, very small eyes with fissures of the iris, shallow supraorbital ridges, and slanted palpebral fissures. His ears are malformed and low set. Both hands have six fingers and a single simian crease, and his feet are shaped like the runner of a rocking chair. There is no family history of congenital abnormalities. At 1 month of age, he dies from heart failure. Which of the following neurologic abnormalities was likely to have been present in this infant?

    (A) Anencephaly

    (B) Encephalocele

    (C) Hydranencephaly

    (D) Holoprosencephaly

    (E) Porencephaly

22. A 4-year-old boy presents to the emergency department with generalized tonic-clonic seizures. On physical examination, the child is noted to be lethargic. His temperature is 37.4° C (99.3° F), blood pressure is 100/60 mm Hg, pulse is 72/min, and respirations are 16/min. His oral mucosa is moist, and there is no peripheral edema. Laboratory tests show:

Blood:

Sodium	120 mEq/L
Potassium	4.2 mEq/L
Chloride	96 mEq/L
Bicarbonate	20 mEq/L
Blood urea nitrogen	9.6 mg/dL
Creatinine	0.4 mg/dL
Glucose	88 mg/dL

Urine:

Sodium	55 mEq/L
Potassium	16 mEq/L
Osmolality	530 mOsmol/kg

Which of the following is the most likely diagnosis?

(A) Acute renal failure

(B) Addison disease

(C) Congestive heart failure

(D) Hyponatremic dehydration

(E) Syndrome of inappropriate antidiuretic hormone secretion (SIADH)

23. A 1-month-old, previously healthy infant develops forceful projectile vomiting. No bile is seen in the vomitus. After the infant feeds, gastric peristaltic waves are visible crossing the epigastrium from left to right. Several minutes later, the projectile vomiting occurs. Which of the following is the most likely diagnosis?

(A) Diaphragmatic hernia

(B) Duodenal atresia

(C) Esophageal atresia

(D) Hypertrophic pyloric stenosis

(E) Meconium plug syndrome

24. A 2-month-old girl presents to her pediatrician's office for well-child care. Her mother complains of excessive tearing of the baby's left eye for the past 4 weeks. Each morning, a yellow crusty discharge is noted along the lashes of the left eye. The conjunctiva appears uninflamed. The right eye is not affected. On physical examination, the infant is otherwise well and achieving adequate weight gain on an exclusive breast milk diet. She is developmentally appropriate, including visually tracking 180 degrees. Which of the following is the most likely diagnosis?

(A) Dacryostenosis

(B) Gonococcal conjunctivitis

(C) Normal infant eye

(D) Viral conjunctivitis

(E) Vitamin A deficiency

25. A term neonate is small for dates and has a small head. Further physical examination of the infant demonstrates small eyes with short palpebral fissures, a flattened nose, and abnormal palmar creases. With which of the following maternal conditions is this presentation most likely associated?

(A) Alcohol abuse

(B) Cirrhosis

(C) Cocaine abuse

(D) Diabetes mellitus

(E) Hypothyroidism

26. A pediatrician is called to the delivery room because a full-term infant has developed cyanosis and respiratory distress immediately after birth. A brief examination of the infant reveals cyanosis on room air not completely relieved by oxygen administered by mask, subcostal and intercostal retractions, absent air entry on the left with audible bowel sounds in the left chest, and poor air entry on the right chest. The heart is best heard in the right hemithorax; the abdomen is flat without organomegaly. Which of the following is the most likely diagnosis?

    (A) Congenital diaphragmatic hernia

    (B) Hyaline membrane disease

    (C) Meconium aspiration

    (D) Pneumonia

    (E) Tracheoesophageal fistula

27. A blood type B infant born to a blood type O mother has clinically significant fetal-maternal blood group incompatibility with mild anemia and a weakly positive Coombs test. The infant develops jaundice a few hours after birth, with a bilirubin (measured at 12 hours after birth) of 12 mg/dL (predominately unconjugated) compared with 3.5 mg/dL in cord blood. The physician is concerned that the rising bilirubin levels will damage the infant's nervous system. Which of the following sites is most vulnerable to this injury?

    (A) Basal ganglia

    (B) Cerebellum

    (C) Cerebral cortex

    (D) Peripheral nerve

    (E) Spinal cord

28. Within 8 hours after birth, an infant has "excessive salivation." Physical examination reveals that she has an imperforate anus, with a small fistula to the vagina. A small, soft nasogastric tube is inserted, and the infant is taken to x-ray. The film shows the tube coiled back on itself in the upper chest, and a normal gas pattern in the gastrointestinal tract. There are no apparent abnormalities of the radius or the vertebral bodies. Which of the following is the most appropriate next step in management?

    (A) Renal sonogram and echocardiogram

    (B) Barium swallow

    (C) Placement of a gastrostomy tube

    (D) Diverting colostomy

    (E) Surgical repair of esophageal atresia

29. An 8-year-old girl is brought to the pediatrician's office for evaluation of new onset swelling around the eyes. Physical examination reveals periorbital, sacral, and pretibial edema; her blood pressure is 96/64 mm Hg. The rest of her physical examination is normal. Which of the following is the most appropriate initial diagnostic study?

    (A) Levels of liver enzymes

    (B) Radiography of the chest

    (C) Transthoracic echocardiography

    (D) Ultrasonography of the kidneys

    (E) Urinalysis

30. A 3-month-old girl is brought to the pediatrician for a scheduled visit. She has been meeting all development milestones but has been vomiting after each feeding. The infant weighed 3 kg (6 lb 10 oz) at birth and now weighs 6 kg (13 lb 3 oz). She does not have diarrhea and is afebrile. The remainder of the physical examination is unremarkable. Which of the following is the most likely cause of this patient's vomiting?

    (A) Adrenogenital syndrome

    (B) Child abuse

    (C) Inborn error of metabolism

    (D) Overfeeding

    (E) Pyloric stenosis

31. A neonate is noted to have aniridia of the right eye on physical examination. He was born by spontaneous vaginal delivery after an uncomplicated full-term pregnancy. The remainder of the physical examination is normal. Which of the following is the most appropriate next step before the infant is released from the hospital?

    (A) An abdominal ultrasound

    (B) An echocardiogram

    (C) A neurology consult

    (D) A rapid plasmin reagin (RPR) test

    (E) IV antibiotics

32. A 3-day-old, full-term baby boy is brought into the emergency department because of feeding intolerance and bilious vomiting. X-rays films show multiple dilated loops of small bowel and a "ground glass" appearance in the lower abdomen. The mother has cystic fibrosis. Which of the following diagnostic tests would also have therapeutic value?

    (A) Barium enema

    (B) Gastrografin enema

    (C) Colonoscopy

    (D) Endoscopic retrograde cholangiopancreatogram (ERCP)

    (E) Full thickness rectal biopsy

33. A 17-year-old girl presents with a 4-week history of intermittent fever, increasing fatigue, generalized myalgia, and swelling of both her knees and ankles. There is a fine erythematous rash on her back, and she has swollen knees and ankles; the remainder of her physical examination is unremarkable. Initial laboratory evaluation shows:

Leukocytes	11,400 cells/mm^3
Hemoglobin	8.8 g/dL
Blood urea nitrogen	4 mg/dL
Creatinine	1.4 mg/dL
Glucose	98 mg/dL
C3 complement	36 mg/dL (normal >80 mg/dL)
Antinuclear antibody titer	1:3,200
Anti-double-stranded DNA titer	1:640
Antineutrophil cytoplasmic antibodies	Negative
Urinalysis	Moderate hematuria (50 RBC/hpf)
	Moderate proteinuria (400 mg/dL)

Which of the following is the most likely diagnosis?

    (A) Giant cell arteritis

    (B) Henoch-Schönlein purpura

    (C) Polyarteritis nodosa

    (D) Systemic lupus erythematosus

    (E) Wegener granulomatosis

34. A 3-year-old boy is admitted for seizure-like activity. He has been a healthy child and has been meeting all development milestones. His immunization schedule is up-to-date. Examination is notable for an erythematous throat and fever. His convulsions require IV administration of a benzodiazepine. Serum analysis reveals a normal white cell count with mild basophilic stippling. The lumbar puncture reveals elevated CSF pressure. Head CT scan is notable for cerebral edema. Which of the following is the next diagnostic step?

    (A) Antistreptolysin O titer

    (B) Electroencephalography

    (C) Protoporphyrin level

    (D) Rapid slide (Monospot) test

    (E) Spinal fluid culture

35. A 2-week postmature neonate exhibits severe respiratory distress immediately after birth. Previously, green-tinged meconium was noted in the amniotic fluid. Which of the following is the most appropriate next step in management?

    (A) Chest x-ray

    (B) Suctioning of the mouth and nasopharynx

    (C) Oxygen supplementation by face mask

    (D) Intubation with mechanical ventilation

    (E) Emergency tracheostomy

36. A 29-year-old woman presents to the delivery room in labor at 35 weeks' gestation with a temperature of 40.0° C (104.0° F). She lives on a dairy farm and is in the habit of drinking unpasteurized milk from her cows before sending it to the dairy. For the past 3 days she has been unable to attend to her chores because of fever, headache, mild diarrhea, and a general feeling of illness. When her amniotic membranes rupture, the fluid is dark, cloudy, and brownish-green. At birth, the infant has no malformations or edema, but is in severe respiratory distress. Which of the following is the most likely diagnosis?

    (A) Congenital syphilis

    (B) Congenital toxoplasmosis

    (C) Fetal hydrops

    (D) Neonatal herpes

    (E) Neonatal listeriosis

37. A 5-year-old girl is brought to medical attention by her parents 12 hours after the onset of generalized tonic-clonic seizures. She never had similar episodes in the past. The girl is otherwise healthy. Her temperature is 37.0° C (98.6° F). Physical examination is unremarkable. There is no evidence that the girl had a fever at the onset of the convulsive episode. The parents fear that seizures may damage the child's brain and may eventually recur. Which of the following is the most appropriate next step in management?

    (A) Provide reassurance to child and family

    (B) Admit patient to the hospital for further evaluation

    (C) Perform electroencephalographic studies

    (D) Perform CT/MRI studies of the brain

    (E) Start antiepileptic medication

38. A neonate is markedly edematous and dies 1 hour after birth. A diagnosis of hydrops fetalis is made after the hematocrit on cord blood is demonstrated to be 5%. The erythrocytes in a smear from the cord blood are markedly hypochromatic. The mother is Rh positive and is known to have alpha-thalassemia trait. The thalassemia status of the father is unknown. Alpha-thalassemia is the suspected cause of the infant's hydrops. Which of the following hemoglobins would most likely be markedly elevated in this infant's blood if this diagnosis were correct?

    (A) HbBarts

    (B) HbC

    (C) HbGlower 2

    (D) HbH

    (E) HbS

39. A 1-year-old girl is brought to the emergency department by her mother because the child's "eyes and feet are dancing." On physical examination, the girl is well developed and in no acute distress. Her temperature 37.0° C (98.6° F), blood pressure is 100/55 mm Hg, pulse is 100/min, and respirations are 20/min. The patient has opsoclonus, myoclonus, and ptosis of the right eye. On history, the mother notes the child was born "looking like a blueberry muffin" and has had a persistent cough since the age of 2 months. Which of the following is the most likely diagnosis?

    (A) Astrocytoma

    (B) Glioblastoma multiforme

    (C) Hyperthyroidism

    (D) Neuroblastoma

    (E) Wilms tumor

40. An otherwise healthy 13-year-old boy has seasonal allergic rhinitis. He complains of excessive rhinorrhea, frequent sneezing, and nasal congestion. He has a nasal voice and breathes with his mouth. He derives some relief from keeping windows closed at home and spending as little time as possible outdoors in periods of high pollen concentration. However, he is excessively bothered by nasal congestion. Which of the following drugs would be most effective in relieving nasal congestion?

    (A) Alpha-adrenergic agents such as phenylephrine

    (B) Antihistamines such as chlorpheniramine

    (C) Antihistamines such as loratadine

    (D) Cromoglycate or similar mast cell stabilizers

    (E) Ipratropium bromide

Items 41-42

A 1-month-old infant is seen in a well-baby clinic. The mother states that the baby is constipated and feeds poorly. On examination, he is jaundiced, exhibits poor muscle tone, and has a large posterior fontanelle and an umbilical hernia. He has gained only 300 g since discharge from the normal newborn nursery.

41. Which of the following is the most likely diagnosis?

    (A) Alpha-1-antitrypsin deficiency
    (B) Biliary atresia
    (C) Congenital hypothyroidism
    (D) Congenital myasthenia gravis
    (E) Pyloric stenosis
    (F) Syphilis
    (G) Werdnig-Hoffmann disease

42. Which of the following would be the most appropriate diagnostic study in this infant?

    (A) Alpha-1-antitrypsin deficiency
    (B) Barium swallow
    (C) Liver and spleen scan
    (D) Measurements of T4 and TSH levels
    (E) Muscle biopsy
    (F) RPR and FTA for syphilis

Items 43-44

A 10-month-old girl is seen in the clinic for a routine check-up. She weighs 10 kg (22 lb) and is 72 cm tall. The mother reports that the infant takes solid foods poorly. Therefore, she is supplementing solid foods with whole cow milk because she can no longer produce breast milk. The mother notes that the infant has increasing lethargy and exhibits less activity compared with other children of the same age. The infant has had three upper respiratory tract infections and one episode of acute otitis media. She is otherwise sleeping well and has met developmental milestones appropriate for her age. On examination, she is found to have pallor of the skin and mucous membranes, good muscle tone, and normal neurologic function. Routine urinalysis is normal, and a peripheral blood smear shows microcytic and hypochromic red blood cells. Complete blood count shows the following:

Mean corpuscular volume (MCV)	77 fL
Mean corpuscular hemoglobin concentration (MCHC)	27 g/dL
Platelet count	445,000/μL
Hematocrit	30%
Red cell distribution width	16.5

43. Which of the following is the most likely explanation for this patient's anemia?

    (A) Acute myelogenous leukemia
    (B) Chronic disease
    (C) Glucose 6-phosphate deficiency (G6PD)
    (D) Hookworm infection
    (E) Hypothyroidism
    (F) Nutritional folic acid deficiency
    (G) Nutritional iron deficiency

44. Which of the following is the most appropriate next step in management?

    (A) Antibiotic therapy
    (B) Bone marrow biopsy
    (C) Dietary advice and oral iron treatment
    (D) Red cell enzyme studies
    (E) Thyroid studies

The response options for items 45-47 are the same. You will be required to select one answer for each item in the set.

(A) Aortic insufficiency

(B) Coarctation of the aorta

(C) Complex congenital heart disease

(D) Congenital heart block

(E) Conotruncal abnormalities

(F) Dextrocardia

(G) Endocardial cushion defects

(H) Patent ductus arteriosus

(I) Supravalvular aortic stenosis

For each patient with a congenital syndrome, select the most likely cardiac defect.

45. A community pediatrician is called to the delivery of an infant girl experiencing fetal distress. After a vaginal delivery with vacuum assist, the infant cries spontaneously but remains acrocyanotic, despite supplemental oxygen delivered by mask. The girl is hypotonic and moves her extremities only in response to noxious stimuli. Physical examination reveals an open mouth with a protruding tongue, upslanting palpebral fissures, low-set ears, and a simian crease across both palms.

46. A 5-year-old girl is referred by her pediatrician to a cardiologist for a newly diagnosed heart murmur. The child is short and overweight, with pointed ears. She has an outgoing and friendly personality, talking to everyone she meets. Her mother describes her as having a "cocktail-party personality." Her medical history is significant for renal stones diagnosed at 10 months of age.

47. A 2-day-old boy is about to be discharged from the hospital with his mother when a nurse witnesses an episode of his eyes rolling upward and his body stiffening. A generalized tonic-clonic seizure ensues. After stabilization, the infant's temperature is 36.5° C (97.7° F), blood pressure is 80/50 mm Hg, pulse is 120/min, and respirations are 50/min. His arterial blood gas in room air is pH 7.37, P_{CO_2} is 40 mm Hg, P_{O_2} is 45 mm Hg, HCO_3^- is 24 mEq/L, and a base deficit is 0.2. Blood chemistries are sodium 145 mEq/L, potassium 5.0 mEq/L, chloride 111 mEq/L, calcium 6.5 mEq/L, magnesium 2.0 mEq/L, and glucose 90 mg/dL. His physical examination is notable for low-set ears, cyanosis in the extremities, and a grade 2 of 6 systolic murmur in the left lower sternal border, with a loud systolic ejection click. On his chest radiograph, a normal heart size and silhouette are noted, but the thymic shadow is absent.

The response options for items 48-50 are the same. You will be required to select one answer for each item in the set.

(A) Appendicitis

(B) Constipation

(C) Gastroenteritis

(D) Henoch-Schönlein purpura

(E) Inflammatory bowel disease

(F) Inguinal hernia

(G) Intussusception

(H) Lactose intolerance

(I) Lead poisoning

(J) Mesenteric adenitis

(K) Pneumonia

(L) Psychosomatic cause

(M) Torsion

(N) Urinary tract infection

For each patient with abdominal pain, select the most likely diagnosis.

48. A 6-year-old boy presents with crampy abdominal pain located in his right lower quadrant for the past four days. There is a recent history of nonbloody diarrhea for 1 week and mild fever. His mother reports no recent changes in appetite. On physical examination, there is mild tenderness to palpation in the right lower quadrant, without guarding or rigidity. His temperature is 38.6° C (101.5° F), and other vital signs are within normal limits. Ultrasound of the abdomen shows enlarged abdominal lymph nodes.

49. A 7-month-old infant is brought to the clinic with fever, nonbilous vomiting, and episodes of inconsolable crying for the past 12 hours. He has a recent history of an upper respiratory tract infection but is otherwise a healthy child who has met all developmental milestones. The mother noticed passage of mucoid stools admixed with blood earlier this morning. On examination, the child appears pale and lethargic. Palpation of the abdomen elicits inconsolable crying, and a small mass is felt in the right upper quadrant.

50. A 6-year-old boy is brought to the clinic with crampy abdominal pain, mild fever, and scrotal pain for the past 12 hours. He developed a maculopapular rash 2 days ago in his lower extremities that appears to be enlarging. On examination, there is joint tenderness in his knees and ankles, diffuse abdominal tenderness to palpation without guarding, and diffuse testicular tenderness with scrotal enlargement. Routine urinalysis reveals microscopic hematuria and 2+ proteinuria.

Pediatrics Test Two:
Answers and Explanations

ANSWER KEY

1.	A		26.	A
2.	D		27.	A
3.	E		28.	A
4.	B		29.	E
5.	D		30.	D
6.	B		31.	A
7.	A		32.	B
8.	A		33.	D
9.	D		34.	C
10.	A		35.	B
11.	B		36.	E
12.	C		37.	A
13.	C		38.	A
14.	C		39.	D
15.	A		40.	A
16.	C		41.	C
17.	C		42.	D
18.	D		43.	G
19.	D		44.	C
20.	A		45.	G
21.	D		46.	I
22.	E		47.	E
23.	D		48.	J
24.	A		49.	G
25.	A		50.	D

1. **The correct answer is A.** Prolonged absence from school is a serious problem. It is important to sort out the reasons why this teenager is not attending school. If she is staying home with her mother's knowledge, then she is probably being kept home by mother to look after another sibling or to keep her mother company. This school refusal may represent separation anxiety, and there could be underlying conflicts of separation. After her illness with strep throat, this teenager may be having difficulties transitioning back to school. Perhaps she dreads going back to a particular class or teacher. It is important to establish whether her school absence is related to something at home or at school. Importantly, everyone needs to help this teenager return to school, even if a contract needs to be made that she will go only for part of the day.

The physician should not write a medical excuse to keep her home for any more days (**choice B**). This is not the answer and may only prolong the problem. Many times in such situations families want a doctor's note in support of keeping the child at home and arranging for a home tutor. This should not be done.

The physician should not report the girl as truant (**choice C**). Truancy is when a student is absent from school but is not at home. Instead the student may be away with peers playing or doing something else. There is no history of truancy in this case. The school is surely aware of the girl's absence from school.

Sending the mother for counseling (**choice D**) is not the best choice. The mother may have underlying separation problems herself. Many mothers of children with school phobia may have a history of depression or have had school phobia themselves during their own childhood. All issues need to be explored over time.

Sending the girl to psychotherapy (**choice E**) seems premature until the physician explores what is going on. At this point, she has not even returned to school. It will take some skill in uncovering the underlying issues and seeing that this teenager gets the help she needs.

2. **The correct answer is D.** Retinoblastoma is the most common intraocular malignancy in infants and children. With early diagnosis and treatment, survival is greater than 90%. However, patients with a germline retinoblastoma mutation have a substantial risk (as high as 70%) for having a second high-grade malignancy. The most common secondary nonocular tumors associated with retinoblastoma is osteosarcoma. Physicians must always have a high index of suspicion of osteosarcoma in these patients when there is a new onset of bone pain or new bony lesions.

Infantile or congenital glaucoma (**choice A**) is associated with other congenital anomalies, such as aniridia, Sturge-Weber syndrome, Marfan syndrome, and neurofibromatosis. There is, however, no association with retinoblastoma.

Other secondary tumors, such as brain tumors (glioblastoma [**choice B**]), malignant melanoma (**choice C**), and squamous cell carcinoma (**choice E**), are also associated with retinoblastoma, but to a much lesser degree than osteosarcoma.

3. **The correct answer is E.** In the neonatal period, midgut volvulus is the most common cause of abdominal obstruction due to malrotation. Green-colored vomitus represents bilious vomiting, which is caused by obstruction of the small bowel. The infant typically has normal feeding and appears to be well in the first few days of life. As the malrotation worsens, the infant starts to develop abdominal fullness, especially in the right upper quadrant. Bilious vomiting soon develops as the small bowel is completely obstructed. If the volvulus is not diagnosed and treated early, intestinal ischemia and necrosis may develop. This can lead to bowel perforation and shock. Volvulus is the most common type of malrotation in newborns. It is caused by failure of the cecum to move into the right lower quadrant. The usual location of the cecum is in the subhepatic area. Because the cecum fails to rotate properly, it does not form the normal broad-based adherence to the posterior abdominal wall. A midgut volvulus is formed when the mesentery, which includes the superior mesenteric artery, is tethered by a narrow stalk and is twisted around itself. In addition, bands of adhesive tissue (Ladd bands) may extend from the cecum to the right upper quadrant, obstructing the duodenum. Midgut volvulus is an emergency in neonates. When an infant is suspected of having this condition, he or she should be stabilized immediately by IV fluids, antibiotics, and nasogastric suctioning. Abdominal radiographs should be taken as soon as possible to evaluate for bowel obstruction. Radiologic findings of volvulus include small bowel dilatation, paucity of air in the intestine, and a corkscrew-like appearance of the duodenum. Emergent surgery is needed to relieve the obstruction. Adhesive tissues should be resected, and the entire intestine should be inspected for anomalies. If segments of ischemic bowel are present, they should be removed. If the viability of the bowel cannot be determined during the surgery, a second surgery 12-36 hours later may be necessary to inspect and remove any ischemic bowel segment. Short bowel syndrome is a dreaded complication if a significant portion of the bowel was nonviable, and thus removed.

Allergic reaction to formula (**choice A**) typically presents between 4 and 6 weeks of age. Reactions rarely present in the neonatal period. Bilious vomiting is also not consistent with an allergic reaction to formula.

Gastroesophageal reflux disease (**choice B**) happens commonly in infants. In fact, the lower gastroesophageal sphincter is poorly developed during infancy. Most cases of reflux are a normal variant, and the parents need not be worried. However, when reflux causes significant problems, such as poor weight gain or apnea, it then needs to be treated. The vomiting in gastroesophageal reflux disease is never bilious.

Hirschsprung disease (**choice C**) results from partial or complete absence of ganglion cells in the colon. It is the most common cause of neonatal obstruction of the colon. Hirschsprung disease is suspected when the infant fails to pass meconium in the first 24 hours of life. Diagnosis becomes more likely when barium enema shows the appearance of a megacolon proximal to the aganglionic segment. It is confirmed with punch biopsy.

Meconium ileus (**choice D**) is most commonly associated with cystic fibrosis. It typically presents at birth or within the first 48 hours. Symptoms include failure to pass meconium, abdominal distention, and vomiting, which may be bilious.

4. **The correct answer is B.** Hypertension happens in children. It is defined as blood pressure higher than the 95th percentile for age on three different measurements. Unlike adults, most cases of hypertension in infants and younger children are secondary hypertension. Children with hypertension usually present with headaches, visual symptoms, easy fatigability, or epistaxis. One of the possible reasons for failure to thrive is hypertension. Seventy to seventy-five percent of children who have hypertension have a renal etiology. Up to 25% of patients have a history of recurrent urinary tract infection secondary to obstructive uropathy or reflux nephropathy. Other renal causes include renovascular disease, glomerulonephritis, and hemolytic uremic syndrome. These children develop hypertension when azotemia occurs because of the underlying disease. Hence, the most appropriate initial laboratory tests are complete blood count, urinalysis, serum electrolytes, blood urea nitrogen and creatinine concentration, and uric acid.

The most common cardiac cause of hypertension is coarctation of the aorta, but this usually presents in infancy. In older patients with good collateral flow, a "machinery" systolic murmur is typically evident on examination, but in younger patients, the murmur is usually short, systolic, and best heard along the lower sternal border at the third and fourth intercostal spaces. Also, the lower extremities blood pressure will be lower than the upper extremities. Femoral pulses would be weak or absent. Other causes of secondary hypertension in children include drugs (especially corticosteroids, oral contraceptives in sexually active adolescents, and

sympathomimetics), lead poisoning, neuroblastoma, and seizure.

Twenty-four-hour urine creatinine clearance and protein (**choice A**) is not indicated for the initial evaluation of a hypertensive child. The purpose of doing this test is to have an accurate measurement of the creatinine clearance, but collection of urine for 24 hours can be very inconvenient to the family. It is also not cost-effective as an initial test.

Plasma and urine catecholamine levels (**choice C**) are used to assess the presence of a catecholamine-producing tumor, such as a pheochromocytoma. Pheochromocytoma usually presents with episodic symptoms of palpitation, headaches, flushing, nausea and vomiting, and urinary frequency. Pheochromocytoma is not suspected in this case; therefore, catecholamine levels are not indicated here.

Serum aldosterone (**choice D**), if elevated, represents either primary or secondary hyperaldosteronism. Clinical manifestations include hypertension, muscle weakness, polydipsia, and polyuria. Laboratory findings include hypokalemia, hypernatremia, and decreased chloride. Therefore, serum electrolytes would be an appropriate initial test for this condition. Serum aldosterone level is not an appropriate initial test in this patient, although it would be indicated later if the patient had the relevant symptoms and characteristic laboratory findings.

Serum cortisol (**choice E**) would be used to assess Cushing syndrome, which is another cause of secondary hypertension in children. In children older than 7 years, the most common cause of Cushing syndrome is bilateral adrenal hyperplasia secondary to a pituitary adenoma or ectopic production of corticotropin (ACTH). Children with Cushing syndrome have characteristic moon facies, double chin, buffalo hump, obesity, masculinization, acne, impaired growth, and hypertrichosis.

5. **The correct answer is D.** Developmental assessment is essential in pediatrics health maintenance. It should be included in every health supervision visit. A developmental screening includes assessment of the following four areas: neurodevelopment, cognitive development, language development, and psychosocial development. The ability to make repetitive consonant sounds, such as "mama" or "dada," is learned by 8-9 months. At that time, the infant can also recognize his or her own name. In terms of social cognition, an infant will seek reassurance from a familiar person, usually parents or caretakers, when frightened. By 9 months, an infant can also wave bye-bye.

At 3 months (**choice A**), neurodevelopment is more important. At this time, an infant can raise his or her head when place on a firm surface. The infant may be able to laugh at pleasurable social contacts.

At 5 months (**choice B**), an infant can often be pulled from a sitting to a standing position. The infant can also support his or her weight on extended legs.

At 7 months (**choice C**), the infant can make repetitive vowel sounds but is not able to recognize his or her own name yet. A prone infant at this age is able to pivot in pursuit of an object.

At 11 months (**choice E**), the infant enjoys playing ball with the examiner. He or she can also use a few words other than "mama" or "dada."

6. **The correct answer is B.** The child has biliary atresia. This condition may either develop prenatally, in which case the gallbladder may be absent, or postnatally, probably after inflammation and scarring of the extrahepatic (and intrahepatic) biliary ducts. The underlying etiology is unclear. The history illustrated in the question stem is typical. In cases in which ultrasound is unrevealing, needle biopsy of the liver can yield tissue that usually excludes alternative diagnoses and can sometimes definitively demonstrate the atresia.

    Alpha-1-antitrypsin deficiency (**choice A**), cystic fibrosis (**choice C**), hepatitis B (**choice D**), and hepatitis C (**choice E**) can all cause hepatitis in infancy but would not cause the gallbladder to be absent.

    Congenital toxoplasmosis (**choice F**) results from a systemic infection with *Toxoplasma gondii*. When found in the newborn, congenital toxoplasmosis is always severe, and neurologic signs are always present. The classic triad is chorioretinitis, hydrocephalus, and intracranial calcifications. Other characteristic features include intrauterine growth retardation, jaundice, hepatomegaly, splenomegaly, lymphadenopathy, and rash.

7. **The correct answer is A.** A child with a known cardiac defect now presenting with fever, seizure, and focal neurologic deficit (anisocoria) is likely to have a brain abscess. Ventricular septal defect (VSD) predisposes the patient to an occult infection in the heart (i.e., endocarditis). Vegetations usually develop around the defect. Seeding of the bacteria may occur, and the patient thus becomes bacteremic. The bacteria may travel to the brain and cause a brain abscess. Common pathogens include *Streptococcus viridans*, *Bacteroides*, Enterobacteriaceae, and *Staphylococcus aureus*. Brain abscess is a life-threatening condition that requires rapid recognition and treatment. CT of the brain is the best diagnostic test for brain abscess. Surgical drainage and IV antibiotics are the treatment of choice. Broad spectrum antibiotics, such as a third-generation cephalosporin with metronidazole, are necessary. Oxacillin or vancomycin can be used if *S.*

aureus is present. If CT scan reveals that the abscess is less than 2.5 cm and the patient is neurologically stable and conscious, it is recommended to just start antibiotics and observe. Otherwise, surgical drainage is necessary.

ECG (**choice B**) is not helpful in the diagnosis of this child. Even though she has a cardiac condition (VSD), it is apparent that her clinical deterioration is secondary to a serious infection and a neurologic condition, rather than an abnormal heart rhythm.

Electroencephalography (**choice C**) is an appropriate initial diagnostic procedure for this critically ill child. It may help to elucidate the kind of seizure that she had. It is not immediately necessary, however, because the confirmation of a brain abscess by a CT scan is more crucial for prompt diagnosis and intervention.

MRI of the brain (**choice D**) can show fine details of the soft tissue. In this case of brain abscess, however, a rapid study such as the CT scan is more appropriate because it is faster and easier to obtain and is adequate to diagnose a brain abscess.

Complete blood count and blood cultures (**choice E**) are helpful but are not diagnostic of brain abscess. An elevated white count is not always present. Multiple blood cultures should be obtained but they are not as helpful as the CT scan.

Lumbar puncture (**choice F**) is contraindicated in this case because the child might have increased intracranial pressure. Brain stem or uncal herniation might occur.

8. **The correct answer is A.** Acute poststreptococcal glomerulonephritis is characterized by hematuria with either no or mild edema and elevated blood pressure. In cooler weather, it is often preceded by a sore throat. During warmer weather, a skin infection, such as impetigo, may be the preceding infection. This illness is thought to be mediated by immune complexes, and serum complement (C3) is reduced. When edema is mild, it is most easily seen in loose, thin tissues, such as the eyelids or scrotum. It is uncommon before 3 years of age.

    Hemolytic-uremic syndrome (**choice B**) is a systemic disease, which often follows an acute diarrheal illness and occurs most frequently in children younger than 4 years. Enteropathogenic *Escherichia coli* strains (O157:H7) have been associated with this illness. Following an attack of gastroenteritis, the child becomes pale and lethargic, and urine output falls. Examination often shows edema, petechiae, and hepatosplenomegaly. It is a major cause of renal failure in children.

    Henoch-Schönlein purpura (**choice C**) is associated with a characteristic petechial or purpuric rash, followed by edema. Some patients have bloody stools and abdominal cramping. Glomerulonephritis may occur 1-2 months after the first symptoms appear and usually presents as asymptomatic hematuria.

The characteristic clinical manifestation of nephrotic syndrome (**choice D**) is edema. In addition, children with nephrotic syndrome have proteinuria, hypoproteinemia, and hyperlipidemia. Although individuals with post-streptococcal glomerulonephritis and Henoch-Schönlein purpura may develop nephrotic syndrome, hematuria is rare in nephrotic syndrome.

Vesicoureteral reflux (**choice E**) is usually discovered during an evaluation for a urinary tract infection. Significant hematuria or edema is uncommon.

9. **The correct answer is D.** In this case, the mechanism of the injury (i.e., that the 3-month-old infant rolled off the sofa and hit her head) is inconsistent with the developmental age of the child. A normal 3-month-old infant is unable to roll. Child abuse is suspected in this scenario. In addition, when a parent seeks medical care for the child with a head injury, he or she usually volunteers the mechanism of injury right away, rather than waiting until a CT scan is done to confirm the injury. Such reluctance to give related history is highly suspicious of child abuse. Other clues of injury secondary to child abuse include a changing history, a conflicting history by different caretakers, and a history that is inconsistent with the severity or the type of the injury. In this case, a skeletal survey is indicated to detect any other skeletal injury and to document the findings for legal purpose. A detailed and well-documented physical examination should also be performed to identify any other injury. Other physical findings that are highly suggestive of child abuse include bruises of buttocks, cigarette burns, circular burns from hot water immersion, human bites, lash marks, spiral fractures of the long bones, subdural hematoma, and multiple bony injuries at different stages of healing. Child abuse continues to be a major problem in this country and is a major threat to the wellness of affected children. Pediatricians should always be advocates of the children; they are required by law to report any suspected case of child abuse.

Discharging the patient home (**choice A**) is inappropriate because a full evaluation of other possible injuries related to child abuse has not been completed. Failure to recognize child abuse may lead to further serious injury of the victim.

The problem with 12-hour monitoring of this child (**choice B**) is similar to the choice above. Further investigation of the child abuse is necessary. If this is not a child abuse case, monitoring may be useful to detect any development of signs of increased cranial pressure, such as worsening vomiting, lethargy, seizure activities, and

Cushing's triad (hypertension, bradycardia, and change in respiration).

Neurosurgical consultation (**choice C**) is not indicated without any evidence of intracranial hemorrhage. A simple linear fracture of the skull does not require immediate surgical intervention.

Repeating the CT scan in 24 hours (**choice E**) is not helpful if the infant remains clinically stable.

10. **The correct answer is A.** The clinical picture is that of intussusception, which occurs in this age group with the presentation given and the classic bloody stools (often referred to as "currant jelly stools") mentioned. A barium enema, water-soluble contrast enema, or air enema are all both diagnostic and therapeutic with a success rate of approximately 80%. Up to 10% may reoccur during the next 24 hours, so it is important to closely monitor the patients.

Colonoscopy (**choice B**) could give the diagnosis (in an expensive and invasive way) but would not help resolve the problem. Colonoscopy is extensively used to decompress a distended colon (such as in Ogilvie syndrome), but it offers no way to push back the ileum.

Reassurance and discharge (**choice C**) is clearly incorrect, as intussusception is a clinical emergency. If the telescoping bowel is not reduced, the affected intestine will become ischemic, which can lead to death.

The upper gastrointestinal tract (**choice D**) is not the seat of the problem. The bloody stools may have lured you into this choice, but in this case the blood comes from the engorged, irritated, and battered intussuscepted bowel.

Exploratory surgery (**choice E**) may eventually be needed to fix a recurring problem, but it is not the first step.

11. **The correct answer is B.** History and physical examination are crucial in the diagnosis of contact dermatitis. The appearance of the erythematous papules and vesicles in a linear fashion on the exposed skin suggests contact dermatitis due to plant allergens. The most common culprits are poison ivy, poison oak, and poison sumac. The chemical found in these plants, urushiol, is a very potent allergen that causes an acute dermatitis that presents as vesicles, bullae, papules, and edema. If the contact dermatitis covers more than 10% to 15% of the body surface area, oral prednisone is indicated for 14-21 days. An initial dose of 1 mg/kg/day may be used, tapered every 3 days to complete the whole course. Taking tepid baths or applying calamine lotions may promote drying when the vesicles rupture.

Oral cephalexin (**choice A**) is an antibiotic and is not indicated in this case because there is no evidence that the dermatitis is complicated with a bacterial infection.

KAPLAN MEDICAL

Topical diphenhydramine (**choice C**) should be avoided because it may cause a secondary dermatitis that complicates the primary process. Oral diphenhydramine may be considered to treat burning and itching.

Topical mupirocin (**choice D**) is a topical antibiotic. Unless secondary bacterial infection is present, a topical antibiotic is not necessary.

Topical 1% hydrocortisone (**choice E**) is a low-potency topical corticosteroid, which is ineffective in treatment of contact dermatitis. If the contact dermatitis is localized to a small area, and if it is mild, a mid-potency topical corticosteroid (e.g., mometasone furoate 0.1% or triamcinolone acetonide 0.1%) may be used instead of oral prednisone.

12. **The correct answer is C.** Intraventricular and/or intraparenchymal intracranial bleeding is a common serious problem among newborns, particularly those born prematurely. This diagnosis should be suspected in infants with apnea, seizures, lethargy, or an abnormal neurologic examination. CT scan or ultrasound of the head can confirm the diagnosis. The usual source of the bleeding is the germinal matrix (a mass of embryonic tissue near the caudate nucleus that is not present in adults), which often has been damaged by episodes of hypotension or hypoxia/ischemia. Depending on the exact sites that start to bleed, the blood may either flow into the ventricles or spread into the adjacent brain tissue, "dissecting" a path (and rupturing neuron axons as it goes). This latter form of hemorrhage, which is considered the most serious (and potentially fatal) form of intracranial hemorrhage in infants, typically develops in the first 3 days of life. Infants with small intraventricular hemorrhages often do well; those with large hemorrhages may either die or be left with severe neurologic defects.

Bridging veins of the skull (**choice A**) can be a source of bleeding and cause subdural hemorrhage. These vessels are damaged in shaken baby syndrome.

The cerebral cortex (**choice B**) may be damaged by dissecting blood but is not the usual site of initial bleeding in these infants.

Bleeding from the middle meningeal artery (**choice D**) results in an epidural hematoma. This typically follows trauma. It is, however, an unusual source of bleeding in newborns.

The thalamus (**choice E**) and other areas in the deeper aspects of the brain can be damaged by dissecting blood but are not the usual site of initial bleeding in these infants.

Bleeding from the vessels of the circle of Willis (**choice F**) causes subarachnoid hemorrhage.

13. **The correct answer is C.** Most cases of meningitis in children will be one of two types: bacterial, usually caused by pneumococci or meningococci, or viral, usually caused by enteroviruses. Analysis of the CSF can be very helpful in differentiating the various types of meningitis. Clinicians should also be familiar with other treatable causes of meningitis. Tuberculous meningitis and fungal meningitis have similar clinical presentations and CSF findings. Affected patients have a subacute presentation, focal neurologic abnormalities (in this case a sixth cranial nerve palsy), a CSF pleocytosis with a predominance of lymphocytes (100-400 cells/mL), a low glucose level (20-45 mg/dL), and an increased protein concentration (100-500 mg/dL). Rapid diagnosis of tuberculous meningitis may be difficult, because most patients will have negative results on acid-fast smear. Results of cerebral CT are usually abnormal, showing enhancement of the cerebral cortex, cerebral edema, infarctions, or obstructive hydrocephalus. Accordingly, the findings in this patient are most consistent with tuberculous meningitis, and mycobacterial culture will be the most helpful CSF test.

The cryptococcal antigen test (**choice A**) has good sensitivity and specificity and has replaced the India ink stain for diagnosis. In approximately 95% of cases of meningitis due to *Coccidioides immitis*, complement-fixing antibodies will be present in the CSF.

Bacterial culture (**choice B**) is important in the work-up of bacterial meningitis. Acute bacterial meningitis is typically characterized by an elevated CSF white blood cell count with a predominance of neutrophils, an elevated CSF protein concentration, a low CSF glucose level, and positive findings on Gram stain and culture. Prior treatment with oral antibiotics does not alter these diagnostic parameters significantly, although the yield of the CSF Gram stain and culture may be somewhat decreased.

Latex agglutination tests (**choice D**) for pneumococcal or meningococcal antigens rarely are helpful. The CSF Gram stain has a much higher likelihood of providing early diagnostic help.

Treponema pallidum (**choice E**) is the cause of syphilis. Clinical manifestations of CNS disease usually appear during the tertiary stages of the disease. A picture of aseptic meningitis can occur rarely and may be confirmed by a reactive CSF Venereal Disease Research Laboratories (VDRL) test. Classic neurosyphilis has an indolent course, and psychiatric or neurologic symptoms will not manifest for decades following the initial infection.

14. **The correct answer is C.** This child most likely has supraventricular tachycardia. To be more specific, it is atrioventricular reentry tachycardia (AVRT), a relatively common cardiac emergency among infants. In this con-

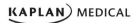

dition, the electric impulse is conducted through the AV node, then reenters the atria via an accessory atrioventricular pathway, producing the arrhythmia. The QRS complexes are narrow, and there are no preceding P waves. The pulse is usually 220-270/min. The best means of converting this rhythm to sinus rhythm is to interrupt the reentry circuit by blocking atrial to ventricular conduction within the AV node. Both vagal maneuvers and drugs that block AV node conduction can be effective treatments. Applying an ice bag to the face is believed to cause a powerful vagal nerve discharge. Most authorities advise using a large plastic bag filled with ice that covers the entire face of the infant; adding some water to the bag appears to achieve the lowest temperature. The face should be covered for only about 5 seconds because the infant will become apneic during the maneuver.

The IV administration of adenosine (**choice A**) is an effective and safe method of blocking AV nodal conduction and converting an AVRT to normal sinus rhythm. However, this therapy requires good IV access because the drug must be administered as a rapid bolus. Following this bolus with a rapid infusion of 5-10 mL normal saline ensures that adenosine will be carried through the central circulation before it is metabolized within seconds. Because obtaining IV access can stress these already compromised infants, adenosine should be administered only if a properly performed ice bag maneuver has failed.

The IV administration of verapamil (**choice B**) effectively blocks AV conduction, but its use in infants younger than 1 year is extremely dangerous and is contraindicated. Serious side effects include asystole, bradycardia, and shock.

Cardiac pacing (**choice D**) is the treatment for bradycardia secondary to third degree or complete AV block. It is required in neonates with ventricular rates less than or equal to 50/min who have evidence of heart failure.

Synchronized direct current cardioversion (**choice E**) should be reserved for the rare infant who presents in a moribund state, because application of an ice bag to the face often can reinstate sinus rhythm even in infants who appear quite ill.

15. **The correct answer is A.** This child has a strawberry hemangioma, which arises when vascular tissue fails to communicate with adjoining tissue. This enlarges and creates a raised erythematous tumor. Strawberry hemangiomas develop after birth and have a benign course if left alone. They enlarge in the first year of life and then regress. In 90% of patients, the strawberry hemangioma resolves by 9 years of age.

These lesions are not inflammatory in nature, and topical steroids (**choice B**) have not been shown to be of benefit in their treatment.

If the hemangioma is pressing on a vital organ, argon laser therapy (**choice C**) may be needed.

These lesions are not malignant; therefore, radiation (**choice D**) is not needed.

Surgical resection (**choice E**) is rarely needed in these cases.

16. **The correct answer is C.** Generalized swelling in a 5-year-old girl with proteinuria, hypoalbuminemia, and hyperlipidemia suggests nephrotic syndrome. In the absence of other pathology, minimal change disease is the most common etiology of primary nephrotic syndrome in childhood. It accounts for 80% to 85% of the cases of nephrotic syndrome. Minimal change disease has a peak occurrence between ages 2 and 8 years. In most of the cases, a viral illness precedes the proteinuria. The initial symptom is typically edema, which can happen around the eyes (periorbital edema) and in the feet (pretibial edema). Both blood pressure and renal function are normal in most patients. Hematuria is absent; complement C3 and C4 levels are normal. Immunosuppressive therapy with steroids is the mainstay of treatment. Minimal change disease is strikingly responsive to steroid therapy, with a 93% success rate with resolution of proteinuria. In cases that are resistant to steroids, cyclophosphamide may be used. In general, the prognosis for minimal change disease is excellent.

Membranoproliferative glomerulonephritis (**choice A**) is the most common cause of primary glomerulonephritis. It often presents in the second decade of life with proteinuria, microscopic or gross hematuria, and hypertension. Renal function is usually normal. Hypocomplementemia is also commonly seen. Renal biopsy is diagnostic. The mainstay of treatment is alternate-day steroids.

Membranous glomerulopathy (**choice B**) is very rare in the pediatric age group. Most cases are asymptomatic. It has been associated with various infections, the most frequent being hepatitis B infection. The diagnosis is confirmed by renal biopsy. The clinical course is very variable in children, but the overall prognosis is excellent, with a 50% to 60% spontaneous remission rate. Alternate-day steroid therapy may improve the prognosis.

Postinfectious acute glomerulonephritis (**choice D**) is a common cause of gross hematuria in children and usually develops 1-2 weeks after a streptococcal infection. Other organisms may also cause this disease. Clinical manifestations vary from asymptomatic microscopic hematuria to gross hematuria to acute renal failure. Tubular casts may be seen on microscopic examination of the urine specimen; C3 levels are decreased. The prognosis is generally good.

Systemic lupus erythematosus (**choice E**) is a systemic rheumatologic disease that usually presents with malar rash, photosensitivity, arthralgia, serositis, neurologic disorders, and immunologic abnormalities. It is associated with positive antinuclear antibodies and anti-double-stranded DNA antibodies. Different forms of glomerulonephritis can occur in patients with this disease.

17. **The correct answer C.** The patient is older than 6 years, and the most common pneumonias in this age group are due to *Mycoplasma pneumoniae* and *Streptococcus pneumoniae*. The girl in this vignette most likely has *Mycoplasma* pneumonia, which is milder than that due to traditional bacteria. It is characterized by gradual onset of fever, headache, and a nonproductive cough. The treatment of choice is erythromycin/azithromycin.

Amoxicillin (**choice A**) would be good coverage for *Streptococcus,* but not for *Mycoplasma.*

Cefazolin (**choice B**) would be a good choice for typical bacteria and for coverage against gram-negative rods, but would not be appropriate for *M. pneumoniae.*

Metronidazole (**choice D**) would provide anaerobic coverage, but would not be appropriate for *M. pneumoniae.*

Trimethoprim-sulfamethoxazole (**choice E**) is good prophylaxis for *Pneumocystis carinii* pneumonia, but this is very unlikely in this presumably immunocompetent patient.

18. **The correct answer is D.** Marfan syndrome is a connective tissue disease with an autosomal-dominant inheritance. Cardinal features of the disorder include tall stature, ectopia lentis, mitral valve prolapse, aortic root dilatation, and aortic dissection. Because cardiovascular disease (aortic dilatation and dissection) is the major cause of morbidity and mortality in these patients, early intervention with beta-adrenergic blocking agents and careful echocardiography screening may help slow aortic dilatation and allow prophylactic aortic root replacement before dissection occurs. The average lifespan of an affected individual is reduced by 50% but is improving because of better recognition and management of cardiovascular abnormalities.

Bone density (**choice A**) is performed in conditions predisposing to secondary osteoporosis, including Cushing syndrome, thyrotoxicosis, hyperparathyroidism, malabsorption syndrome, and long-term steroid use. However, osteoporosis is not associated with Marfan syndrome.

CT scan of the pituitary stalk (**choice B**) is appropriate when evaluating for a pituitary tumor as the source of this child's tall stature. It may also help in identifying a cause of precocious puberty. Most commonly, these pituitary tumors are growth-hormone secreting tumors. However, this patient presents with the characteristic features of Marfan syndrome.

Dexamethasone suppression test (**choice C**) is the screening and confirmatory test of Cushing syndrome. Patients with Marfan syndrome are not at risk for Cushing syndrome.

Electrocardiogram (**choice E**) can identify changes in rhythm and electrical activity, ischemia, and muscular hypertrophy. However, it is not a good method of evaluating the risk for aortic root dilatation and dissection in Marfan syndrome patients.

Glucose tolerance test (**choice F**) is the screening test for diabetes of any cause. Although it is not associated with Marfan syndrome, it can be associated with conditions of growth-hormone hypersecretion (acromegaly and gigantism), Cushing disease, and thyrotoxicosis. Although this child is tall for her age, gigantism is not the cause.

19. **The correct answer is D.** Migraine may affect children as well as adults. It is the most common cause of headaches in children. Migraine in children manifests with symptomatology similar to that observed in adult patients. Certain triggers are easily identified, such as loud noises, bright lights, stress, fatigue, caffeine-containing drinks, and some foods. Parent education on what is known about migraine etiology is essential in management. Treatment consists of the measures that the parents or patients themselves have found to provide relief, plus acetaminophen or a nonsteroidal anti-inflammatory drug (NSAID) if such measures are insufficient. Ergotamine should be reserved for the most severe cases, and sumatriptan is not yet approved for use in children.

Brain tumor (**choice A**) is very unlikely in the presence of classic symptoms of migraine, as in this case. The manifestations of a brain tumor in children are usually accompanied by evidence of increased intracranial pressure.

Cluster headache (**choice B**) is extremely rare in childhood. It manifests as attacks of intense pain occurring at night and is often precipitated by alcohol consumption. Each attack lasts up to 2 hours and recurs daily for a period of up to 8 weeks. These periods are then followed by a headache-free interval that usually lasts 1 year.

Conduct disorder (**choice C**) is a childhood behavioral disorder that is similar to antisocial behavior disorder in adults. The child displays persistent patterns of aggression to animals or people, destruction of property, stealing, and opposition to parental guidance.

Tension headache (**choice E**) is the second most important cause of headache in children and is more common in adolescents. This form of headache manifests as a vise-like tightness around the head and in the neck muscles. Tension headache is frequently a response to stress or fatigue.

20. **The correct answer is A.** The probable diagnosis is peritonsillar abscess, which is the most common complication of pharyngitis or tonsillitis. Patients usually present with fever, dysphagia, and odynophagia (pain when swallowing). Drooling is common. Physical examination findings include erythema of the involved tonsillar pillar, edema of the pillar and soft palate, deviation of the uvula toward the contralateral side, and trismus. The tonsils may be inflamed and exudative.

The most common organisms isolated from peritonsillar abscesses are beta-hemolytic streptococci (**choice A**) and anaerobic bacteria. *Haemophilus influenzae* type b (**choice C**), *Moraxella catarrhalis*, and *Pseudomonas aeruginosa* are cultured less frequently. As is typical for most oral infections, mixed cultures are common. Enterococci (**choice B**), *Staphylococcus aureus* (**choice D**), and *Streptococcus pneumoniae* (**choice E**) generally are not isolated.

Treatment of peritonsillar abscess includes parenteral antibiotics that are active against anaerobes and streptococci, as well as drainage of the abscess. Penicillin remains the drug of choice. In patients who are allergic to penicillin, clindamycin or a cephalosporin can be used as an alternative with the addition of metronidazole. Needle aspiration of the abscess is usually performed in the emergency department. In those in whom needle aspiration fails, subsequent incision and drainage, or tonsillectomy may be necessary.

21. **The correct answer is D.** This is trisomy 13, also known as Patau syndrome. The presentation illustrated is typical. These infants usually die before 1 year of age from multiple congenital anomalies, particularly severe congenital heart defects. Patau syndrome is associated with holoprosencephaly due to a failure of forebrain development and consequent failure to form paired cerebral hemispheres. It is associated with midface developmental abnormalities. Other features include hyperconvex, narrow fingernails, scalp defects, abnormal genitalia, apneic spells, and severe mental retardation.

Anencephaly (**choice A**) is a complete failure of higher brain structures to develop. It is accompanied by a grossly deformed head with virtually no cranial vault.

Encephalocele (**choice B**) is protrusion of brain and meninges due to a developmental defect in the skull.

Hydranencephaly (**choice C**) is an extreme form of porencephaly in which the cerebral hemispheres are destroyed. Unlike in anencephaly, the external head forms normally.

Porencephaly (**choice E**) is a cyst or cavity in the brain that communicates with the ventricles; it may occur as a developmental anomaly or secondary to inflammatory disease or a vascular accident.

22. **The correct answer is E.** Hyponatremia is clinically important because it can cause substantial morbidity and mortality. Although most cases are mild, hyponatremia can cause a generalized seizure. The diagnostic approach to hyponatremia should include a careful history (especially concerning medication), clinical assessment of the extracellular fluid (ECF) volume status, and a thorough neurologic evaluation. The differential diagnosis of hyponatremia is categorized into three different groups: hypovolemic hyponatremia, euvolemic hyponatremia, and hypervolemic hyponatremia.

The ECF volume status of the boy in this clinical vignette appears to be euvolemic. There is no evidence of hypovolemia. His heart rate is normal, his oral mucosa is moist, and there is no evidence of hypervolemia. The differential diagnosis of euvolemic hyponatremia includes syndrome of inappropriate antidiuretic hormone secretion (SIADH), glucocorticoid deficiency, hypothyroidism, and water intoxication. With such increased urinary sodium concentration (55 mEq/L) and concentrated urine (550 mOsmol/kg H_2O), SIADH is the most likely explanation of the etiology of the hyponatremia in this child. In SIADH, the urine concentration is increased with respect to serum in the presence of normal renal function and the absence of dehydration. Patients have hyponatremia, normal potassium, concentrated urine, and urinary sodium concentration more than 20 mEq/L. Symptoms include nausea, irritability, loss of appetite, and lethargy. Stupor and seizures occur in severe hyponatremia. Since the underlying problem is retention of water rather than salt wasting, the treatment for SIADH is restriction of fluid.

The child's renal function is normal, as evidenced by the normal blood urea nitrogen and creatinine levels. Hyponatremia associated with acute renal failure (**choice A**) is usually hypervolemic, not euvolemic.

Addison disease (**choice B**) is adrenal insufficiency secondary to destruction of the adrenal cortex. The most common cause is an autoimmune destruction of the glands. Other causes include tuberculosis, acute adrenal hemorrhage, and congenital adrenal hypoplasia. Patients have hyponatremia, hyperkalemia, and hypovolemia. In severe cases, severe hypotension and shock can occur.

In congestive heart failure (**choice C**), the heart fails to pump enough cardiac output to supply the body's metabolic needs. Signs and symptoms include shortness of breath, lower extremity edema, increased jugular venous pressure, and volume overload. Hyponatremia is a commonly associated with metabolic abnormality.

The child in this clinical vignette has no signs of dehydration. Hyponatremic dehydration (**choice D**) is most commonly due to external losses of sodium through the gastrointestinal tract. Sodium deficit must be replaced over several days to avoid neurologic complications.

23. **The correct answer is D.** This infant has hypertrophic pyloric stenosis, which is characterized by obstruction of the pyloric lumen by pyloric muscular hypertrophy. The hypertrophy develops after birth, and typically presents at 4-6 weeks of life. The presentation illustrated in the question stem is typical. The diagnosis can be confirmed by palpation of a 2- to 3-cm ("walnut-sized") movable mass deep in the right side of the epigastrium. Ultrasound can also demonstrate the hypertrophied pyloric muscle. Surgical correction is with pyloromyotomy, in which the gastric mucosa is left intact but the muscles of the pyloric areas are incised.

Diaphragmatic hernia (**choice A**), in which loops of bowel protrude into the chest cavity, produces respiratory distress with bowel sounds heard over the chest.

Duodenal atresia (**choice B**) also causes projectile vomiting in infants, but the vomitus is bile stained.

Esophageal atresia (**choice C**) causes regurgitation on feeding but not projectile vomiting.

Meconium plug syndrome (**choice E**) causes bowel obstruction in neonates.

24. **The correct answer is A.** Dacryostenosis, or congenital nasolacrimal duct obstruction, occurs in at least 6% of all newborns. It is characterized by unilateral tearing and yellow crusting of the eye each morning, sometimes so thick that the infant cannot open the eyelids. Although uncommon, dacryostenosis can be bilateral. Parents are advised to massage the inner canthus of the eye twice daily to encourage resolution of the obstruction. Resolution occurs by 1 year of age in 90% of infants.

Gonococcal conjunctivitis (**choice B**) is unlikely because perinatal transmission of gonococcus results in conjunctivitis several days after birth. Clinical findings include lid edema, purulent exudate, and corneal ulcerations. Early diagnosis requires Gram staining of the exudate.

Eye discharge is never a normal finding in infants, therefore **choice C** is incorrect.

Viral conjunctivitis (**choice D**) is unlikely without symptoms of upper respiratory infection, such as rhinorrhea, cough, fever, lethargy, or poor feeding. Eye involvement may begin unilaterally but progresses to bilateral involvement within 1-2 days. The major clinical finding is an inflamed or red conjunctiva.

In breast-fed infants, vitamin A deficiency (**choice E**) is extremely unlikely. The major clinical finding of avitaminosis is a thick and hazy cornea (keratomalacia). Bottle-fed infants are also unlikely to have vitamin A deficiency, since commercial formulas contain adequate daily allowances of essential vitamins if they are mixed to the correct concentration. Unfortunately, this is not always the case.

25. **The correct answer is A.** Maternal alcohol abuse is a common cause of teratogenesis. The fetal alcohol syndrome is characterized by potentially severe mental retardation secondary to impaired brain development. Other phenotypic features seen in severely affected infants include growth retardation, microcephaly, microphthalmia, short palpebral fissures, and midfacial hypoplasia. In addition, these infants may have abnormal palmar creases, cardiac defects, and joint contractures. Partial expression in mild cases is common and may make diagnosis difficult.

Maternal cirrhosis (**choice B**) can decrease fertility and cause miscarriages and prematurity, but does not specifically cause fetal malformation.

Maternal cocaine abuse (**choice C**) can cause spontaneous abortion, fetal death, placental abruption, low birth weight, reduced body length, and reduced head circumference.

Maternal diabetes mellitus (**choice D**) can cause large-for-gestational-age infants who tend to be hypoglycemic after birth.

Maternal hypothyroidism (**choice E**) may worsen during pregnancy but usually does not produce prominent fetal effects.

26. **The correct answer is A.** Typically, the abdominal contents herniate into the left hemithorax. This causes displacement of the heart into the right hemithorax and pulmonary hypoplasia. If gas has entered the intestinal tract during resuscitation, bowel sounds may be heard in the chest. The displacement of the abdominal contents renders the abdomen flat. In cases of severe pulmonary hypoplasia, administration of oxygen results in only a poor improvement in oxygenation.

Hyaline membrane disease (**choice B**) is uncommon, if not rare, in full-term infants. Occasionally this form of respiratory distress may occur in infants of diabetic women, but this history is absent in this case.

Meconium aspiration (**choice C**) should be accompanied by a history of fetal stress, meconium-stained amniotic fluid, or meconium-staining of the skin and cord. Physical findings are symmetric, there is no displacement of the heart, and breath sounds are similar bilaterally.

Pneumonia (**choice D**) in the neonate is usually due to either group B beta-hemolytic streptococci or *Escherichia* *coli*, accompanied by a history of maternal fever or prolonged rupture of the amniotic membranes. Breath sounds are symmetrically diminished.

Tracheoesophageal fistula (**choice E**) usually presents with a history of polyhydramnios, cyanosis with feeding, and increased oropharyngeal secretions. It is unusual for this condition to present so soon after birth with severe respiratory distress.

27. **The correct answer is A.** The term kernicterus is used to denote damage to the brain by high bilirubin levels in the perinatal period. The fetal liver is less efficient at conjugating bilirubin compared with the adult liver, and neonates are consequently prone to develop hyperbilirubinemia, particularly unconjugated hyperbilirubinemia. In most cases, there are predisposing conditions, such as hemolytic anemia, polycythemia, prematurity, maternal diabetes, congenital liver or biliary tract disease, sepsis, or intrauterine infections. In contrast to what you might except, the bilirubin is not uniformly poisonous to the nervous system, but instead selectively accumulates in, damages, and stains the basal ganglia and the brain stem nuclei. Early symptoms may include lethargy, poor feeding, and vomiting. Severe kernicterus can cause opisthotonos, oculogyric crisis, seizures, and even death.

    The cerebellum (**choice B**), cerebral cortex (**choice C**), peripheral nerve (**choice D**), and spinal cord (**choice E**) are all much less sensitive to damage by high bilirubin levels than are the basal ganglia and brain stem nuclei.

28. **The correct answer is A.** This infant already has evidence of imperforate anus and tracheoesophageal fistula with the most common configuration (blind esophageal end at the top, and fistula to the tracheobronchial tree at the bottom—that is how gas got into the gastrointestinal tract). Those two anomalies are part of the VACTERL constellation (vertebral, anal, cardiac, tracheoesophageal, renal, and limb abnormalities). The x-ray already ruled out vertebral and radial anomalies, but we still have to rule out cardiac and renal anomalies. For that reason, the infant needs the renal sonogram and the echocardiogram. No surgical repair should be planned until we know the full extent of the problem.

    Barium swallow (**choice B**) is not the first thing we need. If further definition of the esophageal anomaly is desired, a more gentle medium (Gastrografin) should be used to avoid aspiration of barium.

    Gastrostomy (**choice C**) may very well be needed if the full extent of the anomalies delays repair of the tracheoesophageal fistula. Reflux of gastric contents into the tracheobronchial tree will produce chemical damage. However, it does not take that long to do a sonogram of the kidney and an echocardiogram, and if they are nega-

tive, repair of the tracheoesophageal anomaly may be undertaken at once.

Colostomy (**choice D**) is not urgent, because there is a fistula from the end of the gastrointestinal tract to the vagina. A decision as to the type of repair possible now, or to be deferred until later can be made at leisure.

Surgical repair (**choice E**) has to wait until we know the full extent of the anomalies. The idea that diagnosis must precede therapy is well illustrated in this case.

29. **The correct answer is E.** Apparently, the girl in this clinical vignette has generalized edema (i.e., anasarca). The most common causes of swelling are nephrotic syndrome, congestive heart failure, and liver disease. Other causes include hypothyroidism, shock, mineralocorticoid excess, and malnutrition. Since there is no evidence of any abnormal cardiac or hepatic findings, urinalysis is the most appropriate initial diagnostic test to screen for proteinuria. In children with nephrotic syndrome, albumin (a serum protein) is lost in the urine and hence causes the oncotic pressure inside the vessels to decrease. Fluid there shifts from the intravascular space into the interstitial space, causing generalized edema.

    Liver enzymes (**choice A**), chest radiographs (**choice B**), echocardiography (**choice C**), and kidney ultrasound (**choice D**) are not indicated in this case as the initial diagnostic test.

30. **The correct answer is D.** Usually, infants gain an ounce/day during the first 4 months of life. Those who gain more than this and are spitting up are probably being overfed.

    Adrenogenital syndrome (**choice A**), or congenital adrenal hyperplasia, presents in the first week of life with metabolic abnormalities and results in poor weight gain.

    Children being abused (**choice B**) would probably not be overfed.

    Inborn errors of metabolism (**choice C**) present in the first weeks of life and generally lead to poor weight gain.

    Pyloric stenosis (**choice E**) typically presents with projectile vomiting at 2 weeks of age. It is more common in boys.

31. **The correct answer is A.** Aniridia describes the absence of an iris. It can be inherited as an autosomal dominant trait or it can occur sporadically. Approximately one third of sporadic cases are associated with Wilms tumor. Hemihypertrophy is also associated with Wilms tumor in some individuals. It is important to obtain an abdominal ultrasound to investigate for renal abnormalities or Wilms tumor in such cases.

    An echocardiogram (**choice B**) is not indicated.

KAPLAN) MEDICAL

A neurology consult (**choice C**) is not required because aniridia and Wilms tumor are not associated with acute nervous system disease. An ophthalmology consult would be more appropriate.

A rapid plasmin reagin (RPR) test (**choice D**) is not warranted because syphilis is not suggested by the clinical findings or history. Neurosyphilis is associated with the Argyll-Robertson pupil, which irregularly shaped and nonreactive to light.

IV antibiotics (**choice E**) are not indicated because aniridia is not associated with *in utero* or perinatal infection.

32. **The correct answer is B.** Anytime you see an infant with abdominal difficulties plus cystic fibrosis, think of meconium ileus. The vignette did not say that this infant had cystic fibrosis (he has not been diagnosed yet; he is only 3 days old), but the mother provides the connection. A Gastrografin enema will show the unused microcolon and the pellets of inspissated meconium higher up. As the hypertonic solution of Gastrografin draws water into the lumen, the inspissated meconium will be diluted and "unplugged." More complete diagnostic steps and treatment for the cystic fibrosis will follow.

     Barium enema (**choice A**) is a tantalizing distracter because it also serves double duty as diagnosis and therapy, but not in this condition. It does so in intussusception, which we see in chubby 2-year-olds with colicky pain and the famous "currant jelly stool," not in the newborn.

     Colonoscopy (**choice C**) can also do double duty, but it does so in Ogilvie syndrome, the paralytic ileus of the colon that we see in old, immobilized people.

     Endoscopic retrograde cholangiopancreatogram (ERCP; **choice D**) is also a diagnostic test with therapeutic value, but its role is in clearing up an obstructed biliary tract.

     And as for rectal biopsy (**choice E**), save it for the infant suspected of having aganglionic megacolon; it will give you the diagnosis but will not help with the therapy.

33. **The correct answer is D.** Systemic lupus erythematosus (SLE) is a multisystemic rheumatologic disease. Its major clinical manifestations include fever, malaise, arthritis, arthralgia, and rash. Anorexia and weight loss are also common. The malar butterfly rash on the face that extends over the bridge of the nose, but spares the nasolabial fold, is very characteristic but is not present in all patients with SLE. Raynaud phenomenon, polyserositis, hepatosplenomegaly, lymphadenopathy, and renal disease also are frequently associated with SLE. Antinuclear antibodies are found in 97% of patients with SLE, but this finding lacks specificity. Antibodies to double-stranded DNA are more specific, and are

elevated in active disease. Complement C3 and C4 levels are decreased in patients with active SLE. The American Rheumatism Association has published the criteria for the diagnosis of SLE. At least 4 of the 11 criteria must be met to diagnose SLE.

These criteria can be remembered by a mnemonic SOAP BRAIN MD (see below).

Serositis
Oral ulcers
Arthritis
Photosensitivity
Blood (hemolytic anemia, leukopenia, lymphopenia, or thrombocytopenia)
Renal (proteinuria or cellular cast)
ANA
Immunologic (positive LE preparation, antibody to double-stranded DNA, antibody to Sm antigen)
Neurologic (seizure or psychosis)
Malar rash
Discoid lupus

Giant cell arteritis (**choice A**), also known as Takayasu arteritis, primarily affects the aorta and other large arteries. Symptoms include fever, anorexia, weight loss, and arthritis. Laboratory findings include increased sedimentation rate, weakly positive antinuclear antibody titer, and anti-aorta antibodies.

Henoch-Schönlein purpura (**choice B**) is a vasculitis of unknown etiology that occurs most commonly in boys aged between 2 and 8 years. It is characterized by nonthrombocytopenic, palpable purpuras, most commonly in shins, lower extremities, and buttocks. The syndrome also includes arthritis, abdominal pain, and nephritis. The prognosis is good in the absence of significant renal complications.

Polyarteritis nodosa (**choice C**) is a vasculitis that affects small and medium-sized arteries. It can present with diverse symptoms such as fever, malaise, arthritis, abdominal pain, rash, kidney disorder, ischemic heart pain, testicular pain, peripheral nervous system disorders, lethargy, and weight loss. Antineutrophil cytoplasmic antibodies with peripheral staining (p-ANCA) are positive. Complement levels are normal.

Wegener granulomatosis (**choice E**) is characterized by necrotizing granulomatous lesions of the entire respiratory system (airways and lungs). It is also associated with glomerulonephritis. The triad of sinusitis, pulmonary involvement, and glomerulonephritis suggests the diagnosis.

34. **The correct answer is C.** In the differential diagnosis of acute cerebral edema with convulsions in a child,

ingestion of toxic substances, including lead, must be considered early. Lead toxicity is high on the differential, but a history of pica may not be elicited, and basophilic stippling and lead lines may be absent. A lead level is difficult to obtain quickly; however, a free protoporphyrin level may be obtained expediently and is an indication of lead toxicity. Biochemical evidence of lead toxicity includes elevations of blood lead and signs of interference with hemoglobin synthesis, such as an increase in free erythrocyte protoporphyrin.

A positive antistreptolysin O level (**choice A**) is evidence of an infection with *Streptococcus*. Poststreptococcal glomerulonephritis is a frequent cause of nephritic syndrome in young children, but there is no evidence of a nephritic syndrome, and antistreptolysin O titer is unlikely to be helpful.

Electroencephalography (**choice B**) may be helpful to study seizure activity if the initial work-up is negative. Sharp delta waves on the EEG will be indicative of seizure activity.

The patient's white count is normal, and the Monospot test (**choice D**), is unlikely to be helpful. Heterophil antibody kits such as the Monospot test are simple and fairly sensitive. This antibody can reach high titers in patients who have infectious mononucleosis and will cause sheep erythrocytes to agglutinate.

Meningitis must be considered, but the possibility of lead poisoning is more important in this case, given the history and the finding of basophilic stippling. Bacterial meningitis is always high on the differential in such situations, and, if the answer is not obtained promptly, a lumbar puncture for cell count should be done and fluid should be cultured (**choice E**) before presumptive antibiotics are started.

35. **The correct answer is B.** Meconium is the fetal stool, which is mostly composed of desquamated cells from the gastrointestinal tract admixed with enough bile to give the soft stool a greenish color. A distressed fetus will pass meconium into the amniotic fluid and then may aspirate it. These infants often have placental insufficiency as a result of conditions such as maternal preeclampsia, hypertension, or postmaturity. The aspirated meconium is very irritating to the lungs and causes a chemical pneumonitis. Postmature infants are particularly likely to have severe problems, because the meconium is diluted much less in their small amniotic fluid volume. The most important initial step in therapy is prompt suction of the nasopharynx and mouth to remove the meconium before more (or even any) is aspirated. This can be performed even before the infant is fully delivered, as soon as a head coated with meconium emerges from the birth canal.

Neither chest x-ray (**choice A**) nor emergency tracheostomy (**choice E**) is warranted at this point.

Oxygen supplementation by face mask (**choice C**) is deferred until after the nasopharynx and mouth are cleared of meconium.

Intubation with mechanical ventilation (**choice D**) may become necessary if oxygen supplementation by facemask is unsuccessful after the meconium is cleared.

36. **The correct answer is E.** Neonatal listeriosis presents soon after birth, usually within 5 days. The usual neonatal presentation is predominantly that of respiratory distress. Late-onset neonatal listeriosis is more likely to present with meningitis. Maternal infection is commonly acquired by contact with unpasteurized milk (mother works on a farm and drinks unprocessed milk), soft cheeses, deli meats such as hot dogs and pâté, undercooked vegetables, and undercooked poultry. Typical symptoms in adults (exhibited by the mother) include fever, diarrhea, malaise, and a flu-like illness. Once maternal infection has been acquired, it can be transmitted to the fetus either vaginally or transplacentally. Amniotic fluid is often cloudy and discolored.

Mothers with syphilis (**choice A**) typically have a history of chancre or rash. Discolored amniotic fluid, acute fever, and diarrheal illness are not typical. Severely affected infants may have pneumonia and hepatosplenomegaly.

A symptomatic infant with congenital toxoplasmosis (**choice B**) may display such signs as hydrocephalus, microcephaly, cataracts, hepatosplenomegaly, and a petechial and/or "blueberry muffin" rash. Respiratory distress is rare.

Fetal hydrops (**choice C**) is a nonspecific finding that can occur in a wide variety of conditions resulting in severe edema of the fetus. These include *in utero* heart failure, severe anemia, and intrauterine viral or spirochetal infection. In the present case, a typical maternal history compatible with listerial infection is obtained and no other blood or cardiac anomalies are present.

Neonatal herpes (**choice D**) can present with general collapse (associated with severe respiratory distress or liver failure), or as localized disease, including meningitis, ophthalmitis, or rash. The rash in infants is vesicular in its early stages, becoming crusted as the illness progresses. Many mothers do not have symptoms during their first infection; thus, a typical history of maternal genital herpes is not obtained in 70% to 90% of cases. However, the typical prodrome of listerial infection in the mother and lack of signs of neonatal herpes in either the mother or infant make this infection less likely.

37. **The correct answer is A.** After a first seizure, there is a high likelihood (approximately 60% to 70%) that a

child will not experience another seizure episode again. Extensive laboratory examination and hospital admission (**choice B**) are not necessary, unless physical examination reveals some organic disease that may be related to the onset of the seizure. However, the majority of seizures of new onset are idiopathic (i.e., no cause can be identified with the commonly available diagnostic tools). Children developing a first-time seizure do not need antiepileptic drugs. Furthermore, approximately two-thirds of children who develop a second episode will not have additional seizures. Medication may reduce the risk of having a second or third episode but does not affect the long-term outcome (i.e., the probability that a patient will be seizure-free 2-3 years after the first seizure). Thus, the only measure to take in this situation is to provide reassurance to both patient and family by explaining that the child probably will not have any other seizures and that isolated seizures do not cause any damage to the brain.

Electroencephalographic (EEG) studies (**choice C**) would most likely yield no information. In fact, there is not a single test that can diagnose or rule out epilepsy. In addition, continuous EEG monitoring with or without video monitoring is very expensive. It is indicated only when seizures are frequent during the day and it is necessary to establish a relationship between neurologic manifestations and abnormal electrical activity.

CT/MRI studies of the brain (**choice D**) are rarely necessary after a single episode, unless there is some clinical evidence suggesting a focal intracranial lesion.

Starting antiepileptic medication (**choice E**) would be unnecessary following a first episode. In fact, there is still controversy whether it should be started even after a second episode (i.e., once a diagnosis of *epilepsy* is made).

38. **The correct answer is A.** The thalassemias are due to inadequate production of alpha or beta hemoglobin chains. The genes coding for the alpha chain have been duplicated, producing a total of four copies. If all four alpha genes are normal, or if three are normal and one is thalassemic, the person is clinically normal. If two are abnormal, the person has alpha-thalassemia trait with mild hypochromic anemia. If three are abnormal, the patient has HbH disease with hemolytic disease. If all four are abnormal, hydrops fetalis, clinically similar to that produced by Rh disease, is produced. Newborns with alpha-thalassemia trait, HbH disease, or hydrops fetalis produce HbBarts, which corresponds to a tetramer of four gamma chains. Adults with HbH disease, and sometimes those with alpha-thalassemia trait, produce HbH, a tetramer of four beta chains.

HbC (**choice B**) is an abnormal hemoglobin that, like HbS, can be associated with variable degrees of anemia.

HbGlower 2 (**choice C**) is a hemoglobin present in first trimester embryos.

HbH (**choice D**) is seen in adults with alpha-thalassemia (three abnormal genes), but is made in infants.

HbS (**choice E**) is associated with sickle cell anemia and trait.

39. **The correct answer is D.** Neuroblastoma arises from neural crest tissue and occurs in infancy. It is the most common solid tumor in children other than brain tumors. Eighty-five percent of neuroblastoma cases are diagnosed in children younger than 2 years. The clinical presentation varies with the tumor's location. Common signs and symptoms include asymptomatic abdominal mass, Horner syndrome, persistent cough, superior vena cava syndrome, bone pain, cord compression, subcutaneous nodules ("blueberry muffin" lesions), hypertension, opsoclonus ("dancing eyes"), and myoclonus ("dancing feet").

Astrocytoma (**choice A**) and glioblastoma multiforme (**choice B**) are intracranial tumors and are therefore incorrect. The typical presentation of a brain tumor is early morning headache and vomiting, ataxia, cranial nerve palsies, nystagmus, and papilledema.

Hyperthyroidism (**choice C**) does not cause opsoclonus or myoclonus, although it can cause tremor. Other typical features in children are irritability, excessive appetite, weight loss, increased perspiration, tachycardia, and goiter. Of note, hyperthyroidism occurs most frequently in children aged 12-14 years; only 2% of patients present before 10 years of age.

Wilms tumor (**choice E**) occurs in the metanephric cells in the kidney. It is not associated with nervous system involvement.

40. **The correct answer is A.** Nasal congestion, rhinorrhea, sneezing, and itchy nose and eyes are the most characteristic manifestations of allergic rhinitis, whether due to seasonal or perennial triggers. Nasal congestion can be particularly bothersome to patients with this condition. It is due to edema of the nasal mucosa, with resultant narrowing of the nasal passages. Patients are forced to breathe through their mouth, causing nasal speech and snoring. Over time, children will acquire what is known as "adenoidal facies," with flat malar eminences, narrow maxillae, and an arched palate. Pharmacotherapy becomes necessary if avoidance of allergens is not feasible or sufficient to provide satisfactory relief. Alpha-adrenergic drugs, such as phenylephrine and pseudoephedrine, are most effective in relieving nasal congestion because of their vasoconstricting action. Two important side effects are rebound congestion and rhinitis medicamentosa.

Antihistamines such as chlorpheniramine (**choice B**; i.e., first-generation antihistamines) are useful in treating symptoms of rhinitis, especially sneezing, rhinorrhea, and itching, but are less effective in preventing congestion. These drugs cause sedation and anticholinergic side effects.

Antihistamines such as loratadine (**choice C**; i.e., second-generation antihistamines) do not cause sedation and have therapeutic effects similar to first-generation antihistamines.

Cromoglycate, or similar mast cell stabilizers (**choice D**), have therapeutic effects comparable to antihistamines but are not useful in relieving nasal congestion. These drugs are most effective when administered prior to allergen exposure.

Ipratropium bromide (**choice E**) is an anticholinergic agent that blocks cholinergic-mediated mucus secretion and vasodilatation. It can prevent rhinorrhea but is less effective for congestion.

41. **The correct answer is C.** Typical findings of congenital hypothyroidism include constipation (35%), prolonged jaundice (75%), failure to thrive (35%), an enlarged fontanel (33%), and an umbilical hernia (50%). This constellation of findings is typical of the month-old hypothyroid patient.

Alpha-1-antitrypsin deficiency (**choice A**) is an uncommon cause of prolonged jaundice in the neonate. About 10% of infants with this condition present with prolonged neonatal jaundice. It is usually associated with increased conjugated bilirubin. Constipation is not a common feature of this illness in the infant.

Biliary atresia (**choice B**) presents with prolonged jaundice, but is accompanied by pale (acholic) stools. Hepatomegaly and increased venous patterning over the abdomen will appear later.

Congenital myasthenia gravis (**choice D**) is a disorder of the neuromuscular junction with heterogenous causes and which presents with hypotonia at or close to birth. Fatigable muscle weakness is seen most often in the ocular, bulbar, respiratory, and limbs. Deep tendon reflexes are reduced. A decremental repetitive stimulation response is found. Acetylcholine-receptor antibody tests are negative.

Although infants with pyloric stenosis (**choice E**) are often jaundiced, the classic intestinal symptom is projectile vomiting after feedings without any of the other physical signs mentioned. Stool color and consistency are generally unremarkable.

Syphilis (**choice F**) is accompanied by hepato-splenomegaly, a rash, and an elevated direct bilirubin.

Infants may also develop "snuffles," a persistent watery to mucoid nasal discharge.

Werdnig-Hoffmann disease (**choice G**) is a form of spinal muscular atrophy. The earliest feature may be decreased fetal movements during late pregnancy. Despite being alert, the infant is floppy and weak at birth. The weakness is maximal in the shoulder and hip girdle muscles. Muscle fasciculation, especially of the tongue, may be seen. Other features of the disease include deformed chest with seesaw respiration, frog-leg position of the limbs, and absent reflexes.

42. **The correct answer is D.** Measurements of T4 and TSH levels are the most appropriate tests to confirm congenital hypothyroidism.

Alpha-1-antitrypsin genotyping (**choice A**) is used to confirm alpha-1-antitrypsin deficiency.

Barium swallow (**choice B**) will indicate the presence of pyloric stenosis ("string" sign = narrowing of barium stream passing through the duodenum; "umbrella" sign = the holdup of barium in the stomach).

A liver and spleen scan (**choice C**) is useful to indicate the absence of the biliary tree or blockage of the extrahepatic bile ducts and is therefore most useful to confirm biliary atresia.

Muscle biopsy (**choice E**) is used to diagnose myopathic conditions, including Werdnig-Hoffmann disease, muscular dystrophy, and metabolic inclusion diseases.

The RPR and FTA (**choice F**) are serologic tests for syphilis.

43. **The correct answer is G.** The search for a cause of anemia is important in children because it can result in diminished bone growth and learning. Nutritional anemia is the most common anemia in infants of this age. Infants consuming cow milk have a greater incidence of iron deficiency because bovine milk has a higher concentration of calcium, which competes for iron absorption. The major physical finding is pallor. Infants may also be lethargic, irritable, and tired easily. Classic peripheral blood smear findings are described here, and a complete blood count (CBC) characteristically shows decreased mean corpuscular volume (MCV) and mean corpuscular hemoglobin concentration (MCHC). Diagnosis can be further confirmed with iron studies, TIBC, and serum ferritin.

Acute myelogenous leukemia (**choice A**) results in pancytopenia due to bone marrow failure. Neoplastic proliferation of blast cells occurs in the bone marrow and presents clinically with anemia, bleeding, fatigue, nonspecific body aches, and vulnerability to infection. Pancytopenia with circulating blasts is characteristically found on peripheral blood smear.

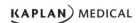

Anemia of chronic disease (**choice B**) can impair erythropoietin production, resulting in decreased red cell production. A normocytic, normochromic pattern is seen on peripheral blood smear and CBC.

Red cell destruction, as seen in glucose 6-phosphate (G6PD) deficiency (**choice C**), can be the cause of anemia. G6PD is a red cell enzyme abnormality that causes intrinsic hemolysis of red blood cells. Bite cells are usually seen on peripheral blood smear.

Anemia due to blood loss can be seen in hookworm infections (**choice D**). Although the anemia found in hookworm infection is due to the loss of bleeding and ultimately iron deficiency, there is nothing in the history to suggest a hookworm infection in this child. The most likely cause of the anemia is the ingestion of whole cow milk that results in the inadequate absorption of nutritional iron.

Hypothyroidism (**choice E**) can cause normochromic, normocytic anemia. Infants with hypothyroidism present with cretinism, whereas children may show lethargy, constipation, dry skin, and mental retardation.

Folic acid deficiency (**choice F**) is a cause of megaloblastic anemia when there is insufficient leafy vegetables in the diet. However, the peripheral blood smear and CBC findings in this case reveal a microcytic anemia.

44. **The correct answer is C.** Because the most likely clinical diagnosis at this time is iron deficiency anemia, it would be appropriate to offer dietary advice (iron-fortified cereal, meat, green vegetables, egg yolk) and provide supplemental iron in the form of drops. A reticulocytosis typically occurs with a peak response in 5 to 7 days, followed by an increase in hemoglobin over the next 1 to 4 weeks. This treatment is both diagnostic and therapeutic.

Antibiotic therapy (**choice A**) may also be used in hookworm infections to prevent further loss of blood and may be useful in the treatment of other concurrent infections, but it will have no effect in this child's nutritional iron deficiency anemia due to cow milk ingestion.

Bone marrow biopsy (**choice B**) is helpful in evaluating the presence of malignant cells and bone marrow failure, in the case of leukemia.

Red cell enzyme studies (**choice D**) are used to diagnose glucose 6-phosphate (G6PD) deficiency and pyruvate kinase as the cause of intrinsic hemolysis and subsequent anemia.

Thyroid studies (**choice E**) can diagnose hypothyroidism as a cause of anemia. However, clinical and laboratory features of this child's anemia suggest nutritional iron deficiency.

45. **The correct answer is G.** Approximately 50% of children with Down syndrome are born with endocardial cushion defects, such as ventricular septal defect, atrial septal defect, or complete atrioventricular canal defect.

46. **The correct answer is I.** Williams syndrome is a deletion of the 7q chromosome, causing short stature, hypercalcemia, or hypercalciuria in infancy; developmental delay; dysmorphic features; overly friendly personality; and supravalvular aortic stenosis. Without surgical correction, the cardiac disease will progress and can cause sudden death.

47. **The correct answer is E.** DiGeorge syndrome is caused by microdeletions in the 22q11 chromosome region. Features include facial dysmorphisms, thymic hypoplasia with resultant hypocalcemia, and conotruncal abnormalities, such as truncus arteriosus or total anomalous pulmonary venous return. The child in this vignette had a hypocalcemic seizure and cyanosis caused by truncus arteriosus. Therapy includes surgical correction of the heart defect and dietary supplementation with calcium and vitamin D.

Aortic insufficiency (**choice A**) is associated with Marfan syndrome. Aortic dissections are also seen in this condition and can be lethal.

Coarctation of the aorta (**choice B**) is seen in 35% of patients with Turner syndrome.

Complex congenital heart defects (**choice C**) is too broad an answer choice and cannot be correlated with one congenital syndrome in particular.

Congenital heart block (**choice D**) can occur in infants born to mothers with systemic lupus erythematosus.

Dextrocardia (**choice F**) is a common finding in patients with Kartagener syndrome.

Patent ductus arteriosus (**choice H**) can be seen in infants with congenital rubella infection. However, it is usually the result of prematurity, sepsis, metabolic acidosis, or pulmonary defects not associated with congenital syndromes.

48. **The correct answer is J.** Mesenteric adenitis is an important cause of right iliac fossa pain in children. It is due to a nonspecific inflammation of mesenteric lymph glands that, in turn, is due to viral and bacterial infections. The most common causes are *Yersinia* species, *Streptococcus viridans*, and *Campylobacter jejuni*. The clinical picture includes abdominal pain, which may be generalized or localized and is usually in the right iliac fossa. There is moderate tenderness but little guarding or rebound. The patient may have mild pyrexia, and there may be diarrhea (with or without vomiting) or there may have been a recent upper respiratory tract infection. Mesenteric

adenitis is, at times, difficult to differentiate from acute appendicitis, but in this case, it is differentiated by the lack of abdominal rebound and guarding and by a normal appetite. Ultrasonography of the right lower quadrant with graded compression has been the mainstay of diagnosis in children.

49. **The correct answer is G.** Intussuscepton causes paroxysms of severe, crampy abdominal pain and early-onset vomiting in children under 5 years old, with peak presentation at 6 months of age. It is caused by the invagination of one portion of the bowel into the lumen of the immediately adjoining bowel. The most common form is ileocolic intussusception. Classic findings on physical examination are a walnut-sized mass palpated abdominally, a high-pitched peristalsis on auscultation, and "currant-jelly" stools on rectal examination. In the absence of treatment, this condition is usually fatal. Barium or air enemas are both diagnostic ("stack of coins" sign) and therapeutic in reducing the invaginated segment. Surgical reduction is performed in some cases.

50. **The correct answer is D.** The cardinal features of Henoch-Schönlein purpura (HSP) are gastrointestinal, joint, and renal manifestations due to widespread vasculitis of the arterioles and small capillaries. The dominant clinical features are shown in this case: cutaneous purpura, arthritis, abdominal pain (gastrointestinal bleeding may also occur), orchitis, and nephritis (hematuria and proteinuria). In up to two-thirds of patients, clinical onset is preceded by an upper respiratory tract infection. In general, HSP is an acute, self-limited illness, but one-third of patients has one or more recurrences. The most feared complication is progressive renal disease. Scrotal involvement is common and may mimic testicular torsion.

The abdominal pain of appendicitis (**choice A**) classically begins as a crampy epigastric or periumbilical pain and progresses to a constant pain in the right lower quadrant. It is associated with vomiting and anorexia. On clinical examination, there are signs of peritoneal inflammation in the right iliac fossa, fever, and tachycardia, and there may be a positive Rovsing, obturator, or psoas sign.

Constipation (**choice B**) may occur at any age and is usually the cause of recurrent, crampy abdominal pain, especially after meals. Constipation may occur if there is inadequate food or fluid intake. Children who drink a lot of milk may have hard stools that are difficult to pass. Feces is often palpable on examination, and there is no associated fever.

The abdominal pain associated with gastroenteritis (**choice C**) is diffuse in nature, with no localized physical signs and with associated diarrhea, nausea, or vomiting and fever. The etiology is usually viral, most often due to rotavirus. The presentation of blood, mucus, and frequent small motions is suggestive of a bacterial cause. With progression, the child may become lethargic and dehydrated, with accompanying acidosis.

Inflammatory bowel disease (**choice E**) is suggested in children with chronic abdominal pain, episodes of diarrhea that may be bloody, fever, and weight loss. One of the most important clues is growth failure, especially in adolescents. Crohn disease is a transmural process that may affect any part of the gastrointestinal tract, whereas in uncomplicated ulcerative colitis, inflammation is confined to the muscosa of the colon.

Inguinal hernia (**choice F**) in infants and early childhood results from a patent processus vaginalis. The defect can be large enough to allow abdominal or pelvic organs to descend. The parents may report that the swelling appears with straining or crying, only to disappear at rest.

Lactose intolerance (**choice H**), in its congenital form, is characterized by severe diarrhea, abdominal pain, and distension that appear soon after birth due to marked lactase deficiency in the small intestine. Lactase normally catalyzes the cleavage of lactose into glucose and galactose. Symptoms disappear with milk withdrawal (the source of lactose). Stool pH is acidic because of the presence of lactic acid resulting from the bacterial fermentation of the ingested lactose.

Colicky abdominal pain and vomiting may be the presenting symptoms of acute lead poisoning (**choice I**) in children. Poisoning due to absorption or ingestion of lead affects the brain, nervous and digestive systems, and blood. Clinical features following ingestion of lead also include encephalopathy (ataxia, drowsiness, convulsions), pica, and papilledema.

Pneumonia (**choice K**) can cause referred abdominal pain, especially when the infection is located in the lower lobes. Look for other symptoms that will suggest pneumonia as the cause of the abdominal pain, including fever, tachycardia, tachypnea, nasal flaring, cough, and crackles on auscultation. A chest x-ray will help with diagnosis.

Nonorganic causes of abdominal pain, the most common of which is psychosomatic (**choice L**), are common causes of recurrent abdominal pain in childhood. Features that suggest nonorganic pain include pain occurring only on school days or certain social circumstances, nonorganic abdominal pain that is usually umbilical, a family history of recurrent abdominal pain of unknown etiology, and distractibility and variability of pain on examination.

Torsion of the testis (**choice M**) is a surgical emergency that typically presents with a tender, swollen scrotum and lower abdominal pain. Although it occurs in all age groups, torsion is most common in adolescents, who have the highest incidence of undescended testes. There may be a history of mild trauma to the testis or a history of episodes of testicular pain due to torsion and untwisting.

A urinary tract infection (**choice N**) is an important cause of lower abdominal pain in children because missing its diagnosis may damage the developing kidney. Presenting features include fever, loin pain and tenderness, dysuria, and urinary frequency. Diagnosis is made on urinalysis with culture and microscopy.

Pediatrics: **Test Three**

1. A 4-week-old male infant has been spitting up his formula feedings for the past few days. He does not vomit bilious material or blood. The spitting up is gradually becoming more frequent, and forceful vomiting ensues. The vomitus seems to shoot straight out and nearly hit the wall. On examination, the baby seems hungry and is chewing his fist. His mucous membranes appear dry. A small, round mass, about the size of an adult thumbnail, is palpated in the upper abdomen. Laboratory data reveal Na^+ of 133 mEq/L, K^+ of 3.5 mEq/L, Cl^- of 93 mEq/L, and HCO_3^- of 29 mEq/L. Which of the following is the most appropriate next step in management?

   (A) Change the feedings to clear liquids or Pedialyte

   (B) Obtain a surgical consult immediately

   (C) Obtain flat plate and upright x-ray films of the abdomen

   (D) Insert a nasogastric tube

   (E) Begin parenteral antibiotics

2. An infant has had repeated pneumonias and middle ear infections that began at about 5 months of age. At 1 year of age, serum electrophoresis demonstrated hypogammaglobulinemia. T cell function was normal. By 2 years of age, the child's infection rate has decreased, and repeat serum electrophoresis is normal. Which of the following immunoglobulins was likely decreased in this child during the period of increased susceptibility to infection?

   (A) IgA

   (B) IgD

   (C) IgE

   (D) IgG

   (E) IgM

3. A 12-year-old, previously healthy girl presents to her physician with a chief complaint of early morning headaches. She states that these headaches wake her up from sleep 2 to 3 days a week. She also complains of some vomiting associated with the headaches. The headaches have been getting progressively worse for the past 2 months. She denies any photophobia, dizziness, or blurred vision. There is no history of a recent respiratory infection, runny nose, or cough. There is no history of recent trauma. In the office, her vital signs are within normal limits. Her examination shows pupils that are equal, round, and reactive, with no maxillary or frontal sinus tenderness. Her tympanic membranes are clear and intact. Her neck is supple with full range of motion. Neurologic examination shows a positive Romberg sign. Which of the following tests would most likely confirm the diagnosis?

   (A) CT of the brain

   (B) MRI of the brain

   (C) Plain film of the skull

   (D) Sinus x-ray film

   (E) Spinal tap

4. A 10-month-old boy develops an upper respiratory tract infection 2 days before presentation. On the day of presentation, he has a generalized tonic-clonic seizure lasting 30 seconds. His temperature is 40.0° C (104.0° F), blood pressure is 90/60 mm Hg, and respirations are 22/min. He is alert and smiling. He has rhinorrhea, and his neck is supple. He has bruises below his knees. Which of the following is the most likely diagnosis?

   (A) Child abuse

   (B) Idiopathic epilepsy

   (C) Infantile spasms

   (D) Meningitis

   (E) Simple febrile seizure

KAPLAN MEDICAL

5. A previously well 3-year-old child presents to the clinic with marked erythema of the cheeks that appeared suddenly overnight. The rash has spread to involve the proximal arms, and it has a reticular erythematous maculopapular appearance. There are no known allergies, and the child has no prior illnesses and has not been exposed to any individuals who are ill. Vital signs are within normal limits. Cervical lymphadenopathy is noted on physical examination. Which of the following is the most likely cause of this child's rash?

(A) Contact dermatitis

(B) Fifth disease

(C) Measles

(D) Roseola

(E) Rubella

(F) Systemic lupus erythematosus (SLE)

6. A premature infant born at 28 weeks' gestation develops respiratory distress shortly after birth. The infant is placed in an incubator with supplemental oxygen and is monitored in the neonatal intensive care unit. Given the severe prematurity of the infant, the physician gives strict instructions for the nursing staff regarding oxygen tension levels. Attempts at oxygen weaning are begun as soon as clinically feasible. Which of the following is characteristic of the eye damage that occurs following prolonged oxygen exposure in preterm neonates?

(A) Blood vessels in the vitreous

(B) Cotton wool exudates in the retina

(C) Microaneurysms of the retinal arterioles

(D) Papilledema of the optic nerve head

(E) Ulcers on the cornea

7. A 7-year-old boy is brought to the clinic by his mother, who states that he has been complaining of abdominal pain for 2 to 3 days. He has been afebrile, with no vomiting or diarrhea. His mother states she brought him to the office today because she noticed a rash on his legs that is getting worse, and he is now complaining of knee pain. On examination, there are palpable purpuric lesions on both legs and buttocks. He has pain around his ankle and knee joints with minimal swelling, and no warmth or erythema. Which of the following is the most likely diagnosis?

(A) Dermatomyositis

(B) Gastroenteritis

(C) Henoch-Schönlein purpura

(D) Juvenile rheumatoid arthritis

(E) Kawasaki disease

8. A previously healthy 12-year-old boy is brought to the physician the day after a nocturnal crisis of difficulty breathing, chest tightness, and cough. He has a history of atopic dermatitis that resolved around 6 years of age. He now has no apparent respiratory distress. His breathing is regular, and his respirations are 12/min. Blood pressure, pulse, and temperature are normal. Chest examination reveals only a few crackles that quickly clear after coughing and mild end-expiratory wheezes. Which of the following is the most appropriate next step in diagnosis?

(A) Arterial blood gas analysis

(B) Bronchial provocation test with histamine or methacholine

(C) Complete blood count

(D) Chest x-ray examination

(E) Spirometry before and after administration of a bronchodilator

9. A 7-year-old boy is brought to the physician because of persistent nasal obstruction for 6 months. There is no personal or family history of allergic disorders. Examination of the nasal fossae reveals bilateral ethmoidal polyps that protrude into the middle meatus and nasal cavity. Which of the following is the most appropriate next step in diagnosis?

   (A) Cutaneous allergen testing

   (B) Excisional biopsy

   (C) Nasal provocation testing

   (D) Pilocarpine iontophoresis sweat test

   (E) Radioallergosorbent test (RAST)

10. A neonate is very small for gestational age and shows hypotonia and marked skeletal muscle and subcutaneous fat hypoplasia. During delivery, a large volume of amniotic fluid was released at rupture of membranes. The placenta was small, and only a single umbilical artery was noted. The face has a pinched appearance with hypoplastic orbital ridges, short palpebral fissures, and a small mouth and jaw. The head is small with prominence of the occiput. The ears are low set and malformed. The infant's fists are clenched, with overlapping of the third and fourth fingers. The feet are clubbed, and the great toe is shortened. Which of the following is most likely diagnosis?

   (A) 47,XXY

   (B) Triple X

   (C) Trisomy 13

   (D) Trisomy 18

   (E) Trisomy 21

11. A 2-year-old girl is taken to a pediatrician because she has developed a rash and seems unusually unsteady when she tries to walk. Physical examination demonstrates a diffuse rash on body parts exposed to sun. Also noted are short stature, possible mental retardation, and ataxia. Screening studies demonstrate increased total amino acids in the urine. Which of the following is the most likely diagnosis?

   (A) Alkaptonuria

   (B) Cystinuria

   (C) Hartnup disease

   (D) Fanconi syndrome

   (E) Phenylketonuria

12. A 1-year-old child is brought in for a regular "well baby" check-up. The child appears to have strabismus. The reflection of a bright light from the ceiling of the examination room comes from a different place in each eye. The family explains that the child has always looked that way, and there has been no recent change in the appearance of his eyes. Which of the following is the most effective management?

   (A) No treatment unless the condition has not resolved spontaneously by age 7

   (B) Corrective lenses

   (C) Each eye patched for a month at a time, alternating sides

   (D) Surgical correction whenever he is old enough to decide whether he wants it for cosmetic reasons

   (E) Surgical correction as soon as it is practical to do it

13. A 6-year-old boy presents in clinic for a routine visit. Examination reveals coarse, dark pubic hair, an enlarged penis and testes, and acne of the face and upper back. His mother notes that he has a body odor similar to that of her teenage son after playing sports. The child is in the 99th percentile of height for his age group. Which of the following is the most likely diagnosis?

   (A) Congenital adrenal hyperplasia

   (B) Hypothalamic tumor

   (C) Klinefelter syndrome

   (D) Male pseudohermaphroditism

   (E) XYY syndrome

14. A 10-year-old girl is brought to a pediatrician because her mother notices that she stumbles frequently at night, even with adequate lighting. Visual field testing demonstrates a relatively narrow mid-peripheral ring scotoma. Ophthalmoscopy demonstrates dark pigmentation in a bone spicule configuration involving the equatorial retina. Additional findings include a waxy yellow appearance to the disk and narrowed retinal arteries. Which of the following is the most likely diagnosis?

   (A) Cataract

   (B) Central retinal artery occlusion

   (C) Retinal detachment

   (D) Retinitis pigmentosa

   (E) Uveitis

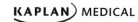

15. A 5-year-old child develops left-sided ear pain, but her mother is too busy to take her to the pediatrician. There is no improvement in the child's condition, and the mother has noticed painful, swollen, red areas behind the pinna. At this point, the child is brought to the emergency department, where the physician notes the presence of a creamy discharge in the left ear canal and a temperature of 38.6° C (101.5° F). Tuning fork tests localize hearing better on the left ear when placed on apex of head, and bone conduction is greater than air conduction in the left ear. Which of the following is the most likely diagnosis?

    (A) Acute mastoiditis

    (B) Barotitis media

    (C) Cholesteatoma

    (D) Chronic otitis media

    (E) Ménière disease

    (F) Myringitis

    (G) Otitis externa

    (H) Secretory otitis media

16. A 3-year-old girl is believed to have swallowed a marble. She presents to the emergency department unable to speak and begins to become cyanotic. Initial attempts at endotracheal intubation are unsuccessful. Which of the following is the most appropriate next step in management?

    (A) Continued attempts at endotracheal intubation

    (B) Cricothyroidotomy (surgical)

    (C) Face mask 100% O_2 with succinylcholine

    (D) Formal tracheostomy

    (E) Needle cricothyroidotomy

17. A 24-month-old girl is brought to the pediatrician's office for evaluation because her mother noticed a yellowish discharge on the girl's underwear for the past 3 days. She had no fever, but her mother said she has been fussier recently. On physical examination, the girl is appears excessively anxious about contact with the physician. Her introitus is inflamed, and the hymeneal edge is jagged at the 8 o'clock position. A vaginal culture is taken. Which of the following organisms, if isolated from the vaginal vault, would constitute the most definitive evidence of sexual abuse?

    (A) *Candida albicans*

    (B) *Chlamydia trachomatis*

    (C) *Gardnerella vaginalis*

    (D) *Pseudomonas aeruginosa*

    (E) *Neisseria gonorrhoeae*

18. A premature neonate develops respiratory distress syndrome several hours after birth. The infant is placed on a respirator and given other appropriate care. However, when the infant reaches a corrected gestational age of 36 weeks, he does not tolerate weaning from the ventilator. A chest x-ray film demonstrates alternating areas of hyperaeration and pulmonary scarring, resulting in parenchymal streaks and hyperexpanded areas. Which of the following is the most likely diagnosis?

    (A) Apnea of prematurity

    (B) Bronchopulmonary dysplasia

    (C) Cystic fibrosis

    (D) Persistent pulmonary hypertension of the newborn

    (E) Transient tachypnea of the newborn

19. Approximately 19 days after having had a severe sore throat, a 10-year-old girl is taken to a pediatrician because she is complaining that her arms and legs hurt. The mother reports that before the extremity pain began, the child had a rash with irregular boundaries that lasted about a day. Physical examination demonstrates mild fever, as well as swelling and erythema around several large joints. Laboratory studies show an elevated erythrocyte sedimentation rate, and ECG demonstrates a prolonged PR interval. Which of the following is the most likely explanation for these findings?

    (A) Antigenic mimicry

    (B) Bacterial infection of valves

    (C) Parasitic infection of myocytes

    (D) Toxin production

    (E) Viral infection of myocytes

20. A 5-year-old boy is scheduled for a medical checkup and MMR booster before beginning the school year. All of his vaccinations are up to date, but his mother reports that he had a reaction to the first MMR shot, which was given at 12 months of age. The reaction involved a cough, red eyes, and a rash over the skin that resolved in about 1 week. The mother reports that the child is presently resolving from a "mild case of the flu," with mild fever, coughing, and rhinorrhea, that has kept him awake during the last couple of nights. Past medical history is significant for anaphylaxis to previously administered amoxicillin and neomycin. There is no history of major illnesses. Which of the following is a contraindication to the administration of MMR vaccine in this patient?

   (A) Anaphylaxis to amoxicillin

   (B) Anaphylaxis to neomycin

   (C) Pregnancy in the mother

   (D) Previous febrile reaction to the MMR vaccine

   (E) Upper respiratory tract infection with low-grade fever

21. A 15-year-old boy is seen in the pediatrician's office for a health maintenance physical examination. The boy reports a heavy, dragging sensation in his left scrotum. The sensation is more pronounced after exercise. He denies any scrotal pain. He is not sexually active. Examination of his genitalia indicates Tanner stage 4. There is a palpable fullness over his left scrotum. Both testes are normal in size and smooth in contour. Which of the following is the most likely explanation of these findings?

   (A) Hydrocele

   (B) Inguinal hernia

   (C) Orchitis

   (D) Testicular tumor

   (E) Varicocele

22. A 5-year-old child undergoes a school entrance physical examination. The pediatrician notices gray-brown pigmentation on the skin of his forehead, hands, and pretibial regions. Subconjunctival areas near the corneoscleral junction show wedge-shaped, yellow-brown discoloration (pingueculae). Enlargement of both the spleen and the liver are noted on abdominal examination. Needle biopsy of the spleen demonstrates the presence of unusually large (20- to 100-mm diameter) reticuloendothelial histiocytes with a "crumpled-silk" appearance. Bone marrow biopsy demonstrates the presence of the same type of cells. Which of the following is the most likely diagnosis?

   (A) Abetalipoproteinemia

   (B) Fabry disease

   (C) Gaucher disease

   (D) Niemann-Pick disease

   (E) Tangier disease

23. A 12-year-old boy presents to his pediatrician with frequent episodes of headache, nausea, blurry vision, and sweating. On physical examination, his temperature is 37.4° C (99.3° F), blood pressure is 148/94 mm Hg, pulse is 92/min, and respirations are 18/min. The rest of his examination is unremarkable. His 24-hour urinary vanillylmandelic acid (VMA) and metanephrines are increased. An abdominal CT reveals an extrarenal mass above the left kidney. Which of the following is the most appropriate pharmacotherapy?

   (A) Alpha-adrenergic blocker

   (B) Angiotensin-converting enzyme inhibitor

   (C) Beta-adrenergic blocker

   (D) Calcium channel blocker

   (E) Diuretics

24. A 12-year-old girl with mild asthma comes to the office for a health maintenance visit. Her mother states that she is using her albuterol inhaler two to three times a week and that she has a cough that wakes her up at night about three times a month. On physical examination, she has diffuse inspiratory and expiratory wheezes. She has no accessory muscle use. Pulse oximetry shows 95% oxygen saturation on room air. Which of the following is the most appropriate treatment for her at this time?

   (A) Albuterol nebulized treatment

   (B) Cromolyn sodium nebulized treatment

   (C) Oxygen via nasal cannula

   (D) IV steroids

   (E) Subcutaneous epinephrine

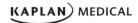

25. The 1-year-old brother of a child with known abeta-lipoproteinemia is evaluated by a pediatrician for the disease. The 1-year-old has been exhibiting steatorrhea and ataxia. Which of the following would most strongly support the suspected diagnosis?

    (A) Acanthocytes on peripheral smear

    (B) "Crumpled silk" histiocytes on bone marrow biopsy

    (C) Globoid cells on brain biopsy

    (D) Metachromatic deposits on sural nerve biopsy

    (E) "Sea-blue" histiocytes on bone marrow biopsy

26. A 6-year-old boy is brought to the emergency department because of the acute onset of headache, nausea, and vomiting. On arrival, physical examination reveals marked nuchal rigidity and funduscopic evidence of papilledema. A head CT scan reveals a solid tumor in the posterior fossa, centered in the cerebellar vermis and extending to the fourth ventricle. An emergency craniotomy is performed, during which a small sample of the tumor is sent to the pathologist for a frozen section consultation. Which of the following is the most likely diagnosis?

    (A) Ependymoma

    (B) Glioblastoma multiforme (GBM)

    (C) Hemangioblastoma

    (D) Medulloblastoma

    (E) Oligodendroglioma

    (F) Pilocytic astrocytoma

27. A 3-month-old infant with a history of chronic constipation presents with fulminant, watery diarrhea over 2 days. The infant is brought to the emergency department with signs of severe dehydration and a distended abdomen. His history is significant for delayed passage of meconium after birth and failure to thrive. Plain x-ray films of the abdomen reveal a massively dilated transverse colon, with the presence of gas in the distal colon. Which of the following is the most likely diagnosis?

    (A) Congenital hypothyroidism

    (B) Meconium ileus

    (C) Necrotizing enterocolitis

    (D) Toxic enterocolitis

    (E) Volvulus

28. A mother brings her 9-month-old daughter to the pediatrician with complaints of a rash. The mother states that the infant had a high fever (temperature up to 40.0° C [104.0° F]) for 3 days prior to developing the rash, but is now afebrile. The mother also says that the infant has had a runny nose and a slight cough for the past 3 days. On examination, there is a fine macular rash on the infant's trunk and neck. The examination is otherwise within normal limits, and the infant is playful and smiling. Which of the following is the most likely diagnosis?

    (A) Erythema infectiosum

    (B) Roseola

    (C) Rubella

    (D) Rubeola

    (E) Varicella

29. An infant is born with a craniofacial abnormality. There is a patch of very white skin on the midline forehead, above which is a white forelock of hair. The remainder of the hair is dark brown. The eyes are also abnormal, with color variations from brown to blue within the irises. The medial canthi are displaced laterally. The infant does not respond to sound. Which of the following is the most likely diagnosis?

    (A) Beckwith-Wiedermann syndrome

    (B) Fragile X syndrome

    (C) Goldenhar syndrome

    (D) Pierre Robin syndrome

    (E) Treacher Collins syndrome

    (F) Waardenburg syndrome

30. A 15-month-old boy is brought into the clinic with a 1-day history of fever, decreased oral intake, and runny nose. His vital signs are within normal limits except for a temperature of 39.5° C (103.1° F). He is active and in no distress. His ears are clear bilaterally. There is a clear nasal discharge. Multiple small (1 to 2 mm) vesicular lesions are noted on the mucosa of the anterior tonsillar pillars and posterior palate. The rest of his examination is within normal limits. Which of the following is the most likely diagnosis?

    (A) Aphthous stomatitis

    (B) Hand-foot-and-mouth disease

    (C) Herpangina

    (D) Kawasaki disease

    (E) Stevens-Johnson syndrome

31. A nurse notices that a 1-week-old, premature infant in the neonatal unit is experiencing migratory jerks of the extremities. She picks the infant up and can feel that the muscle jerks continue to happen, even when she holds an involved extremity still. After about 5 minutes, the jerking movements stop. Which of the following is the most appropriate first step in diagnosis?

    (A) CT scan of head
    (B) Electroencephalography
    (C) Serum chemistries
    (D) Skull x-rays
    (E) Ultrasound of head

32. A female neonate is undergoing an examination after birth. She was born to a 33-year-old primigravid mother at term via a normal spontaneous vaginal delivery. The pregnancy was uncomplicated, except for a positive maternal group B *Streptococcus* culture at 36 weeks' gestation, for which the mother received penicillin during labor. The infant's APGAR scores are 8 at 1 minute and 9 at 5 minutes. The mother notices that the infant has prominent labia and a dull pink vaginal epithelium. Which of the following is the most likely cause of the appearance of the infant's genitalia?

    (A) Exposure to maternal estrogen
    (B) Exposure to penicillin
    (C) Infection with *Chlamydia*
    (D) Infection with group B *Streptococcus*
    (E) Sexual abuse

33. A 3-year-old girl is brought to the pediatrician with complaints of abdominal pain and fever. Her mother states that the fever started 2 days ago, with the highest temperature being 39.0° C (102.2° F). She has had no vomiting or diarrhea. The mother states that her daughter has been complaining of pain on urination. On examination, she is tender in her lower abdomen, and there is some right-sided costovertebral angle tenderness. A urinalysis confirms the suspicion of a urinary tract infection. This is the patient's second urinary tract infection. Which of the following would be the most appropriate diagnostic procedure?

    (A) Cystoscopy
    (B) Dimercaptosuccinic acid (DMSA) scan in 1 to 2 months
    (C) Intravenous pyelogram
    (D) Voiding cystourethrogram (VCUG) now
    (E) VCUG in 1 to 2 months

34. A neonate has an obviously abnormal foot. The foot is in a markedly plantar flexed position, with the sole facing the adjacent leg in a position of marked adduction. No other anomalies are noted on physical examination. Which of the following is the most likely diagnosis?

    (A) Epispadias
    (B) Hypospadias
    (C) Talipes calcaneovalgus
    (D) Talipes equinovarus
    (E) Torticollis

35. A new mother complains that her 6-week-old infant frequently regurgitates small volumes of formula during and after feedings. Physical examination demonstrates a happy baby who has gained half a pound since his last visit. No abdominal masses are noted. Which of the following is the best next step in management?

    (A) Change the baby's formula
    (B) Change the bottle's nipple
    (C) Monitor the baby carefully
    (D) Order abdominal x-rays
    (E) Order CT of the abdomen

36. A 3-year-old girl presents to the pediatrician's office. The mother states that the girl has been having big, bulky stools that float in the toilet. She also has intermittent diarrhea. On examination, her height is 88 cm (34.6 in, <5th percentile) and weight is 15.8 kg (34.8 lb, <5th percentile). In addition, she has an uncle who died of recurrent lower respiratory infections. Which of the following would be most effective for alleviating the gastrointestinal symptoms of this patient?

    (A) Avoidance of dairy products
    (B) Elimination of dietary fat
    (C) Ketogenic diet
    (D) Oral metronidazole
    (E) Pancreatic enzyme replacement

37. A 2-year-old boy presents to the emergency department with fever, irritability, and a skin rash 5 days after the onset of an upper respiratory infection. On examination, his temperature is 39.8° C (103.6° F), and his pulse is 94/min. There is an erythematous skin rash that involves his face, chest, back, and upper extremities. His skin is very tender to touch. Rubbing the skin causes separation of the epidermal layer. Which of the following is the most likely diagnosis?

    (A) Kawasaki disease

    (B) Staphylococcal scalded skin syndrome

    (C) Streptococcal scarlet fever

    (D) Toxic epidermal necrolysis

    (E) Toxic shock syndrome

38. A frantic mother telephones the pediatric office. She reports that her 10-year-old boy accidentally splashed Drano (a strongly corrosive, alkaline drain cleaner) on his face, and he is screaming in pain complaining that his right eye hurts terribly. Which of the following is the best advice to give to the mother?

    (A) Apply antibiotic ointment to the eye and make an appointment with an ophthalmologist

    (B) Bring the boy to the hospital right away

    (C) Pry the eye open and drip vinegar over it until the pain goes away

    (D) Pry the eye open and swipe it clean with a tissue before bringing the boy in for further evaluation

    (E) Pry the eye open, hold it under running cold water for about 30 minutes, and then bring the boy to the hospital

39. The mother of a 4-year-old child takes her daughter to a pediatrician because she is "scratching all the time." Physical examination demonstrates multiple areas of excoriation, which are worst on the shoulders, buttocks, and abdomen. In the areas where the scratching has occurred, scattered tiny red punctate lesions are also seen. Careful examination of the clothing reveals small, ovoid, grayish-white structures attached to threads on the seams. Which of the following is the most likely causative agent?

    (A) *Ancylostoma braziliense*

    (B) *Corynebacterium minutissimum*

    (C) *Pediculus humanus corporis*

    (D) *Sarcoptes scabiei*

    (E) *Trichophyton rubrum*

40. An 8-year-old boy is brought to the emergency department with a head injury. He hit his head on the ground when he fell off his bicycle. He was not wearing a helmet at the time. There was no loss of consciousness. He vomited two times after the accident and now complains of a right-sided headache and inability to hear with his right ear. There is no photophobia or diplopia. On physical examination, his blood pressure is 110/72 mm Hg, pulse is 104/min, and respirations are 22/min. He is alert and oriented and responds appropriately to questions. There is a round hematoma on the right side of his head. Bloody drainage is noted from his right ear. Which of the following injury is most consistent with these findings?

    (A) Concussion

    (B) Epidural hematoma

    (C) Subdural hematoma

    (D) Temporal bone fracture

    (E) Tympanic membrane perforation

41. A 16-year-old girl comes to the physician's office because she has not begun menstruating yet. Both her mother and an older sister started menstruation at age 12. She takes no medication and denies strenuous exercise or excessive dieting. Her height is at the 50th percentile for age; her weight is at the 60th percentile. Both her breast and pubic hair development are at Tanner stage 4. Pelvic ultrasonography reveals a normal uterus and ovaries. Which of the following is the most likely diagnosis?

    (A) Imperforate hymen

    (B) Physiologic pubertal delay

    (C) Prolactinoma

    (D) Testicular feminization syndrome

    (E) Turner syndrome

42. A 3-week-old infant is being evaluated for hematochezia. His mother states that the infant passed stools that contain both blood and mucus. There were no complications during her pregnancy, and the infant has been otherwise healthy. On physical examination, his temperature is 37.1° C (98.9° F), pulse is 110/min, and respirations are 18/min. He appears well, and his fontanelle is flat and level. Abdominal examination reveals normal active bowel sounds; his abdomen is nontender to palpation and there is no mass. His diaper contains stool that has bright red blood on it with mucus. Which of the following is the most likely explanation of his hematochezia?

    (A) Food allergy-induced colitis
    (B) Meckel diverticulum
    (C) Necrotizing enterocolitis
    (D) Rectal fissure
    (E) Ulcerative colitis

43. A 7-year-old boy is brought to the physician because of a persistent mucopurulent nasal discharge for 2 weeks following a common cold. The mother also reports that the child has had frequent cough during the day and occasional temperatures up to 38.0° C (100.5° F). The child does not appear critically ill, but he complains of mild pain in the maxillary region and nasal obstruction. Rhinoscopic examination reveals a rivulet of purulent fluid coming from the inferior meatus. The rest of the physical examination is normal. Which of the following is the most likely diagnosis?

    (A) Acute bacterial sinusitis
    (B) Acute otitis media
    (C) Acute viral rhinitis
    (D) Allergic rhinosinusitis
    (E) Asthma

44. A 10-year-old girl comes to medical attention because of recurrent attacks of wheezing and dyspnea. The attacks occur mostly at home or, if outdoors, soon after exercise. Exacerbations are noted in springtime. The severity of symptoms is mild. Pulmonary function tests show that peak expiratory flow (PEF) and forced respiratory volume per second (FEV_1) are reduced during an attack but are relatively normal during symptom-free intervals. Height and weight are in the 60th percentile. Complete blood count shows 8% eosinophils; all other parameters are normal. Cutaneous testing shows the patient to be allergic to a variety of allergens, including dust mites, animal dander, and several pollens. Which of the following is the most effective step in management?

    (A) Avoidance of exercise
    (B) Avoidance of respiratory irritants, such as cigarette smoke
    (C) Use of a humidifier at home
    (D) Use of air cleaners at home
    (E) Administration of multiple-drug regimens
    (F) Immunotherapy against identified allergens

45. A 3-year-old child is evaluated for possible causes of her mental retardation. Physical examination demonstrates elfin facies. The child has a history of stenosis of the aortic valve and transient hypercalcemia in infancy. Genetic microdeletion studies are performed. The lesion most likely involves which of the following genetic loci?

    (A) 7q11.23
    (B) 20p12
    (C) 22q11.21
    (D) Maternal chromosome at 15q11
    (E) Paternal chromosome at 15q11

46. A term neonate is healthy at birth and receives routine perinatal care. The infant is discharged from the hospital on day 3. Ten days after delivery, the infant develops severe erythema and edema in both eyelids. There is an associated watery discharge that soon became copious and mucopurulent, with presence of pseudomembranes. Which of the following conditions is this infant most at risk for?

    (A) Corneal ulceration
    (B) Encephalitis
    (C) Pneumonia
    (D) Sepsis
    (E) Silver toxicity

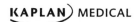

47. A 3-month-old, previously well male infant presents to the emergency department in January with a 2-day history of clear rhinorrhea, low-grade fever, and poor appetite, but no cough. On physical examination, there are mild subcostal retractions, coarse breath sounds heard throughout the lung fields, and scattered expiratory wheezes. The child receives an intravenous fluid bolus in the emergency department and is admitted for observation. Which of the following is the most severe, life-threatening complication of this child's illness?

    (A) Apnea

    (B) Congestive heart failure

    (C) Dehydration

    (D) Hypoxemia

    (E) Wheezing

48. A 14-year-old boy has pain in his left leg. An x-ray shows a tumor and a biopsy reveals histopathologic features characteristic of neural origin. Which of the following is the most likely diagnosis?

    (A) Chondroblastoma

    (B) Ewing sarcoma

    (C) Neuroblastoma

    (D) Osteosarcoma

    (E) Rhabdomyosarcoma

49. A 2-year-old child is brought to the emergency department because of generalized convulsions that last 15 minutes. He has had a fever for 24 hours, and his current temperature is 39.5° C (103.0° F). He also has a sore throat, but otherwise looks healthy. His father also had several episodes of febrile seizures in his childhood. Which of the following is the most important factor that will increase the risk of recurrence of febrile seizures?

    (A) Age older than 18 months

    (B) Duration of seizure longer than 5 minutes

    (C) Family history of febrile seizures

    (D) Fever of long duration before onset of seizure

    (E) Temperature higher than 39.0° C

50. A concerned mother brings her 2-month-old daughter to the clinic because of constipation. The mother had appropriate prenatal care but decided to deliver her child at home with the help of a midwife. The child has not received any medical attention since birth. Examination reveals jaundice, an umbilical hernia, and poor muscle tone. Which of the following is the most appropriate diagnostic study?

    (A) Alpha-1-antitrypsin genotyping

    (B) Liver and spleen scan

    (C) Measurements of T_4 and TSH

    (D) Barium swallow

    (E) RPR and FTA for syphilis

Pediatrics Test Three:
Answers and Explanations

ANSWER KEY

1.	B	26.	D
2.	D	27.	D
3.	B	28.	B
4.	E	29.	F
5.	B	30.	C
6.	A	31.	C
7.	C	32.	A
8.	E	33.	E
9.	D	34.	D
10.	D	35.	B
11.	C	36.	E
12.	E	37.	B
13.	B	38.	E
14.	D	39.	C
15.	A	40.	D
16.	E	41.	B
17.	E	42.	A
18.	B	43.	A
19.	A	44.	B
20.	B	45.	A
21.	E	46.	C
22.	C	47.	A
23.	A	48.	B
24.	A	49.	C
25.	A	50.	C

1. **The correct answer is B.** This infant has the classic presentation of pyloric stenosis. It occurs more commonly among first-born males, particularly white males. The cause of pyloric stenosis is unknown. It usually presents with nonbilious vomiting at 3-6 weeks of age. It progresses from intermittent vomiting to increasing numbers of episodes with more and more forceful vomiting. The infant acts hungry afterward, but as the vomiting continues there is loss of fluids and electrolytes resulting in hypochloremic metabolic alkalosis. Abdominal examination usually reveals a pyloric lump that feels like an olive-size mass. Treatment for pyloric stenosis is surgical; therefore, immediate consultation with the surgeon is necessary. The surgeon will preoperatively correct the metabolic alkalosis and surgically perform a pyloromyotomy.

    Changing the feedings to clear liquids and a solution, such as Pedialyte (**choice A**), will not relieve this obstruction and will only delay the needed surgical treatment.

    Obtaining abdominal x-ray films (**choice C**) will not delineate the specific problem. Appropriate x-ray films in this situation include either a barium swallow, which will reveal a large stomach with only thin streaks of barium in the pylorus due to the hypertrophied pylorus, or an ultrasound, which will reveal a doughnut appearance of the pyloric area.

    Insertion of a nasogastric tube (**choice D**) will relieve an overdistended stomach, but will not treat the underlying problem.

    Treating the infant with parenteral antibiotics (**choice E**) is not indicated. This is not an infectious condition, and prophylactic antibiotics are not used in conjunction with the surgery.

2. **The correct answer is D.** The condition is called transient hypogammaglobulinemia of infancy. It is due to exhaustion of maternally supplied IgG (the only antibody to cross the placenta in significant amounts) before the infant has begun to produce significant amounts of his own antibodies. Affected infants typically go through several months to years of being very vulnerable to infection, and then improve as their immune systems mature and they are able to produce more IgG. The condition does not present in the neonatal period because maternal IgG can cross the placenta during the third trimester of intrauterine life. The maternally supplied IgG is usually exhausted by about the fourth to sixth month of life.

    IgA (**choice A**) is found in secretions and in serum but does not cross the placenta.

    IgD (**choice B**) is a transiently produced antibody during B cell development that is present in trace amounts in serum.

    IgE (**choice C**) is the antibody associated with allergic reactions; it does not cross the placenta.

    IgM (**choice E**) is a large antibody found in serum that does not cross the placenta.

3. **The correct answer is B.** The early morning headaches associated with vomiting and getting progressively worse, along with the presence of a positive Romberg sign, suggest the presence of a space-occupying lesion (a brain tumor). An MRI of the brain would be the best diagnostic test to rule out brain tumors, posterior fossa tumors, which are of clinical concern in children.

    CT of the head (**choice A**) would be a good first test in most cases, except when you are looking for a brain tumor in children because it may not show a posterior fossa tumor. For investigation of an intracranial bleed, a CT would be an appropriate test, although there is no recent history of trauma to suggest this diagnosis.

    A plain skull x-ray film (**choice C**) would provide information regarding any fracture or lytic lesions, both unlikely in this example.

    Sinus films (**choice D**), although rarely used, would be helpful in the diagnosis of sinusitis, which could relate to chronic headaches. However, this patient had vomiting with headaches, no sinus tenderness, and no history of chronic rhinitis, so sinusitis would be an unlikely diagnosis.

    A spinal tap (**choice E**) would reveal increased intracranial pressure or an infection of the cerebrospinal fluid. However, it would not be the first test to do before ascertaining whether there was a space-occupying lesion in the brain.

4. **The correct answer is E.** The most frequent cause of a short generalized tonic-clonic seizure is a simple febrile seizure. The patient must be treated with antipyretics, but prognosis is excellent. Febrile seizures are not considered to be epileptic since they are provoked events. This seizure type is seen typically in children aged 6 months to 3 years, but may occur until 6 years.

    Given the high proportion of child abuse (**choice A**) cases seen in emergency departments, child abuse should always be on the differential. However, this patient's history suggests other causes.

    Idiopathic epilepsy (**choice B**) is also called the benign focal epilepsy of childhood. The age of onset is 4-10 years, and the disorder is not associated with underlying cerebral abnormalities.

    Infantile spasms (**choice C**) are massive myoclonic seizures with either forceful flexion or extension of the trunk. The spasms occur in clusters, and the child may cry or be extremely irritable during these periods.

    Meningitis (**choice D**) should be considered, but a lumbar puncture is not essential in this infant, who is alert and smiling and showing no meningeal signs on examination, although miningeal signs may not always be evident at this age.

5. **The correct answer is B.** Fifth disease, or erythema infectiosum, is caused by infection with human parvovirus B19. The rash of erythema infectiosum starts on the

cheeks, giving a "slapped cheek" appearance. The rash may disappear and recur.

Contact dermatitis (**choice A**) presents with a history of contact with an allergen. The skin is inflamed and itchy, with weeping and vesiculations. The site of involvement is often suggestive: e.g., the ear lobes and nape of neck (from nickel in jewelry), wrist (watch straps, bracelets), and feet (dyes in socks, tanning agents, glues in shoes). Typically, the dermatitis does not spread because the reaction is limited to the areas of contact.

The rash of measles (**choice C**) begins on the head and spreads down the body. It is erythematous and maculopapular, becoming confluent with progression.

Roseola (**choice D**) is caused by human herpesvirus 6 and has an incubation period of 9 days. The rash is maculopapular and develops 3 to 4 days after fever.

Rubella (**choice E**) produces a maculopapular rash that has no prodrome in children. Lymphadenopathy develops. The rash starts on the face and then becomes generalized.

Systemic lupus erythematosus (SLE; **choice F**) is a multisystem autoimmune disease. An erythematous facial butterfly rash can result with or without sun exposure. Diagnosis requires symptoms from multiple organ systems (e.g., hematologic, joints, pulmonary, nervous system, renal, gastrointestinal).

6. **The correct answer is A.** The physician is trying to prevent retinopathy of prematurity, also known as retrolental fibroplasia. This is a cause of permanent blindness in premature neonates with respiratory distress syndrome who are treated with high oxygen levels. The pathophysiology of this condition is related to the fact that the premature infant's retinas are not yet fully vascularized, and the direction in which the vessels grow is partly in response to changes in oxygen tension. When the infant's eyes are not protected from increased environmental oxygen levels, the vitreous of the eye develops a higher oxygen tension than the retina, and the blood vessels grow abnormally into the vitreous (where they block the light) rather than staying on the retina. Shielding the neonate's eyes prevents this from happening and reduces the incidence of the complication of visual loss.

Cotton wool exudates in the retina (**choice B**) indicate vascular leakage, which is not a feature of this condition.

Microaneurysms of the retinal arterioles (**choice C**) are relatively specific for diabetic retinopathy, which is seen in adults rather than in neonates.

Papilledema of the optic nerve head (**choice D**) suggests increased intraorbital or intracranial pressure.

Ulcers on the cornea (**choice E**) are seen in gonorrhea ophthalmia and other serious conjunctival diseases.

7. **The correct answer is C.** Henoch-Schönlein purpura is a syndrome of small blood vessel vasculitis that presents as a triad of purpuric ("palpable purpura") rash, intermittent abdominal pain, and arthritis. The rash usually affects the lower extremities, buttocks, and lower back. The abdominal pain is crampy, and there are often guaiac positive stools. The arthritis can be transient, most commonly affecting the knees and ankles.

Dermatomyositis (**choice A**) is an inflammation of striated muscle and skin. Most patients have fatigue, weight loss, anorexia, and fever. There is progressive weakness of proximal muscles.

Gastroenteritis (**choice B**) would be characterized by vomiting and diarrhea, often accompanied by fever. Gastroenteritis would not be associated with a purpuric rash or arthritis.

Juvenile rheumatoid arthritis (**choice D**) presents with polyarthritis. Fatigue, fever, weight loss, morning stiffness, and refusal to walk may be presenting complaints. It is unlikely to present with a purpuric rash and abdominal pain.

Kawasaki disease (**choice E**) is characterized by prolonged fever, bilateral nonpurulent conjunctivitis, cervical lymphadenopathy, fissuring of mucous membranes, desquamation of extremities, and truncal rash. None of these symptoms are present in this case.

8. **The correct answer is E.** The chest examination may be normal or nearly normal between attacks in patients with mild asthma. A positive personal or family history of other allergic disorders (such as atopic dermatitis in childhood) is frequently found in those with allergic asthma. To confirm a clinical diagnosis, spirometric tests are particularly useful. These should be performed before and after administration of a short-acting bronchodilator to demonstrate that there is airflow obstruction and that this is promptly reversible. Airflow obstruction is supported by finding a forced expiratory volume in 1 second/forced vital capacity (FEV_1/FVC) ratio of <75%.

Arterial blood gas analysis (**choice A**) is not informative in the diagnosis of asthma, and the results may even be normal during mild exacerbations.

A bronchial provocation test with histamine or methacholine (**choice B**) may be used if spirometry is not diagnostic and asthma is strongly suspected. It must be performed in a specialized setting.

A complete blood count (**choice C**) may reveal blood eosinophilia, which is frequently present in chronic allergic disorders but would not support the specific diagnosis of asthma.

Chest x-ray examination (**choice D**) is necessary only when other disorders that mimic asthma, such as pulmonary infections or pneumothorax, are likely.

9. **The correct answer is D.** Nasal polyps are not neoplasms, but rather a florid hyperplastic response of nasal and

paranasal mucosa to chronic inflammation. Allergic rhinitis/sinusitis is the most common underlying condition. However, presence of polyps in children should raise the possibility of *cystic fibrosis*. This should be promptly investigated by a pilocarpine iontophoresis sweat test, which would show elevated sweat chloride in patients with cystic fibrosis. Up to 20% of cystic fibrosis patients ultimately develop nasal polyps.

Cutaneous allergen testing (**choice A**) and detection of allergen-specific serum IgE by in vitro RAST (**choice E**) constitute the proper course of action when there is clinical evidence of an allergic nature of nasal polyps. These methods allow identification of triggering allergen(s) and subsequent institution of appropriate therapy (i.e., allergen avoidance and/or desensitization treatments).

Excisional biopsy (**choice B**) is necessary only when nasal polyps have not regressed with pharmacologic therapies, namely topical application of steroids (beclomethasone) or a short course of oral prednisone. Histopathologic examination of removed nasal polyps usually confirms the allergic, inflammatory nature of the process by demonstrating chronic inflammatory infiltration and tissue eosinophilia.

Nasal provocation testing (**choice C**) is a direct allergen challenge performed by inhalation of allergens through the nose. This test may allow identification of involved allergens in case of a positive reaction.

10. **The correct answer is D.** This is trisomy 18, also known as Edwards syndrome and trisomy E. The phenotype described in the question stem is typical. Both club feet and rocker bottom feet are common. These infants often have multiple congenital anomalies, which may involve heart, lungs, diaphragm, abdominal wall, or urinary tract. Hernias and cryptorchidism may also occur. Most affected individuals die by 1 year of age; the few survivors usually show marked developmental delay.

47,XXY (**choice A**), or Klinefelter syndrome, causes males with tall stature and is usually not diagnosed in infancy.

Triple X (**choice B**) causes apparently phenotypically normal women and is usually not diagnosed in infancy.

Trisomy 13 (**choice C**), or Patau syndrome, produces many midline defects, including holoprosencephaly, cleft lip, cleft palate, microphthalmia with colobomas of the iris, scalp defects, and dermal sinuses; other defects are present as well.

Trisomy 21 (**choice E**), or Down syndrome, is characterized by laterally upward slanting eyes, Brushfield spots of the irises, simian creases, and cardiac anomalies.

11. **The correct answer is C.** This is Hartnup disease, which is an autosomal recessive condition that produces a neutral aminoaciduria with increased renal clearance of alanine, asparagine, glutamine, histidine, isoleucine, leucine, phenylalanine, serine, threonine, tyrosine, valine, and tryptophan. This is accompanied by malabsorption of other amino acids, notably tryptophan, but also phenylalanine and methionine. The resulting tryptophan deficiency produces pellagra-like symptoms (tryptophan is used to synthesize nicotinamide) with photosensitive skin lesions, ataxia, and neuropsychiatric disturbances. Hartnup disease can be effectively treated (early diagnosis is important to limit neurologic manifestations) with good nutrition supplemented with nicotinamide.

Alkaptonuria (**choice A**) leads to urinary secretion of homogentisic acid (causing urine that turns black on standing) and causes arthritis and dark coloration of cartilage.

Cystinuria (**choice B**) principally produces urinary tract calculi.

Fanconi syndrome (**choice D**) produces a generalized dysfunction of the proximal tubules with glucosuria, generalized aminoaciduria, and hypophosphatemia (with bony abnormalities).

Phenylketonuria (**choice E**), which is characterized by excess phenylalanine in urine, is an important cause of mental retardation in young children. Most affected children have pale skin, blond hair, and blue eyes.

12. **The correct answer is E.** This is not an emergency, but strabismus must be corrected as soon as possible to enable the brain to learn to process images from both eyes. Otherwise, images from one side are suppressed; by age 7, permanent cortical blindness will occur in the suppressed side (amblyopia).

Spontaneous correction (**choice A**) does not occur. It is an often-quoted myth, probably stemming from the fact that some children with a broad base of the nose appear to be cross-eyed and then "grow out of it." They never had strabismus, and, if properly examined, the corneal reflection of a bright light would be seen coming from the same place in each eye.

Corrective lenses (**choice B**) are the treatment for a different type of strabismus: if a child has had normal alignment until he reaches an older age, and then gets "cross-eyed" whenever he focuses on a nearby object. This type of patient has an accommodation problem that can be corrected with appropriate lenses.

Eye patches (**choice C**) are used to force the brain to process images from the "bad eye" while preparations are made for surgical correction. Only the "good eye" is patched, and the notion of alternating patches would not be effective and could not be the only treatment.

Delayed correction for cosmetic purposes only (**choice D**) would be appropriate if the strabismus had not been diagnosed or treated during infancy, so that when the patient was first seen (after the age of 7), he already had irreversible cortical blindness.

13. **The correct answer is B.** The child is exhibiting isosexual precocious development. The enlarged gonads indicate that he has an increased exposure to gonadotropins, which may be the result of precocious release. Thus, increased testosterone is not the primary abnormality but is secondary to increased exposure to gonadotropins. In boys, a hypothalamic tumor can be found in an appreciable percentage of cases.

    An ectopic source of androgenic hormones, such as congenital adrenal hyperplasia (**choice A**), causes gonadotropins to be shut off and the testes to be small.

    Klinefelter syndrome (**choice C**) is a common cause of primary hypogonadism.

    Male pseudohermaphroditism (**choice D**) refers to infants who are 46,XY males with testes but appear to have incomplete masculinization, including hypospadias. This can be the result of defects in testosterone synthesis, metabolism, or action at the cellular level.

    The XYY syndrome (**choice E**) is associated with acne and tall stature but not with precocious puberty.

14. **The correct answer is D.** Retinitis pigmentosa is an often hereditary progressive degenerative disease of the retina. Patients present with progressive night blindness, visual field constriction with a ring scotoma, and loss of acuity. Characteristically, the rods in the equatorial retina are affected first, producing a mid-peripheral ring scotoma that can be detected with visual field testing. The ophthalmoscopic findings illustrated in the question stem are typical; additional manifestations include cataracts, myopia, and opacities in the vitreous humor. Some patients also have hearing loss. The condition is slowly progressive (usually leading to complete blindness over a period of several decades) and is at the moment untreatable, although fetal retinal transplants show some promise.

    A cataract (**choice A**) is an opacity of the lens of the eye.

    Central retinal artery occlusion (**choice B**) causes sudden, painless, unilateral blindness, and is associated with pallor of the macula.

    In the case of retinal detachment (**choice C**), ophthalmoscopy reveals a raised area in one retina and would not selectively affect night vision.

    Uveitis (**choice E**) is an inflammation of the iris, ciliary body, or choroid, and may cause visual loss secondary to "floaters" in the vitreous humor.

15. **The correct answer is A.** This child has acute mastoiditis, which can complicate untreated (and occasionally treated) cases of acute otitis media, especially when caused by bacteria. This is a dangerous complication because the mastoid process is adjacent to the brain, and this destructive infection can spread to cause a purulent meningitis. CT scans can be very helpful in defining the extent of the infection. Initial treatment is with intravenous forms of the antibiotics

used to cover acute otitis media; coverage is then switched after cultures demonstrate specific antibiotic sensitivities.

Barotitis media (**choice B**) is middle ear damage caused by rapid pressure changes, as in airplane descent or deep sea diving.

Cholesteatoma (**choice C**) is a benign condition in which stratified squamous keratinizing epithelium grows in the middle ear. It results in a smelly discharge from the ear, hearing loss, vertigo, headache, and facial nerve palsy. Local expansion may result in damage to adjacent structures, and the condition can be fatal if left untreated.

Chronic otitis media (**choice D**) is the term used for chronic ear drum perforation and the infection that accompanies it.

Ménière disease (**choice E**) causes the cluster of vertigo, tinnitus, and fluctuating hearing loss.

Myringitis (**choice F**) is inflammation of the tympanic membrane and is associated with *Mycoplasma* or viral respiratory infections. Myringitis bulbosa occurs when there are painful vesicles on the tympanic membrane. Herpes zoster of the eardrum presents with a similar condition.

Otitis externa (**choice G**) is a diffuse inflammation of the skin lining the external auditory meatus. There is either scanty discharge or no discharge. The condition is typically painful upon movement of the pinna.

Secretory otitis media (**choice H**) occurs when the eustachian tube is blocked and (initially noninfectious) serous fluid accumulates in the middle ear.

16. **The correct answer is E.** In any emergency situation, the first step is to secure an airway and verify breathing (the ABCs: airway, breathing, circulation). Because endotracheal intubation was unsuccessful, a surgical airway must be secured. There are two types of cricothyroidotomy: needle and surgical. Needle cricothyroidotomy is the procedure of choice in children younger than 12 years. A patient can be ventilated for 30 minutes this way, allowing time for a more secure airway. In addition, enough pressure may be generated to expel a foreign body in the glottic area.

    Intubation (**choice A**) has already failed, and the patient is becoming cyanotic and needs oxygenation.

    Surgical cricothyroidotomy (**choice B**) is reserved for patients older than 12 years.

    A face mask with 100% O_2 plus succinylcholine (**choice C**) is incorrect because there is complete obstruction, which must be bypassed for oxygenation to be successful.

    Formal tracheostomy (**choice D**) is reserved for long-term management of the airway. In this acute setting, a rapid, temporary airway is essential.

17. **The correct answer is E.** The physical examination findings, in particular a posterior tear of the hymen, in this

24-month-old girl are highly suggestive of sexual abuse. However, physical findings alone are not enough to prove a sexual abuse case. Cultures taken from the vaginal vault of the suspected victim are essential in diagnosis and documentation. Of all the pathogens associated with sexual abuse, *Neisseria gonorrhoeae* provides definitive evidence.

Candida albicans (**choice A**) is a common infection of the diaper area for both boys and girls. Vaginal candidiasis can occur in a 24-month-old child.

Chlamydia trachomatis (**choice B**) can be vertically transmitted to the infant from the mother at birth, and persists for 3 years. It could be associated with sexual abuse but cannot be confirmatory in this case, when it is isolated from a 24-month-old girl.

Gardnerella vaginalis (**choice C**) presents as vaginitis with discharge. It is uncommon in young girls but does not confirm sexual abuse.

Pseudomonas aeruginosa (**choice D**) rarely causes vaginitis and is not associated with sexual abuse.

18. **The correct answer is B.** This infant has bronchopulmonary dysplasia, which is an important chronic lung disorder that can complicate respiratory distress syndrome of the newborn. Damage to the lungs by mechanical ventilation produces alternating areas of emphysema and scarred lungs. The smooth muscles of bronchioles and arterioles may also be hypertrophied. The modern trend is to try to prevent this complication by using the smallest amount of mechanical ventilation that still adequately aerates the infant's lungs. Management of significant degrees of bronchopulmonary dysplasia is problematic, and therapeutic regimens vary from neonatal unit to neonatal unit.

Apnea of prematurity (**choice A**) causes transient interruptions in breathing.

The lung problems of cystic fibrosis (**choice C**) are usually not present at birth, but develop after the child has repeated bouts of pneumonia.

Persistent pulmonary hypertension of the newborn (**choice D**) is due to a persistence of fetal type circulation (typically due to either a patent foramen ovale or a persistent patent ductus arteriosus), which clinically causes severe hypoxemia.

Transient tachypnea of the newborn (**choice E**) causes 2 or 3 days of difficult breathing in neonates who are slow to reabsorb amniotic fluid trapped in the lungs.

19. **The correct answer is A.** The child has acute rheumatic fever. Jones criteria for diagnosing rheumatic fever includes using both "major" criteria (carditis, polyarthritis, chorea, erythema marginatum, subcutaneous nodules) and "minor" criteria (arthralgia, fever, erythrocyte sedimentation rate elevation, C-reactive protein elevation, prolonged PR interval). Either two major criteria or one major plus two minor criteria can be used for diagnosis. Typically, by the time the acute rheumatic fever develops, the preceding streptococcal sore throat has healed, and the patient is no longer infected. The damage that is produced is immunologically mediated, based on antigenic mimicry of bacterial antigens for human ones. A number of specific targets have been proposed, including Lancefield group A antigen mimicking mitral valve glycoprotein, part of the M protein antigen mimicking helical proteins such as myosin, protoplast membrane mimicking myocardial sarcolemma or neuronal tissue, and bacterial hyaluronate capsule mimicking hyaluronate-containing articular tissues.

Although streptococci, staphylococci, and other bacteria can infect cardiac valves (**choice B**), causing endocarditis, this would not be associated with arthritis and erythema marginatum.

Parasitic infection of myocytes (**choice C**) can occur with either trichinosis or Chagas disease. Neither of these conditions would present with sore throat followed by arthritis.

Toxic damage to the heart (**choice D**) can occur with diphtheria but would accompany the sore throat, not be delayed by weeks.

Viruses can cause myocarditis (**choice E**), but arthritis and erythema marginatum would not be present.

20. **The correct answer is B.** It is important to know the contraindications to childhood immunizations. The true contraindications to the MMR vaccine include anaphylactic reaction to the vaccine or any of its components (neomycin, gelatin), immunodeficiency, pregnancy, and untreated and active tuberculosis. Precautions are given in cases of moderate or severe illness, recent administration of immunoglobulin containing blood products, and thrombocytopenia or thrombocytopenic purpura.

Anaphylaxis to amoxicillin (**choice A**) is not a contraindication to MMR vaccination because it is not a component of the vaccine. Components of the vaccination to which patients may be allergic include neomycin and gelatin.

MMR vaccination is contraindicated in pregnant women due to its possible effects on fetal development. However, MMR vaccination is not contraindicated in persons who are in contact with pregnant women (**choice C**).

Previous febrile reaction to the MMR vaccine (**choice D**) is not a contraindication to vaccination. Some patients can develop measles-like infection with cough, cold, red eyes, and rash. However, it typically lasts 2 to 5 days and is self-limiting. An anaphylactic reaction to a previous vaccination, however, is a contraindication to repeat doses.

Febrile respiratory illness or any other active febrile infection (**choice E**) is not a contraindication. However, the Advisory Committee on Immunization Practices (ACIP) for the Centers for Disease Control (CDC) has recommended that vaccines be administered to persons with minor illnesses, such as diarrhea, mild upper respiratory infection with or without low-grade fever, and other low-grade febrile illnesses.

21. **The correct answer is E.** The findings in the history and physical examination are most consistent with the diagnosis of varicocele, which is an abnormally dilated pampiniform venous plexus. Varicocele is very common; it is found in 15% to 20% of male adolescents and is usually asymptomatic. Patients with symptomatic varicocele usually describe a heavy, dragging sensation in the groin or the scrotum on the affected side. Palpation along the spermatic cord often reveals the classic "bag of worms" mass above the testis. The size of the varicocele increases with Valsalva maneuver and decreases with lying down.

Hydrocele (**choice A**) is the presence of fluid within the tunica vaginalis. It may be noncommunicating, when the mass is confined to the scrotum, or communicating, when there is continuity from the tunica vaginalis to the peritoneum. Hydroceles are typically asymptomatic, although a large hydrocele may interfere with ambulation.

Inguinal hernia (**choice B**) usually presents with an increase in scrotal size. It occurs more commonly in males than in females. Surgical repair is indicated to prevent complications.

Orchitis (**choice C**) is inflammation of the testis. It can be caused by sexually transmitted diseases, such as gonorrhea or chlamydia, or by viruses, such as Epstein-Barr virus, influenza, varicella, or coxsackieviruses. Orchitis usually presents with a painful and enlarged testicle.

Testicular tumor (**choice D**) usually presents as a painless mass that is firm, hard, and inseparable from the testis.

22. **The correct answer is C.** This is Gaucher disease, which is a familial autosomal recessive disorder of lipid metabolism. The disease is caused by a lack of glucocerebrosidase activity, which normally hydrolyzes glucocerebroside to glucose and ceramide, and occurs in three major clinical forms. All three types are characterized by prominent splenomegaly and accumulation of abnormal glucocerebrosides in reticuloendothelial cells in many organs (spleen, liver, bone marrow, and brain in more severe cases), producing the pathognomonic "crumpled-silk" histiocytes. This case is an example of the type 1, or the adult chronic nonneuronopathic, form. Type 1 is the most common form and actually presents frequently in childhood, although the most serious manifestations are often deferred to adulthood. Type 1 has an increased frequency in Ashkenazi Jews and manifests with hypersplenism, splenomegaly, and bone lesions. The pingueculae and brown skin pigmentation noted in the question stem may be helpful clues on physical examination. Type 2, the acute infantile neuronopathic form, causes splenomegaly, severe neurologic abnormalities, and death

in early childhood. Type 3 is a juvenile form and has features intermediate to types 1 and 2.

Abetalipoproteinemia (**choice A**) is characterized by absent beta-lipoproteins, steatorrhea, acanthocytes, retinitis pigmentosa, ataxia, and mental abnormalities.

Fabry disease (**choice B**) is characterized by angio-keratomas, corneal opacities, burning extremity pain, and involvement of kidneys, heart, and brain.

Niemann-Pick disease (**choice D**) may clinically resemble Gaucher disease, but is characterized by "sea-blue" rather than "crumpled-silk" histiocytes.

Tangier disease (**choice E**) may resemble Gaucher disease, with hepatosplenomegaly and neurologic disease, but a helpful distinctive feature is orange-yellow tonsillar hyperplasia.

23. **The correct answer is A.** The clinical presentation of this patient is consistent with pheochromocytoma; this impression is confirmed by the increased levels of urinary catecholamines and metabolites, and an extrarenal mass on abdominal CT. Pheochromocytoma arises from the chromaffin cells in the adrenal medulla or the abdominal sympathetic chain. Clinical manifestations include headache, sweating, nausea, vomiting, palpitation, blurry vision, nervousness, and hypertension. In fact, pheochromocytoma is one of the important causes of secondary hypertension. In a 12-year-old boy with a blood pressure of 148/94 mm Hg, the differential diagnosis of secondary hypertension should be triggered in every clinician's mind. If pheochromocytoma is suspected, a 24-hour collection of urine for catecholamines and metabolites (vanillylmandelic acid and metanephrines) can be checked. If these substances are elevated, the diagnosis of pheochromocytoma is confirmed. CT scan of the abdomen may be done to locate the tumor. Most pheochromocytomas are benign. When hypertension is present, as in this clinical vignette, it should be treated promptly, even before surgical resection of the tumor. An alpha-adrenergic blocker, such as phenoxybenzamine, is the drug of choice because it has been shown to effectively decrease blood pressure in patients with pheochromocytoma.

Angiotensin-converting enzyme inhibitor (**choice B**) does not play any role in controlling blood pressure in children with pheochromocytoma.

A beta-adrenergic blocker (**choice C**) is actually contraindicated in the initial treatment of hypertension in pheochromocytoma because it causes an unopposed alpha effect that would result in a paradoxical rise of blood pressure. However, labetalol, which is a combined alpha and beta blocker, can be used in some patients with efficacy similar to phenoxybenzamine.

Calcium channel blockers (**choice D**) and diuretics (**choice E**) are not used for treatment of hypertension in patients with pheochromocytoma.

24. **The correct answer is A.** This child has mild asthma, requiring an albuterol treatment but no other urgent treatment at this time. Albuterol is used as a "rescue" medicine for someone having an acute attack.

Cromolyn sodium (**choice B**) is used as a daily medicine to control asthma and has no benefit in situations requiring an immediate effect. It is not used in acute attacks.

Oxygen via nasal cannula (**choice C**) is unnecessary at this time since she has an oxygen saturation greater than 92%.

IV steroids (**choice D**) would not be necessary since the patient is experiencing only mild symptoms. If the patient were thought to need steroid treatment, oral steroids would suffice.

Subcutaneous epinephrine (**choice E**) is rarely needed except in life-threatening situations, such as patients with severe asthma in status asthmaticus.

25. **The correct answer is A.** Numerous acanthocytes (erythrocytes with spiny membrane projections) on peripheral smear are a feature of abetalipoproteinemia, which is caused by a mutation in the gene for microsomal triglyceride transfer protein. Abetalipoproteinemia is a rare, usually autosomal recessive, congenital disorder characterized by a complete absence of beta-lipoproteins, steatorrhea, blindness due to retinitis pigmentosa, ataxia, and mental retardation. The complete absence of beta-lipoproteins means that neither chylomicrons nor VLDL is formed. Massive-dose vitamin A and E therapy has delayed neurologic deterioration in some cases.

"Crumpled silk" histiocytes on bone marrow biopsy (**choice B**) suggest Gaucher disease.

Globoid cells on brain biopsy (**choice C**) suggest Krabbe disease.

Metachromatic deposits on sural nerve biopsy (**choice D**) suggest metachromatic leukodystrophy.

"Sea-blue" histiocytes on bone marrow biopsy (**choice E**) suggest Niemann-Pick disease.

26. **The correct answer is D.** The most common posterior fossa tumors in children include medulloblastoma, ependymoma, and pilocytic astrocytoma. Medulloblastoma, an anaplastic neoplasm thought to derive from primitive neuroectodermal precursors, belongs to the group of *primitive neuroectodermal tumors* (PNET). It originates from the cerebellar vermis and grows into the fourth ventricle, often producing signs and symptoms of increased intracranial pressure. The histologic features are those of other small round cell tumors.

Ependymoma (**choice A**) usually derives from the ependymal cells lining the central canal. Childhood ependy-momas typically develop in the fourth ventricle and may present with increased intracranial pressure. In contrast to medulloblastoma, however, ependymoma appears on CT/MRI as a mass that fills the fourth ventricle and secondarily involves adjacent structures.

Glioblastoma multiforme (GBM; **choice B**) is a rare tumor in children of this age, and the cerebellum is a rare location at any age. Furthermore, GBM grows in a diffuse fashion within the white matter without involving the ventricular cavities.

Hemangioblastoma (**choice C**) is a vascular tumor of uncertain histologic origin. The cerebellar hemisphere is its most common location, and it often appears as a cystic mass with a mural nodule. Its association with von Hippel-Lindau syndrome is noteworthy.

Oligodendroglioma (**choice E**) is a slow-growing tumor of adults that usually develops in the white matter of a cerebral hemisphere. Calcifications within the tumor are frequently detected on x-ray films or CT scan, and seizures are often the presenting sign.

Pilocytic astrocytoma (**choice F**) is a low-grade, well-circumscribed astrocytoma of children and young adults. Cerebellar pilocytic astrocytoma often presents as a cyst with a mural nodule (like hemangioblastoma) within a cerebellar hemisphere. Surgical resection is usually curative.

27. **The correct answer is D.** The most likely cause of this infant's presentation is toxic enterocolitis (toxic megacolon), which is most often seen in the setting of Hirschsprung disease. The disease is suggested in this infant by the delayed passage of meconium, chronic constipation, and the failure to thrive. When unrecognized, putrefaction and development of colitis can occur. In its severest form, it presents as toxic megacolon. The resultant diarrhea, with potentially fatal fluid loss, is due to bacterial overgrowth in the dilated bowel with resulting production of bacterial toxins. Although fluid replacement and antibiotics are important in the management of the these cases, the most helpful therapeutic intervention is prompt surgical resection of the involved bowel with formation of a colostomy.

Infants with congenital hypothyroidism (**choice A**) have a history of constipation. However, other features of hypothyroidism are lacking in this case. Classic features include prolonged jaundice, umbilical hernia, macroglossia, hypotonia, and failure of the posterior fontanelle to close.

Meconium ileus (**choice B**) occurs in infants with cystic fibrosis who fail to pass meconium in the first few days of life.

Necrotizing enterocolitis (**choice C**) is a feared complication of the newborn period, with abdominal distension and sepsis.

Volvulus neonatorum (**choice E**) is usually due to a defect in the normal rotation of the bowel in which the caecum remains high, often with a congenital band passing across the duodenum. This results in an intestinal obstruction and vessel occlusion at the base of the mesentery. Clinically, the features of intestinal obstruction predominate, with vomiting, abdominal pain, and constipation. Abdominal radiograph shows a "comma sign" or "beak sign" with absence of distal bowel gas.

28. **The correct answer is B.** Roseola is a virus that causes an exanthem (exanthem subitum). It typically affects children between 6 months and 3 years of age. Most cases manifest with a fever (temperature often up to 40-40.5° C) that lasts for 2-3 days; there is often mild erythema of the pharynx and congestion. The discrete, macular rash typically erupts on the trunk with an abrupt end to the fever.

Erythema infectiosum (**choice A**), also known as fifth disease, is caused by parvovirus B19. This virus usually affects children aged 5-14 years. There is usually a non-specific febrile illness with malaise and myalgias lasting 2-3 days. The rash of erythema infectiosum is characterized by a red rash on the cheeks ("slapped" cheeks) and a erythematous maculopapular rash on the extremities and trunk described as a "lacy" reticular pattern.

Rubella (**choice C**), also known as German measles, is characterized by a low-grade fever (temperature usually less than 39° C), erythematous maculopapular rash, and lymphadenopathy.

Rubeola (**choice D**), or measles, is characterized by 3-5 days of increasing fever, coryza, cough, and conjunctivitis. Koplik spots (white lesions on a red mucosa) appear in the mouth. There is a discrete, erythematous, maculopapular rash that begins on the face and moves downward, covering the trunk and upper and lower extremities.

Varicella (**choice E**), or chickenpox, begins with a period of malaise and low-grade fever. The lesions begin as macules and progress to fluid filled vesicles that then crust; the crust eventually falls off. The fever is usually gone by the end of the first week of the rash.

29. **The correct answer is F.** The child most likely has Waardenburg syndrome, which is one of the more common craniofacial abnormalities. Defects of this type are related to maldevelopment of the first and second vertebral arches that form the face. The defects usually begin during the second month of gestation. The features illustrated in the question stem are typical. On a practical basis, you should remember that children with white forelocks (partial albinism) should be tested for hearing loss.

Beckwith-Wiedermann syndrome (**choice A**) is characterized by macroglossia, a large fontanelle, and a linear fissure in the external ear. Organomegaly of both the pancreas and kidney is common, and omphalocele may be seen at birth.

Clinical features of fragile X syndrome (**choice B**) include mental retardation, large testicles, a prominent jaw, large ears, and a large head. The syndrome is caused by a dominant X-linked trinucleotide repeat gene with only a 50% penetrance in females. Features are most prominent in affected males.

Goldenhar syndrome (**choice C**) produces an asymmetric face, malformed ears, small eyes, hearing loss, a large mouth, a small mandible, and vertebral anomalies.

Pierre Robin syndrome (**choice D**) produces micrognathia, glossoptosis, and cleft palate.

Treacher Collins syndrome (**choice E**) is characterized by malformation of the external ear, deafness, micrognathia, antimongoloid eye slanting, and coloboma of the lower eyelids.

30. **The correct answer is C.** Herpangina is a caused by coxsackievirus and usually manifests with dysphagia and vesicles on the anterior tonsils and palate. There is typically a history of fever and viral symptoms (runny nose, cough). Diagnosis is made by the presence of small vesicular lesions on the anterior tonsils and posterior palate.

Aphthous stomatitis (**choice A**) usually presents with ulcers on the buccal mucosa. There is no associated fever, and the patient does not usually complain of pain.

Hand-foot-and-mouth disease (**choice B**) is also caused by coxsackievirus and presents with small vesicles in the mouth, but there are also vesicles on the hands and feet. Commonly, a maculopapular rash is also present.

Kawasaki disease (**choice D**) is associated with a history of prolonged fever (more than 5 days), conjunctival erythema, cracked lips, maculopapular rash, cervical lymphadenopathy, and swollen hands.

Stevens-Johnson syndrome (**choice E**) is a systemic disease that presents with ulcers over the entire mouth and lips. There usually is a confluent rash on the body as well. The child will appear very ill.

31. **The correct answer is C.** The infant is having neonatal seizures, which can take a variety of forms. In addition to the migratory clonic jerks described in the question stem, these infants may alternatively experience alternating hemiseizures or primitive subcortical seizures. The latter may take the form of respiratory arrest, chewing motions, eye deviations, or changes in muscle tone. True grand mal seizures are usually not seen, possibly because the immaturity of the brain makes it difficult to transmit a seizure to all sites. Neonatal seizures can be seen in a variety of settings, which can be roughly subclassified as primary CNS versus metabolic. The metabolic causes are common, and screening chemistry studies can identify potentially correctable hypoglycemia, hypocalcemia, hypomagnesemia, hypernatremia, or hyponatremia. Consequently,

the earliest diagnostic step is to order these appropriate serum screening tests, usually on a STAT basis.

CT scan of head (**choice A**), EEG (**choice B**), skull x-rays (**choice D**), and ultrasound of the head (**choice E**) can all be very useful in offering diagnostic clues to true CNS problems, but should be deferred until after the child's metabolic status is established.

32. **The correct answer is A.** At birth, a neonate will typically exhibit some signs of exposure to maternal estrogen. Two of these signs include prominent labia and a dull pink vaginal epithelium. As estrogen levels fall, the labia will become less prominent and the vagina will take on a brighter red appearance. In the absence of other signs or symptoms of disease, these findings are normal and do not require further evaluation.

    Exposure to penicillin (**choice B**) will almost never cause findings isolated to the labia and vagina.

    Infection with *Chlamydia* (**choice C**) can lead to neonatal pneumonia and eye infection.

    Infection with group B *Streptococcus* (**choice D**) can cause respiratory distress, pneumonia, meningitis, and sepsis in the newborn. It does not typically cause findings isolated to the genitalia.

    Sexual abuse (**choice E**) almost always must be considered whenever there are complaints or findings regarding an infant's genitalia. In this case, however, the infant is newborn—only minutes old. Therefore, sexual abuse would not be in the differential diagnosis.

33. **The correct answer is E.** A voiding cystourethrogram (VCUG) is the appropriate test to run to evaluate the lower urinary tract and the presence of any reflux of urine into the kidney. It is appropriate to first wait until the acute infection is over, since there may be some degree of reflux present during an infection. The usual procedure is to wait 1-2 months after treatment to perform the VCUG to evaluate for reflux.

    Cystoscopy (**choice A**) is not indicated in the evaluation of urinary tract infection.

    Dimercaptosuccinic acid (DMSA) scan (**choice B**) is a radionuclide renal imaging scan. It might be an appropriate test to diagnosis acute pyelonephritis, but it is not indicated as a first test in evaluating reflux in a urinary tract infection 2 months after the infection. It is the most accurate test to diagnose acute pyelonephritis.

    Intravenous pyelogram (**choice C**) is rarely used in the pediatric population to evaluate for a urinary tract infection.

    Performing a VCUG now (**choice D**) would not be appropriate since there might be some degree of reflux present during an acute infection.

34. **The correct answer is D.** This is talipes equinovarus, which is the most common form of clubfoot abnormality. The term talipes is used for any deformity of the foot that involves the talus bone. The term equinus refers to a permanent extension of the foot so that only the ball rests on the ground. The term varus refers to a permanent inversion of the foot, so that only the outer side of the sole touches the ground. Talipes equinovarus is best corrected with repetitive casting of the foot beginning at a young age; this approach slowly brings the foot to a more normal position.

    Epispadias (**choice A**) and hypospadias (**choice B**) are urethral abnormalities.

    Talipes calcaneovalgus (**choice C**) is associated with a flat and dorsiflexed foot.

    Torticollis (**choice E**) is head tilt, which can be present at birth as a result of neck trauma.

35. **The correct answer is B.** Regurgitation of small volumes (usually less than 5-10 mL) is common among babies and is usually of no clinical significance unless the baby is failing to grow normally. It is of concern to some mothers, and switching to a firmer nipple bottle with a smaller hole will slow the rate that the baby is drinking and often reduce the amount of swallowed air.

    Changing the baby's formula (**choice A**) does not usually alter the amount of regurgitation.

    Careful monitoring of the baby (**choice C**), abdominal x-rays (**choice D**), and CT scan (**choice E**) are not warranted for this benign condition.

36. **The correct answer is E.** This 3-year-old girl has steatorrhea, recurrent diarrhea, and failure to thrive. There is a family history of an uncle who died of recurrent lower respiratory infections. This patient most likely has cystic fibrosis (CF). The gastrointestinal system is significantly affected by CF. Gastrointestinal manifestations are caused by pancreatic exocrine insufficiency, which occurs in more than 85% of patients with CF. The mutation of the CF gene causes inspissation of pancreatic secretions and obstruction of the ductules. It causes the malabsorption of protein and fat, resulting in steatorrhea. Untreated pancreatic insufficiency results in malnutrition and failure to thrive. The treatment is to replace the missing pancreatic enzymes by oral supplementation of purified pancreatic enzymes (pancrelipase) with food. Several capsules are taken with each meal and snack. Even with pancreatic enzyme replacement, however, there might still be mild steatorrhea. Fat-soluble vitamins, such as A, D, E, and K, are also supplemented in these patients to avoid fat-soluble vitamin deficiency. Successful nutritional management is an important part of the overall management of CF, because good nutritional status improves the overall prognosis and decreases the frequency of pulmonary infections.

Avoidance of dairy products (**choice A**) is useful in diarrhea caused by lactose intolerance but not in CF.

Elimination of dietary fat (**choice B**) is inappropriate. In fact, the intake of fat should be encouraged because the fat content increases palatability and provides high calories to the patient's body. Dietary fat is also essential for the absorption of fat-soluble vitamins.

A ketogenic diet (**choice C**) has no role in the management of CF. It is sometimes used to control epilepsy.

Oral metronidazole (**choice D**) is effective against anaerobic bacterial infection. It can be useful in bacterial overgrowth in the intestine and in *Clostridium difficile* colitis, but it has no role in the treatment of pancreatic insufficiency.

37. **The correct answer is B.** The boy in this clinical vignette has staphylococcal scalded skin syndrome (SSSS). It is characterized by fever, malaise, and a generalized fine erythematous rash. It is then followed by crusty, sometimes exudative, lesions around the mouth and eyes. It is usually preceded by an upper respiratory infection. The skin is tender to touch. With gentle rubbing, the epidermal layer can exfoliate, which is the characteristic Nikolsky sign. This syndrome is caused by an exfoliative toxin secreted by certain strains (55 and 71) of *Staphylococcus aureus*. Sometimes, injection of the conjunctiva and fissuring of the lips can happen and might be confused with Kawasaki disease. The differential diagnosis includes toxic shock syndrome, scarlet fever, and toxic epidermal necrolysis. Nafcillin or oxacillin can be used to treat SSSS.

Kawasaki disease (**choice A**) involves vasculitis of epicardial coronary vessels, with possible development of coronary aneurysm. The clinical syndrome presents with fever longer than 5 days, bilateral conjunctival injection, mucosal change in the oral pharynx, erythema of hands and feet with desquamation, and cervical lymphadenopathy. Transient arthritis may also occur.

Streptococcal scarlet fever (**choice C**) usually presents with an erythematous sandpaper-like rash with fever and "strawberry tongue." It is caused by erythrogenic exotoxins secreted by group A *Streptococcus*. It is usually associated with streptococcal pharyngitis.

Toxic epidermal necrolysis (**choice D**) is a dermatologic emergency characterized by widespread epidermal necrosis and desquamation after formation of blisters and bullae. It is caused by a severe hypersensitivity reaction, usually to a drug. Major complications include sepsis, dehydration, and shock. Patients should be treated as if they have a generalized severe burn.

Toxic shock syndrome (**choice E**) is caused by an exotoxin (TSST-1) of *Staphylococcus aureus,* or less commonly, *Streptococcus pyogenes*. Patients present with high fever, myalgia, pharyngitis, abdominal pain, vomiting, diarrhea, headache, and a diffuse, sunburn-like rash. Severe cases are complicated by hypotension, shock, and renal failure.

38. **The correct answer is E.** Alkaline burns are extremely destructive, and the process of destruction continues as long as the agent is in contact with the tissues. Immediate removal is essential, and the best way to do it is with massive irrigation. In the emergency department, sterile saline would be used; at home, tap water will do.

Antibiotics (**choice A**) do not help, and a leisurely approach will guarantee loss of the eye.

Rushing to the hospital (**choice B**) might seem like the thing to do for all kinds of emergencies, but in this case immediate first aid is more important. If the corrosive substance remains in the eye during the trip to the emergency department, the eye will be destroyed by the time the patient arrives.

"Playing chemist" (**choice C**) is never acceptable because of the possibility of causing an exothermic reaction.

Swiping with a tissue (**choice D**) would be better than nothing, but not by much. Swiping has a role, but not as the first thing to do. After massive irrigation, little particulate matter may remain, which may then have to be mechanically swiped away.

39. **The correct answer is C.** The child has body lice, *Pediculus humanus corporis*, which live in the clothing and cause itchy bites. The structures on the clothing seams are the eggs. The lice themselves can also often be seen. The lice are confined to the skin surface, and, unlike scabies mites, do not burrow into the skin. The patient, family members, and social contacts (such as other daycare children) should all be treated at the same time with permethrin cream, 5%. Clothing and bedding should also be washed.

Ancylostoma braziliense (**choice A**) causes cutaneous larva migrans, which produces long itchy burrows on the legs and buttocks.

Corynebacterium minutissimum (**choice B**) causes erythrasma, characterized by pink to brown itchy patches in moist areas of skin.

Sarcoptes scabiei (**choice D**) causes scabies, which is diagnosed by finding fine white lines up to 1 cm in length (burrows) in the skin, with an often invisible mite at the end of them.

Trichophyton rubrum (**choice E**) is a fungus that can cause ringworm of the body.

40. **The correct answer is D.** Bleeding from the ear following an injury to the skull is pathognomonic of a temporal bone fracture. The bleeding can be medial to an intact tympanic membrane, from the middle ear through a rupture of the tympanic membrane, or from a fracture line in the ear canal.

Hemotympanum gives the tympanic membrane a blue-black color. Usually, there is a communication with the subarachnoid space through the fracture line. Often, there is cerebrospinal fluid otorrhea. Cleaning of the ear canal should be avoided for fear of introducing microorganisms. The immediate danger to the patient is the development of meningitis. Prophylactic antibiotic therapy has to be initiated immediately.

Most fractures of the temporal bone are longitudinal (80%) to the long axis of the petrous pyramid. Only 20% are transverse. Longitudinal fractures usually extend through the middle ear into the ear canal, causing rupture of the tympanic membrane. Approximately 35% of longitudinal fractures produce a sensorineural hearing loss, and approximately 15% produce facial paralysis. Transverse fractures extend across the cochlea and fallopian canal, causing a profound, permanent sensorineural hearing loss and a facial paralysis. These fractures are usually well demonstrated with CT.

Concussion (**choice A**) is a syndrome of alteration of consciousness secondary to head injury, typically brought about by a sudden change in the momentum of the head. Its usual manifestations include loss of consciousness, temporary respiratory arrest, and loss of reflexes.

Epidural hematomas (**choice B**) are blood clots that form between the inner table of the skull and the dura. Eighty percent are associated with skull fractures across the middle meningeal artery or across a dural sinus. The high arterial pressure of the bleeding vessel dissects the dura away from the skull, permitting the formation of the hematoma. The incidence of skull fractures in children with epidural hematomas is lower than in adults because of the elasticity of the skull.

Subdural hematoma (**choice C**) usually results from trauma involving acceleration or deceleration head injury and is commonly associated with parenchymal brain injury.

Tympanic membrane perforation (**choice E**) most commonly happens after an object is inserted into the ear canal and perforates the eardrum.

41. **The correct answer is B.** Primary amenorrhea is defined as the absence of menses by the age of 16, or 4 years after thelarche (the onset of breast development). The prevalence of primary amenorrhea is 1% to 2%. In this country, the median age of menarche is 12.5 years. Most girls have menarche about 2 years after thelarche.

Primary amenorrhea is different from secondary amenorrhea, which is defined as the absence of menses for three menstrual cycles or a maximum of 6 months in women who previously had normal menstruation. Primary amenorrhea has a vast differential diagnosis and is usually divided into three categories: 1) outflow tract anomalies (e.g., imperforate hymen, transverse vaginal septum, vaginal agenesis, testicular feminization); 2)

end-organ disorders (e.g., ovarian failure, gonadal agenesis with 46,XY chromosomes); and 3) central disorders (e.g., hypothalamic disorders, pituitary disorders).

The age of the adolescent girl in this scenario is consistent with primary amenorrhea. Her sexual maturation is progressing appropriately. It is most likely that she has physiologic pubertal delay because the pelvic ultrasonography is normal. She probably has not completed her pubertal development.

Imperforate hymen (**choice A**) does not allow egress of menses. Patients usually present with pelvic pain from the accumulation of menses and dilatation of the uterus. Physical examination reveals a bulging membrane across the introitus and a midline pelvic mass.

Prolactinoma (**choice C**) can cause headache, decreased growth rate, galactorrhea, delayed puberty, primary or secondary amenorrhea, gynecomastia, and visual field defects.

Testicular feminization syndrome (**choice D**) is caused by either dysfunction or total absence of the testosterone receptor and results in a phenotypical female with 46,XY chromosomes. Patients with testicular feminization will have normal breast development but lack pubic hair. Pelvic ultrasound would reveal agenesis of the vagina and uterus.

In Turner syndrome (45,XO; **choice E**), the ovaries undergo rapid atresia; by puberty, there are no primordial oocytes.

42. **The correct answer is A.** Food allergy-induced colitis is a clinical syndrome of enterocolitis usually presenting between 1 week and 3 months of age. The dietary proteins implicated are generally cow's milk or soy proteins. Although diarrhea and emesis are the most prominent symptoms, rectal bleeding, protein-losing enteropathy with edema, and dehydration with metabolic acidosis are also prominent. The diarrhea is relatively acute and progressive to the point of dehydration if the etiologic protein is not eliminated. The stools contain mucus, polymorphonuclear leukocytes, and eosinophils. Rectal bleeding progresses from occult to increasingly gross bleeding and anemia. Whereas the diarrhea is most consistent with an inflammatory colitis, stools may also contain reducing sugars, suggesting a small intestinal component as well. Approximately one-third of infants with severe diarrhea will develop metabolic acidosis. Hypotension may complicate the presentation in younger infants but is more commonly seen following protein challenge, especially with soy.

Irritability, emesis, and abdominal distention are also prominent with acute manifestations. When a more indolent clinical course is encountered, the infant will manifest failure to thrive, edema from enteric protein loss, and anemia. Food refusal, a feature of eosinophilic esophagitis and enteropathy, is also common.

The diagnosis is confirmed when symptoms resolve within 72-96 hours after the elimination of the offending protein from the diet, and subsequent oral challenge provokes both symptoms and a measurable inflammatory response. More than 90% of the infants will respond to initiation of an extensively hydrolyzed casein-based formula. From 15% to 50% of infants sensitive to cow's milk will also be sensitive to soy-based formula.

Meckel diverticulum (**choice B**) is the most common congenital malformation of the gastrointestinal tract, occurring in about 1.5% of the general population, most of whom experience no symptoms. The mucosa is often gastric, and the acid secreted may cause ulceration and bleeding, which is usually painless.

Necrotizing enterocolitis (**choice C**) affects premature infants and usually occurs as a complication of respiratory distress syndrome or patent ductus arteriosus. It manifests as abdominal distention, tenderness, bilious vomiting, and occult or frank blood in stool.

Rectal fissure (**choice D**) is one of the most common causes of rectal bleeding in young children. There is usually a history of constipation, with passage of large and hard stools.

Ulcerative colitis (**choice E**) is an inflammatory bowel disease primarily affecting the colon. It causes abdominal pain, hematochezia, diarrhea, weight loss, and fever.

43. **The correct answer is A.** Acute otitis media and acute sinusitis are among the most common infectious conditions of childhood. Acute sinusitis usually follows a common cold and is due to bacterial infection of the maxillary sinuses. It manifests with persistent mucopurulent discharge, daytime coughing *without* wheezing, and nasal obstruction. The diagnosis is based on a temporal criterion, with such manifestations present for at least 10 days. The 10-day mark allows differentiation of acute sinusitis from acute viral rhinitis (**choice C**), which should resolve within a week or so. If nasal discharge and obstruction persist for more than 30 days, the diagnosis is subacute sinusitis. High fever, swelling of eyelids, and pain on slight pressure over the sinuses indicate a severe sinus infection that needs prompt evaluation and aggressive antibiotic treatment. Most cases of acute sinusitis resolve after antibiotic treatment with amoxicillin or a macrolide, plus topical vasoconstrictors and nasal saline lavage for symptomatic relief.

Acute otitis media (**choice B**) usually follows an upper respiratory infection. It is characterized by otalgia (especially in older children) and the otoscopic findings of bulging and fullness of the tympanic membrane. Acute otitis media is more frequent between 6 months and 3 years of age.

Allergic rhinosinusitis (**choice D**) manifests with chronic *clear* nasal discharge, without fever or pain. There is usually an accompanying history of allergies.

Asthma (**choice E**) is characterized by paroxysmal attacks of respiratory distress with tachypnea and wheezing. Cough and increased nasal secretion may be present.

44. **The correct answer is B.** The most crucial step in the management of *asthma* is avoidance of triggering factors (e.g., allergens). Unfortunately, it is difficult to avoid specific types of allergens, such as pollens. Specific measures to eliminate or reduce exposure to dust mites and animal dander at home lead to reduced frequency of attacks and hospitalization rates. Regardless of the allergens involved, elimination of respiratory irritants, especially *cigarette smoke,* is of crucial importance. The bronchial tree of asthmatic patients is highly reactive to any form of chemical or physical irritation. Thus, exposure to passive smoke should be absolutely avoided.

Avoidance of exercise (**choice A**) is not an appropriate measure, although exercise frequently triggers asthmatic attacks. The efficacy of antiasthma measures can be evaluated by observing how the child can sustain adequate forms of exercise.

Use of a humidifier at home (**choice C**) will favor growth of dust mites and consequently increase the concentration of these allergens in the environment.

Use of air cleaners at home (**choice D**) has not been shown to be uniformly effective in getting rid of dust mites.

Administration of multiple-drug regimens (**choice E**) is not a recommended strategy in the pharmacologic treatment of asthma. In fact, the fewest number of drugs at the lowest effective doses should be used. Typically, a regimen of one drug (a bronchodilator or a inhaled corticosteroid) for mild-moderate cases or two drugs for more severe cases is sufficient to control asthma exacerbations.

Immunotherapy against identified allergens (**choice F**) is of some benefit when a single allergen is involved, but not with multiple airborne allergens.

45. **The correct answer is A.** Mental retardation associated with abnormal facial features may be related to abnormal genetics. As our skill with DNA analysis has improved, we have identified a number of microdeletion syndromes involving contiguous genes on a single chromosome that are associated with mental retardation and often distinctive clinical presentations. The case illustrated is Williams syndrome, which involves 7q11.23.

20p12 (**choice B**) is associated with Alagille syndrome, characterized by lack of bile ducts, cardiac abnormalities, butterfly vertebrae, and eye abnormalities.

22q11.21 (**choice C**) is associated with DiGeorge syndrome, which is characterized by thymus and parathyroid abnormalities, heart defects, cleft palate, and mental retardation.

Involvement of the maternal chromosome 15 at 15q11 (**choice D**) is associated with Angelman syndrome, which is characterized by seizures, puppet-like movements, outbursts of laughter, and severe mental retardation.

Involvement of the paternal chromosome 15 at 15q11 (**choice E**) is associated with Prader-Willi syndrome, which is characterized by obesity, small hands and feet, and mental retardation.

46. **The correct answer is C.** This infant has neonatal chlamydial infection that was acquired during birth from an infected mother. The major manifestation presented in this case is chlamydial ophthalmia, which occurs in about 30% to 40% of infants born to infected mothers. The severity of chlamydial ophthalmia can range from mild conjunctivitis to the severe pattern described in the question stem. Follicles are not present in the conjunctiva; they appear in in older children and adults. Chlamydial ophthalmia becomes evident 5 to 14 days after birth. Many of these infants also have nasopharyngeal colonization with *Chlamydia*, and neonatal pneumonia is common in patients who have clinically developed conjunctivitis. Symptoms of chlamydial pneumonia typically occur within 2 to 19 weeks, with an insidious onset of staccato cough.

Gonorrheal ophthalmia produces an acute purulent conjunctivitis that appears 2 to 5 days after birth or earlier with premature rupture of membranes. It can rapidly lead to corneal ulceration (**choice A**) and perforation if treatment is delayed.

Serious systemic complications, such as encephalitis (**choice B**), can result from herpes simplex keratoconjunctivits because these infants have poor immunologic response to the generalized herpes infection.

Sepsis (**choice D**) can be a complication of conjunctivitis, but it is less specific to chlamydial ophthalmia compared with other types of bacterial conjunctivitis. The risk for chlamydial pneumonia is more significant in this patient.

A chemical conjunctivitis may result from prophylactic silver nitrate use in neonates. It usually appears within 6 to 8 hours after installation and disappears spontaneously within 24 to 48 hours. Silver toxicity (**choice E**) is not typical of prophylactic silver nitrate use, and it is unrelated to chlamydial ophthalmia.

47. **The correct answer is A.** Apnea can be a life-threatening complication of RSV infection in infants younger than 1 year. For this reason, infants with respiratory distress and either laboratory confirmation or a clinical picture suggestive of RSV infection are often admitted to the hospital for supportive care and monitoring.

Congestive heart failure (**choice B**) is not associated with RSV infection in a child with normal cardiac function.

Infants are obligate nose-breathers and may have difficulty feeding because of nasal congestion. In the face of respiratory distress, infants have increased insensible fluid losses

and are at risk for dehydration (**choice C**). Dehydration, however, is not the most severe risk for this child.

Hypoxemia (**choice D**) and cyanosis may result from mucous plugging of the lower bronchial tree, atelectasis, and $\dot{V}/\dot{Q}$ mismatch in infants with acute RSV infection. The hypoxemia is usually transient and not life-threatening. Hypoxemia is readily corrected with supplemental oxygen administration.

Wheezing (**choice E**) is a very common sign of RSV infection. It signifies inflammation of the bronchioles, but it is not life-threatening.

48. **The correct answer is B.** Ewing sarcoma (ES) is the second most common bone cancer in childhood and adolescence. It has a peak age incidence during adolescent years. It rarely occurs in blacks and is more prevalent in boys than girls. ES may have histopathologic features characteristic of neural differentiation; ES is thought to be a tumor of neural origin, whereas most bone tumors are thought to be of mesodermal origin. The tumor category of ES has recently been expanded to include more neural tumors, such as peripheral primitive neuroectodermal tumor (PNET). Like other bone tumors, ES is associated with a consistent chromosomal translocation, t(11;22)(q24;q12), which occurs in about 90% to 95% of cases.

Chondroblastoma (**choice A**) is a very rare bone tumor that most often occurs in the pelvis. Histopathology reveals cartilaginous tumor tissue with malignant spindle cells.

Neuroblastoma (**choice C**) is a common solid tumor of childhood that typically occurs during the first few years of life. Histologically it is a small round cell tumor with characteristic Homer-Wright rosettes. It displays neural differentiation and therefore might initially be confused with ES, but it is not a bone tumor. It usually occurs in the neck, thorax, abdomen, or flank.

Osteosarcoma (**choice D**) is the most common bone cancer of childhood and adolescence. Like ES, osteosarcoma may involve the bones of the leg, especially the femur, and frequently metastases to the lungs. Osteosarcoma is known to be associated with certain genetic conditions, such as osteogenic imperfecta, and there is an increased occurrence of osteosarcoma in children with retinoblastoma. It occurs in all races. Pathologically, neural differentiation is not observed.

Rhabdomyosarcoma (**choice E**) is the most common soft tissue sarcoma of childhood. It does occur more frequently among males and whites, but it is usually found in the head and neck areas and the genitourinary tract. Like neuroblastoma and ES it is a small round cell tumor. It does not display neural differentiation. It may first be noticed after trauma as in this case, but there is no bony involvement.

49. **The correct answer is C.** Febrile seizures are common events. This form of *benign* manifestation affects approximately 3% to 4% of children. Since epilepsy is defined as at least two seizures occurring *without* an identifiable trigger, febrile seizures do not constitute epilepsy even if they recur. Fever, in fact, is the identifiable trigger. Most children who have an episode of febrile seizure will not have a recurrence. Risk factors that do increase the likelihood of recurrence include family history, age younger than 18 months (**choice A**), and temperature less than 39.0° C (**choice E**) when seizure occurred. Overall, children with a first febrile seizure will have a recurrence in 25% of cases by 1 year and in 30% by 2 years.

    The duration of the first seizure (**choice B**) will not influence the likelihood of recurrence, but recurrences will likely also be prolonged if the first episode lasted for more than 15 minutes.

    Fever of long duration (**choice D**) is negatively correlated to the probability of recurrences.

50. **The correct answer is C.** Measurements of T4 and TSH levels are the most appropriate tests to confirm congenital hypothyroidism.

    Alpha-1-antitrypsin genotyping (**choice A**) is used to confirm alpha-1-antitrypsin deficiency.

    A liver and spleen scan (**choice B**) is useful to indicate absence of the biliary tree or blockage of the extrahepatic bile ducts and is therefore most useful to confirm biliary atresia.

    Barium swallow (**choice D**) will indicate the presence of pyloric stenosis ("string" sign = narrowing of barium stream passing through the duodenum; "umbrella" sign = the hold-up of barium in the stomach).

    The RPR and FTA (**choice E**) are serologic tests for syphilis.

Psychiatry: **Test One**

1. A 39-year-old African American man is an inpatient on a psychiatric ward. He was admitted because of concerns that his neighbors are spying on him and devising ways to kill him. He states that the neighbors have inserted cameras in several rooms of his house to monitor his activities. He claims to hear them through the walls saying they are going to kill him. The patient's wife called the police when he bought a gun stating that he was going to kill the neighbors "in self-defense." Which of the following is the most appropriate pharmacologic treatment?

   (A) Benztropine

   (B) Diazepam

   (C) Fluoxetine

   (D) Lithium

   (E) Risperidone

2. A 61-year-old man is brought to a physician for evaluation of his behavior. His family states that recently he has been yelling, spitting, and pulling other people's noses or ears unexpectedly. He was always a fine man and devoted husband but now uses foul language and is openly promiscuous. He has no significant medical or psychiatric history. The family recalls that the patient's uncle displayed similar behavior and was placed in a nursing home, where he quickly died. On examination, memory and visuospatial functions are intact, but the patient exhibits some word-finding difficulties. During the examination, the patient keeps repeating the doctor's command and giggling inappropriately and loudly. Which of the following is the most likely diagnosis?

   (A) Alzheimer disease

   (B) Dementia pugilistica

   (C) Multi-infarct dementia

   (D) Neurosyphilis

   (E) Pick disease

3. While on the Psychiatry Consult-Liaison Inpatient Service, a psychiatry intern is called to assess a patient on a general medical floor who has developed a muscle spasm causing her neck to twist uncontrollably to the left. She is also having difficulty speaking and is upset. The intern evaluates the patient's list of medications and concludes that her new symptoms may be due to one of them. Which of the following medications is most likely responsible for the patient's symptoms?

   (A) Aspirin

   (B) Digoxin

   (C) Erythromycin

   (D) Fluoxetine

   (E) Metoclopramide

4. A 29-year-old woman was attacked, held at gunpoint, robbed, and beaten after leaving a restaurant in the evening. Despite this, she managed to report the incident to police and continue with her daily activities. Two months later, she seeks psychiatric help because she has been having difficulty going to work and participating in other activities. Which of the following constellation of symptoms would she most likely report to her psychiatrist?

   (A) Confusion and disorientation

   (B) Depression and suicidal thoughts

   (C) Euphoria and racing thoughts

   (D) Flashbacks and increased arousal

   (E) Hyperphagia and hypersomnia

KAPLAN MEDICAL

5. A 25-year-old man presents to the emergency department (ED) with a sore arm and difficulty using his hand. He has been evaluated multiple times in the ED for multiple somatic complaints, but medical evaluation has been consistently unrevealing. He also has a history of cocaine abuse, for which he was admitted to various substance abuse rehabilitation facilities. Often, his trips to the hospital coincided with scheduled court appearances after violating probation. Physical examination of the man's arm does not show obvious injury or focal abnormalities, and an x-ray of the arm is normal. A urine toxicology screen is negative. The patient was offered ice, anti-inflammatory medication, and information concerning the benign nature of his pain. The patient was then told that he was to be discharged from the ED, at which point he stated that his pain was too great for him to leave the hospital and he demanded admission. Which of the following is the most likely diagnosis?

(A) Conversion disorder

(B) Dissociative identity disorder

(C) Factitious disorder

(D) Malingering

(E) Rheumatoid arthritis

6. A 23-year-old man is taking classes at a local community college. He had finished high school without difficulties and was voted "most popular" by his classmates. Three months ago, he started skipping classes after he had a "special revelation" that the "holy spirit" had a more important mission for him. He began worshipping computers, believing them to be sending him special, secret messages from the "holy spirit." His family, alarmed by the change in his behavior, brings him to the local emergency department. His past history is significant for occasional alcohol and marijuana use. A urine toxicology screen is negative. The patient is admitted to the psychiatric ward of the hospital for further evaluation. In which of the following ways does this person's presentation preclude a diagnosis of schizophrenia?

(A) Age of onset

(B) Duration of symptoms

(C) Presence of a mood disorder

(D) Severity of symptoms

(E) Type of auditory hallucinations

7. A 37-year-old man has a 2-year history of major depression that is managed with sertraline. Several attempts at discontinuing therapy resulted in relapses with major depressive symptoms and strong suicidal ideation. The man visits his psychiatrist to discuss management options. In particular, he discusses problems with his marriage because of sexual dysfunction. He describes a lack of libido that started when he began antidepressant therapy, and he believes that it is destroying his marriage. He discloses the presence of nocturnal erections but a lack of interest in sexual intimacy with his wife. Their relationship is otherwise well, and he doesn't know what he should do. Which of the following medications is an appropriate antidepressant alternative for relieving his symptoms of sexual dysfunction?

(A) Amitriptyline

(B) Bupropion

(C) Fluoxetine

(D) Paroxetine

(E) Sildenafil

8. A 28-year-old, malodorous woman in dirty clothing is brought by police into a psychiatric community crisis response center after being found shouting in the middle of a busy street. The woman reportedly was yelling about the end of the world coming soon and that all cars must be abandoned to save the earth from eternal destruction. She screamed at the police who brought her into custody, calling them "evil." She visibly shook when taken by police car, crying out that "cars are the means to destruction." Further, she was noted to stare off into the distance and talk to herself during the car ride. On her arrival at the crisis center, her behavior quickly escalated. She became belligerent, shouting obscenities and trying to hit everyone around her. To calm her down and in an attempt to speak with her in a less agitated fashion, the psychiatric intern on call ordered an intramuscular medication to be administered. Which of the following medications is the best choice for rapid tranquilization in this agitated patient?

(A) Clozapine

(B) Haloperidol

(C) Lithium

(D) Quetiapine

(E) Perphenazine

9. An emergency department physician orders a 5-mg haloperidol injection for a psychotic 30-year-old man. Six hours later, the patient's temperature is 39.4° C (103.0° F), and there is diffuse muscular rigidity and diaphoresis. Over the next 24 hours, the patient becomes increasingly obtunded. He is put on a cardiac monitor, and his blood pressure is noted to fluctuate from 100/70 mm Hg to 170/96 mm Hg. Which of the following is the most likely diagnosis?

   (A) Catatonia

   (B) Malignant hyperthermia

   (C) Neuroleptic malignant syndrome

   (D) Serotonin syndrome

   (E) Tardive dyskinesia

10. A 22-year-old college student presents to her physician complaining of increasing apathy and lethargy over the past several weeks. She has also been eating and sleeping more, and her grades have begun to drop. She also states that some of her classmates find her a bit overbearing and irritating, particularly when she goes for days at a time without sleeping while participating in her many student activities. She states that her alcohol intake is limited to two or three beers on occasional weekends while socializing with friends, and she denies any other substance use. Around 6 months ago, she spent almost $1,000 on clothing and other gifts for her boyfriend, and she spent another large amount of money on a computer to use to write her latest novel. She states that she was put on paroxetine as a teenager and she "didn't sleep for days." Which of the following is the most appropriate single agent to use for pharmacotherapy in this case?

    (A) Alprazolam

    (B) Amitriptyline

    (C) Bupropion

    (D) Fluoxetine

    (E) Lithium carbonate

11. Parents of a 3-year-old boy take their child to the pediatrician for evaluation of what they consider to be "abnormal" behavior. They describe their son as never wanting to be held, even as a baby, not making good eye contact with anyone, crying whenever he is bathed, and having no interest in playing with other children. He does not have any favorite toys, security play items, or any known make-believe friends. He has minimal ability to speak in a coherent language, although the parents believe that they can understand him when he is trying to communicate. The pediatrician observes the boy in the office playroom. He is sitting alone in the corner of the playroom, carefully piling blocks one on top of the other. He is noted to make occasional circular gestures with his left hand. There are four other children, aged 2-4 years, waiting to be seen by the pediatrician; these children are playing together, apart from the boy. In which of the following areas is this boy most likely to have difficulty?

    (A) Attention

    (B) Concentration

    (C) Intelligence

    (D) Interpersonal relations

    (E) Urinary incontinence

12. A 15-year-old boy is brought in by his mother to see a psychiatrist for "strange behavior." She reports that her son is often late for school because he spends more than an hour in the shower every morning. When asked about this, he says that he takes a long time because he feels compelled to wash himself in a certain manner, and has to repeat the whole process if he makes a mistake. He knows it sounds ridiculous, and that it makes him late for school and other activities, but he cannot seem to stop himself. In addition, he has found it difficult to fall asleep at night because he needs to constantly check that he has set his alarm for the morning. Which of the following is the most likely diagnosis?

    (A) Attention deficit/hyperactivity disorder

    (B) Bipolar disorder

    (C) Generalized anxiety disorder

    (D) Major depressive disorder

    (E) Obsessive-compulsive disorder

13. A 75-year-old woman experiences several episodes of syncope. She is evaluated and found to have critical aortic stenosis. She is otherwise healthy and, with the advice of her cardiologist, decides to undergo valve replacement surgery. Three days after the surgery the patient is found to be irritable, have a labile mood, and be awake for much of the night. She yells at the nurses at 4 A.M. one morning for not helping her get into her street clothes; however, the next morning at 8 A.M., when the surgical intern came to see her, she was calm and cooperative. She did not remember the events of the previous night. The patient had no known psychiatric history and got a 30/30 on the Folstein Mini-Mental State Examination 1 week prior to the surgery. Which of the following is the most likely diagnosis?

    (A) Adjustment disorder

    (B) Cyclothymia

    (C) Delirium

    (D) Dementia

    (E) Malingering

14. A 52-year-old man is seen for the first time by a psychiatrist. He states that he always feels "keyed up" and "on edge" and has been having nightmares about combat experience from the Vietnam War, from which he is a veteran. He states that he witnessed several of his fellow soldiers get killed in combat and he has since experienced what he describes as "movies of it all happening over again" while awake. He reports that he has difficulty discussing these events because they are so distressing. Prior to Vietnam, he was happily married and had several friends; now he feels that he cannot get close to other people and often gets angry with people for no apparent reason. Which of the following is the most likely diagnosis?

    (A) Acute stress disorder

    (B) Generalized anxiety disorder

    (C) Posttraumatic stress disorder

    (D) Schizoid personality disorder

    (E) Sleep terror disorder

15. A 20-year-old woman with bipolar disorder, who is currently in a manic state, responds to many emergency department interview questions with flight of ideas. The patient is asked how she got to the hospital. Which of the following statements by the patient is the best example of this form of thought disturbance?

    (A) "I drove here myself."

    (B) "I was reading a great book at home and, after I finished it, I drove here myself."

    (C) "I really like history books and I was reading one at home today while eating tuna fish."

    (D) "I started driving but was thinking about my history. History books are great. I once wrote a paper on Alexander the Great. I do well in college."

    (E) "The spy in the book I was reading is real, and he was watching me through the pages. He knew who I was."

16. A 45-year-old man is admitted to the ICU for trauma-related injuries sustained in a car accident. Thirty-six hours after admission he becomes agitated. He is pulling at his IV access lines and is disoriented to place and time. His blood pressure is 190/110 mm Hg, and his pulse is 114/min. A reliable history from the patient's son reveals that the patient is alcohol dependent. Which of the following is the most appropriate next step in management?

    (A) Haloperidol

    (B) Lithium

    (C) Lorazepam

    (D) Propranolol

    (E) No medication

17. A 29-year-old woman consistently meets "the man of her dreams" only to have the relationships fail after a month or two. She views herself as unworthy of being loved and often hurts herself after these relationships fail. She feels depressed if she has no weekend plans and has difficulty controlling both her anger and sadness if she knows she will be alone. When frustrated, she often acts out, impulsively drinking alcohol and having sex with men whom she does not know well, only to find herself feeling empty afterward. Further, she is unhappy in her job and thinks that she could "do better." Which of the following is the most characteristic defense mechanism used by people who have this personality disorder?

    (A) Displacement

    (B) Idealization

    (C) Intellectualization

    (D) Reaction formation

    (E) Splitting

18. A 51-year-old Vietnam veteran who has been treated for several months with antidepressants for posttraumatic stress disorder (PTSD) recently began taking a new sleep medication for insomnia. After several days, he calls his doctor complaining of a prolonged and painful erection. The doctor instructs him to stop the medication and immediately come into the emergency department. Which of the following medications is most likely causing this condition?

    (A) Chlordiazepoxide

    (B) Hydroxyzine

    (C) Mirtazapine

    (D) Trazodone

    (E) Zolpidem

19. A 32-year-old man has chronic paranoid schizophrenia and a history of mild tardive dyskinesia. His psychiatrist recently switched his medication to olanzapine taken at bedtime. The patient smokes approximately a pack of cigarettes daily, weighs 70 kg (154 lb) at a height of 178 cm (5 feet 10 inches), and does not drink alcohol. Which of the following would be the most common adverse side effect of olanzapine in this patient?

    (A) Gastrointestinal complications

    (B) Orthostatic hypotension

    (C) Sedation

    (D) Tardive dyskinesia

    (E) Weight gain

20. A 34-year-old man has had a significantly increased appetite, gained 10 lb, and required increased sleep over the past several months. He has felt severely fatigued during the same time period and describes a heavy feeling in his arms and legs. His brother, a psychiatrist, visits him, notes the complaints, and feels that the sensation he described in his arms and legs is pathognomonic for "leaden paralysis." This is a characteristic feature of which of the following diagnoses?

    (A) Conversion disorder

    (B) Major depression with atypical features

    (C) Schizophrenia, catatonic type

    (D) Schizotypal personality disorder

    (E) Somatoform disorder

21. Available clinical evidence indicates that individuals who are homozygous for the Apo E4 gene are at increased risk of developing Alzheimer disease. However, laboratory testing aimed at the identification of Apo E4 carriers does not appear adequate as a screening test for early detection of this risk factor. Which of the following is the most commonly suggested reason for not using Apo E allele determination as a screening test?

    (A) The disease does not have a preclinical (asymptomatic) stage

    (B) The disease is not preventable or treatable

    (C) The disease is not sufficiently prevalent

    (D) The disease is not sufficiently serious

    (E) The test is not sufficiently accurate

    (F) The test is not sufficiently sensitive

22. A teacher calls the parents of an 8-year-old boy to discuss his poor adjustment to the second grade. He has difficulty sitting still for group activities and needs constant reminders from the teacher not to hit his classmates. He has problems listening in class and does not complete assignments without several reminders. These multiple reminders and behavioral reprimands do not seem to be leading to any improvement. His parents have also been noticing similar problems at home. The boy is sent to a child psychiatrist, who notes increased psychomotor activity with restlessness during the evaluation. The testing revealed no learning disability, and the boy was diagnosed with attention-deficit hyperactivity disorder. This boy is at a higher risk than the normal population to have which of the following comorbid disorders?

    (A) Asperger disorder

    (B) Autistic disorder

    (C) Anxiety disorder

    (D) Oppositional defiant disorder

    (E) Schizophrenia, undifferentiated type

23. A 22-year-old female student presents to her physician after collapsing in the cafeteria following loud joking and laughter with her friends. She describes loss of muscle tone after she fell but no loss of consciousness. On further examination, she reveals a 4-month history of increased daytime sleepiness, with several episodes of falling asleep during her classes. She believed that the episodes were related to poor sleep because of vivid dreams she had on falling asleep. Which of the following is the most likely diagnosis?

    (A) Catalepsy

    (B) Kleine-Levin syndrome

    (C) Narcolepsy

    (D) Periodic paralysis

    (E) Primary hypersomnia

24. A 27-year-old woman, after undergoing elective cosmetic breast augmentation surgery, presents to her surgeon dissatisfied with the results and requesting more surgery, even though she has received compliments from both her friends and her boyfriend concerning her new appearance. She has had no medical complications from the procedure. The patient, who weighs about 110 pounds, tells her surgeon that she has been preoccupied with her breast size since she was a teenager and that she has had difficulties in relationships with previous boyfriends because she felt that they viewed her as inadequately feminine. She describes that she has also had difficulties dating in the past because of the excessive amount of time she spends working out at the gym and jogging to maintain her figure. Which of the following would be the most appropriate diagnosis in this patient?

    (A) Adjustment disorder with disturbance of emotion

    (B) Body dysmorphic disorder

    (C) Borderline personality disorder

    (D) Hypochondriasis

    (E) Somatoform disorder, not otherwise specified

25. A concerned mother asks a child psychiatrist whether her child's behavior is abnormal. She describes the child as typically happy: she smiles often at her parents, is a good eater, and is mostly a good sleeper, able to sleep through the night without waking. However, when the parents leave her with a baby-sitter on occasional weekend nights, the child reportedly screams uncontrollably. The baby-sitter finds it difficult to feed her, and likewise she rarely falls asleep without a hysterical crying outburst. Which of the following is the most likely age of this child?

    (A) 1 week

    (B) 3 months

    (C) 8 months

    (D) 18 months

    (E) 24 months

26. A 35-year-old woman, who was hospitalized 6 months ago and diagnosed with bipolar disorder, mixed type, arrives for a follow-up appointment. She feels that she is stable on her medication but has noticed an increased appetite with significant weight gain, as well as hair loss, since her discharge. Her physical examination and laboratory tests, including a thyroid panel, are unremarkable. Her physician concludes that her medication is the cause of her problems. Which of the following medications is this patient most likely taking?

    (A) Clonazepam

    (B) Divalproex

    (C) Gabapentin

    (D) Lithium

    (E) Olanzapine

27. A breast cancer patient starts to feel nauseated as she exits the hospital corridor leading to the chemotherapy treatment area and enters the waiting room. After she opens the waiting room door, she feels even more nauseated. As she waits in line to check herself in for her eighth of ten chemotherapy treatments, she vomits. This reaction is an example of which of the following learning theories?

    (A) Classical conditioning

    (B) Covert sensitization

    (C) Habituation

    (D) Learned helplessness

    (E) Operant conditioning

28. A 6-year-old boy learns how to paint with watercolors in his first-grade art class. He likes to learn new skills and works hard at painting a picture of himself outside his house. Despite gross irregularities in the sizes and shapes of the objects in the picture, he is very proud of himself and feels competent. He brings the picture home from school and announces to his mother, "Mommy, look at the beautiful picture I made!" According to Erik Erikson, this child is at which of the following stages of development?

    (A) Autonomy vs. shame and doubt

    (B) Identity vs. role confusion

    (C) Industry vs. inferiority

    (D) Initiative vs. guilt

    (E) Trust vs. mistrust

29. A 17-year-old girl is caught stealing three lipsticks from a local convenience store. The security guard takes her to the back of the store and gathers information from her. The girl hands over her driver's license, and the guard calls the police with her identifying information. He learns that this girl has been caught stealing several times before, with reports from convenience, clothing, and food stores. The police come to the store and arrest her. Which of the following attributes is likely to be absent in this individual?

    (A) Delusional thinking

    (B) Displeasure at the thought of being caught in the act of the theft

    (C) Failure to resist impulses to steal

    (D) Increasing tension before the theft

    (E) Pleasure at the time of committing the theft

30. A 24-year-old, unemployed man is brought to the hospital by police after he was found sleeping on chairs at a departure gate in the airport. When awakened by the police and asked to leave the premises, the man insisted that he be allowed to stay in that specific location, since he was able to pick up on "special radiowave signals" emanating from that airline's planes arriving between 1 P.M. and 3 P.M. He spoke of being part of a secret mission with spies from an unidentified foreign country and stated that he was concerned that the police were working with his enemy. The police were able to calmly bring the man into the nearest psychiatric emergency department, where he was evaluated. He was taking no medications at the time, and a urine toxicology screen was negative. Which abnormality is most consistently seen in CT scans of the brains of persons who have the disorder suggested by the history and findings?

    (A) Atrophic changes in the cerebellar vermis

    (B) Bilateral hypodensities in the orbitofrontal region

    (C) Hydrocephalus

    (D) Increased ventricle-to-brain ratio

    (E) Significant sulcal widening

31. A 59-year-old woman is brought to a psychiatrist because her family has been worried about her worsening behavior. The family reports prominent changes in personality and in the way in which she has recently been relating to others. They report that she has recently become sexually provocative in her attire and demeanor, she does not know how to hold socially appropriate conversations anymore, and she lacks the insight that she once had. She has a new grandchild and has recently become indifferent to him, and occasionally sits still, stares ahead, and seems mute. She is found to have mild memory and cognitive dysfunction, perseveration, and an inability to plan and organize. She has a positive glabellar sign. This patient most likely has dysfunction of which of the following regions of the brain?

    (A) Basal ganglia
    (B) Frontal lobe
    (C) Hypothalamus
    (D) Temporal lobe
    (E) Ventricular obstruction

32. A 34-year-old Caucasian woman presents to the emergency department with thoughts of suicide. She states that she was feeling "fine" until a week ago, when she began to feel very depressed. In addition, she states that she has not slept very much in the past few days and has been experiencing rapidly shifting extremes of mood, one day feeling "on top of the world" and the next feeling "tired and down in the dumps." She claims that she has thoughts of jumping in front of a train to kill herself. When asked about illicit drug use, she becomes rather indignant, stating that she is being accused of being a drug addict. A urine drug screen is positive for cocaine metabolites. Which of the following is the most likely diagnosis?

    (A) Bipolar disorder, manic
    (B) Dysthymic disorder
    (C) Histrionic personality disorder
    (D) Major depressive disorder
    (E) Substance-induced mood disorder

33. A 33-year-old salesman returns from work following a meeting with his boss. The man demanded a raise because of his increased sales. He was told that there were other people who deserved it more. He comes back home and starts yelling at his son for watching TV after he had finished his homework. Which of the following most appropriately describes this man's reaction?

    (A) Acting out
    (B) Displacement
    (C) Projection
    (D) Reaction formation
    (E) Sublimation

34. A 28-year-old Caucasian man is referred to a psychiatrist for management of anxiety. The patient reports that, in the past year, he has had "anxiety attacks," during which he experiences an intense feeling of anxiety, chest pain, difficulty breathing, numbness and tingling in his hands and feet, and sweating. The attacks usually last for about 5 to 10 minutes and are unprovoked. The episodes used to occur only once or twice a month, but have been increasing in frequency to several times per day. He has been evaluated a number of times at an emergency department because he thought he was having a heart attack. Each emergency visit revealed no cardiac or other medical explanation for his symptoms. There is no family history of cardiac disease, and his physical examination is unremarkable. Which of the following is the most likely diagnosis?

    (A) Generalized anxiety disorder
    (B) Histrionic personality disorder
    (C) Hypochondriasis
    (D) Panic disorder
    (E) Somatization disorder

35. A 23-year-old African American man with a diagnosis of schizophrenia, paranoid type, has been maintained on a low dose of haloperidol for the past 3 years. For the past month, his symptoms of paranoia and auditory hallucinations have been more prominent, and his psychiatrist decides to increase his dose of haloperidol. The patient's mother calls the psychiatrist, concerned that he seems slower than usual and has a fine resting tremor of his upper extremities. Furthermore, he seems to be drooling and complains of being stiff. Which of the following is the most likely diagnosis?

    (A) Benign essential tremor

    (B) Neuroleptic-induced parkinsonism

    (C) Neuroleptic malignant syndrome

    (D) Parkinson disease

    (E) Tardive dyskinesia

36. A 48-year-old African American woman is brought to the emergency department by her mother because of "infestation." The patient states that she is infested with mites and points to areas on her arms. She reports that her house became infested with mites and other bugs about 3 months ago, and she has called an exterminator several times to have the house sprayed with a chemical. Further, she has been spraying herself with a pest-control agent daily because "the bugs are coming out of every part of my body, my eyes, my nose, and my mouth. I think my kids are getting infested, too!" She does not report auditory hallucinations. She denies any past psychiatric or medical history. Physical examination is remarkable for several scattered excoriated areas, but there is no evidence of infestation. Laboratory studies, including a urine drug screen, are negative. Which of the following is the most likely diagnosis?

    (A) Delirium tremens

    (B) Delusional disorder

    (C) Hypnagogic hallucination

    (D) Obsessive-compulsive disorder

    (E) Paranoid personality disorder

    (F) Schizophrenia

37. A 33-year-old man being treated for bipolar disorder develops gradual slowing of cognition, with concomitant development of a gravelly voice, constipation, dry skin, and hair loss. Examination is normal, except for a lag in the relaxation phase of the ankle jerk reflex. His only medication is lithium, and a lithium level is within normal limits. Which of the following tests should most likely be ordered next?

    (A) BUN and creatinine

    (B) Liver function tests

    (C) Serum sodium

    (D) Thyroid function tests

    (E) Urine electrolytes

38. A 30-year-old woman comes to her physician with multiple complaints. She has had insomnia, loss of appetite, and anxiety for 6 months. She also reports intestinal symptoms, such as epigastric pain and bloating. She has thought of quitting her work as a secretary because her husband wants her to stay at home to take better care of their 3-year-old boy. Physical examination reveals multiple bruises on her trunk. On further questioning, the patient admits that she has been physically abused by her husband. The violence has been increasing in frequency and severity over the past few months. Which of the following is the most appropriate next step in short-term management?

    (A) Express doubts about the patient's account but document lesions carefully

    (B) Express indignation against the perpetrator

    (C) Instruct the patient on how and when to leave her husband

    (D) Provide emotional support and ensure the patient's safety

    (E) Refer both the victim and her husband for marriage counseling

    (F) Try to persuade the patient's husband to quit abusing his wife

39. A 45-year-old, obese woman presents to a psychiatrist with depression. She describes two previous similar episodes that occurred in the past 2 years that were milder and resolved with the support of her family. Her symptoms are much worse now, and she is prepared to do anything to help herself. On the basis of her information, the psychiatrist decides to start her on phenelzine for treatment of atypical depression. Which of the following features was likely present in the patient's history to lead to the diagnosis of major depressive disorder with atypical features?

    (A) Decreased appetite

    (B) Depression worse in the morning and better in the evening

    (C) Leaden paralysis

    (D) Negativism

    (E) Psychomotor agitation

40. A 63-year-old woman with a 9-year history of Parkinson disease has developed worsening problems with visual hallucinations. In particular, she complains of seeing cats crawling along the floors in her house. She is taking L-dopa/carbidopa (Sinemet) and has had significant improvement in her rigidity. Which of the following drugs would be most appropriate for her psychosis?

    (A) Chlorpromazine

    (B) Clomipramine

    (C) Clozapine

    (D) Haloperidol

    (E) Pergolide

41. A 29-year-old Caucasian man is brought into the emergency department by ambulance. He was found unresponsive in an alleyway by a passerby. On arrival to the emergency department, the patient is responsive to deep pain only, respirations are slow and shallow, and the pupils are pinpoint. There are track marks noted on the upper and lower extremities. Which of the following is the most appropriate next step in management?

    (A) Chlordiazepoxide

    (B) Flumazenil

    (C) Methadone

    (D) *N*-Acetylcysteine

    (E) Naloxone

    (F) Naltrexone

42. A 22-year-old woman with a history of depression is brought to the emergency department by her friend, who found her groggy and minimally responsive at home. On examination, she is mildly obtunded and complains of blurry vision. She has enlarged, minimally reactive pupils, but no focal deficits. A cardiac monitor demonstrates frequent premature ventricular contractions and tachycardia to 120 beats per minute. A Foley catheter is inserted, with passage of 800 mL of urine. An overdose is presumed. Which of the following drugs did the patient most likely take?

    (A) Bupropion

    (B) Fluoxetine

    (C) Nortriptyline

    (D) Phenelzine

    (E) Sertraline

43. A 19-year-old man presents to the emergency department after a car accident in which he was driving drunk. He was wearing a seat belt and sustained only minor cuts and bruises. When questioned about his history of drinking alcohol, he states that he has driven while intoxicated before and that his drinking has caused him to miss work on a few occasions. He was arrested twice for driving under the influence (DUI). He says that his drinking caused his parents to force him out of the house last month. When questioned further, he states that in the past it took him a few shots of vodka to get drunk, but now it takes up to a pint of liquor. Which of the following factors in the patient's history suggests a diagnosis of substance dependence rather than substance abuse?

    (A) Continued substance use despite persistent familial problems

    (B) Failure to fulfill work obligations because of substance use

    (C) Increased amount of alcohol necessary to achieve intoxication

    (D) Recurrent alcohol-related legal problems, like a DUI arrest

    (E) Recurrent substance use while driving

44. A 31-year-old woman has had panic attacks for almost 15 years. She recalls that they first occurred when she was sitting in large crowds at her high school's sporting arenas. She remembers feeling trapped on the football bleachers and feeling that her world was closing in on her. Her heart began racing, and she became sweaty and had to lie down to avoid fainting. She thereafter stopped attending large events; however, the panic attacks resumed when she went to college and had to wait in long cafeteria lines. After college, she became very nervous traveling on both the subways and public buses to get to work. She had several panic attacks and opted to quit her job and find another one within walking distance from her home. Shortly thereafter, she began having panic attacks entering her new work office building. These were unprecedented, uncontrollable, and very frightening to her. She left this job and for the past 3 years has not left her home. She allows her family to visit her, bring her food, and do errands for her, but she refuses to leave her house. Which of the following behavioral therapies has been shown to most effectively treat this condition?

    (A) Biofeedback

    (B) Flooding

    (C) Gradual exposure

    (D) Learning new habits

    (E) Relaxation therapy

45. A 20-year-old woman is brought to the emergency department by paramedics. She is very anxious and appears frightened; her speech is slurred and dysarthric. She is extremely labile emotionally, and she has been thrashing about and scraping herself inadvertently, requiring restraint. Her blood pressure is 180/95 mm Hg, and her pulse is 120/min. On examination, she has horizontal nystagmus in both eyes. Which of the following is the most likely diagnosis?

    (A) Alcohol withdrawal

    (B) Lithium intoxication

    (C) Neuroleptic malignant syndrome

    (D) Paranoid schizophrenia

    (E) Phencyclidine intoxication

46. An 83-year-old woman is brought from her nursing home residence to the local psychiatric emergency evaluation center. She was diagnosed with Alzheimer type dementia 4 years ago. She is described as usually being calm and pleasantly confused (disoriented to place, date, and time). She had been stable, but for the past 3 nights she woke up in the middle of the night, shouting out incoherent statements and apparently hallucinating. In the daytime of the past 3 days, she has been eating less and occasionally napping (which is unusual for her), with episodes of agitation during which she has tried to hit other nursing home residents. She has also had a low-grade fever. In the psychiatric emergency evaluation center, she appears excited and is asking for her husband, who has been deceased for 12 years. Which of the following is the most appropriate initial step in management?

    (A) Inquire about her medications, including any recent changes

    (B) Obtain vital signs and an ECG

    (C) Protect the patient from unintentional harm

    (D) Request a medicine consult

    (E) Administer intramuscular haloperidol

47. A 26-year-old man claims that he was smoking crack cocaine at a party and became intensely paranoid. He thought that his mother was trying to kill him and that his girlfriend was plotting to have him imprisoned for treason against the U.S. In addition, he experienced the sensation of bugs crawling under his skin. On examination, the patient appears somewhat anxious, but is able to make himself well understood. He currently denies auditory or visual hallucinations, and the paranoia, albeit present, is milder and less distressing. Physical examination is unremarkable, and laboratory studies are significant only for a urine drug screen positive for cocaine metabolites. Overactivity at which of the following receptors best explains this patient's presenting symptoms?

    (A) Acetylcholine

    (B) Dopamine

    (C) GABA

    (D) Glutamate

    (E) Glycine

48. A 77-year-old woman is admitted to the hospital late in the afternoon for the treatment of urosepsis. The on-call resident is paged in the middle of the night to evaluate the patient because of a mental status change. The patient is heard yelling that she is in prison and states that she is covered with insects. Her primary nurse says that the patient has been alternating between periods of overt agitation and lethargy over the past 12 hours since she has been on the ward. Which of the following is the most likely diagnosis?

    (A) Amnestic disorder not otherwise specified

    (B) Delirium

    (C) Major depressive disorder, with psychotic features

    (D) Parkinson dementia

    (E) Senile dementia, Alzheimer type

49. A 29-year-old white man visits an emergency department complaining that "black women are putting spells on me and are trying to rape me." He reports that for the past 6 years he has had held the firm belief that women he encounters are hypnotizing him and then raping him. The patient also states that he can hear voices of women in his head talking "dirty" to him. His mental status examination is remarkable for the delusions and hallucinations noted above. His thought process is goal-oriented, and his affect is constricted. Physical examination and laboratory studies, including a drug screen, are unremarkable. Which of the following is the most likely diagnosis?

    (A) Bipolar disorder

    (B) Brief psychotic disorder

    (C) Major depressive disorder with psychotic features

    (D) Posttraumatic stress disorder

    (E) Schizophrenia

50. A forensic psychiatrist is evaluating a patient before a criminal trial. The suspect is a 17-year-old girl who is accused of fatally stabbing her stepfather while he was asleep. There is substantial forensic evidence against the suspect, including a murder weapon with the suspect's fingerprints. The suspect states that she does not remember stabbing her stepfather. However, she feels no sense of loss that her stepfather is dead because of a long history of being sexually abused by him. During the assessment, the suspect's facial expression and voice rapidly change. She says that she is now the "adopted older brother" of the suspect and that he stabbed the suspect's stepfather without her knowledge. For the remainder of the interview, the psychiatrist is unable to speak to the suspect directly. Which of the following is the most likely diagnosis?

    (A) Depersonalization disorder

    (B) Dissociative fugue

    (C) Dissociative identity disorder

    (D) Major depressive disorder, with psychotic features

    (E) Schizophrenia, paranoid type

Psychiatry Test One:
Answers and Explanations

ANSWER KEY

1.	E		26.	B
2.	E		27.	A
3.	E		28.	C
4.	D		29.	A
5.	D		30.	D
6.	B		31.	B
7.	B		32.	E
8.	B		33.	B
9.	C		34.	D
10.	E		35.	B
11.	D		36.	B
12.	E		37.	D
13.	C		38.	D
14.	C		39.	C
15.	D		40.	C
16.	C		41.	E
17.	E		42.	C
18.	D		43.	C
19.	C		44.	C
20.	B		45.	E
21.	B		46.	C
22.	D		47.	B
23.	C		48.	B
24.	B		49.	E
25.	C		50.	C

KAPLAN) MEDICAL

1. **The correct answer is E.** This clinical vignette illustrates an individual with a primary psychotic disorder, probably schizophrenia. Risperidone, an atypical antipsychotic, would treat symptoms of paranoid delusions and auditory hallucinations.

   Benztropine (**choice A**) is an anticholinergic medication that is generally used with the typical antipsychotics (such as haloperidol) for the prophylaxis of extrapyramidal symptoms. It has no antipsychotic properties.

   Diazepam (**choice B**) is a long-acting benzodiazepine that would be appropriate in the management of an anxiety disorder. Shorter-acting benzodiazepines, such as lorazepam, are often used adjunctively in psychotic individuals for acute agitation.

   Fluoxetine (**choice C**) is a selective serotonin reuptake inhibitor (SSRI) used in depressive illnesses.

   Lithium (**choice D**) is used in bipolar disorder. Although individuals with bipolar disorder may have delusions, they are usually of a grandiose quality. In such individuals, antipsychotic medications like risperidone are often given as well, because lithium takes approximately 10 days to have a beneficial effect. This patient has profound paranoid delusions, suggestive of schizophrenia.

2. **The correct answer is E.** Pick disease is one in the spectrum of frontotemporal dementias. Unlike most other dementias, which present initially with cognitive changes, Pick disease presents insidiously with behavioral changes related to atrophy in frontotemporal regions. The cause is unknown. It is more common in men, especially those with an affected first-degree relative. In the early stages, it is more often characterized by personality and behavioral changes, such as disinhibition, impulsivity, repetitive behaviors, hypersexuality, and hyperorality. Treatment relies on behavior management.

   Alzheimer disease (**choice A**) is a progressive dementia with associated risk factors that include age, positive family history, head trauma, and Down syndrome. Typical first symptoms are a subtle loss of short-term memory, language difficulties, and apraxias, followed by impaired judgment and personality changes. Psychiatric symptoms are often prominent in the course of the illness. Treatment targets specific symptoms and includes psychosocial interventions and pharmacologic therapy.

   Dementia pugilistica (**choice B**) is a posttraumatic dementia that develops after blunt head trauma. It often occurs as a result of motor vehicle accident injuries and sports related traumas. The clinical symptoms are dependent on the areas affected most (cortical versus subcortical). After a period of amnesia and recovery, the most common symptoms are decreased attention, slowed information processing, increased distractibility, and problems with memory. Behavioral changes include impulsivity, depression, aggression, and personality changes. Treatment is targeted at controlling the symptoms.

   Multi-infarct dementia (**choice C**), or vascular dementia, accounts for 20% of the cases of dementia. Typical features include progression of cognitive deficits and associated motor or sensory neurologic deficits. Risk factors are associated with vascular disease, vasculitis, or embolic disease. Treatment is focused on addressing risk factors.

   Neurosyphilis (**choice D**) is a dementia of infectious origin, which is potentially reversible if diagnosed and treated early. It appears 10-15 years after the primary infection. It generally affects the frontal lobes, resulting in personality changes, poor judgment, irritability, and decreased care for oneself. Delusions of grandeur are seen in 10% to 20% of affected patients. The disease progresses into dementia with neurologic symptoms, such as tremor, Argyll-Robertson pupils, dysarthria, and hyperreflexia. Cerebrospinal fluid tests confirm the diagnosis. Treatment targets the infection and includes administration of IV penicillin G.

3. **The correct answer is E.** Metoclopramide is used as a gastric motility agent, often in patients with diabetes who have gastric paresis. It has antidopaminergic properties and can cause acute dystonic reactions such as are occurring in this patient. A dystonia is a spontaneous contraction of individual muscles. Treatment includes cessation of the metoclopramide and providing an anticholinergic agent, such as benztropine, or an antihistamine, such as diphenhydramine, both of which are usually given in IM or IV form for immediate effect.

   Aspirin (**choice A**) is an analgesic, antipyretic, anti-inflammatory, and antiplatelet agent. It is widely used and does not cause acute dystonic reactions.

   Digoxin (**choice B**) is a cardiac medication, specifically a steroid glycoside, used in the treatment of certain heart diseases, especially congestive heart failure. It does not cause acute dystonic reactions.

   Erythromycin (**choice C**) is a macrolide antibiotic and does not cause acute dystonic reactions.

   Fluoxetine (**choice D**) is an antidepressant medication. It is a selective serotonin reuptake inhibitor and has not generally been associated with acute dystonic reactions.

4. **The correct answer is D.** The patient is experiencing symptoms of acute posttraumatic stress disorder. The event is persistently reexperienced in flashbacks, nightmares, increased arousal, and avoidance of stimuli associated with the trauma. The symptoms are of less than 3 months' duration for the acute course, and the

disturbances cause significant social or occupational impairment.

Confusion and disorientation (**choice A**) are symptoms usually seen in cognitive disorders (delirium, dementia) but can also be seen as a part of psychotic disorders.

Depression and suicidal thoughts (**choice B**) are symptoms seen in various mood disorders and in the depression associated with psychosis. They can also be associated with anxiety disorders and substance-induced mood disorders.

Euphoria and racing thoughts (**choice C**) are usually symptoms of bipolar disorder (manic or mixed type) or schizoaffective disorder. These symptoms can also be seen with substance abuse.

Hyperphagia and hypersomnia (**choice E**) are symptoms of major depressive disorder with typical features along with sensitivity to rejection and a heavy leaden feeling in limbs. They can also be symptoms of several medical conditions.

5. **The correct answer is D.** This patient is malingering. He appears to be intentionally producing symptoms of arm pain in an attempt to gain admission to the hospital. His pattern has been such that his behavior is motivated by the external incentive of avoiding his legal responsibilities. His urine toxicology screen was negative, thereby making it less likely that he was experiencing a substance-induced mood disorder. Further, there is a clear discrepancy between the patient's complaint of arm pain and the objective physical examination and radiologic findings. This is characteristic of malingering.

Conversion disorder (**choice A**) differs from malingering in that the symptom is not intentionally produced and there is no obvious external incentive. In conversion disorder, one's voluntary motor or sensory function is affected, and the symptom suggests a neurologic or other general medical condition. Further, unlike malingering, relief of symptoms can be obtained by suggestion.

Dissociative identity disorder (**choice B**) involves the presence of two or more distinct, recurrent identities or personality states and the condition of being unable to recall extensive and meaningful personal information. This patient does not show features of this.

Factitious disorder (**choice C**) does involve the intentional production of symptoms, but the motivation is to assume the sick role and not to gain external incentive.

Rheumatoid arthritis (**choice E**) is a chronic, systemic inflammatory disease affecting synovial membranes of multiple joints. It causes inflammation and characteristic symmetric joint swelling, with associated stiffness, warmth, tenderness, and pain. Although any joint may be affected, the proximal interphalangeal and metacarpo-

phalangeal joints of the fingers are most often involved. Of all the laboratory tests, x-ray changes are the most specific. The earliest changes occur in the wrists or feet and demonstrate soft tissue swelling and juxta-articular demineralization. Later changes include uniform joint space narrowing and erosions.

6. **The correct answer is B.** This patient has schizophreniform disorder. Except for its duration of symptoms, schizophreniform disorder is similar to schizophrenia in diagnostic criteria. Whereas the symptoms must be present for at least 6 months to establish a diagnosis of schizophrenia, an episode of schizophreniform disorder lasts at least 1 month but less than 6 months. Also, social and occupational dysfunction is not required to meet the diagnosis, although it may occur during some point in the illness. In its typical presentation, schizophreniform disorder is a rapid-onset psychotic disorder without a significant prodrome. It is estimated that 60% to 80% of persons diagnosed with schizophreniform disorder are later diagnosed with schizophrenia. Schizophreniform disorder can be differentiated from brief psychotic disorder by the latter's duration of more than 1 day but less than 1 month.

The average age of onset (**choice A**) for persons with schizophreniform disorder is the same as that for persons with schizophrenia. Typically, both begin in the mid-teens to the twenties.

One cannot simultaneously have a mood disorder (**choice C**) in the context of schizophreniform disorder. Only in schizoaffective disorder are symptoms that meet criteria for a mood disorder present. In schizoaffective disorder, the affective symptoms are present for much of the duration of the illness.

The symptoms of schizophreniform disorder and schizophrenia may be of equal and indistinguishable severity (**choice D**).

The frequency, character, and description of auditory hallucinations (**choice E**) may be identical in schizophreniform disorder and schizophrenia. There are no reports of differences in the types of auditory hallucinations and features of commands, multiple voices, unfamiliar voices, and voices talking to one another.

7. **The correct answer is B.** Antidepressant-induced sexual dysfunction is a common condition and can be a major obstacle to long-term therapy for major depression. The most common antidepressant medications associated with sexual dysfunction include selective serotonin reuptake inhibitors (SSRIs), tricyclic antidepressants, and monoamine oxidase inhibitors (MAOIs). Bupropion, a reuptake inhibitor of norepinephrine and dopamine, is an appropriate alternative to the major classes of

antidepressants because it has a low-to-zero risk for sexual dysfunction. Mirtazapine and nefazodone are also appropriate alternative antidepressants indicated for this purpose.

Substitution of sertraline with a drug in the tricyclic antidepressant family, such as amitriptyline (**choice A**), is unlikely to alleviate the symptoms due to a similarly high risk for sexual side effects.

Substitution of sertraline with another drug in the SSRI class, such as fluoxetine (**choice C**) or paroxetine (**choice D**), is unlikely to change the symptoms of sexual dysfunction in this patient.

Sildenafil (**choice E**) is used for erectile dysfunction and may help reverse sexual dysfunction from antidepressant use in both men and women. However, it does not heighten sexual interest, the major complaint in his patient. Additionally, substitution with this drug neglects the patient's ongoing need for antidepressant therapy.

8. **The correct answer is B.** This patient is clearly psychotic and shows evidence of a formal thought disorder. Her acute presentation in the crisis center demonstrates the agitation that often accompanies acute psychosis. Often, after calming a patient down with medication and perhaps allowing her to sleep for a short while, the patient is much more calm, cooperative, and redirectable. This not only enables the psychiatric intern to have an easier time with the interview, diagnosis, and immediate treatment planning, but also provides the most safety for the patient. Haloperidol is a typical high-potency antipsychotic: it has a quick onset of action, is reliably administered in all of its forms (i.e., PO, IM, and IV), and can temper the agitation of acute psychosis. It is not unusual for haloperidol to be given in conjunction with IM lorazepam in severe acute agitation.

Clozapine (**choice A**) is not used in acutely agitated patients, and is associated with more frequent seizures unless the initial daily dose is minimal. This antipsychotic is very effective in patients who have treatment-resistant psychotic disorders, most often schizophrenia. It has been used to treat aggression in some patients with a broad variety of neuropsychiatric disorders, including traumatic brain injury and mental retardation, but is not used in acute, agitated psychosis as in this scenario.

Lithium (**choice C**), an antimanic medication, is the most widely used treatment for the bipolar disorders. It has proved useful in the treatment of acute episodes of mania and depression and, perhaps most significantly, in the long-term prophylaxis of the bipolar disorders. It is not effective acutely.

Quetiapine (**choice D**) is not used in acute psychosis because of its delayed onset of action compared with haloperidol. This is mostly because quetiapine is not available in an IM formulation.

Perphenazine (**choice E**) is a medium-potency, typical antipsychotic that is not used in the acute treatment of agitated psychosis. Like olanzapine, it is not available in IM form. Likewise, it is effective in first-episode and chronic schizophrenia. However, because of several undesirable side effects, it is not currently considered a first-line drug in the treatment of schizophrenia, including acutely agitated psychotic patients.

9. **The correct answer is C.** Neuroleptic malignant syndrome is a life-threatening adverse reaction to antipsychotic medications. It typically develops early in the course of treatment, although it can occur at any point, including after prolonged treatment. It is believed to be caused by impairment of CNS dopamine systems, either from dopamine receptor blockade or following treatment with a presynaptic dopamine depleting-agent like tetrabenazine. In addition to fever, muscle rigidity, and mental status changes, patients may develop autonomic instability, tremor, or dystonia. The most common laboratory abnormality is an elevated creatine kinase. Treatment involves discontinuation of the drug and supportive care, usually in an intensive care unit. Dopamine agonists, such as bromocriptine, are often given in conjunction with dantrolene, which acts as a muscle relaxant. Mortality can be as high as 25% without specific treatment. Symptoms resolve within 10 days.

Catatonia (**choice A**) is characterized by mutism and stupor, and may be present in patients with schizophrenia or other psychotic disorders. It may also include bizarre motor behavior, such as sustained postures and stereotypies. Catatonia may respond acutely to treatment with benzodiazepines or electroconvulsive therapy.

Malignant hyperthermia (**choice B**) follows administration of general anesthetic agents, not neuroleptics. It is believed to be caused by excessive release of calcium by the sarcoplasmic reticulum, resulting in severe, sustained muscle contraction. Dantrolene is also used to treat this disorder.

Serotonin syndrome (**choice D**) is a potentially lethal reaction due to excess serotonin activity associated with combined use of a selective serotonin reuptake inhibitor (SSRI) and an MAO inhibitor or overdosage with an SSRI. It shares certain features of the neuroleptic malignant syndrome, including confusion and diaphoresis. Patients may also be hypertensive and tachycardic.

Tardive dyskinesia (**choice E**) presents as a movement disorder developing many months to years after chronic antipsychotic use. It would not develop acutely and would not have any effect on temperature or mental status. Involuntary movements classically involve the oro-buccal-lingual musculature in this condition.

10. **The correct answer is E.** The most likely diagnosis is bipolar disorder, most recent episode depressed. The patient's recent symptoms suggest that she previously had an episode of mania, and this is supported by her description of disinhibition when started on a traditional selective serotonin reuptake inhibitor (SSRI) as a teen-ager—an event that is sometimes reported when patients with bipolar disorder are started on these agents. Lithium carbonate is more effective in treating bipolar disorder than is an SSRI, particularly in dealing with the cycles of depression and mania. Her hypersomnia and atypical symptoms of depression, combined with her gender, younger age of onset, and history of a manic episode, point to the depression of bipolar disorder rather than major depressive disorder. Therefore, lithium would be the most effective treatment.

Alprazolam (**choice A**) is a short-acting benzodiazepine, which is not used to treat depression.

Amitriptyline (**choice B**) is a tricyclic antidepressant, which would not treat the mood instability that the patient describes previously having.

Bupropion (**choice C**) is a dopamine-norepinephrine reuptake inhibitor used to treat major depressive disorder, not as a single agent in the depression of bipolar disorder.

Fluoxetine (**choice D**) is an SSRI similar to paroxetine used to treat depression, and would not be appropriate as a single agent in this case to treat a patient with a history of mania.

11. **The correct answer is D.** This boy likely has autistic disorder, which affects 3-5 per 10,000 persons. The male to female ratio is 3:1. This boy demonstrates a qualitative impairment in social interaction as manifested by nonverbal behaviors, such as poor eye contact and lack of desire to be touched. He has failed to develop peer relationships appropriate to his developmental level and does not seek enjoyment or shared pleasure with any-one. He lacks emotional reciprocity to his parents, has a marked delay in the development of spoken language, and demonstrates a stereotyped and repetitive manner-ism. These are all attributes of autism. Also, since the boy's behavior was described as chronic, his impairments cannot be better accounted for by childhood disintegra-tive disorder. Children with autistic disorder do not know how to regulate social interaction. They often are not interested in others, cannot accurately interpret the facial expressions and body postures of others, and do not understand social reciprocity.

Difficulty in attention (**choice A**) is not prototypical for children with autistic disorder. Their attention span is

variable and more often is affected by intelligence level rather than the autistic disorder itself.

Inability to concentrate (**choice B**) is also not a charac-teristic marker of children with autistic disorder. Such children are often preoccupied with aspects of their inner world and with one or more stereotyped and restricted patterns of interest. This is often abnormal either in intensity or in focus. They may concentrate more on one area of focus than another, but this is common for normal children as well and is not viewed as a diagnostic component of autistic disorder.

Intelligence (**choice C**) is variable in autistic disorder. Children can be high or low functioning depending on several variables, including intelligence, ability to com-municate, and severity of repetitive behaviors, as well as other symptoms. Seventy percent of affected children have IQs measured below 70, and 50% have IQs below 50. Autistic disorder is considered to have an organic basis with no specific site of organic damage. The autis-tic character portrayed by Dustin Hoffman in the movie "Rainman," an idiot savant with talents at the genius level, is very rare.

Urinary incontinence (**choice E**) is no more prevalent in children with autistic disorder than in normal children.

12. **The correct answer is E.** In obsessive-compulsive dis-order (OCD), patients may either experience intrusive thoughts (obsessions) or perform ritualized activities (compulsions), or do both. Obsessions with cleanliness and orderliness, as illustrated by the patient's showering ritual, are common in OCD. Obsessions and compul-sions (such as clock checking) can be so severe that they impact on functions of daily living.

Although OCD and attention deficit/hyperactivity dis-order (ADHD; **choice A**) may coexist, this vignette does not demonstrate ADHD, which is characterized by an inability to maintain focus, easy distractibility, and dif-ficulty with behavioral control.

Bipolar disorder (**choice B**) is a mood disorder charac-terized by sustained extremes of mood states (depres-sion and mania). Obsessions and compulsions are not features of bipolar disorder.

Although OCD is categorized as an anxiety disorder, it is distinct from generalized anxiety disorder (**choice C**), which is characterized by excessive worry about several different events and activities. These patients may worry about things that elicit anxiety, but they do not experi-ence obsessions or perform compulsions.

Patients with major depressive disorder (**choice D**) have either depressed mood or anhedonia (loss of inter-est) and a constellation of other symptoms, including change in appetite, disturbance in sleep, loss of energy,

KAPLAN) MEDICAL

and decreased concentration. Many patients with OCD develop major depressive disorder, and pharmacotherapy is the same in most cases; however, the case illustrated above is not consistent with major depression.

13. **The correct answer is C.** This patient is delirious. Delirium is a transient disorder of brain function that results in global cognitive impairment and other behavioral phenomena. It is a common disorder, with its main features being impairment of consciousness, attentional deficit, and a fluctuating course. An estimated 10% to 15% of general medical inpatients are delirious at any given time, and studies show that as many as 30% to 50% of acutely ill geriatric patients become delirious at some point during their hospital stay. Risk factors for delirium include new or worsened medical illness, older age, and baseline cognitive impairments, usually secondary to dementia. The syndrome of delirium is almost always due to an identifiable cause, such as systemic or cerebral disease or drug intoxication or withdrawal.

Adjustment disorder (**choice A**) is characterized by the development of emotional or behavioral symptoms, often related to anxiety or depression, in the context of a psychosocial stressor. The symptoms resolve when the stressor ends, or when the patient learns to adapt to them better. Symptoms of severe confusion, as were present in this patient, are unusual in adjustment disorders, as is the sudden resolution of symptoms despite the continuing stressor.

Cyclothymia (**choice B**) is a disorder characterized by symptoms that have occurred for at least 2 years. This patient has been suffering for only 3 days. In cyclothymia, there are numerous periods of hypomanic, but not manic, symptoms and of depressive symptoms that do not meet criteria for a major depressive episode. By definition, the person has not been symptom-free for more than 2 months at a time.

Dementia (**choice D**) is characterized by the development of multiple cognitive deficits manifested by memory impairment, and by one or more of the following features: aphasia (language disturbance), apraxia (impairment in carrying out motor activities), agnosia (failure to recognize or identify objects), or disturbance in executive functioning. The onset is usually gradual and cannot occur exclusively during the course of a delirium. As stated above, a person with dementia is more susceptible to delirium.

The characteristic feature of malingering (**choice E**) is the intentional production of false or markedly exaggerated physical or psychological symptoms as motivated by external incentives. This woman is unlikely to be producing her symptoms intentionally, and there is no obvious external incentive to do so.

14. **The correct answer is C.** The patient describes classic symptoms of posttraumatic stress disorder (PTSD), which is relatively common in patients who have combat exposure. In addition to having witnessed a traumatic event, patients also complain of flashbacks, nightmares, persistent avoidance of stimuli associated with the trauma, and symptoms of increased arousal/anxiety.

Acute stress disorder (**choice A**) is similar to PTSD; however, symptoms are resolved within 4 weeks of the associated event.

In generalized anxiety disorder (**choice B**), there is excessive worry about a number of things and there often are somatic manifestations of the anxiety, such as irritability and restlessness. Nightmares, flashbacks, and an identifiable traumatic event are not prominent features.

Schizoid personality disorder (**choice D**) is characterized by a pervasive detachment from social relationships. There often is an indifference on the patient's part with regard to establishing relationships with others. The patient described above is obviously distressed that he can no longer seem to form a connection with others.

Patients with sleep terrors (**choice E**) often do not report nightmares. They have the sensation of fear and autonomic hyperactivity on sudden awakening, and there is unresponsiveness to efforts of others to comfort them during the episode.

15. **The correct answer is D.** Flight of ideas is non-goal-directed speech that reflects a rapid jumping of thoughts through a series of weakly related ideas. "I started driving but was thinking about my history. History books are great. I once wrote a paper on Alexander the Great. I do well in college," demonstrates this process. The sentences are abruptly and tenuously connected. The "great" in "history books" is the topic for the reference to "Alexander the Great," which was the subject of a paper. The paper was likely an assignment written in college, which led to the reference to "do[ing] well in college." The patient did not answer the question she was asked.

"I drove here myself" (**choice A**) is a goal-directed, linear statement.

"I was reading a great book at home and, after I finished it, I drove here myself" (**choice B**) is an example of circumstantiality. The answer is overly detailed, but the question is ultimately answered. The mention of the book is vaguely related to the patient's driving herself to the emergency department.

"I really like history books and I was reading one at home today while eating tuna fish" (**choice C**) is an example of tangentiality. The question is not answered; however, proper words and grammar are used, and ideas flow from a train of thought.

"The spy in the book I was reading is real, and he was watching me through the pages. He knew who I was" (**choice E**) is an example of looseness of association. There is a disintegration of a meaningful connection of ideas. In addition, this statement describes paranoia and a delusion of reference and likely also of persecution.

16. **The correct answer is C.** This patient is likely beginning to exhibit alcohol withdrawal. Even without full-blown delirium tremens (DTs), alcohol withdrawal can be serious and should be treated. Tremulousness usually develops 6-8 hours after the cessation of drinking. Perceptual symptoms often begin after 8-12 hours, seizures in 12-24 hours, and DTs after 72 hours. Benzodiazepines are the primary medications for the control of alcohol withdrawal symptoms. Benzodiazepines, such as lorazepam, help with anxiety, shakiness, tachycardia, hypertension, diaphoresis, seizure activity, and delirium. In this situation, lorazepam has advantages over other benzodiazepines in that it can be administered in PO, IM, and IV forms and is not hepatotoxic.

Haloperidol (**choice A**) will help with some perceptual disturbances of alcohol withdrawal, and may cause a calming effect on agitated behavior, but it will not address the sympathetic hyperactivity, seizures, or alcohol-withdrawal delirium.

Lithium (**choice B**) is an antimanic agent used in bipolar disorders and will not treat alcohol withdrawal symptoms.

Propranolol (**choice D**) helps block the symptoms of sympathetic hyperactivity; it is not an effective drug for seizures or delirium.

No medication (**choice E**) is incorrect because alcohol withdrawal, especially DTs, is a medical emergency that can result in significant morbidity and mortality. Even with treatment, DTs have a mortality rate of approximately 15%. Although this patient is not described as having DTs, treatment with lorazepam will help prevent them from occurring.

17. **The correct answer is E.** This patient meets the DSM-IV criteria for borderline personality disorder. She has a pervasive pattern of unstable interpersonal relationships, poor self-image, and lack of control of her affect. Her behavior is marked by impulsivity. She feels sad during weekends when she is alone and imagines herself as being abandoned. Her unstable relationships are characterized by alternating between extremes of idealization ("the man of her dreams") and devaluation. She appears to have a very poor sense of self, with an inability to find a suitable partner and job. She is impulsive in substance abuse and sexual activity, both of which are potentially self-damaging, and she shows lability of affect because

of a marked reactivity of mood. The question did not indicate whether this person is suicidal, although she quite possibly would be; some of the described behaviors of hurting herself may include suicide gestures. One of the most characteristic defense mechanism associated with borderline personality disorder is splitting, which means that the person psychologically separates positive attributes into one individual and negative attributes into another. Splitting occurs because the person is not able to tolerate her ambivalent feelings toward another individual. Usually, the person is unconscious of her ambivalence toward another and does not realize the extremes of her reaction.

Displacement (**choice A**) occurs when the feelings associated with a psychologically unacceptable object, idea, or situation are transferred to another object, idea, or situation. The latter one is often symbolically related to the former. For instance, a woman who is raped by her husband may become angry at the prosecutor who is handling the case because he was 10 minutes late for a meeting.

Idealization (**choice B**) occurs when a person unrealistically attributes strictly positive characteristics to another person or situation. In the above example, the person with borderline personality disorder repeatedly believed that she had met the "man of her dreams"; however, this idealization was only shortly lived and was quickly replaced with devaluation.

Intellectualization (**choice C**) is the transformation of emotionally disturbing events into cognitive challenges that do not recognize the emotional stress. For example, a person who has been rejected for a job she wanted very much says that this is simply a problem of getting her resume into a better format.

Reaction formation (**choice D**) occurs when an unacceptable feeling or thought is transformed into its opposite. This often occurs when hate is transformed into love or fear is transformed into empowerment. For instance, a battered woman who has managed to leave her abusive home situation may become involved in work with her local battered women's shelter.

18. **The correct answer is D.** Priapism is persistent penile erection accompanied by severe pain. It can occur with antidepressants or antipsychotics, but it is most frequently seen with trazodone use (1 in 1,000 men). It is medical emergency that requires evaluation by a urologist.

Chlordiazepoxide (**choice A**) belongs to the group of long-acting benzodiazepines and is usually used for detoxification from sedative hypnotics because of its long half-life. It is not used for the treatment of insomnia. Side effects include sedation, amnesia, psychomotor retarda-

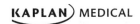

tion, decreased respiratory response to carbon dioxide, and a potential withdrawal syndrome.

Hydroxyzine (**choice B**) is a piperazine derivative that exerts antihistaminic, anticholinergic, mild sedative, and bronchodilator effects. It is used as premedication in anesthesia and in management of pruritic syndromes. It exerts a mild antianxiety effect. It is not used as a hypnotic. Its side effects include drowsiness and dry mouth.

Mirtazapine (**choice C**) is a novel antidepressant. It has sedative properties related to its antihistaminic activity; in lower doses, it can be used for treatment of insomnia. It is mainly indicated for treatment of depression. Side effects include dizziness, weight gain, and increases in serum lipids and transaminases.

Zolpidem (**choice E**) is a nonbenzodiazepine hypnotic used for short-term treatment of insomnia. Its most common side effects include headache, dizziness, drowsiness, gastrointestinal symptoms, generalized pain, and myalgias.

19. **The correct answer is C.** Approximately 30% of patients taking the usual maintenance dose of olanzapine experience sedation, making it the most common side effect of the choices listed. The reason that the medication is given at bedtime is to reduce adverse effects of sedation as much as possible. Other much less common side effects of olanzapine include prolactinemia, dizziness, and akathisia.

Gastrointestinal complications (**choice A**), particularly constipation, are known to be associated with olanzapine use, but are not as common as sedation.

Orthostatic hypotension (**choice B**) is also a complication of olanzapine use. Patients who take olanzapine should be cautious when rising in the morning or nighttime hours, or when rising from a sitting position, so that they do not lose consciousness or become unsteady. However, orthostatic hypotension is less common than sedation with olanzapine.

Tardive dyskinesia (**choice D**), a syndrome of abnormal involuntary movements associated with neuroleptic use, has not yet been reported in patients taking olanzapine.

Weight gain (**choice E**) is a recognized complication of olanzapine use but is not as common as sedation.

20. **The correct answer is B.** Major depression with atypical features is characterized by mood reactivity, in which the patient's mood brightens in response to actual or potentially positive events, and two or more of the following features: leaden paralysis, significant weight gain or increase in appetite, hypersomnia, or a long-standing pattern of interpersonal rejection sensitivity that results in significant social or occupational impairment. This type of depression differs from other types in that its characteristic psychomotor disturbances are opposite those of others. In other depressions, there is a lack of reactivity to usually pleasurable stimuli. Affected patients do not feel much better, even temporarily, when something good happens. Likewise, in other types of depression, there is usually anorexia and weight loss, and early morning awakening commonly marks the sleep pattern. Further, there typically are no complaints of either a heavy feeling in one's arms or legs or a sensitivity-based concern of rejection. Atypical depression responds especially well to MAOIs.

Conversion disorder (**choice A**) is a disturbance of bodily functioning that does not conform to the current concepts of the anatomy and physiology of the central or peripheral nervous systems. It is characterized by one or more symptoms affecting voluntary motor or sensory function that suggest a neurologic or medical condition but cannot be explained by one. It typically occurs in a setting of stress and tends to transform the psychic energy of the turmoil of acute conflict into a personally meaningful metaphor of bodily dysfunction. The symptom is not intentionally produced, as in a factitious disorder or malingering.

Schizophrenia, catatonic type (**choice C**), is marked by at least two of the following features: immobility suggestive of either catalepsy or stupor, excessive and apparently purposeless motor activity, extreme negativism, peculiar voluntary movement such as posturing, stereotypy, mannerisms, grimacing, echolalia, or echopraxia. There are no common somatic complaints, and leaden paralysis is not typical of this disorder.

Schizotypal personality disorder (**choice D**) is in the cluster A category of personality disorders. It is marked by a pervasive pattern of social and interpersonal deficits characterized by acute discomfort with, and reduced capacity for, close relationships. There also are cognitive or perceptual distortions and eccentricities of behavior that begin by early adulthood. Furthermore, there must be five of the following features: ideas of reference, odd beliefs that influence behavior, unusual perceptual experiences, odd thinking and speech, suspiciousness, inappropriate affect, eccentric behavior, and lack of close friends. As in schizophrenia, there are no common somatic complaints, and leaden paralysis is not typical of this disorder.

Somatoform disorder (**choice E**) is not a disorder in and of itself. There are five specific somatoform disorders: somatization disorder, conversion disorder, pain disorder, hypochondriasis, and body dysmorphic disorder.

21. **The correct answer is B.** There are three allelic forms of this gene, *e2*, *e3*, and *e4*. Clinical studies have shown that the allele *e4* of *apolipoprotein E* (Apo E) increases the

risk for late-onset Alzheimer disease (AD), especially in homozygous individuals. However, its use as a screening tool to identify individuals who have an increased risk of developing AD is highly controversial, mainly because there are no known effective methods to prevent AD or cure it once it manifests. The clinical usefulness of a screening test for early detection of diseases or predisposing factors is based on a number of criteria, including the following: the disease must be sufficiently serious, prevalent, treatable, or preventable, and the test should be sufficiently accurate (i.e., sensitive and specific). Furthermore, a presymptomatic stage should precede the onset of the disease to allow preclinical or early detection.

AD has a long preclinical stage (compare with **choice A**) before its earliest manifestations.

The prevalence of AD is very high (compare with **choice C**). Approximately 6% of persons older than 65 have varying degrees of AD.

AD is a severe form of dementing disorder and ultimately leads to death within an average of 7-10 years following clinical onset (compare with **choice D**).

Testing for Apo E phenotype is both sensitive (compare with **choice F**) and specific (compare with **choice E**).

22. **The correct answer is D.** The most common comorbid disorders found in both clinical and epidemiologic samples of children with attention-deficit hyperactivity disorder (ADHD) are oppositional defiant disorder (ODD) and conduct disorder (CD). Typically these children display argumentative behavior and attitudes, temper tantrums, defiance of authority and rules, and aggressive, antisocial behavior in addition to the symptoms of ADHD. The rate of concurrent ADHD and ODD is 35%; the combination of concurrent ODD or CD and ADHD is 50% to 60%. Interestingly, school-aged children with ODD or CD almost invariably meet criteria for ADHD; yet, it is more common for adolescents with ODD or CD to not have a concurrent diagnosis of ADHD. Other influences that seem to correlate ODD and CD with ADHD include greater symptom severity, reading disorder, lower socioeconomic status, and parental alcoholism. Short-acting psychostimulants are the first-line treatment for the pharmacotherapy of ADHD, mostly because of their ability to improve both behavioral and cognitive problems in 70% to 80% of affected children. However, behavioral improvements do not always lead to complete remission of symptoms. There often is significant residual ADHD symptomatology, as well as peer and academic problems, even after treatment.

Asperger disorder (**choice A**) is a pervasive developmental disorder characterized by qualitative impairment in social interaction, restricted and repetitive stereotyped patterns of behavior, and no clinically significant lan-

guage or cognitive delay. Persons with this disorder do not have difficulty in the development of age-appropriate self-help skills or adaptive behavior that children with ADHD often have. Rather, children with Asperger disorder often do not play with others and are seen more as aloof, introverted, and bizarre in comparison to the disruptive and extroverted behavior of children with ADHD.

Autistic disorder (**choice B**), like Asperger disorder, is a pervasive developmental disorder. It causes impairment in social interaction, often with the use of multiple nonverbal behaviors, failure to develop peer relationships, and lack of social or emotional reciprocity. There is a problem in communication, often with delay or total lack in the development of spoken language and stereotyped behavior that may encompass an inflexible adherence to a preoccupation with a specific, nonfunctional routine. Autistic persons often have low IQs and cannot tolerate standard classroom environments. They do not present similarly to children with ADHD.

Anxiety disorder (**choice C**) is incorrect. Nonetheless, significant comorbidity exists with ADHD and anxiety disorders. The average comorbidity is 25%. With the early onset of ADHD, most diagnoses of anxiety disorders are made after the emergence of ADHD. This suggests that some instances of ADHD-anxiety disorder comorbidity are possibly secondary to the experience of enduring the chronic disorder of ADHD itself. Some differences in patterns of performance on cognitive tasks and reduced cognitive improvement with stimulants distinguish children with ADHD plus anxiety and those without anxiety.

Schizophrenia, undifferentiated type (**choice E**) is incorrect. There is no known correlation between ADHD and schizophrenia of any type.

23. **The correct answer is C.** Narcolepsy is diagnosed by irresistible attacks of refreshing sleep that occur during the day over at least 3 months. It is characterized by the presence of cataplexy (brief episodes of sudden loss of muscle tone throughout the body mostly in association with intense emotion) or recurrent intrusions of REM sleep in transition between sleep and wakefulness, as manifested by hypnagogic or hypnopompic hallucinations. Narcolepsy occurs most frequently before the age of 30. Sleep paralysis, characterized by the inability to move in the presence of preserved consciousness, is another typical symptom on waking up.

Catalepsy (**choice A**) is a term for motoric immobility maintained voluntarily and is most commonly seen as a part of schizophrenic symptomatology.

Kleine-Levin syndrome (**choice B**) is a rare, self-limiting condition consisting of recurrent episodes of prolonged sleep lasting one to several weeks. It begins in childhood, and the wakeful periods are marked by social withdrawal, irritability, confusion, and frank psychotic symptoms, such as delusions or hallucinations.

Periodic paralysis (**choice D**) is a group of hereditary muscle disorders inherited in autosomal-dominant fashion; it develops in early childhood and adolescence. Attacks occur at rest following heavy exercise or meals rich in carbohydrates. During the attacks, patients are unable to move their limbs. Serum levels of potassium can be below, at, or above normal limits, depending on the type of disorder. Treatment is directed at controlling serum potassium and preventing attacks.

Primary hypersomnia (**choice E**) is a syndrome of excessive sleepiness for at least 1 month, as evidenced by prolonged sleep or daytime sleep episodes. It causes clinically significant impairment in social functioning. It does not occur secondary to the effects of substance abuse or a general medical condition and does not happen during the course of another sleep disorder.

24. **The correct answer is B.** Body dysmorphic disorder involves a preoccupation with an imagined defect in appearance, which causes clinically significant distress or impairment in social, occupational, or other important areas of functioning. The preoccupation is not better accounted for by another mental disorder, such as the dissatisfaction with body shape and size found in anorexia nervosa. The fact that this patient has had social difficulties because of her perception of her body shape points to body dysmorphic disorder as the most appropriate diagnosis.

Adjustment disorder with disturbance of emotion (**choice A**) requires both a recent stressor and some symptoms of depression, which this patient does not report.

The patient does not have evidence of borderline personality disorder (**choice C**), as she does not have an unstable self-image or sense of self, and she does not have any recurrent suicidal behavior or gestures required for this diagnosis.

Hypochondriasis (**choice D**) requires a preoccupation with fears of having a serious disease based on the person's misinterpretation of bodily symptoms. The belief is not restricted to a circumscribed concern about appearance (as in body dysmorphic disorder).

Somatoform disorder, not otherwise specified (**choice E**), includes false beliefs (e.g., that one is pregnant when actually not) or disorders that involve unexplained physical complaints (such as fatigue or body weakness) of less than 6 months' duration that are not due to another mental disorder.

25. **The correct answer is C.** A number of child psychiatrists have written about various theories of child development. Multiple models exist that concern the organization of cognition, attachment, learning, aggression, social skill development, and individuation. The child in this question is in a normal stage of development and is experiencing stranger anxiety. A fear of strangers is usually first noted in infants at about 26 weeks of age, but does not develop fully until about the age of 32 weeks, or 8 months. When a stranger approaches an 8-month-old infant, he will often cry and cling to his mother. Infants exposed to many caretakers, most often in an extended family or a daycare setting, are less likely to have stranger anxiety than those infants exposed to only one caretaker. Stranger anxiety is believed to be a result of an infant's increasing ability to distinguish caretakers from all other persons. Separation anxiety, which usually occurs between 10 and 18 months of age, is related but not identical to stranger anxiety. Separation from the person to whom the infant is attached instigates separation anxiety, whereas stranger anxiety occurs even when the infants is in his mother's arms. In separation anxiety, an infant learns to crawl or walk away from his mother but often looks back at her to reassure himself that she is still there.

26. **The correct answer is B.** Divalproex, a preparation of valproic acid, is an anticonvulsant medication that has also been approved by the FDA for treatment of manic episodes. Its common side effects include nausea, sedation, weight gain, and transitory hair loss, as well as a transitory increase in liver function tests. Rare side effects include hepatitis and pancreatitis, as well as a possible decrease in platelets or platelet dysfunction.

Clonazepam (**choice A**) is a benzodiazepine that is used in place of or in conjunction with an antipsychotic to treat acute manic agitation. It is used for short-term treatment of anxiety, insomnia, or catatonia associated with mania or depression. It can also be used as adjunctive maintenance treatment along with mood stabilizers, but lacks specific antimanic, antidepressant, or mood stabilizing properties. Clonazepam is also used as an anticonvulsant. Side effects include drowsiness and ataxia.

Gabapentin (**choice C**) is a new antiseizure medication that has been approved as adjunctive therapy for treatment of refractory partial seizures. In some cases, it has been used as adjunctive medication for treatment of refractory bipolar disorder. Its mood stabilizing properties have not been confirmed. The most common side effects include somnolence, dizziness, and ataxia.

Lithium (**choice D**) is the treatment of choice for bipolar I disorder. It is less effective in mixed bipolar disorder. Symptoms of lithium toxicity include diarrhea, severe tremor, polyuria, ataxia, confusion, seizures, gastric distress, weight gain, tremor, fatigue, and cognitive deficits. Other side effects involve the kidneys, heart, thyroid gland, and skin.

Olanzapine (**choice E**) is an atypical antipsychotic that also has some mood stabilizing properties. It has also been used recently in the treatment of bipolar disorders. Its most common side effects include postural hypotension, constipation, weight gain, and dizziness. However, hair loss is not one of the side effects of this medication.

27. **The correct answer is A.** Classical conditioning is learning that takes place when two events occur closely together in time. According to this theory, learning occurs when an initially neutral stimulus, the conditioned stimulus, is paired with a stimulus that naturally elicits a response, the unconditioned stimulus (chemotherapy). In this example, the conditioned stimulus is the entrance into the waiting room. The response (nausea and vomiting) elicited by the unconditioned stimulus is called the unconditioned response. After repeated and contiguous pairing of the two stimuli (in this instance, eight pairings of the waiting room and nausea and vomiting), the conditioned stimulus elicits the unconditioned response, which then is called the conditioned response. The learning theory of classical conditioning has been influential in the conceptualization of certain clinical disorders, as well as in developing some treatment methods. It is particularly useful in understanding and treating phobic disorders, appreciating stress responses that were not part of one's initial trauma, and cueing exposure treatment for alcoholics and drug addicts.

Covert sensitization (**choice B**) is a method of reducing the frequency of behavior by associating it with the imagination of unpleasant consequences. This is a treatment method used in circumstances during which a patient wants to decrease the amount of an unwanted behavior. An example of this is a smoker who wishes to quit smoking and is trained to imagine herself lying on a hospital bed after being diagnosed with lung cancer, gasping for air and permanently attached to an oxygen tank in order to breathe.

Habituation (**choice C**) is a simple form of learning in which the response to a repeated stimulus lessens over time. An example of this is a psychotherapy patient who initially feels very anxious entering the door to her therapist's office and then, after several therapy sessions, feels less anxiety and is more comfortable at the door.

Learned helplessness (**choice D**) describes the cognitive experience of a person who perceives unpredictable and uncontrollable events as the basis for feeling helpless and powerless. Studies of rats who were put in mazes with no possible exit demonstrated this theory, showing that after

repeated efforts of unsuccessful escape, the rats gave up and no longer tried to escape.

Operant conditioning (**choice E**) is a form of learning in which behavioral frequency is altered through the application of positive and negative consequences. Learning is thought to occur as a consequence of one's actions. An example of this is placing a hungry cat in a cage with a latching device that, when accurately manipulated, allows the cat access to a separate cage with food. As the cat learns how to maneuver the device, effective behaviors are reinforced by the cat's experiences of successes and failures.

28. **The correct answer is C.** Erikson conceptualized eight stages of ego development across the life cycle. Each stage represents a point along a continuum of development in which physical, cognitive, instinctual, and sexual changes combine to create an internal crisis whose resolution results in either psychosocial regression or growth. The boy in this example is in Erikson's psychosocial stage of industry vs. inferiority. This stage occurs at approximately 5 to 13 years, during which time the child discovers the pleasures of productivity and the feelings of competency. He develops industry by learning new skills and taking pride in things made. If the child is not ready for this stage, either by lack of resolution of a previous stage or by a problem that he is experiencing, the child may develop a sense of inferiority and inadequacy.

Autonomy vs. shame and doubt (**choice A**) occurs from about age 18 months to 3 years. While the toddler is developing speech and sphincter control, he practices holding on and letting go and, according to Erikson, experiences the beginning of his will. At this stage, a toddler is learning to develop his own internal controls and is learning the consequences of his lack of self-control or judgment. He is learning to have self-certainty as opposed to self-consciousness and, if successful in this stage, will learn not to find shame in and doubt himself.

Identity vs. role confusion (**choice B**) occurs from about 13 to 21 years. During the phase of puberty and its associated physiologic and social changes, the adolescent becomes focused on the question of identity. The formation of cliques and the intolerance of individual differences are methods of dispelling a sense of identity loss. According to Erikson, during this psychosocial stage, a person's goal is to develop a more sharply focused identity and develop a sense of faithfulness to one's idea of self. Role confusion occurs when the adolescent is unable to attain a sense of self and belonging.

Initiative vs. guilt (**choice D**) occurs from about 3 to 5 years of age. In this stage, Erikson describes the child as increasing his mastery over locomotor and language skills, stimulating curiosities of the outside world. The child is naturally active and intrusive and, if successful at this stage, learns the basis for the subsequent development of realistic ambition and the purpose of virtue. If the child is unsuccessful, however, he has overwhelming guilt over the drive for conquest and anxiety over anticipated punishment.

Trust vs. mistrust (**choice E**) is the first of Erikson's stages, occurring from birth to approximately 18 months. The task of the infant is to trust his surroundings. This occurs most easily if there is a mother available who is able to anticipate and respond to her baby's needs in a consistent and timely manner. If the baby does not acquire a sense of trust and pleasantness in his world, he will feel hopeless and will tend to isolate himself and be distrustful of others.

29. **The correct answer is A.** The most likely disorder that might be responsible for this girl's behavior is kleptomania, an impulse-control disorder. Kleptomania is characterized by a recurrent impulse to steal objects that are not needed for personal use or monetary value. According to the DSM-IV, the stealing is not due to anger or revenge, is not associated with a delusion or hallucination, and is not due to conduct disorder, a manic episode, or antisocial personality disorder. Pathologic stealing is estimated to occur in 6 per 1,000 persons. Fewer than 5% of shoplifters actually have kleptomania. There seems to be a preponderance of female kleptomaniacs; however, these data may be skewed since, in general, women are more likely than men to present for psychiatric evaluation. Similarly, women are more likely to be referred for psychiatric evaluation by the courts, as opposed to men who are more often sent to jail. At first presentation, the average age for women is 35; for men, 50. A high rate of pathologic stealing occurs in bulimia nervosa, and, given that kleptomania is at least somewhat responsive to serotonergic agents, these conditions may actually have a common pathophysiologic connection. Delusional thinking is absent because among the criteria listed in the DSM-IV is that the person cannot be responding to a delusion or hallucination when stealing.

Persons with kleptomania experience displeasure at the thought of being caught in the act of the theft (compare with **choice B**). They do not want to get caught, as there is no associated thrill. The only pleasure felt is at the time of the actual stealing, and this is not related to the consequences of the act.

This girl is unable to resist impulses to steal (compare with **choice C**). She may know on some level that stealing is morally wrong, as well as illegal, but she cannot resist because her impulse to steal is overwhelmingly strong.

The quality of an increasing sense of tension immediately before the theft (compare with **choice D**) is a necessary criterion for the diagnosis of kleptomania.

Feeling pleasure at the time of committing the theft (compare with **choice E**) is a necessary criterion for the diagnosis of kleptomania.

30. **The correct answer is D.** Schizophrenia occurs in 1% of the population, equally affecting males and females. It is characterized by psychosis and disruption in one's ability to function socially. Presenting complaints may include auditory hallucinations, strange belief systems, paranoia, lack of motivation, decrease in self-care, and peculiar mannerisms. In schizophrenia, neuropathologic volumetric analyses suggest a loss of brain weight, specifically of gray matter. CT studies may show a compensatory enlargement of the lateral and third ventricles, thereby increasing the ventricle-to-brain ratio. The temporal lobes appear to lose the most volume when compared with those of persons without schizophrenia. The frontal lobes may likewise have abnormalities; however, these are not related to the volume of the lobes but rather to the level of activity detected by functional MRIs.

Atrophic changes in the cerebellar vermis (**choice A**) are not typical for CT scans of patients with schizophrenia. The cerebellum is responsible for the regulation and control of muscular tone, the coordination of movement, and the control of posture and gait. Specifically, the vermis is the narrow middle zone between the two hemispheres of the cerebellum; it is unrelated to any dysfunction related to schizophrenia.

Bilateral hypodensities in the orbitofrontal region (**choice B**) are not typically seen in schizophrenic patients. Damage to the orbitofrontal region of the brain usually results in impaired social judgment. One criterion for the diagnosis of schizophrenia is social/occupational dysfunction. Often this is characterized by a disturbance in interpersonal relations. This is not thought to be due to an error in social judgment; likewise, it is not due to abnormalities in the orbitofrontal region of the brain.

Hydrocephalus (**choice C**) is a condition marked by an excessive accumulation of fluid, which leads to dilation of the ventricles and elevated intracranial pressure. There are several types of hydrocephalus, including but not limited to communicating, noncommunicating, normal pressure, and congenital. This condition is not related to schizophrenia.

Significant sulcal widening (**choice E**) is often seen as a result of atrophic changes consistent with aging and the dementias. Mild sulcal widening may be seen in scans of patients with schizophrenia, but significant changes are not characteristic.

31. **The correct answer is B.** Frontal lobe dementia is characterized by damage to the frontal lobes and includes marked personality and behavioral changes as described in the question. The age of onset is most often between 50 and 60, and the condition is often progressive. Frontal lobe dementia is usually characterized by disproportionate impairment in tasks related to frontal lobe function, such as deficiency in abstract thinking, attentional shifting, or set formation. Disinhibition is also a key finding. CT or MRI reveals atrophy of the frontal lobe, especially early in the disease process. At present, the definitive diagnosis of any degenerative dementia is based on postmortem neuropathologic examination. Only one type of frontal lobe dementia, Pick disease, is associated with distinctive histopathologic abnormalities that allow for certain diagnosis. The patient's glabellar sign is one of several signs elicited in a neurologic exam of a patient with frontal lobe dysfunction.

The basal ganglia (**choice A**) consist of deep subcortical nuclei responsible for movement disorders. The basal ganglia are composed of the caudate nucleus, putamen, globus pallidus, subthalamic nucleus, and substantia nigra. Certain movement disorders that result from basal ganglia dysfunction include Parkinson disease and hemiballism. The basal ganglia are not involved in this woman's symptoms.

The hypothalamus (**choice C**) helps to maintain homeostasis through the secretion of hormones, central control of the autonomic nervous system, and the development of emotional and motivational states. The hypothalamus also interacts with limbic structures and the reticular formation for the maintenance of arousal.

Temporal lobe dysfunction (**choice D**) can occur in several ways; however, the resultant problems would be different. Temporal lobe seizures include simple partial seizures characterized by olfactory and gustatory hallucinations and complex partial seizures characterized by impairment of consciousness, repetitive psychomotor movements, and automatic behavior. Tumors in the temporal lobe may cause memory disturbances, superior quadrantanopsia, and, if the dominant temporal lobe is involved, aphasia. Disruption of the temporal lobe can involve limbic structures and tends to cause psychosis. Further, mania can be associated with temporal lobe lesions, especially on the right side.

Ventricular obstruction (**choice E**) results in hydrocephalus, which is an increase in the volume of cerebrospinal fluid within the skull. It can occur with or without an increase in pressure. Most commonly, there is an increase in pressure; this type of hydrocephalus can be divided into obstructive and communicating hydrocephalus. Many types of pathology can cause obstructive

hydrocephalus, including brain tumors, inflammatory processes, and developmental abnormalities. Increased intracranial pressure may not be present in normal pressure hydrocephalus, which can cause a reversible dementia, but the characteristics of this dementia are not congruent with this woman's symptoms.

32. **The correct answer is E.** The key to this case is that the patient's mood was "fine" until 1 week prior to presentation. Thereafter, her symptoms of mood lability and dysphoria with suicidal thoughts can be attributable to cocaine use and/or withdrawal. Once cocaine use stops, the mood symptoms generally improve within a few days, and suicidal ideation often resolves.

In bipolar disorder, manic (**choice A**), elevated or irritable mood states generally last for days on end, even in so-called rapid cyclers. It would be difficult to make the diagnosis of bipolar disorder in this patient because of the positive urine drug screen and the fact that all of her symptoms can be ascribed to cocaine use.

Dysthymic disorder (**choice B**) is characterized by the presence of depressive symptoms that do not meet the full criteria for major depression, with a duration of at least 2 years. Rapidly shifting extremes of mood and acute suicidal impulses are not characteristic.

Although individuals with histrionic personality disorder (**choice C**) have rapidly shifting expressions of emotion and may have chronic dysphoria, the key feature of this disorder is the need and constant quest for attention from others.

Major depressive disorder (**choice D**) requires at least a 2-week history of a constellation of depressive symptoms. This diagnosis cannot be reliably made when symptoms can be otherwise explained, such as in this case of drug use.

33. **The correct answer is B.** In displacement, feelings that are otherwise unacceptable or dangerous are transferred or redirected onto a more acceptable (and usually less threatening) substitute object. In this way, their open expression is still allowed.

Acting out (**choice A**) refers to a defense mechanism by which the individual deals with unacceptable emotional conflict by actions rather than by reflection or expression of feelings.

Projection (**choice C**) is a defense mechanism that allows the individual to deal with emotionally conflicting issues by falsely attributing his or her own unacceptable thoughts, feelings, or impulses to another person.

Reaction formation (**choice D**) is a way individuals deal with emotional conflict by substituting diametrically opposed thoughts or feelings with their own unacceptable ones.

KAPLAN) MEDICAL

Sublimation (**choice E**) is a defense mechanism in which an individual deals with emotional conflict by channeling potentially maladaptive impulses or feelings into socially acceptable behaviors.

34.   **The correct answer is D.** Panic disorder is characterized by recurrent unprovoked panic attacks that have occurred for at least a month and cause significant distress in areas of daily functioning. Such patients often describe symptoms not dissimilar to a myocardial infarction, which obviously must be ruled out. The first-line treatment for panic disorder is a selective serotonin reuptake inhibitor. Benzodiazepines can be used to abort an attack. Alprazolam and clonazepam are benzodiazepines that are used for long-term management when SSRIs are ineffective or contraindicated, but carry with them the disadvantages of withdrawal and dependency, so long-term use is not recommended.

Generalized anxiety disorder (**choice A**) is characterized by excessive worry about several events or activities. Panic attacks are not the sole distressing symptom.

An individual with histrionic personality disorder (**choice B**) shows a pervasive pattern of excessive emotionality and attention seeking. He may exhibit an exaggerated expression of emotion; however, anxiety *per se* is not a defining feature.

In hypochondriasis (**choice C**), there is the preoccupation with having a serious disease, but overt pathology is not evident. Although anxiety may be associated with this disorder, panic attacks typically are not.

People with somatization disorder (**choice E**) have various somatic complaints, which are chronic and do not occur in acute attacks.

35.   **The correct answer is B.** Neuroleptic-induced parkinsonism, which is clinically indistinguishable from Parkinson disease, occurs in the context of neuroleptic use. It is caused by decreased dopaminergic activity in the substantia nigra resulting from dopamine receptor antagonism. It will often appear in neuroleptic-naïve patients or in patients whose dose of neuroleptic has been increased, as in this case.

In benign essential tremor (**choice A**), the only clinical feature is tremor. Other symptoms of parkinsonism, such as sialorrhea (drooling), stiffness, shuffling gait, and bradykinesia, are not features.

Neuroleptic malignant syndrome (NMS; **choice C**) is characterized by rigidity, fever, altered mental status, and autonomic dysfunction. It is a rare complication of neuroleptic use. Other than rigidity, symptoms of parkinsonism are not present.

Parkinson disease (**choice D**) is idiopathic and often occurs late in life. It is clinically indistinguishable from

drug-induced parkinsonism, but the fact that the presentation occurred in the context of an increased dose of haloperidol suggests drug-induced parkinsonism as the clear correct choice.

Tardive dyskinesia (**choice E**) is a late complication of typical neuroleptic use. (Its association with the atypical neuroleptics has not been established.) It is a hyperkinetic movement disorder characterized by abnormal choreoathetoid movements often affecting the face and mouth. Parkinsonism, a hypokinetic movement disorder, is an entirely different entity.

36.   **The correct answer is B.** This patient has delusional disorder of the somatic type. In this delusional disorder, there is the presence of a single delusion of having some general medical condition; other criteria for a primary psychotic disorder, such as schizophrenia, are not met. Hallucinations, if present, are not a primary feature and are congruent with the delusion (such as seeing the mites). This disorder tends to have an onset in middle age and responds poorly to treatment.

Delirium tremens (**choice A**) is a severe withdrawal reaction that occurs in alcohol users following heavy ingestion and rapid reduction of alcohol consumption. Clinical features include delirium, sympathetic overactivity, electrolyte disturbances, and hallucinations that are commonly of the visual type. Delirium tremens can result in seizures, but improvement usually occurs in 36 hours. This patient has no history of alcohol use and displays a hallucination disorder that is over a long period of time (3 months).

Hypnagogic hallucinations (**choice C**) describe hallucinations that occur when one is falling asleep. They are usually short, auditory hallucinations, such as a ringing bell, and are a feature of narcolepsy.

In obsessive-compulsive disorder (OCD; **choice D**), patients experience intrusive thoughts that are generally considered inappropriate and may feel compelled to engage in compulsions. The thoughts, although intrusive and inappropriate, are not delusional in nature, and hallucinations are clearly not a feature.

Individuals with paranoid personality disorder (**choice E**) have pervasive mistrust toward others; however, somatic delusions and hallucinations are not present.

Schizophrenia (**choice F**) is incorrect. It would be highly unlikely for its onset to be in the fifth decade, whereas this would not be unusual for delusional disorder. In addition, to make the diagnosis of schizophrenia, symptoms need to present for at least 6 months.

37.   **The correct answer is D.** This patient has several classic symptoms of hypothyroidism. Lithium inhibits secretion by the thyroid gland and may result in hypothyroidism

and a nontoxic goiter. Decreased secretion of thyroid hormone should be reflected by low levels of thyroid hormone, and by an increased serum TSH. This can be treated with thyroid replacement and does not necessarily mean that lithium should be discontinued.

BUN and creatinine (**choice A**) may be elevated secondary to any one of a number of renal complications from lithium treatment, including diabetes insipidus (see explanation for **choice C** below), interstitial fibrosis, or focal renal necrosis. With the exception of slowed cognition, however, the patient's symptoms are not suggestive of uremia.

Liver function tests (**choice B**) are not frequently elevated by lithium therapy and, even if elevated, would not produce the clinical picture described in this case.

Serum sodium (**choice C**) may be elevated in patients taking lithium who develop diabetes insipidus (DI). Lithium causes a nephrogenic form of DI in which the renal tubules do not respond to antidiuretic hormone, with resultant loss of free water. Hypernatremia may cause mental status changes but none of the other symptoms.

Urine electrolytes (**choice E**) would also be helpful in making a diagnosis of nephrogenic DI. In DI, the urine electrolytes should be diluted by the excess free water in the urine. Symptoms of DI will usually remit with discontinuation of lithium or sometimes simply with decreased dosage.

38. **The correct answer is D.** The prevalence of domestic violence (partner or spousal abuse) is high. Approximately 12% to 28% of women report having suffered physical abuse by their husbands or partners, according to recent statistics. Although domestic violence is a definite medical diagnosis (code 995.81 of the *International Classification of Disease*, 9th ed.), it is often unrecognized by primary care physicians. Most victims of domestic violence come to clinical attention because of seemingly unrelated problems, including anxiety, depression, and various physical complaints. Identification of cases of domestic violence relies on two general strategies: *universal screening* (if generic questions on domestic violence are asked in the context of history taking) and *case finding* (when specific evidence of physical abuse is observed during physical examination). Once a victim of domestic violence has been identified, such as in this example, the next steps include providing emotional support and information about social resources, ensuring safety, documenting injuries carefully, and scheduling follow-up appointments.

There are a number of mistakes that should be avoided:

Expressing doubts about the patient's account (**choice A**) will most likely cause the victim to cease seeking help. Furthermore, studies have shown that the great majority of victims' accounts regarding domestic violence are accurate.

Expressing indignation against the perpetrator (**choice B**) may result in losing rapport with the victim. Usually, a victim of spousal abuse has a conflicting relationship with the perpetrator of violence. She both loves and fears him, and the physician's outrage may offend her.

Instructing the patient on how and when to leave her husband (**choice C**) is a mistake. Victims are at greatest risk of suffering injury and death precisely when they try to leave a relationship with the abuser.

Referring both the patient and her husband for marriage counseling (**choice E**) is another common mistake. Referral to counseling implies breaching of confidentiality and may expose the victim to increased abuse.

Trying to persuade the patient's husband to stop abusing her (**choice F**) should never be attempted, even if the victim expresses consent. This action entails breaching of confidentiality and usually results in retaliatory abuse by the perpetrator.

39. **The correct answer is C.** In major depressive disorder with atypical features, mood reactivity is a response to potential or actual positive events, with at least two significant symptoms present: significant weight gain or increase in appetite (cravings for sweets at times), hypersomnia, heavy feeling in arms and legs ("leaden paralysis"), and increased sensitivity to interpersonal rejection resulting in social dysfunctioning.

Decreased appetite (**choice A**) and weight loss are more common, but not specific, features of several psychiatric disorders and medical conditions. They are not features of atypical depressive disorder.

Worsening of depression in the morning with some improvement of mood in the evening (**choice B**) is typically seen in major depressive disorder with melancholic features and is defined as diurnal variation of mood.

Negativism (**choice D**) is manifested by maintenance of rigid posture or resistance to commands and instructions. It can be seen as a part of normal childhood development and in a variety of psychiatric disorders.

Psychomotor agitation (**choice E**) is a symptom that can be seen in several acute psychiatric disorders, including affective disorders, psychotic disorders, substance-induced disorders, and cognitive disorders like delirium and dementia.

40. **The correct answer is C.** All the new atypical antipsychotics have reduced extrapyramidal side effects, and

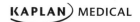

clozapine has the least effect on the basal ganglia. It works predominantly as an antagonist to D1, D3, and D4 dopamine receptors. Of all the antipsychotics, it has the lowest activity against D2 receptors, which is the best measure of a drug's potential to cause extrapyramidal side effects. Clozapine appears more effective in the mesolimbic dopamine pathways, which are disrupted in psychotic states and less effective in the nigrostriatal systems crucial to fluid movement. The main limitation to using clozapine is the risk of agranulocytosis (1% to 2%), which requires weekly leukocyte counts for the first 6 months of treatment, then every 2 weeks thereafter.

Chlorpromazine (**choice A**) is an example of a typical antipsychotic. It is considered a low-potency antipsychotic and has less of a tendency to cause extrapyramidal side effects than do the high-potency antipsychotics. It is still more likely than any of the atypical antipsychotics to worsen this patient's parkinsonism and should be avoided here.

Clomipramine (**choice B**) is a tricyclic antidepressant. In addition to its inhibition of norepinephrine reuptake, it is a strong serotonin reuptake inhibitor, making it a good choice for treatment in obsessive-compulsive disorder (OCD) when SSRIs are poorly tolerated. It has no role in the treatment of psychosis.

Haloperidol (**choice D**) is one of the high-potency antipsychotics, and it may produce prominent extrapyramidal side effects. It would very likely improve this patient's psychosis but would also worsen her parkinsonian symptoms. In general, haloperidol is never used in patients with Parkinson disease.

Pergolide (**choice E**) is a dopamine agonist and may be used as adjuvant therapy in Parkinson disease to lessen the daily Sinemet requirement. It would tend to produce the same CNS side effects as Sinemet, including dyskinesias and visual hallucinations.

41. **The correct answer is E.** Overdose of opiates, such as heroin, causes CNS and respiratory depression and miosis. Naloxone is a short-acting opioid antagonist that reverses the signs and symptoms of opiate overdose. Because it has a short half-life, it may need to be administered repeatedly.

Chlordiazepoxide (**choice A**) is a long-acting benzodiazepine that is used in treatment of alcohol withdrawal. It would likely exacerbate this patient's condition.

Flumazenil (**choice B**) is a benzodiazepine antagonist that can reverse respiratory and CNS depression from severe benzodiazepine overdose, although its use in benzodiazepine addicted patients can induce seizures.

Methadone (**choice C**) is a synthetic compound with a similar action to that of morphine and heroin, and it is almost equal to them in addiction liability. It is used as a method of long-term opiate withdrawal by monitored administration and gradual tapering. It, however, has no effect in the immediate management of opiate overdose.

N-Acetylcysteine (NAC; **choice D**) protects against liver damage in early acetaminophen poisoning by production of cysteine, which acts as a glutathione precursor. NAC also acts by supplying additional thiol groups that bind directly with the reactive metabolites of acetaminophen. It has no place in the therapy of opiate overdose.

Naltrexone (**choice F**) is also an opioid receptor antagonist; however, it is the incorrect choice because its onset of action is too slow to be useful in acute overdose. It has indication in the treatment of both alcohol and opiate dependence to assist with craving.

42. **The correct answer is C.** Nortriptyline is a tricyclic antidepressant. Like most tricyclics, it has prominent anticholinergic properties, which would explain the patient's lethargy, blurry vision with mydriasis, urinary retention, and tachycardia. The tricyclics may be lethal in overdose because of their tendency to cause arrhythmias; therefore, the patient should continue to be observed on a cardiac monitor.

Bupropion (**choice A**) is a second-generation antidepressant without anticholinergic side effects. It can cause seizures in up to 0.5% of patients when taken at high doses. It is therefore contraindicated in patients with epilepsy.

Fluoxetine (**choice B**) and sertraline (**choice E**) are selective serotonin reuptake inhibitors (SSRIs). This class of antidepressants is considered relatively safe in overdose. It also has only minimal anticholinergic effects. One side effect that limits compliance with this class of drugs is sexual dysfunction.

Phenelzine (**choice D**) is a monoamine oxidase inhibitor. This class of drug may induce a life-threatening hypertensive crisis when patients eat foods containing tyramine. They may also precipitate a serotonin syndrome when taken in excess or combined with an SSRI.

43. **The correct answer is C.** The fact that it takes more alcohol to achieve intoxication is indicative of tolerance, a diagnostic criterion that makes substance dependence more likely than substance abuse. Any history of withdrawal from a substance also more strongly suggests substance dependence.

Choices A-D are all DSM-IV criteria for substance abuse, provided they occur within a 12-month period and there is no indication of tolerance or withdrawal.

44. **The correct answer is C.** This patient has panic disorder with agoraphobia, which is characterized by anxiety about being in places or situations from which escape

may be difficult or in which help may not be available in the event of having an unexpected or situationally predisposed panic attack. Agoraphobia itself is a fear of open spaces. Gradual exposure is often used for agoraphobia, specific phobia, and obsessive-compulsive disorder. It involves exposure to situations, specifically open spaces for patients with agoraphobia, organized along a hierarchy of gradually more fear-inducing situations. It is usually performed in small steps at a time, with the experiencing of anticipatory anxiety in smaller, more tolerable exposures. The patient is monitored and in the presence of the therapist throughout the gradual exposure.

Biofeedback (**choice A**) involves the recording and display of small changes in the feedback parameter. The display may be visual, such as a bar of lights, or auditory. Patients are instructed to change the levels of the parameter, using the feedback from the display as a guide. The treatment was based on the discovery that laboratory animals could control their autonomic function by using biofeedback under stringent conditions that appeared to eliminate possible mediation by skeletal muscle activity. On the basis of these findings, biofeedback has been used with certain patients, such as those with urinary incontinence, who can use biofeedback to regain control over their pelvic musculature. It can be used by itself or in conjunction with relaxation and breathing retraining.

Flooding (**choice B**) involves exposure to a maximally fear-inducing situation, which can be real or contrived. It may seem traumatizing, but usually flooding therapy sessions are long and consist of continually decreasing levels of anxiety.

Learning new habits (**choice D**) is useful in many preventive health behaviors that ought to become regular occurrences. This is more practical in behaviors such as using seat belts, brushing teeth, and taking prescribed medications. To build a new habit, one can identify regularly occurring behaviors and use the stimuli from these behaviors to prompt the new habit. This is not a way to help with agoraphobic patients, however.

Relaxation therapy (**choice E**) is used either as a component of treatment programs (i.e., biofeedback or systematic desensitization) or as its own treatment. It is characterized by immobility of the body, control over the focus of attention, low muscle tone, and cultivation of a specific, contemplative frame of mind. If done properly, muscle tension, respiratory rate, heart rate, and blood pressure decrease. Indications are for any conditions thought to be related to adrenergic stress responses. Patients with agoraphobia may find some benefit in relaxation therapy, but alone it will not treat the fear of open spaces.

45. **The correct answer is E.** The patient's symptoms of hypertension, tachycardia, nystagmus, dysarthria, impulsiveness, and psychomotor agitation are all indicative of phencyclidine intoxication.

Alcohol withdrawal symptoms (**choice A**) do not include nystagmus. Instead, tremor, seizures, or hallucinations are common.

Lithium intoxication (**choice B**) is associated with symptoms of coarse tremor, impaired consciousness, and, most importantly, myoclonus, seizures and coma. Nystagmus is not associated with lithium toxicity.

Neuroleptic malignant syndrome (**choice C**) is a life-threatening complication of antipsychotic treatment. The symptoms include muscular rigidity and dystonia, akinesia, mutism, obtundation, and agitation. The autonomic symptoms include high fever, sweating, and increased blood pressure. This patient does not have fever, nor is there any indication of antipsychotic use.

Paranoid schizophrenia (**choice D**) is a chronic condition characterized by frequent auditory hallucinations of more than 6 months' duration. The acute nature of this patient's symptoms and her physical findings make this an unlikely diagnosis.

46. **The correct answer is C.** This patient with dementia probably also has delirium. Dementia, delirium, amnestic disorder, and other cognitive disorders are usually grouped together under the category of organic mental disorders. The term "organic" implies brain dysfunction. The patient's change in mental status from being calm and pleasant to being disruptive and agitated is indicative of a likely delirium. Also, a low-grade fever in an elderly person should not be taken lightly. It is often more difficult for the elderly to mount a substantial fever, so any temperature above normal is considered abnormal and may be serious. By definition, delirium is an acute reversible mental disorder characterized by confusion and some impairment of consciousness. It is usually associated with emotional lability, hallucinations (more commonly visual than auditory), and often violent behavior. The most important first step in treating this patient is protecting her from unintentional harm. It would be quite unfortunate for this patient to hurt herself in the context of an acute delirium. Calming her with words, holding her hands, removing potentially dangerous objects, and possibly putting her in a restrictive posey vest, if necessary, should be the first steps taken to ensure this patient's safety.

Inquiring about this woman's medications, including any recent changes (**choice A**), is very important and should be among the initial steps in history gathering after the patient is restricted from hurting herself and is medically and psychiatrically evaluated. Often the patient herself will be unable to report this information, and a treating staff member from the nursing home should be contacted.

Obtaining vital signs and an ECG (**choice B**) is important, but should be done after safety measures are taken. Any changes in vital signs or in an ECG from the patient's baseline should be carefully attended to and treated as necessary.

It may be necessary to request a medicine consult (**choice D**), but this can be determined only after the patient's condition is understood and evaluated better. Safeguarding the patient, evaluating her condition, and determining the problems at hand should be performed prior to any thought of asking for a medicine consult.

Administering intramuscular haloperidol (**choice E**) is too aggressive to be taken as a first step. It is better to avoid medications in this patient to get a clearer picture of what her presentation is really like and also to avoid further sedation. Moreover, the elderly tend to be very sensitive to medications. If haloperidol were required, it would be judicious to use the smallest dose possible.

47.   **The correct answer is B.** Cocaine blocks dopamine reuptake at the dopamine transporter, increasing dopamine concentration at the D1 and D2 receptors, which appear to mediate many of the symptoms of psychosis. The dopamine system is also implicated in schizophrenia, which is characterized by psychotic symptoms, such as hallucinations and delusions.

Medications that block acetylcholine (**choice A**) are used in psychiatry for neuroleptic-induced movement disorders. Furthermore, acetylcholinesterase inhibitors, such as donepezil, are used in Alzheimer type dementia.

Benzodiazepines and barbiturates are sedative-hypnotics that act at GABA (**choice C**) receptors. These drugs are not associated with psychosis.

If the patient admitted to phencyclidine (PCP) use, and PCP were detected on the urine drug screen, glutamate might be an appropriate answer. PCP inhibits the NMDA receptor, which uses glutamate (**choice D**) as a neurotransmitter. Given the information, cocaine is the most likely drug involved; therefore, **choice B** is correct.

Glycine receptors (**choice E**) are largely located in the spinal cord. Strychnine, a glycine antagonist, causes convulsions.

48.   **The correct answer is B.** The patient has a mental disturbance characterized by alterations in cognition, attention, alertness, and perception. Delirium is, by definition, caused by a separate physiologic condition such as illness or substance intoxication/withdrawal. Essential features of the diagnosis of delirium include the development of symptoms over a short period of time and a fluctuating clinical presentation.

Amnestic disorders (**choice A**) are conditions in which there is gross impairment in memory, but level of alertness and other cognitive problems are not evident. The most striking feature of this patient's presentation includes disturbances in cognition and perception.

The patient in question evidences no depressive complaints and the abrupt production of symptoms and their waxing and waning course are not consistent with a depression. Therefore, **choice C** is incorrect.

The patient does not have a known history of Parkinson disease and there is no report of the neurologic symptoms of Parkinson disease in this patient. A diagnosis of Parkinson dementia is not tenable in this patient. Therefore, **choice D** is incorrect.

The diagnosis of senile dementia, Alzheimer type (**choice E**) requires an extensive history of difficulties in memory, language, motor behaviors, recognition of people or objects, and disturbances in executive functioning. Alzheimer dementia cannot be diagnosed in the context of a delirium.

49.   **The correct answer is E.** The presence of delusions of persecution and auditory hallucinations are the hallmarks of paranoid type schizophrenia. The disorder requires symptoms that meet criteria for schizophrenia be present for greater than 6 months (psychotic symptoms themselves need be present for only 2 weeks, incidentally); therefore, brief psychotic disorder (**choice B**), in which psychotic symptoms resolve between 1 day and 1 month, is incorrect.

Although individuals with bipolar disorder (**choice A**) may have delusions, they are usually but not always of a grandiose quality. Furthermore, an individual with acute mania would have a thought process marked by loosening of associations or flight of ideas. In addition, the affect of a bipolar patient would likely be rather animated, not constricted, as in this case.

Major depressive disorder with psychotic features (**choice C**) is incorrect because the psychotic symptoms associated with this disorder tend not to be bizarre, as they are in this individual. It is also a time-limited disorder and would not endure for an entire 6 years without some degree of remission. If this had been the correct answer, there should have been other symptoms of depression.

Although rape is a recognized stressor that may predate posttraumatic stress disorder (PTSD; **choice D**), the preoccupation in this case is clearly delusional since the patient reports that women are putting spells on him. In addition, auditory hallucinations are not a feature of PTSD. Again, one would look for other classic symptoms of PTSD, such as hypervigilance, increased startle reflex, and avoidance behavior, to make the diagnosis.

50. **The correct answer is C.** Patients with dissociative identity disorder manifest multiple distinct personalities that assume control of the patient's awareness of the environment and behavior. Common comorbidities for patients with dissociative identity disorder include borderline personality disorder, posttraumatic stress disorder, and physical or sexual abuse.

    Depersonalization disorder (**choice A**) is defined by the perception that one is detached from his/her mental processes or body. It is not characterized by the assumption of multiple personalities.

    Dissociative fugue (**choice B**) is a rare dissociative disorder involving abrupt travel and an amnesia for events that may include the circumstances preceding arrival at one's destination and one's identity. The etiology of dissociative fugue is unknown, though a possible correlation between dissociative fugue and recent life stressors may exist. The condition is usually self-limited.

    This patient does not report symptoms consistent with a major depressive disorder (**choice D**), such as depressed mood or neurovegetative signs of depression.

    The patient in question has periods of dissociation involving the assumption of another personality. This is not to be confused with a chronic psychotic state such as found in schizophrenia, chronic paranoid type (**choice E**). Patients with schizophrenia typically evidence a disorganization of thought process and reality testing mechanisms that are inadequate. Patients with dissociative identity disorder have a fragmentation of actual conscious functions with intact reality testing.

KAPLAN) MEDICAL

Psychiatry: **Test Two**

1. A 35-year-old married man presents to his primary care physician 1 month after a recent hospitalization for a car accident, which left him with limited use of his arm and hand. The patient, who is a local contractor building houses, was instructed to avoid any gripping, arm raising, and other strenuous activities that his work had previously required. He continues to oversee his workers on the job but now complains that he finds himself anxious and despondent at times, with episodes of irritability and tearfulness and a decreased interest in his work. He still enjoys coaching his son's baseball team, and he has had no sleep or appetite changes. He also feels that his sexual desire has diminished. The patient has no prior personal or familial history of a mood disorder or psychiatric disorder. Which of the following is the most likely diagnosis?

   (A) Adjustment disorder with depressed mood

   (B) Bipolar disorder, most recent episode depressed

   (C) Conversion disorder

   (D) Dysthymic disorder

   (E) Major depressive disorder

2. A 57-year-old Asian American man, accompanied by his wife, presents to a psychiatrist. The patient has no significant past medical or psychiatric history. He admits to depressed mood, decreased appetite, a 10-pound weight loss, initial insomnia, decreased ability to concentrate, and mild memory problems for the past 3 weeks. On further questioning, he states that he feels hopeless and helpless. On mental status examination, the patient appears calm and is cooperative. He has a sad affect. There is no evidence of a thought disorder. Which of the following would be the most appropriate next step in management?

   (A) Assessment of suicidality

   (B) Cognitive-behavioral therapy

   (C) Initiation of a selective serotonin reuptake inhibitor

   (D) Initiation of a benzodiazepine

   (E) Urine drug screen

3. A 47-year-old Asian American man visits his physician for problems falling asleep. The man says he goes to bed every night at 11 P.M. and arises at 6 A.M.; however, he does not fall asleep until about 60 minutes after going to bed. He denies depressed mood or recent psychosocial stressors. When asked about his daily routine, he reports that he takes a brisk walk every morning and then goes to work. On the way to work, he drinks one cup of coffee, but denies any other caffeine intake during the remainder of the day. At around 9:30 P.M., he eats dinner and then watches television until 11 P.M., at which time he drinks 1 ounce of whiskey before retiring. Which of the following would be the best advice for this patient?

   (A) Decrease the intensity of the morning exercise

   (B) Eat dinner earlier in the evening

   (C) Exercise vigorously just prior to going to bed

   (D) Increase the amount of alcohol drunk before retiring

   (E) Use zolpidem at bedtime as needed

4. A 15-year-old high school sophomore is brought to the emergency department by his father because of bizarre behavior during the past week. Two weeks earlier, the patient's twin brother was killed in a car accident. After the funeral, while helping to go through his brother's things, the boy began screaming and flailing about wildly, saying that his brother's guardian angel was coming to get him for not taking better care of his brother. The patient had been an excellent student and a popular athlete, with no previous psychiatric history. Which of the following is the most likely diagnosis?

   (A) Brief psychotic disorder

   (B) Delusional disorder

   (C) Drug intoxication

   (D) Grief reaction

   (E) Schizophrenia

5. A 62-year-old Iranian American man is seen for the first time by a physician for complaints of abdominal pain. The patient states that the pain has been present for more than a year, is localized to the lower abdomen, and is "sharp and crampy" in character. He has brought with him a rather sizable stack of medical records. A careful review of the records reveals that the patient has had the same complaint for approximately 3 years, and several extensive and redundant evaluations by various physicians for pathology have been uninformative. When the physician asks the patient what he believes to be responsible for the pain, he replies, "I don't *believe* it's anything—I *know* it's cancer." When confronted with the contents of his medical records, which reveal no malignancy, the patient states, "Colon cancer runs in my family. I know that if you run another test, it'll show something serious." Which of the following is the most likely diagnosis?

   (A) Body dysmorphic disorder

   (B) Conversion disorder

   (C) Hypochondriasis

   (D) Schizophrenia

   (E) Somatization disorder

6. A 68-year-old Latina is seen in the emergency department because of complaints of anxiety. She states she has been taking medication for anxiety for the past 10 years; however, she ran out of medication 2 days ago. She denies the use of any illicit drugs or alcohol. She does not know the name of the medication she has been taking. Laboratory studies are remarkable for a urine drug screen positive for benzodiazepines. The physician should be most concerned about withdrawal from which of the following medications?

   (A) Alprazolam

   (B) Buspirone

   (C) Chlordiazepoxide

   (D) Clonazepam

   (E) Diazepam

7. A mother brings her 4-year-old boy to the pediatrician because he has had trouble relating to children in his new preschool. His birth history was unremarkable, but he has been slow to develop language and has required speech therapy. In the office, the child rarely makes eye contact, and he flaps his hands. When given a doll, he does not engage in imaginary play. He has no dysmorphic features, and the rest of his examination is normal. Which of the following is the most likely diagnosis?

   (A) Asperger syndrome

   (B) Autism

   (C) Dyslexia

   (D) Fragile X syndrome

   (E) Rett syndrome

8. A 43-year-old African American woman is discharged from a 4-week-long alcohol dependence treatment program. At the end of this program, the patient discusses with her physician possible pharmacologic modalities that may assist in preventing relapse. It is decided that she begin a trial of disulfiram (Antabuse™). She is told that she must avoid ingestion or dermal contact of any substances containing alcohol. The patient asks how the medication works and is told that disulfiram inhibits an enzyme that then causes accumulation of a noxious metabolite. Inhibition of which of the following enzymes accounts for the clinically significant effect of disulfiram?

   (A) Acetylcholinesterase

   (B) Alcohol dehydrogenase

   (C) Aldehyde dehydrogenase

   (D) Cytochrome P450

   (E) Tyrosine hydroxylase

9. On Halloween, a group of teenagers decides to go to a new haunted house that they heard had extraordinary "scary" effects. At the entrance, they laugh loudly and tease each other. This is an example of which of the following types of behavior?

   (A) Counterphobic behavior

   (B) Denial

   (C) Reaction formation

   (D) Regression

   (E) Undoing

10. A 40-year-old man presents to the emergency department complaining of abdominal pain. He lives alone and states that he was otherwise healthy before this episode. He undergoes emergency abdominal surgery for the removal of a ruptured appendix. Three days after surgery, the patient becomes delirious, with fluctuations in his level of consciousness, but is afebrile. Which of the following would be the most likely source of this patient's delirium?

    (A) Delirium tremens

    (B) Infection

    (C) Pain medications

    (D) Postoperative depression

    (E) Stress of surgery

11. A 40-year-old Caucasian man with chronic paranoid schizophrenia presents to his primary care physician's office for his yearly physical examination. The physician notes that the patient currently weighs 220 pounds, whereas the previous year he weighed 197 pounds. The patient explains to the physician that his psychiatrist switched his medication about 5 months earlier, from risperidone to a new medication called olanzapine. The patient states that over the past few months, he has had a decrease in auditory hallucinations but has had some difficulty because he was laid off from his job and has been having increasing strain in his marriage. He states also that he has been drinking more alcohol lately, up to a case of beer a week. Which of the following is the most likely cause of this patient's increase in weight?

    (A) Alcohol use

    (B) Decreased auditory hallucinations leading to increased appetite

    (C) Discontinuation of risperidone

    (D) Initiation of olanzapine

    (E) Overeating due to familial stress

12. A fourth-year medical student is interviewing a 38-year-old woman who has schizophrenia, disorganized type. As part of the mental status examination, the student asks the patient to name the floor of the hospital she is on. In response, the patient begins to discuss the last hospital she was admitted to, the quality of the food while she was a patient there, and how attractive she thought her last physician was. Her speech is intelligible and normal in tone, and her vocabulary is good, but she never answers the student's question. Which of the following best describes this patient's behavior?

    (A) Circumstantiality

    (B) Tangentiality

    (C) Thought blocking

    (D) Verbigeration

    (E) Word salad

13. A 35-year-old woman is admitted to the psychiatric unit for treatment. After a few days on medication, she complains of diarrhea, a metallic taste in her mouth, and polyuria. While examining her, the psychiatrist observes a fine intention tremor of her hands. The patients also complains that her psoriasis has flared up. Which of the following medications most likely caused these symptoms?

    (A) Carbamazepine

    (B) Fluoxetine

    (C) Haloperidol

    (D) Lithium carbonate

    (E) Valproic acid

14. A 47-year-old Caucasian man is seen by a psychiatrist for treatment of refractory depression. He has a 10-year history of severe depression, which has been treated with several different medications, as well as with electroconvulsive therapy. After careful consideration, the psychiatrist and the patient decide that he should try a monoamine oxidase inhibitor (MAOI). The psychiatrist gives him a list of foods and medications to avoid while taking the MAOI. Which of the following adverse outcomes is the psychiatrist trying to avoid?

    (A) Agranulocytosis

    (B) Hypertensive crisis

    (C) Pigmentary retinopathy

    (D) Priapism

    (E) Serotonin syndrome

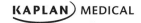

15. A 16-year-old girl is brought to the psychiatrist by her mother, who had noticed that her daughter pulls her hair and chews it. It is more evident now that she has several bald patches on both sides of her head. The daughter says that pulling her hair provides some sense of relief when she feels nervous or upset. She is doing well at school and denies any other symptoms. She has seen a dermatologist, who ruled out any medical causes for the alopecia. Which of the following is the most likely diagnosis?

    (A) Bulimia nervosa

    (B) Factitious disorder

    (C) Major depressive disorder

    (D) Obsessive-compulsive disorder

    (E) Trichotillomania

16. A 30-year-old Caucasian man has been treated with antipsychotic medications for the past 6 years. He has a chronic delusion that the FBI is constantly monitoring him through hidden cameras in his apartment and listening devices in his telephone. He also claims to hear the voice of the devil telling him not to eat certain foods because his neighbors are trying to poison him. Despite several hospitalizations and multiple trials of different antipsychotic medications, his symptoms are continuously present and are very distressing. Accordingly, his psychiatrist decides to start him on clozapine. Which of the following laboratory studies should be monitored at regular intervals?

    (A) Complete blood count

    (B) Prolactin level

    (C) Serum glucose level

    (D) Serum urea nitrogen and creatinine levels

    (E) Thyroid stimulating hormone

17. A 22-year-old African American woman visits a psychiatrist for "violent mood swings." She reports that she experiences intense periods of "utter contentment" followed, often within minutes to hours, by intense feelings of depression. During these episodes, she feels she is useless and unloved by her parents and boyfriend. In addition, despite desperate attempts to engage in a long-term romantic relationship, she regrets that she can never seem to stay involved with anyone for very long, as she feels "no one understands me." In assessing past thoughts of harm to herself, she admits that she has had more than 10 suicide attempts, usually involving superficial cuts to her wrists. The patient offers that "sometimes I feel so numb, I cut myself just to feel something." Which of the following is the most likely diagnosis?

    (A) Attention deficit/hyperactivity disorder

    (B) Bipolar disorder

    (C) Borderline personality disorder

    (D) Intermittent explosive disorder

    (E) Major depression

18. A 38-year-old African American man with schizophrenia, chronic undifferentiated type, is evaluated by a psychiatrist. On mental status examination, he has a notable poverty of speech, along with poor eye contact, inattentiveness during testing, thought insertion, and flat affect. He does not appear to be actively responding to auditory hallucinations. Which of the above is the only positive symptom of schizophrenia in this patient?

    (A) Flat affect

    (B) Inattentiveness during testing

    (C) Poor eye contact

    (D) Poverty of speech

    (E) Thought insertion

19. A 27-year-old man is brought to the emergency department in an agitated state by police. The man had been talking to himself and threatening people in the street, stating he was the son of God. On the psychiatric unit, he refuses to take medication. However, after engaging in several altercations with other patients, he is given an injection of haloperidol. The haloperidol is then ordered "as needed" in case of agitation over the next few days. The staff reports that he has started pacing down the hall and cannot sit still for more than 5 minutes. Which of the following disorders is this patient most likely experiencing?

    (A) Akathisia

    (B) Akinesia

    (C) Festination

    (D) Stereotypic movement disorder

    (E) Tardive dyskinesia

20. The 12th grade teacher of a 17-year-old girl is concerned about the girl's behavior over the past school year. She has been talking to herself while looking off into the distance, isolating herself from her classmates, and wearing the same clothes daily for several weeks likely without washing them. However, she has been completing her homework assignments. The teacher calls the girl's parents, who admit that she has been "acting strangely" for quite a while. The parents ask their daughter if anything is bothering her. She replies, "I want to save Swedish children from persecution by the devil." According to data from the National Institute of Mental Health Sponsored Epidemiologic Catchment Area, what is the lifetime prevalence of this girl's disorder?

    (A) 0.01%

    (B) 0.1%

    (C) 1%

    (D) 5%

    (E) 10%

21. A 28-year-old pregnant woman attempts to drown herself and her three young children. She is brought to the emergency department, and her children are taken to their grandmother's house. The woman is offered admission but she refuses, saying, "It doesn't matter. It's all going to end sooner or later." Which of the following is the most appropriate next step in management?

    (A) Admit her to a day program and order 15-minute observation checks there

    (B) Admit her as an involuntary patient to an inpatient unit with high observation

    (C) Arrange for outpatient follow-up to begin the following morning

    (D) Create a contract with her to ensure that she agrees not to harm herself

    (E) Call the police to report her as having endangered her children and unborn fetus

22. A 40-year-old woman presents to the emergency department after having cut her arm on a knife. She states that she sleeps with a knife for protection from her neighbors, who she thinks are conspiring to rob her. The patient also tells the physician that she cannot hold a job because everywhere she works, her coworkers conspire to slander her for her political beliefs. Which of the following is the most likely diagnosis?

    (A) Capgras syndrome

    (B) Delirium

    (C) Delusional disorder, persecutory type

    (D) Paranoid schizophrenia

    (E) Shared psychotic disorder

23. A 24-year-old physics student with a history of bipolar disorder presents to a clinic. He is dressed in new white suit and is wearing a hat. He goes around the waiting room, flirting with female patients, laughing, and talking loudly. Which of the following delusions is most consistent with his condition?

    (A) "I created the bomb that killed people in Vietnam; I don't deserve to live."

    (B) "I know that my family is going bankrupt; we won't have anything to eat."

    (C) "I heard them talking about me on TV; they clearly said my name."

    (D) "My brain is melting inside; I know it."

    (E) "NASA called me to be the director of their new space program."

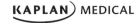

24. A 31-year-old man describes himself as "on top of the world" to strangers whom he meets in the street or on public transportation. He is considering running for president of the United States, since he views himself as more intelligent, handsome, and charismatic than anyone he knows. He has engaged in sexual activity with eight different women over the past 8 nights. He thinks his talents are unique and are the envy of all. He has been prescribed lithium by his treating psychiatrist, yet he has opted not to take the medication because he feels that it limits his creativity and genius. Which of the following symptoms would be seen in such a person during a manic episode but not during a major depressive episode?

    (A) Anhedonia
    (B) Decreased sleep
    (C) Distractibility
    (D) Flight of ideas
    (E) Impairment of functioning

25. A 52-year-old woman with a history of mitral valve prolapse, myocardial infarction, and diabetes returns to her primary care physician's office after having been recently diagnosed by her psychiatrist as having panic disorder. She is obese, has a history of alcohol dependence, and frequently has episodes of hypoglycemia due to poor control of blood glucose. Which of the following conditions has a demonstrated association with panic disorder?

    (A) Alcohol dependence
    (B) Diabetes
    (C) Hypoglycemia
    (D) Mitral valve prolapse
    (E) Obesity

26. An 87-year-old Hispanic man is accompanied by his daughter for evaluation of memory problems. The daughter explains that, for the past year, her father has been getting increasingly forgetful. He misplaces personal items, such as his house keys, and it often takes him a while to come up with the words for simple objects. Furthermore, he has been acting suspicious toward his wife, whom he suspects is having an affair even though she is bedridden. Last week, he insisted that his apartment had been broken into because he discovered that the entry door was unlocked one morning when he awoke. When his wife suggested that he might have forgotten to lock it, he became very angry and said, "it was probably that man you've been going around with!" Physical examination is unremarkable, and laboratory studies, including a thyroid stimulating hormone (TSH) level, are within normal limits. Which of the following is the most likely underlying pathology that accounts for this patient's symptoms?

    (A) Bilateral necrosis of the globus pallidus
    (B) Focal demyelination and gliosis of periventricular white matter
    (C) Focal hemorrhage and necrosis of the mammillary bodies
    (D) Loss of pigmented cells in the substantia nigra
    (E) Neurofibrillary tangles and senile plaques in the temporoparietal cortex

27. A 32-year-old archeologist has been fighting with his wife because of his drug abuse. His wife is threatening to divorce him and take their child unless he quits using drugs. To keep his family together, he decides to stop using drugs right away, without going to treatment. Soon afterward, he has cramps and diarrhea, is sneezing and yawning, and stays wrapped in the blanket feeling chills and aches all over his body. Which of the following drugs was this man most likely taking?

    (A) Alprazolam
    (B) Amphetamines
    (C) Cocaine
    (D) Heroin
    (E) Nicotine

28. A 32-year-old man is diagnosed with obsessive-compulsive disorder by his psychiatrist, and is started on daily sertraline. Which of the following is the most common compulsion in patients with this disorder?

    (A) Avoiding social situations

    (B) Incessant checking

    (C) Overwhelming need to repeat work tasks

    (D) Repetitive washing

    (E) Striving for completeness

29. A 76-year-old Caucasian male, accompanied by his wife, presents at a psychiatrist's office. The man has a 5-year history of depression and has tried several antidepressant medications without satisfaction. At the advice of his primary care physician, the patient was referred to the psychiatrist to be evaluated for electroconvulsive therapy (ECT). After a thorough discussion regarding the treatment, including its efficacy, risks, and benefits, the patient's wife asks whether there are any absolute contraindications to ECT. Which of the following is the most appropriate response?

    (A) "Anyone who has ever had a heart attack should not receive ECT."

    (B) "Only pregnant patients should not receive ECT."

    (C) "Patients with a seizure disorder are not candidates for ECT."

    (D) "There are no absolute contraindications to receiving ECT."

    (E) "Very elderly patients should not receive ECT."

30. A young woman has been in psychotherapy twice a week for several months. She feels "used" by others and gets frustrated when she is unable to refuse to do favors for people, even though she knows that they do not deserve her help. On one occasion, her psychotherapist is very late for the session because of an urgent situation. At the next session, the patient brings him a small gift. Which of the following mechanisms is most likely present in this situation?

    (A) Blocking

    (B) Displacement

    (C) Inhibition

    (D) Isolation

    (E) Reaction formation

31. The family of a 42-year-old violinist brings her to a psychiatrist for evaluation. She tells the psychiatrist that a famous Italian conductor is in love with her and is planning to leave his wife so they can be married. She had met him once at a reception while on tour in Milan with the philharmonic orchestra. She further tells the psychiatrist that, during his concerts, he gives her signals that he loves her. In addition, the family reports that she somehow got his e-mail address and has been sending him messages. Which of the following types of delusional disorder does this patient most likely have?

    (A) Erotomanic

    (B) Jealous

    (C) Grandiose

    (D) Persecutory

    (E) Somatic

32. A 20-year-old male college student is brought to the emergency department by his roommate for increasingly odd behavior. The patient has grown increasingly isolated over the past 6 months, with little interest in socializing. Four weeks ago, he began accusing his roommate of trying to "steal thoughts" from his head. His schoolwork has become increasingly disorganized, and he has missed several deadlines for papers. On the day of admission, the roommate heard the patient talking loudly to himself. His initial examination and a head CT are unremarkable. On psychiatric evaluation, he is noted to have a bizarre affect and reports hearing voices. Which of the following is the most likely diagnosis?

    (A) Bipolar disorder

    (B) Delusional disorder

    (C) Depression with psychotic features

    (D) Schizophrenia

    (E) Schizophreniform disorder

33. A 42-year-old teacher at a local school is brought to the emergency department by her husband and brother because she suddenly lost her voice. The day before, she learned about her husband's affair with his secretary. While the physician is asking questions and talking to her and the family members, she seems unconcerned with this sudden onset of illness. Which of the following terms is typically used to describe her lack of concern?

    (A) Denial
    (B) Depersonalization
    (C) Displacement
    (D) Dissociation
    (E) La belle indifference

34. A 43-year-old man with a history of paranoid schizophrenia presents to his psychiatrist for a yearly medication check. He is currently taking haloperidol at bedtime. The psychiatrist notices worsening tardive dyskinesia since last year, with an increase in abnormal involuntary movements in the hands and perioral area. Which of the following would be the most effective treatment in controlling this patient's tardive dyskinesia?

    (A) Addition of an anticholinergic drug
    (B) Addition of a dopamine receptor antagonist
    (C) Making no changes in the patient's antipsychotic medication
    (D) Stopping the patient's antipsychotic medication
    (E) Substituting a serotonin-dopamine antagonist for the haloperidol

35. A 27-year-old woman, after being examined by her psychiatrist to rule out other medical conditions, has been given a diagnosis of panic disorder with agoraphobia. She currently has no known drug allergies, is taking no medications, and denies any illicit drug use. Given her present diagnosis, which of the following is the most appropriate medication to prescribe?

    (A) Diazepam
    (B) Haloperidol
    (C) Lithium carbonate
    (D) Paroxetine
    (E) Temazepam

36. A 45-year-old, homeless Caucasian man is brought into the emergency department by EMS after having been found stuporous in a park. He is known by the emergency department staff to be alcohol dependent, as he has been treated on several occasions for alcohol withdrawal seizures. He is awake but somnolent and complains of abdominal pain and hazy vision. Examination is remarkable for mild bilateral papilledema and generalized abdominal tenderness. Significant laboratory studies suggest an anion gap acidosis. Which of the following is the most appropriate therapy for this patient?

    (A) Activated charcoal
    (B) Disulfiram
    (C) Fomepizole
    (D) Flumazenil
    (E) Naloxone

37. A 25-year-old woman is admitted to the psychiatric unit following an overdose of sleeping pills. She seems very angry for being held in the hospital, since she just wanted to "show her boyfriend" (who had broken up with her) how upset she was. She tells the intern on the unit that he is so caring and competent and that she has never met such a doctor. She complains that no one understands her and that the only one who can really help her is the intern. The intern feels flattered, without realizing that the patient is using a defense mechanism. Which of the following defense mechanisms is the patient most likely using?

    (A) Displacement
    (B) Distortion
    (C) Primitive idealization
    (D) Projection
    (E) Splitting

38. A 38-year-old African American woman visits a psychiatrist for recurrent depression. She states that she has been taking medication for depression for several years, but is now interested in starting St. John's wort for her current episode. Her psychiatrist conducts a literature search and discovers an article about the use of St. John's wort for depression. The article describes six randomized, placebo-controlled trials comparing St. John's wort with placebo; the data obtained from these studies were pooled to generate new data. Which of the following research designs was used in the study described?

(A) Case-control

(B) Case report

(C) Cohort

(D) Cross-sectional survey

(E) Meta-analysis

39. A 62-year-old man with a diagnosis of schizophrenia, paranoid type, has been stable on medication for years. Prior to that, he had several severe exacerbations that led to prolonged inpatient treatment of several months' duration. During an appointment with his psychiatrist, he complains of declining vision. He is referred to an ophthalmologist, who diagnoses pigmentary retinopathy. Which of the following medications would most likely have caused this complication?

(A) Clozapine

(B) Haloperidol

(C) Pimozide

(D) Thioridazine

(E) Thiothixene

40. A 71-year-old Caucasian man is brought to the physician by his wife for evaluation. The patient has a history of Parkinson disease, diagnosed by another physician 6 years ago, for which he takes L-dopa/carbidopa four times a day. His medical history is also significant for congestive heart failure, which is treated with digoxin and metoprolol, and depression, which is treated with fluoxetine. The man describes his mood as generally good, but he is particularly disturbed by visual hallucinations described as "people and small animals" that he is certain are not there and by thoughts that his wife is trying to kill him. These symptoms have been intermittently present for several months but are now getting much worse. He has not been to his internist for more than 5 years, but he assures you he has been taking his medications exactly as prescribed. Which of the following is the most likely explanation for his delusions?

(A) Delusional disorder

(B) Depression with psychotic features

(C) Digoxin toxicity

(D) L-dopa/carbidopa toxicity

(E) Schizophrenia

41. A 45-year-old Asian American female nurse is brought to the emergency department by ambulance after having been discovered unresponsive by her husband 30 minutes earlier. En route to the hospital, paramedics determine her serum glucose to be 13 mg/dL. After infusion of dextrose, the patient regains consciousness. On interview, the patient claims that she has a long history of severe hypoglycemia that often requires visits to the emergency department and, occasionally, admission to the hospital. Review of the chart reveals 10 such visits in the past year. Repeated work-ups for hypoglycemia have been negative. Questioning of her husband reveals that these episodes began to occur after the death of the patient's mother from cancer. Physical examination and routine laboratory tests are unremarkable. Which of the following is the most likely diagnosis?

(A) Factitious disorder

(B) Ganser syndrome

(C) Hypochondriasis

(D) Malingering

(E) Anorexia nervosa

42. A 39-year-old Caucasian woman visits her primary care physician for a routine examination. She denies any physical or psychiatric complaints, and her physical examination is within normal limits. Her physician advises her of the importance of eating a well-balanced diet and exercising on a regular basis. He then asks whether she has any questions before he sees his next patient. She suddenly becomes tearful and says, "Actually, yes. My 17-year-old son just told me he is gay, and I don't know what to do. I've always been taught that homosexuality is wrong, but he is my son and I love him. What should I do?" Which of the following would be the most appropriate response?

    (A) "Experimenting with homosexuality is completely normal behavior in adolescents. I'm sure this is a phase that will pass with time."

    (B) "Homosexuality is considered a normal variant of human sexuality. However, I can see that you are concerned. Let's talk about what's on your mind."

    (C) "These things need to be discussed with a psychiatrist. I can make a referral."

    (D) "Your son's sexual life is his private business and he needs to discuss that with his own physician."

    (E) "You seem rather upset. What is it that you don't like about gay people?"

43. A 12-year-old boy has been sent from his school to a psychiatrist for evaluation. During the past several months, the teacher has observed that the boy has been restless and fidgety. He repeatedly clears his throat and needs to spit. Recently, he distracted the whole class by making loud, barking noises. The parents have observed that he sometimes has facial tics and blinking, and shakes his head on one side. He has been otherwise doing well academically and is very neat. Which of the following is the most likely diagnosis?

    (A) Attention deficit/hyperactivity disorder

    (B) Autistic disorder

    (C) Huntington disease

    (D) Oppositional defiant disorder

    (E) Tourette syndrome

44. A 61-year-old woman has slowly been developing movement abnormalities. She finds herself moving more slowly and stiffly and she notices a tremor in her hands that was not there a year ago. Her husband thinks that she is slower when she starts to move but has trouble slowing down after she gets going. Once she is moving, her steps seem more like a shuffle than a walk. He also thinks that her facial expressions seem blunted, that she does not blink as much, and that the tone of her speech has become more monotonous. This woman is at the highest risk of having which of the following psychiatric disturbances?

    (A) Anxiety

    (B) Auditory hallucinations

    (C) Dementia

    (D) Depression

    (E) Insomnia

45. A patient taking haloperidol for the first time experiences an involuntary twisting of her neck. She is given benztropine for relief. This medication may cause which of the following side effects?

    (A) Diaphoresis

    (B) Diarrhea

    (C) Fevers

    (D) Insomnia

    (E) Mydriasis

46. A 31-year-old woman has refused to leave her home for the past 4 months. She had been on a crowded subway train when she felt lightheaded and nervous, had a headache, and felt like she could not breathe. She felt tingling in her left arm and left side of her head. Since then, she has been afraid of going out on her own, worried that another attack would happen and no one would help her. She has no prior medical history, and the attacks do not occur at home. Which of the following is the most likely diagnosis?

    (A) Agoraphobia

    (B) Avoidant personality disorder

    (C) Dependent personality disorder

    (D) Somatization disorder

    (E) Specific phobia

47. A 29-year-old Asian American woman is seen for the first time by a psychiatrist. She complains of depressed mood, decreased appetite, lack of interest in her usual social activities, decreased energy, and a difficult time concentrating at work for the past 3 months. Occasionally, she feels too fatigued to go to work. Although she denies thoughts of wanting to kill herself, she claims that sometimes she feels that she would be "better off dead." The psychiatrist prescribes medication for her and asks her to return in 6 weeks. On the return visit, she reports that her symptoms are significantly improved. If this patient did not improve and she reported other complaints, such as dry skin, constipation, intolerance to cold temperatures, and hoarse voice, which of the following diagnostic tests would be most appropriate?

    (A) Follicle stimulating hormone (FSH) level
    (B) Thyroid stimulating hormone (TSH) level
    (C) Urinalysis
    (D) Urinary hCG level
    (E) Venereal Disease Research Laboratory (VDRL) test

48. A 38-year-old woman is brought to the emergency department by her husband because of her "odd" behavior over the past day. She seems confused and is unable to recall her name, address, birthday, or age. She is also unable to recall anything about her personal history from the previous 2 months. She and her husband deny any stressful life events or trauma that may have contributed to this. The patient appears appropriately concerned and her mood and affect are congruent with her thought content. Her speech is normal and her thought is organized and goal directed. She denies any use of over-the-counter medication, alcohol, or drugs. Her husband confirms all of the information that she provides. Physical and neurologic examination, blood chemistry, urine toxicology, MRI of the head, lumbar puncture, and EEG are all within normal limits. This patient is most likely suffering from which of the following conditions?

    (A) Anterograde amnesia
    (B) Confabulation
    (C) Dissociative amnesia
    (D) Hypermnesia
    (E) Transient global amnesia

49. A 22-year-old Native American woman sees a psychiatrist for the first time shortly following the dissolution of a 3-year relationship with her boyfriend. She states that she is intensely upset and depressed and experiences frequent crying spells. For the past few days, she has found it difficult to go to work because she cannot seem to shift her focus away from the breakup. Although she can usually find comfort from talking things over with her mother, she notes that she seems to direct her anger at her mother and she feels guilty about this. Which of the following psychotherapeutic interventions is most appropriate?

    (A) Cognitive-behavioral therapy
    (B) Hypnosis
    (C) Psychoanalysis
    (D) Social skills training
    (E) Supportive psychotherapy

50. A 37-year-old man is brought to the emergency department by police after he was found wandering around naked and shouting obscenities. The patient is approached by a female nurse and becomes very agitated. He begins to shout at her and threatens to kill her. He is given an intramuscular injection of haloperidol. Ten minutes later, he complains that his tongue feels thick and that he has difficulty moving because his muscles are stiff. Vital signs are stable. Breathing is unlabored and physical examination is remarkable for diffuse muscular rigidity. Which of the following medications would effectively treat this condition?

    (A) Bromocriptine
    (B) Carbidopa/L-dopa
    (C) Carisoprodol
    (D) Diphenhydramine

Psychiatry Test Two:
Answers and Explanations

ANSWER KEY

1.	A	26.	E
2.	A	27.	D
3.	B	28.	D
4.	A	29.	D
5.	C	30.	E
6.	A	31.	A
7.	B	32.	D
8.	C	33.	E
9.	A	34.	E
10.	A	35.	D
11.	D	36.	C
12.	B	37.	C
13.	D	38.	E
14.	B	39.	D
15.	E	40.	D
16.	A	41.	A
17.	C	42.	B
18.	E	43.	E
19.	A	44.	D
20.	C	45.	E
21.	B	46.	A
22.	C	47.	B
23.	E	48.	C
24.	D	49.	E
25.	A	50.	D

1. **The correct answer is A.** The best diagnosis is adjustment disorder with depressed mood, as the patient had several stressors including a recent hospitalization, a debilitating injury, and an inability to perform his job duties as he had done previously. As a result of these changes, the patient developed some of the symptoms of depression without a full set of symptoms, such as insomnia or anorexia.

The patient does not have any history of manic episodes, which means bipolar disorder, most recent episode depressed (**choice B**), is not a possibility.

Conversion disorder (**choice C**) is a psychiatric disorder in which one or more physical symptoms or deficits affect voluntary motor or sensory function. The diagnosis requires that a symptom or deficit cannot be fully explained by a general medical condition, which is not the case for this patient.

Dysthymic disorder (**choice D**) is a disorder in which mood is depressed for most of the day, for more days than not, for at least 2 years. This diagnosis is not a possibility because the patient's depressive symptoms are limited to the past month.

Major depressive disorder (**choice E**) is not the appropriate diagnosis, as his symptoms have not lasted for more than a few weeks, and the patient does not have the full vegetative set of symptoms of major depressive disorder.

2. **The correct answer is A.** The patient has symptoms suggestive of major depressive disorder, and assessment of suicide risk is paramount in interviewing him. Depressed patients have a significantly higher risk of attempting and completing suicide compared with the general population. Therefore, determining whether a depressed patient is at high risk is essential early in their management.

Although cognitive-behavioral therapy (**choice B**) may be an important adjunct in treating depression, it is not the most appropriate next step in this patient's management.

Although a selective serotonin reuptake inhibitor (SSRI; **choice C**) would be an acceptable pharmacologic intervention in this patient with depression, assessing suicidality takes precedence.

A benzodiazepine (**choice D**) may be acceptable on a short-term basis in an individual who is acutely agitated or has significant symptoms of anxiety. This patient, however, appears calm and cooperates with the examiner, and there is no suggestion for the need for acute use of a benzodiazepine.

A urine drug screen (**choice E**) may prove helpful in differentiating a major depressive episode from a substance-induced mood disorder. However, even patients with a substance-induced mood disorder are at higher risk for suicide than the general population, and assessment of suicidality must occur early in management.

3. **The correct answer is B.** The first step in evaluating insomnia in a patient, after ruling out a mood disorder, is to review the "sleep hygiene" activities that affect the sleep-wake cycle, such as going to bed and waking up at the same time every day. In this case, eating a large meal before retiring might be the reason why this patient is having difficulty falling asleep. Encouraging him to eat an earlier dinner would be an appropriate adjustment in his routine.

Increasing the intensity of the morning workout would likely improve his sleep; decreasing it would prove unhelpful (**choice A**).

Vigorous exercise just prior to going to bed (**choice C**) would likely exacerbate the insomnia.

Although a nightcap (**choice D**) may help the patient fall asleep initially, its effect on sleep architecture would likely keep him from feeling rested on awakening. Increasing his alcohol intake prior to retiring will probably exacerbate this problem.

The use of medication, such as zolpidem (**choice E**), is reserved for situations in which adjustments in sleep hygiene prove ineffective. In addition, hypnotics are intended to be used on a short-term basis only.

4. **The correct answer is A.** Brief psychotic disorder is a diagnosis that requires the sudden onset of a florid psychotic episode immediately after a marked psychosocial stressor in the absence of increasing psychopathology before the stressor.

Delusional disorder (**choice B**) is incorrect because this disorder requires nonbizarre delusions of at least 1 month's duration, which has not occurred in this case.

Drug intoxication (**choice C**) often can present with symptoms similar to brief psychotic disorder, but there is no indication of substance use in this case.

Grief reaction (**choice D**) is an expected and *normal* reaction to the loss of a loved one. The patient's behavior and psychosis are not within the realm of a normal reaction.

Schizophrenia (**choice E**) requires symptoms of psychosis for at least 6 months.

5. **The correct answer is C.** In hypochondriasis, the patient has the firm conviction of having a serious illness, despite repeated evidence to the contrary. Even when presented with definitive evidence, these patients remain convinced that they are ill. Oftentimes these patients make multiple visits to different physicians and undergo repeated diag-

nostic studies, but still remain certain that they have a serious affliction.

In body dysmorphic disorder (**choice A**), the preoccupation has to do with physical appearance, not a physical illness.

In conversion disorder (**choice B**), a deficit or symptom of voluntary motor or sensory function suggests a neurologic disease, which is not present.

Schizophrenia (**choice D**) involves delusions and/or hallucinations, and onset is usually much earlier in life.

Somatization disorder (**choice E**) is characterized by multiple somatic complaints. In hypochondriasis, there is the fear that one has a particular disease.

6. **The correct answer is A.** Of the four benzodiazepines listed, alprazolam has the shortest half-life and the greatest potential for precipitating withdrawal. Benzodiazepine withdrawal, which is indistinguishable from alcohol withdrawal, can be life-threatening.

    Buspirone (**choice B**) is not a benzodiazepine and is not associated with a known withdrawal syndrome. It has FDA approval for generalized anxiety disorder.

    Chlordiazepoxide (**choice C**), clonazepam (**choice D**), and diazepam (**choice E**) are all benzodiazepines with long half-lives. Although abrupt cessation of these medications may precipitate withdrawal, it would be less likely. Therefore, given the choices listed, one would choose the benzodiazepine with the shortest half-life as being the medication most likely to be of concern to the physician.

7. **The correct answer is B.** The diagnosis of autism requires impairment in social interaction and language combined with repetitive or stereotyped patterns of behavior such as hand flapping. There must also be a history of delayed development, occurring prior to age 3 years, in one of the following domains: social interaction, communication, or imaginative play. The etiology is currently unknown, but studies of monozygotic twins suggest a strong genetic component. The most common genetic cause of autism is the fragile X syndrome.

    Asperger syndrome (**choice A**) is similar to autism but spares language function. A patient must have normal language development in the presence of both repetitive or stereotyped behaviors and impaired social interaction.

    Dyslexia (**choice C**) is a language disorder predominantly affecting reading. It may be heralded by a history of language delay in children who are not yet old enough to read, as in this case, but there should be no repetitive behaviors or impaired social interaction.

    Fragile X syndrome (**choice D**) is a common X-linked recessive disorder involving a trinucleotide repeat. It affects boys much more severely than girls, who are usually normal or minimally impaired. It is a common genetic cause of both mental retardation and autism. In addition to symptoms of these two conditions, boys with fragile X often have dysmorphic features, most commonly a long face and enlarged ears.

    Rett syndrome (**choice E**) shares many features of autism, but it affects only girls. In addition to the autistic features, girls with this disorder develop deceleration of head growth between 5 and 48 months of age, lose previously acquired hand skills, and show poor coordination of gait or trunk movements on exam.

8. **The correct answer is C.** Disulfiram inhibits aldehyde dehydrogenase, which causes a marked increase in levels of acetaldehyde after consumption of alcohol, which in turn causes a wide range of unpleasant effects, such as vomiting, headache, and dyspnea. Its success is predicated on the degree of motivation on the part of the patient to abstain from alcohol, as its efficacy is entirely dependent on compliance.

    Acetylcholinesterase (**choice A**) inhibitors used in psychiatry include donepezil and tacrine. These are used to treat Alzheimer type dementia.

    Alcohol dehydrogenase (**choice B**) catalyzes the metabolism of ethanol to acetaldehyde. Disulfiram does not inhibit this first step in alcohol metabolism.

    Several medications affect the cytochrome P450 (**choice D**) system, necessitating appropriate adjustments in dosing. Disulfiram's mechanism of action, however, is at the site of the aldehyde dehydrogenase enzyme.

    Tyrosine hydroxylase (**choice E**) converts tyrosine into DOPA, a neurochemical conversion unrelated to the mechanism of action of disulfiram.

9. **The correct answer is A.** Counterphobic behavior refers to seeking out situations or objects that are or were feared. The person actually takes a position of actively attempting to confront and master what he or she fears.

    Denial (**choice B**) is the avoidance of awareness of a painful aspect of reality by negating sensory data and thus abolishing external reality. Denial may be seen in both normal and pathologic states.

    Reaction formation (**choice C**) transforms an unacceptable impulse into its opposite. It is used in all stages of development and is typically seen in obsessive disorders.

    Regression (**choice D**) is a type of behavior through which a person attempts to avoid tension and conflict at a present level of development by going to an earlier libidinal phase of functioning. It can be normal or can reflect the need to gain easier gratification at a less developed stage.

Undoing (**choice E**) is a secondary defensive operation that a person uses to undo or prevent the consequences that are anticipated irrationally as a result of unacceptable thought or impulse. It is mostly seen in obsessive disorders.

10. **The correct answer is A.** Delirium tremens is the most common cause of delirium in a patient who is suddenly admitted to the hospital for an unrelated condition and no longer has access to alcohol. It is a medical emergency, with a 15% mortality rate if left untreated. It usually occurs within 1 week after the patient stops drinking.

    Infection (**choice B**) is a complication leading to delirium after surgery, but it is commonly associated with a high fever.

    Pain medications (**choice C**) can cause delirium, but usually in elderly patients whose metabolic functions are compromised.

    Postoperative depression (**choice D**) is not a known cause of delirium.

    The stress of surgery (**choice E**) is a cause of postoperative delirium, but it is less common and usually occurs in procedures such as organ transplants.

11. **The correct answer is D.** Olanzapine, an atypical antipsychotic, has been demonstrated to lead to weight gain in many patients with schizophrenia, with studies showing a gain of up to 27 pounds in the course of a year. Olanzapine affects the $5HT_2$ serotonin receptor in the brain, which is also thought to control satiety, in addition to decreasing auditory hallucinations and controlling mood symptoms.

    Alcohol use (**choice A**) can lead to weight gain but would not have caused the significant gain in this patient, as he only recently began drinking more.

    Decreased auditory hallucinations (**choice B**) have not been shown to have a significant correlation to appetite and subsequent weight gain.

    There is no increase in appetite or weight associated with the discontinuation of risperidone (**choice C**).

    Although some patients do overeat in response to stress, this activity is more common in female than in male patients. In addition, this patient describes his familial problems (**choice E**) as more recent in their onset; therefore, this would not be the most likely cause for his weight gain.

12. **The correct answer is B.** Tangentiality is a disturbance in communication characterized by a lack of goal-directed association of thoughts. Patients cannot mentally get from a desired starting point to a desired goal (in this case an answer as to which floor of the hospital the patient is on), but instead jump from one topic to another.

Circumstantiality (**choice A**) is speech in which a patient eventually reaches the answer to a question, but frequently digresses along the way before arriving back at the central idea.

Thought blocking (**choice C**) is an abrupt interruption in a patient's logical progression of thought before an idea or thought is finished.

Verbigeration (**choice D**) is the meaningless repetition of specific words or phrases.

Word salad (**choice E**) is a completely incoherent mixture of words and phrases that have no grammatical meaning in language.

13. **The correct answer is D.** This patient is experiencing side effects associated with therapeutic or lower levels of lithium carbonate. These side effects are often troublesome and include sedation, cognitive difficulties, dry mouth, hand tremor, increased appetite, polydipsia and polyuria, nausea, diarrhea, psoriasis, and acne.

    The most common side effects associated with carbamazepine (**choice A**) include dizziness, ataxia, sedation, dysarthria, nausea, hyponatremia, and cardiovascular conduction problems. Its most serious side effects are aplastic anemia and agranulocytosis. Rarely, it can cause rash and exfoliation.

    Fluoxetine (**choice B**) causes nausea, dyspepsia, tremor, nervousness, and increased anxiety during the initial phase of treatment. It has no effect on fluid intake or worsening of dermatologic diseases.

    Side effects associated with haloperidol (**choice C**) typically are a consequence of the blockade of dopaminergic D2 receptors. Apart from a spectrum of extrapyramidal symptoms, side effects include sedation, weight gain, hyperprolactinemia, and possible neuroleptic malignant syndrome.

    Valproic acid (**choice E**) most commonly causes short-term nausea, vomiting, diarrhea, sedation, dizziness, and tremor. Alopecia and weight gain are long-term side effects.

14. **The correct answer is B.** The monoamine oxidase inhibitors (MAOIs) used to treat depression inhibit the A form of the enzyme, which results in increased concentrations of norepinephrine, serotonin, and dopamine wherever the enzyme is present. Dietary tyramine, which is present in foods such as aged cheeses as well as in red wine, can enter the circulation unmetabolized (as alimentary MAO-A is also inhibited) and act as a pressor. If a patient on an MAOI eats foods rich in tyramine or takes certain medications bearing similarities to biogenic amines, a life-threatening hypertensive crisis could develop.

Agranulocytosis (**choice A**) is an idiosyncratic adverse event associated with clozapine, among other drugs.

Pigmentary retinopathy (**choice C**) has been reported in patients taking high (>800 mg/day) doses of thioridazine.

Priapism (**choice D**) is associated with trazodone use.

Serotonin syndrome (**choice E**) can occur in individuals taking a serotonin-altering medication (such as an SSRI) in addition to an MAOI. This potentially life-threatening syndrome is characterized by autonomic instability and motor and behavioral abnormalities.

15. **The correct answer is E.** Trichotillomania is an impulse control disorder. It is usually seen in childhood or adolescence and is most common in girls. It is manifested by repetitive pulling of one's hair from any part of the body. The tension before pulling is usually relieved afterward. The disturbance is related to impulsive urges, making it different from goal-directed obsessional ideas. The disorder is not due to a general medical condition or the effects of any substance.

Bulimia nervosa (**choice A**) refers to episodes of binge eating characterized by a sense of lack of control. During those episodes patients take in an amount of food larger than most people would eat. It occurs at least twice a month for 3 months and includes inappropriate behavior to prevent weight gain, such as misuse of laxatives or self-induced vomiting. Bulimia may be comorbid with trichotillomania but does not include hair eating itself.

Factitious disorder (**choice B**) is intentional production of or feigning of symptoms of illness to assume the sick role. External motivation, like economic gain or avoidance of legal responsibility, is absent.

Major depressive disorder (**choice C**) requires symptoms of anhedonia and/or depressed mood every day for at least 2 weeks, along with associated symptoms of depression such as low energy, insomnia, weight loss, poor appetite, and poor concentration. It can be comorbid with trichotillomania.

Obsessive-compulsive disorder (**choice D**) is defined by recurrent intrusive thoughts or impulses that cause marked distress. The person tries to ignore or suppress them or to neutralize them with some action. The patient is aware that those ideas are the product of his or her mind and are unreasonable.

16. **The correct answer is A.** There is a 1% to 2% risk of agranulocytosis in patients treated with clozapine. This idiosyncratic event can occur at any time in the course of treatment but is most likely to occur within the first 6 months. Subsequently, periodic examination of a white blood cell count with differential is essential while treating with clozapine.

Clozapine has no effect on prolactin levels (**choice B**) or serum glucose levels (**choice C**).

There is the possibility of renal toxicity (**choice D**) and hypothyroidism (**choice E**) with lithium treatment, not clozapine.

17. **The correct answer is C.** One of the hallmark characteristics of borderline personality disorder is affective instability, recognized as rapidly shifting mood states. Other symptoms include unstable and intense interpersonal relationships, chronic feelings of emptiness, and recurrent suicidal thoughts and gestures, often dramatic and attention-seeking in character.

Attention deficit/hyperactivity disorder (ADHD; **choice A**) is associated with impulsivity, as is intermittent explosive disorder (**choice D**); however, mood swings and recurrent suicidality are not essential features.

Bipolar disorder (**choice B**) is also associated with extremes of mood; however, mood states usually last for days to weeks.

Major depression (**choice E**) is often comorbid in patients with borderline personality disorder; however, there is insufficient evidence to make such a diagnosis here.

18. **The correct answer is E.** There is a clinical distinction in patients with schizophrenia between positive (or productive) symptoms of schizophrenia and negative (or deficit) symptoms. Although not accepted as part of the DSM-IV classification, the clinical distinction of the two types has significantly influenced psychiatric research. Positive symptoms of schizophrenia include delusions, hallucinations, thought insertion, and thought broadcasting.

Negative symptoms include affective flattening (**choice A**), deficits in attention (**choice B**), poor eye contact (**choice C**), and alogia, which is the lack of ability to produce normal fluent speech (**choice D**).

19. **The correct answer is A.** Akathisia denotes a state of extreme motor restlessness. The patient cannot sit still and is constantly walking, shifting weight, and pacing. It is seen in encephalitic illnesses and as a complication of neuroleptic treatment.

Akinesia (**choice B**) is a term that refers to a failure of the patient to engage the limbs in customary activities. It results in poverty of movement, including small automatic postural adjustments, as well as in volitional movements. It is seen in Parkinson disease and related disorders.

Festination (**choice C**) is a gait disorder characteristic of Parkinson disease. The patient's trunk is bent forward, the arms are slightly flexed, the legs are bent at knees, and steps are short and shuffling. With walking, the upper body advances ahead of the lower and steps become increasingly rapid to "catch up."

Stereotypic movement disorder (**choice D**) is repetitive nonfunctional motor behavior (rocking, head banging, self-biting, picking) lasting at least 4 weeks. It is usually seen in mental retardation or pervasive developmental disorder, and it significantly interferes with normal activities.

Tardive dyskinesia (**choice E**) is a late-appearing disorder of involuntary, choreoathetoid movements of the orofacial region or trunk and limbs, following neuroleptic treatment. The movements are present at least 4 weeks. The neuroleptic treatment must last at least 3 months, or the movements must develop within 4 weeks after withdrawal from treatment.

20. **The correct answer is C.** This girl has schizophrenia, which has a lifetime prevalence of 0.6% to 1.9% (1% is most often cited as the average lifetime prevalence). About 0.025% to 0.05% of the total population is treated for schizophrenia in any single year. It is equally prevalent in men and women; however, the onset and course of illness differ between the sexes. Onset is earlier in men than in women. The peak age for men is 15-25 years, and the peak age for women is 25-35 years. In general, the outcome for patients with schizophrenia is better for women than for men; some studies have suggested that men are more likely to be impaired with negative symptoms and have poorer social functioning. Interestingly, the use of psychotherapeutic drugs, the deinstitutionalization of state hospitals, the emphasis on rehabilitation, and the community-based care for schizophrenic patients have led to an increase in the marriage and fertility rates among people with schizophrenia. Because of this, the number of children with at least one schizophrenic parent recently doubled.

The lifetime prevalence for major depressive disorder is 10% to 25% for women and 5% to 12% for men. The lifetime prevalence for dysthymic disorder is 6%. The lifetime prevalence for bipolar I disorder is 0.4% to 1.6%; for bipolar II disorder, it is 0.5%. The lifetime prevalence for cyclothymic disorder is 0.4% to 1.0%.

21. **The correct answer is B.** For a patient to be admitted involuntarily to an inpatient psychiatric unit, she must show evidence of either being harmful to others or to herself (either by a suicide attempt, self-mutilation, or self-neglect). This patient has clearly acted as a danger not only to herself but also to others. She may be suffering from depression, bipolar disorder, psychosis, substance abuse, obsessive-compulsive disorder, posttraumatic stress disorder, or other psychiatric conditions. She needs a thorough evaluation on a highly monitored inpatient psychiatry unit to better understand her condition.

Choices A and C are unacceptable because it is too dangerous for this patient to leave the hospital. Ultimately she may benefit from a day program and/or from outpatient care but certainly not at this point. Also, if the clinician believes that a patient is dangerous enough to require observation checks at the frequency of every 15 minutes, the patient most likely needs around-the-clock inpatient care.

Studies have shown that written contracts with psychiatric patients (**choice D**) are usually worthless. Their only consistently demonstrated value is for the evaluation of a patient who states that she is unable to contract for safety. Under these circumstances, it is made clear to the staff that the person does not trust herself to stay safe.

Calling the police to report her as having endangered her children and unborn fetus (**choice E**) may be necessary at some point, but the priority in the emergency department is to ensure the patient's safety, and this must be through an involuntary hospitalization.

22. **The correct answer is C.** The listed symptoms are suggestive that this woman has delusional disorder, persecutory type, as her beliefs are not outside the realm of reason but are probably not based in reality. Her feelings that other people are out to hurt or injure her put the delusional disorder in the realm of persecutory type.

Capgras syndrome (**choice A**) is the delusion that others, or oneself, have been replaced by impostors. It typically follows the development of negative feelings toward the other person or self that the subject cannot accept and instead attributes to an impostor. The syndrome is frequently found in organic brain disease.

Delirium (**choice B**) requires an alteration of the state of consciousness, which this patient does not have.

Paranoid schizophrenia (**choice D**) is a diagnosis that requires that the patient have some of the symptoms of schizophrenia, including auditory hallucinations, thought blocking, or blunted affect. The patient's age and her ability to obtain employment make schizophrenia an unlikely diagnosis in this case.

In shared psychotic disorder (**choice E**), the patient has a system of disordered thought that is assumed by another person. In most cases, this disorder is found among spouses; typically the spouse with the psychotic disorder is more dominant in the social relationship.

23. **The correct answer is E.** The patient is presenting with a full-blown mania, in which delusions of grandeur are common and congruent with euphoric elevated mood.

Delusions of self-accusation (**choice A**) are false feelings of remorse and guilt frequently seen in depressive disorder with psychotic features.

Delusions of poverty (**choice B**) are false beliefs that one is bereft or will be deprived of all the material possessions.

Delusions of reference (**choice C**) are false beliefs that one is being talked about by others and that events or people have unusual significance in relationship to oneself.

Somatic delusion (**choice D**) is a false belief involving the function of one's body and can be seen in psychotic disorders of schizophrenic spectrum, as well as in depressive disorder with psychotic features.

24. **The correct answer is D.** This patient has bipolar disorder. He is currently in a manic episode, characterized by at least a week (at least 8 days in his case) of inflated self-esteem, pressure to talk, and a goal-directed focus on a grandiose wish to be president. He also has engaged in excessive involvement in sexual indiscretions without regard for the potential dangerous outcomes. Further, although not described in the question, the patient likely has a decreased need for sleep, likely has a subjective feeling that his thoughts are racing, and likely has a wavering attention span. Flight of ideas is characteristic of mania but not of depression. A flight of ideas is a rapid jumping of thoughts through a series of tenuously related ideas that make more sense to the manic patient than to the examiner.

Anhedonia (**choice A**) is characteristic of depression but not mania. Anhedonia is characterized by the absence of pleasure from other persons, situations, or things that would ordinarily be pleasurable. During a manic episode, persons often experience the opposite of anhedonia by finding pleasure in things that do not typically evoke such a contented response.

Decreased sleep (**choice B**) is usually characteristic of both mania and depression. In mania, persons often do not feel as though they need a lot of sleep. In depression, persons have difficulty in both falling asleep and staying asleep. Early morning awakening with an inability to fall back asleep is very common in depression. The net result for both mania and depression typically is decreased sleep.

Distractibility (**choice C**) can be an attribute of both mania and depression. In manic individuals, their attention is often too easily drawn to unimportant or irrelevant external stimuli. In depressed individuals, they are usually unable to focus on completing any one task, since all tasks are often perceived as too difficult to complete. These people are often distracted by their own sad moods.

Impairment of functioning (**choice E**) is among the DSM-IV list of criteria for both a manic episode and a major depressive episode.

25. **The correct answer is A.** Panic disorder is characterized by the spontaneous, unexpected occurrence of panic attacks. Panic disorder is often accompanied by agoraphobia, the fear of being alone in public places. Alcohol and other substance dependence occurs in about 20% to 40% of all patients with panic disorder.

Diabetes (**choice B**) and hypoglycemia (**choice C**) are incorrect because neither low nor high blood sugar levels are known to cause psychiatric disorders, although many patients believe that panic disorder is caused by hypoglycemia.

Mitral valve prolapse (**choice D**) is incorrect because, although many people believe that mitral valve prolapse leads to panic disorder, there is no evidence that panic disorder is more prevalent in patients with mitral valve prolapse than in the general population.

There is no established correlation between the incidence of obesity (**choice E**) and the incidence of panic disorder in the general population.

26. **The correct answer is E.** The clinical vignette is illustrative of dementia of the Alzheimer type. Not only are there typical signs of memory loss, but there may also be evidence of paranoid ideation or delusions, especially as the disease advances. Microscopic examination of postmortem brain tissue reveals the presence of neurofibrillary tangles and senile plaques, which are present to a lesser extent in the brains of nondemented elderly individuals. It is the correlation between the patient's presentation and the abundance of these microscopic features that ensures the diagnosis.

Necrosis of the globus pallidus (**choice A**) is suggestive of carbon monoxide poisoning, which is acute in presentation and may result in an amnestic syndrome with affective disturbance. Laboratory test shows elevated carboxyhemoglobin levels.

Focal demyelination and gliosis of periventricular white matter (**choice B**) are consistent with multiple sclerosis. Initially, symptoms of paresthesias, gait disturbance, motor weakness, and visual effects generally begin before the age of 55, and women are slightly more often affected than are men.

Involvement of the mammillary bodies is consistent with Wernicke encephalopathy (**choice C**), which results from severe thiamine deficiency and is most often associated with chronic alcoholism. Wernicke encephalopathy is characterized by the triad of confusion, ataxia, and nystagmus leading to ophthalmoplegia.

Parkinson disease is microscopically characterized by loss of pigmented cells in the substantia nigra (**choice D**). Clinically, it is characterized by tremor, rigidity, hypokinesia, and abnormal gait and posture.

27. **The correct answer is D.** Opioid withdrawal follows cessation or reduction of prolonged and heavy opioid use and includes at least three of the following symptoms: dysphoric mood, nausea or vomiting, muscle aches, yawning, diarrhea, lacrimation, rhinorrhea, piloerection, pupillary dilatation, sweating, fever, and insomnia. The symptoms cause significant distress in social or occupational functioning and are not due to a general medical condition.

Alprazolam (**choice A**) is a benzodiazepine. Withdrawal starts after a reduction or cessation of prolonged alprazolam use. Symptoms may include autonomic hyperactivity, increased hand tremor, insomnia, nausea and vomiting, transient hallucinations, psychomotor agitation, grand mal seizures, or anxiety.

Amphetamine (**choice B**) withdrawal follows a cessation of prolonged and heavy amphetamine use. The symptoms include dysphoric mood and physiologic changes, such as fatigue, unpleasant dreams, insomnia or hypersomnia, increased appetite, psychomotor retardation, or agitation.

Cocaine (**choice C**) withdrawal follows a cessation of heavy and prolonged cocaine use. The symptoms include dysphoric mood and physiologic changes, such as fatigue, increased appetite, psychomotor retardation or agitation, insomnia or hypersomnia, or vivid unpleasant dreams.

Nicotine (**choice E**) withdrawal starts within 24 hours after abrupt cessation of nicotine use. Withdrawal signs include dysphoric mood, insomnia, irritability, difficulty concentrating, anxiety, restlessness, decreased heart rate, and increased appetite.

28. **The correct answer is D.** The most common compulsion associated with obsessive-compulsive disorder (OCD) is excessive or ritualized hand washing, showering, bathing, toothbrushing, or grooming, with a reported rate of nearly 60% of all patients. The typical pharmacologic treatment for OCD is a selective serotonin reuptake inhibitor (SSRI) such as sertraline.

Avoidance of social situations (**choice A**) is not a compulsion. It is more a symptom of avoidant personality disorder than of OCD.

Incessant checking (**choice B**) occurs in about 32% of all OCD patients.

Repeating rituals (**choice C**) occurs in about 36% of all OCD patients.

Striving for completeness (**choice E**) is a nonpathologic trait that is not indicative of psychiatric illness in the general population.

29. **The correct answer is D.** It is generally accepted that there are no absolute contraindications to receiving electroconvulsive therapy (ECT). There are situations in which risk is increased and close monitoring is prudent; however, any patient is a potential candidate for ECT.

Although patients who have had a recent myocardial infarction (**choice A**) are at higher risk for complications from ECT, this risk is significantly reduced 3 months after the event. Therefore, it would be inappropriate to say that any patient who has ever had a myocardial infarction should never receive ECT.

Pregnancy (**choice B**) is incorrect; in fact, ECT may be the most appropriate treatment for a variety of disorders in a first-trimester pregnant patient, for whom certain medications may pose a teratogenic risk to the fetus.

Although, ideally, a patient should discontinue anticonvulsants during ECT, patients with a seizure disorder on anticonvulsants can safely be treated with ECT (**choice C**), often with excellent results. In fact, one indication for ECT is for intractable seizures. The thought is that repeated seizures actually increases seizure threshold.

Age itself (**choice E**) is not an absolute or relative contraindication to ECT. ECT may, in fact, be the only reasonable option in an elderly patient who may otherwise not tolerate psychotropic medications. ECT is frequently used and is very safe in geriatric populations.

30. **The correct answer is E.** Reaction formation is a defense in which an unacceptable impulse or feeling becomes transformed into its opposite. It is mostly seen in obsessive behavior but can be seen in other forms of neurosis.

Blocking (**choice A**) is a temporary inhibition of thinking. It also applies to affect and impulses. It is similar to repression, except that the patient feels tense once blocking of thoughts, feelings, or impulses is inhibited.

Displacement (**choice B**) occurs when an emotion is shifted from one idea or object to another. It permits symbolic representation of the original idea in a way that causes less distress than the original.

Inhibition (**choice C**) is a conscious process by which ego evades anxiety arising from conflicts with instinctual impulses, the superego, or external stressors.

Isolation (**choice D**) is the separation of an idea from the affect that accompanies it. The affect remains repressed while the patient talks freely about the idea.

31. **The correct answer is A.** In the erotomanic type of delusional disorder, the central delusion evolves around the patient's belief that a famous person or a superior is intensely in love with the patient. Erotomanic patients usually harass public figures (objects of their delusion) through letters, calls, gifts, or visits. The disorder is more

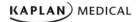

frequent in women who are single and have had limited intimate contacts and a modest, isolated way of life. The onset is usually after the age of 40, but can be earlier.

In jealous type delusional disorder (**choice B**), the central delusion concerns the fidelity of the spouse. Men are more affected, and the disorder can lead to significant abuse, following a search "for evidence." At times, the accusation of infidelity results in the murder of the "accused" spouse. There is frequent association with alcoholism.

Grandiose delusions (**choice C**) are associated with megalomania and mostly involve the belief of having made important discoveries, or having unrecognized talents. At times they may have a religious content, and the patients become leaders of religious cults.

Persecutory delusions (**choice D**) are the most common type and involve the single idea of being conspired against, spied on, followed, or obstructed in achievement of long-term goals. As a result of their delusion, patients may become angry and violent.

The somatic type delusional disorder (**choice E**) is also known as monosymptomatic hypochondriacal psychosis. Patients are convinced that they have a presumed illness, most commonly infection, or some body odor. The disorder is seen in both sexes and is differentiated from hypochondriasis by the degree of conviction.

32. **The correct answer is D.** The diagnosis of schizophrenia requires that at least two of the following symptoms be present for at least a 1-month period: delusions, hallucinations, disorganized speech, disorganized or catatonic behavior, or flattened affect. In addition, a milder degree of these symptoms must be present for at least 6 months. Symptoms must be severe enough to interfere with work or school performance. The peak age of onset for men is 15-25. Imaging is typically normal but may show enlarged lateral ventricles.

Bipolar disorder (**choice A**) may have a similar age of onset and may present with psychotic features, but there is no indication of prominent manic or depressive behavior in this case.

Patients with delusional disorder (**choice B**) report less bizarre delusions (i.e., "people at work are doctoring my reports to get me fired") than are typically reported in schizophrenia. The delusions in this disorder occur in isolation, so that other symptoms of schizophrenia (e.g., disorganized behavior, hallucinations) should be absent.

Depression with psychotic features (**choice C**) can present with prominent auditory hallucinations and delusions but on a background of major depression. Typically, patients have a substantial history of depression prior to developing psychotic features.

Schizophreniform disorder (**choice E**) is diagnosed when a patient meets all criteria for schizophrenia but has had symptoms for only 1-6 months. Most of these patients go on to develop schizophrenia.

33. **The correct answer is E.** The outward lack of concern for a physical illness is called la belle indifference. The term was introduced by Pierre Janet and is mostly seen in conversion disorder.

Denial (**choice A**) is the avoidance of the awareness of a painful aspect of reality by negating sensory data and thus abolishing external reality. Denial may be seen in normal as well as in pathologic states.

Depersonalization (**choice B**) is characterized by persistent recurrent episodes of feeling detached from one's self or body, like feeling mechanical or in a dream. Reality testing remains intact during those episodes. It can happen in depersonalization disorder or as a part of other mental disorders.

Displacement (**choice C**) occurs when an emotion is shifted from one idea or object to another. It permits symbolic representation of the original idea in a way that causes less distress than the original.

Dissociation (**choice D**) is a way that an individual deals with emotional conflict or stressors with a breakdown in the integrated functions of consciousness, memory, or perception of self or environment.

34. **The correct answer is E.** Tardive dyskinesia is a syndrome of abnormal involuntary movements often associated with long-term neuroleptic use. Risk factors for tardive dyskinesia include long-term treatment with dopamine receptor antagonists (typical neuroleptics), female sex, presence of a mood disorder, or increasing age. Serotonin-dopamine antagonists, also known as atypical antipsychotics, are associated with a lower risk of development of tardive dyskinesia than typical antipsychotics, so substituting a serotonin-dopamine antagonist might help to limit the abnormal movements without worsening the progression of tardive dyskinesia.

Addition of an anticholinergic drug (**choice A**) has not been found to be beneficial in most cases, because tardive dyskinesia does not appear to result directly from disruption of the nigrostriatal dopamine pathway.

Although addition of a dopamine receptor antagonist (**choice B**) can suppress tardive dyskinesia temporarily, it can cause a rebound effect of more intense tardive dyskinesia at a later time and is not recommended.

Making no changes (**choice C**) is contraindicated, as tardive dyskinesia will continue to progress on the same medication.

Stopping the patient's antipsychotic medication (**choice D**) usually makes tardive dyskinesia worse.

35. **The correct answer is D.** Panic disorder with agoraphobia is a disorder characterized by recurrent unexpected panic attacks with associated agoraphobia (fear of crowds or public places). The current treatment of choice for this disorder is an antidepressant, usually a selective serotonin reuptake inhibitor (SSRI) such as paroxetine, although tricyclic antidepressants (TCAs) and monoamine oxidase inhibitors (MAOIs) have also been demonstrated to have efficacy.

Diazepam (**choice A**) and temazepam (**choice E**) are benzodiazepines, which must be used in higher than typical doses in treating panic disorder.

Haloperidol (**choice B**) is an antipsychotic and is not indicated in panic disorder.

Lithium carbonate (**choice C**) is a treatment for mania and bipolar disorder but is not indicated in panic disorder with agoraphobia.

36. **The correct answer is C.** This case illustrates poisoning by methanol. A history of known alcohol dependence (such individuals may use methanol as a substitute for ethanol), visual disturbances, and examination findings of altered mental status, papilledema, and abdominal pain suggest the diagnosis. Methanol is converted to formaldehyde by alcohol dehydrogenase, and formaldehyde is further metabolized to formic acid by formaldehyde dehydrogenase. It is formic acid that is primarily responsible for the visual disturbances and metabolic acidosis experienced with methanol poisoning. Fomepizole is a competitive inhibitor of alcohol dehydrogenase eliminating the production of formaldehyde and therefore eliminating the production of formic acid. Fomepizole is expensive. Before the advent of fomepizole, intravenous ethanol was administered to patients with methanol poisoning because methanol and ethanol compete for the enzyme alcohol dehydrogenase, which prefers ethanol. Unfortunately this led to long periods of difficult ethanol drip titrations, and many hospitals had difficulties with the ethanol being "borrowed" from the pharmacy by medical students.

Activated charcoal (**choice A**) is used for decontamination of several toxic substances by adsorption to the toxin in the gastrointestinal tract. Activated charcoal has not been shown to adsorb methanol; therefore, it is not useful in methanol poisoning.

Disulfiram (**choice B**) is an aldehyde dehydrogenase inhibitor. It is used in alcohol dependence as a deterrent to alcohol consumption. Inhibition of aldehyde dehydrogenase by disulfiram causes an increased concentration of acetaldehyde when ethanol is consumed, producing

unpleasant effects. Inhibition of aldehyde dehydrogenase in a person who ingested methanol would lead to accumulation of formaldehyde, which is quite toxic.

Flumazenil (**choice D**) is a benzodiazepine receptor antagonist and has no place in the therapy of methanol overdose.

Naloxone (**choice E**) is an opioid receptor antagonist and is used in opiate overdose only.

37. **The correct answer is C.** In primitive idealization, external objects are unrealistically endowed with great power and are either "all good" or "all bad." All good objects are ideal and omnipotent; the badness of the others is also greatly inflated.

Displacement (**choice A**) occurs when an emotion or a drive is shifted from one idea or object to another that resembles the original. This allows the symbolic representation of the original idea in a less threatening way.

Distortion (**choice B**) is a defense in which external reality is reshaped to suit inner needs. Unrealistic beliefs, delusions, and hallucinations are used to sustain the feelings of superiority or entitlement.

Projection (**choice D**) is a mechanism by which a person attributes his or her intolerable feelings or affects to another person. It is usually seen in psychotic states, especially in paranoid syndromes.

Splitting (**choice E**) is a defense in which external objects are divided into "all good" and "all bad," accompanied by abrupt shifting of an object from one category to another or sudden reversal of feelings about the same person.

38. **The correct answer is E.** A meta-analysis makes use of data from prior studies to synthesize new data and determine more precise statistical information for a particular question. The article described pools the data from six studies concerned with the use of St. John's wort in depression to make broader generalizations than could be made from a single study.

Case-control studies (**choice A**) compare patients with a particular disease or condition with individuals ("controls") who have similar demographics but do not have the disease in question. Case-controls do not pool data from other studies as meta-analyses do.

A case report (**choice B**) describes the medical history of one particular patient.

In cohort studies (**choice C**), two or more groups of individuals with similar characteristics, who differ on the basis of exposure to a particular agent, are followed over time to determine how many individuals in each of the groups develop a particular disease.

In cross-sectional surveys (**choice D**), data are collected at a given time-point but may refer to past medical history. As in the other incorrect choices, these data are used to produce a single study, which may be used in a meta-analysis at some later point.

39. **The correct answer is D.** Thioridazine belongs to the phenothiazine group of antipsychotics that can cause pigmentary retinopathy when doses higher than recommended are given. Clinically, the patient experiences diminished visual acuity, brownish coloring of vision, and impaired night vision. Funduscopic examination discloses the deposits of pigment. The condition is listed as a psychiatric emergency. Remaining within recommended dose limits could reduce the risk of complications.

Clozapine (**choice A**) is a dibenzodiazepine derivative that can cause diverse side effects, such as agranulocytosis, orthostatic hypotension, hepatitis, fever, seizures, pulmonary embolism, and hyperglycemia. The most common gastrointestinal side effect is constipation. Hypersalivation is also very common.

Haloperidol (**choice B**) belongs to butyrophenone group and is a potent antipsychotic. Its side effects are related to dopaminergic D2 blockade, but it can also cause cardiovascular and gastrointestinal side effects and autonomic reactions. Cataracts, visual disturbances, and retinopathy have been very rarely described.

Pimozide (**choice C**) belongs to diphenylbutylpiperidine group. It can cause tardive dyskinesia and neuroleptic malignant syndrome like other antipsychotics, but most commonly it causes sedation and drowsiness, gastrointestinal symptoms, and ECG changes with prolongation of the QT interval. It can rarely cause blurred vision and cataracts.

Thiothixene (**choice E**) is a thioxanthene derivative that is effective in the management of psychotic disorders. Adverse reactions involving the CNS (drowsiness, extrapyramidal symptoms), cardiovascular system (hypotension, tachycardia), and liver (elevated hepatic enzymes) have been reported. Other side effects include the ones usually produced by other phenothiazines; pigmentary retinopathy is not one of them.

40. **The correct answer is D.** Sinemet, which is a combination drug composed of L-dopa and carbidopa, is not infrequently implicated in emergence of psychotic symptoms in patients with advanced Parkinson disease who require frequent dosing. Increased load of L-dopa causes overactivity of dopaminergic cells in the mesolimbic and mesocortical tracts, which are believed to be involved in producing psychotic symptoms.

In delusional disorder (**choice A**), hallucinations are absent.

Although depression with psychotic features (**choice B**) may be associated with visual hallucinations and delusions, this man describes his mood as "generally okay."

Digoxin toxicity (**choice C**) may affect vision; however, it is not associated with frank psychosis.

New-onset schizophrenia (**choice E**) would be exceedingly rare in a 71-year-old man.

41. **The correct answer is A.** In factitious disorder, the patient intentionally produces or feigns signs or symptoms, although the motivation behind such action is largely unconscious and often serves to place the patient into the sick role. In this case, the patient may be surreptitiously injecting insulin or taking oral hypoglycemics. It is not uncommon for the affected individual to be a member of the health care community who may be familiar with the presentation of certain disease states.

Ganser syndrome (**choice B**) is perhaps best classified as a subtype of malingering, commonly seen in prison inmates, and is characterized by the use of approximate, but completely inappropriate, answers. For example, when asked what the middle color of a traffic light is, one might reply "blue." The deception is advertent in an attempt to minimize criminal culpability by feigning mental illness.

Hypochondriasis (**choice C**) is the preoccupation with fears of having a serious physical illness based on a person's misinterpretation of bodily symptoms. In this vignette, the patient intentionally creates a physical disease within herself so as to unconsciously achieve secondary gain. In hypochondriasis, there is no apparent unconscious motivation for believing to be ill.

Malingering (**choice D**) is the voluntary production of physical or psychological symptoms for external gain, such as to attain admission to the hospital for the sole purpose of shelter or to make a workers' compensation claim. The difference between malingering and factitious disorder is that, in malingering, both the production of and motivation behind displaying symptoms of illness are conscious.

In anorexia nervosa (**choice E**), there is an intense fear of gaining weight, and weight reduction is achieved through either severely restricting dietary intake or binge eating followed by purging. Intentional production of hypoglycemia would not be consistent with a diagnosis of anorexia nervosa.

42. **The correct answer is B.** Sexuality, in general, and sexual preference, in particular, are subjects that many physicians are uncomfortable addressing; however, they are important aspects of human life and have medical and psychosocial ramifications. Although homosexuality is no longer considered a mental illness, the discovery of

one's own sexual preference may cause significant distress in that person and in other family members. Accordingly, physicians are charged with the responsibility to identify these concerns and address them with any involved.

Although experimentation with homosexual behavior, particularly in adolescence (**choice A**), is much more common than lifelong homosexuality, it would be inappropriate to assume that any such behavior is mere experimentation. Disseminating such information would likely serve to mitigate the discomfort felt by both the physician and the patient in this case; however, it would be misleading.

Any physician should feel comfortable discussing issues of sexuality, not just psychiatrists (**choice C**). Such disclosure should be treated with the same degree of sensitivity and confidentiality as any other personal information.

Although the patient's son's private affairs are his own business, it would not be considered a breach of confidentiality to discuss the content matter that the patient has disclosed (compare with **choice D**). In fact, refusing to discuss the issue, and thereby dismissing the patient's distress, would be considered inappropriate.

Although it is appropriate to acknowledge a patient's feelings, it is not acceptable to make assumptions as to why she may feel upset; therefore, **choice E** is incorrect. At no point did the patient state she did not like gay people, and it is wrong for the physician to assume such.

43. **The correct answer is E.** Tourette syndrome belongs to the group of tic disorders with onset before age 18. It is most common in boys. Multiple motor and vocal tics are present many times a day, every day, for more than a year, with no tic-free period greater than 3 months. Coprolalia and echolalia occur later.

Attention deficit/hyperactivity disorder (**choice A**) is more frequently seen in males and is characterized by inattention, hyperactivity, or impulsivity persisting at least 6 months. It is not due to any pervasive developmental disorder or other mental disorder.

Autistic disorder (**choice B**) is a pervasive developmental disorder starting in early childhood. It is characterized by qualitative impairment in social interaction and communication, as well as restricted repetitive and stereotyped patterns of behavior or interests. Delay or abnormal functioning with onset prior to 3 years is seen in the areas of social interaction, language, and communication or symbolic play.

Huntington disease (**choice C**) is a dominantly inherited disorder that begins in mid-adult life and is characterized by a hyperkinetic movement disorder and intellectual decline. Involuntary choreiform movements typically affect the limbs or trunk. Intellectual decline usually progresses into dementia of the subcortical type.

Oppositional defiant disorder (**choice D**) occurs in childhood and consists of a pattern of negativistic, hostile, and defiant behavior lasting at least 6 months. During this period, at least four of the following symptoms must be present: loss of temper, arguments with adults, blaming others for own mistakes, deliberately annoying others, and refusing to comply with rules.

44. **The correct answer is D.** This woman has Parkinson disease (PD), which is an idiopathic subcortical degenerative disease that predominantly affects cells containing dopamine. The typical age of onset is 50-60 years, and the clinical course is chronic and progressive, with severe disability usually after 10 years of illness. Subcortical diseases in general affect the "three M's": movement, mentation, and mood. In PD, all three are affected but not necessarily uniformly. The movement abnormalities are prototypically tremor, rigidity, and bradykinesia. Disorders of mentation or cognition affect people in various ways. Most patients complain of slowed thinking, and about 20% to 30% are found to have dementia, with a higher likelihood in those with late-onset disease (i.e., after age 70). Mood disorders are common in PD, with the mean frequency of depression reported at 40%. No relation has been shown to exist between the frequency and severity of depression and the patient's current age, age of onset, or severity of PD symptoms and response to medication. It is postulated that depression is a primary manifestation of brain deterioration and not a reactive psychologic response to disability and chronic illness.

There is no known increased incidence of anxiety (**choice A**) among PD patients when compared with the general age-matched population.

Psychosis as part of PD has been reported in the context of mood disorders, for example in psychotic depression, but this is not particularly common. Visual, but not auditory (**choice B**), hallucinations are a neuropsychiatric feature of dementia with Lewy bodies. This is a type of dementia related to the presence of Lewy bodies in the brain stem and cerebral cortex. It is characterized by a progressive course, visual hallucinations, delusions, fluctuating attention, difficulty with executive functioning, and cognitive deficits. Mood changes are common as well.

As stated above, about 20% to 30% of patients with PD are found to have dementia (**choice C**), with a higher likelihood in those with late-onset disease (i.e., after age 70). About 40% of nondemented PD patients demonstrate some neuropsychological impairment, mostly in visuospatial abilities.

Insomnia (**choice E**) is not characteristic of PD. Often, if a patient with PD does have sleep disturbances, it is in the context of depressive symptomatology.

45. **The correct answer is E.** Benztropine is an antimuscarinic agent given to relieve symptoms of acute dystonic reactions. Blockade of cholinergic transmission produces blurred vision, confusion, constipation, dry skin, hallucinations, mydriasis, and urinary retention.

Diaphoresis (**choice A**) and diarrhea (**choice B**) occur with cholinergic, not anticholinergic, drugs.

Fevers (**choice C**) and insomnia (**choice D**) are not side effects observed with either cholinergic or anticholinergic drugs.

46. **The correct answer is A.** Agoraphobia is a fear of being in public places, away from home or without company. It refers to the fear of being in a situation or place from which there is no easy escape, such as in a theater, on public transportation, or in stores. The symptoms are usually the same as the ones seen in panic attacks, developing abruptly and lasting several minutes. Some of the symptoms include palpitations, sweating, paresthesias, dizziness, feeling of choking, trembling, chest pain, derealization, chills, and fear of losing control or dying.

Avoidant personality disorder (**choice B**) is a pervasive pattern of social inhibition and hypersensitivity to negative evaluation beginning in early adulthood. It is characterized by such symptoms as inhibition in new interpersonal situations, viewing oneself as inept, preoccupation with being criticized, and unwillingness to get involved with people unless sure of being liked.

Dependent personality disorder (**choice C**) is a pervasive need to be taken care of that leads to clinging behavior. At least five symptoms, including difficulty expressing disagreement, difficulty making decisions, feelings of helplessness when alone, fear of taking responsibility for major areas in life, and fear of being left alone to take care of oneself, are typically present.

Somatization disorder (**choice D**) begins before age 30. Typically, there is significant impairment present in major areas of functioning secondary to symptoms. Symptoms include four pain symptoms: one pseudoneurologic, one sexual, and two gastrointestinal.

Specific phobia (**choice E**) is marked, excessive fear that is cued by the presence or anticipation of a specific object or situation. Exposure to the feared object or situation results in an anxiety response, and the person is aware that the fear is unreasonable. The symptoms can cause significant impairment in everyday functioning.

47. **The correct answer is B.** The differential diagnosis of major depression includes hypothyroidism; a TSH level is a good screening test for this condition. This question could have been answered independently of the clinical vignette because the classic symptoms of hypothyroidism are present.

Measurement of follicle stimulating hormone levels (**choice A**) has utility in psychiatry in perimenopausal women to rule out depression secondary to menopause. The patient's young age and presence of symptoms suggestive of hypothyroidism would make this test inappropriate.

A urinalysis (**choice C**) is performed to rule out a urinary tract infection, which may be responsible for delirium in certain predisposed patients (elderly, demented, medically compromised). The above patient's symptoms, however, are strongly suggestive of hypothyroidism.

A urine hCG test (**choice D**) would be helpful in diagnosing pregnancy, not hypothyroidism.

The Venereal Disease Research Laboratory (VDRL) test (**choice E**) is used to screen for primary and secondary syphilis. Neurosyphilis, characterized by personality changes, irritability, and psychosis, is diagnosed by performing a VDRL on the CSF.

48. **The correct answer is C.** Once the differential diagnosis of acute memory loss is done, and delirium, dementia, trauma, and substance use are ruled out, the diagnosis of dissociative amnesia can be established. It usually has a circumscribed nature, and the patient's perplexity, confusion, and amnesia following traumatic events last for a discrete period of time. It is characterized by the inability to recall personal identification that is deeply embedded information and that is only destroyed in very advanced stages of Alzheimer disease.

Anterograde amnesia (**choice A**) is defined by a specific short-term memory deficit in which patients are unable to recall new information or events that happened in the previous minutes before the blackout. During the blackout, remote memory is intact, as is ability to perform tasks. This can be caused by alcohol, medications, drugs, or trauma.

Confabulation (**choice B**) can be seen in chronic alcoholics with dementia, and is characterized by gaps in memory that are filled with events that never happened.

Hypermnesia (**choice D**) describes an exaggerated degree of retention and recall.

Transitory global amnesia (**choice E**) is characterized by the inability to remember new information, such as date and location. Personal information is, however, retained. This discrepancy separates it from dissociative amnesia. Electroencephalogram can show spikes. The cause may be a vascular abnormality that leads to temporary ischemia.

49.　**The correct answer is E.** Supportive psychotherapy is used to help patients through difficult situations. It may incorporate the philosophies underlying other types of insight-oriented psychotherapy, but the main goal is to show sympathy, concern, and interest. When the current crisis has passed, other types of therapies may be appropriate.

Cognitive-behavioral therapy (CBT) (**choice A**) is concerned with repairing cognitive distortions and changing maladaptive behaviors. It may be useful in conditions such as dysthymia or anxiety disorders.

Hypnosis (**choice B**) may be helpful in dissociative and conversion disorders. An adjustment disorder, such as that described above, is most amenable to a supportive approach.

Psychoanalysis (**choice C**) is relatively contraindicated in this case. In psychoanalysis, the therapist maintains a neutral attitude; doing so in this situation may be perceived as rejection and would serve to alienate the patient, not comfort her.

Social skills training (**choice D**) focuses on developing abilities in relating to others and is reserved for patients with severe mental illness, such as schizophrenia.

50.　**The correct answer is D.** The patient is experiencing an acute dystonic reaction as a result of the extrapyramidal side (EPS) effects of antipsychotic medication. This condition is best treated with injectable diphenhydramine.

Bromocriptine (**choice A**) is a dopamine agonist that can be used in neuroleptic malignant syndrome (NMS), a condition associated with antipsychotic use and characterized by autonomic instability, altered mental status, and muscular rigidity.

Carbidopa/L-dopa (Sinemet; **choice B**) is used in idiopathic parkinsonism (Parkinson disease). It has no place in the treatment of EPS.

Carisoprodol (Soma; **choice C**) is a muscle relaxant often used for acute or chronic musculoskeletal conditions and ankylosing spondylitis. EPS is treated with an agent that has prominent anticholinergic or antihistaminergic properties.

Surgery: **Test One**

1. A 22-year-old man is stabbed in the right chest with a 5-cm-long knife blade. On arrival at the emergency department, he is wide awake and alert. He is speaking with a normal tone of voice but complaining of shortness of breath. The right hemithorax is hyperresonant to percussion and has no breath sounds; the rest of the initial survey is negative. His blood pressure is 110/75 mm Hg, pulse is 86/min, and central venous pressure is 3 cm H_2O. Pulse oximetry shows a saturation of 85%. Which of the following is the most appropriate next step in patient care?

   (A) Infusion of 2 L Ringer's lactate

   (B) Securing an airway by orotracheal intubation

   (C) Immediate insertion of a needle into the right pleural space

   (D) Chest x-ray and insertion of a chest tube

   (E) Sonographically guided evacuation of the pericardial sac

2. A 35-year-old man comes to the physician because of persistent dull perineal pain and dysuria for 6 months. The patient denies urinary tract infections or urethral discharge. His temperature is 37.0° C (98.6° F). On digital rectal examination, the prostate is slightly tender and boggy but not enlarged or indurated. Urinalysis is normal. Expressed prostatic secretions show the following:

Leukocytes	30 cells/high power field
Bacteria	None

   Cultures of prostatic secretion and urine are negative for bacteria. Which of the following is the most likely diagnosis?

   (A) Acute cystitis

   (B) Acute prostatitis

   (C) Chronic bacterial prostatitis

   (D) Chronic nonbacterial prostatitis

   (E) Prostatodynia

3. An otherwise healthy 28-year-old man comes to his physician because of painless enlargement of the right testis. He began to feel a sensation of heaviness in the right hemiscrotum approximately 6 months ago. Physical examination reveals diffuse enlargement of the right testis, but it is difficult to determine whether this is due to an intratesticular or extratesticular lesion. Which of the following is the most appropriate next step in diagnosis?

   (A) CT scanning

   (B) Serum levels of hCG, alpha-fetoprotein, and LDH

   (C) Scrotal ultrasonography

   (D) Needle biopsy

   (E) Inguinal orchiectomy

4. A man involved in a high-speed, head-on automobile collision arrives at the emergency department in a deep coma. His pupils react poorly to light but are of equal size. An airway is placed, and the patient is sent for CT scan of the head with extension to the neck. The study shows no cervical spine fractures, but does reveal an 8-cm, crescent-shaped hematoma on the right side, with moderate, leftward deviation of the midline structures. Which of the following is the most appropriate next step in management?

   (A) High-dose steroids

   (B) Hyperventilation, diuretics, and fluid restriction

   (C) Systemic vasodilators and alpha blockers

   (D) Surgical evacuation of his epidural hematoma

   (E) Surgical evacuation of his subdural hematoma

KAPLAN MEDICAL

5. A 19-year-old gang member is shot in the abdomen with a .38 caliber revolver. The entry wound is in the epigastrium, to the left of the midline. The bullet is lodged in the psoas muscle on the right. He is hemo-dynamically stable, and the abdomen is moderately tender. Which of the following is the most appropriate next step in diagnosis?

   (A) Close clinical observation

   (B) Emergency ultrasound

   (C) CT scan of the abdomen

   (D) Diagnostic peritoneal lavage

   (E) Exploratory laparotomy

6. A multiple trauma patient receives 14 units of packed red cells and several liters of Ringer's lactate solution during a laparotomy for multiple intra-abdominal injuries. The surgeons note that blood is oozing from all dissected raw surfaces, as well as from his IV line sites. His core temperature is normal. Which of the following is the most appropriate next step in management?

   (A) Proceed with surgery and give blood transfusions as needed

   (B) Obtain a stat coagulation profile to guide specific therapy

   (C) Empiric administration of fresh frozen plasma and platelet packs

   (D) Abort the operation and close the abdomen with towel clips

   (E) Leave the abdomen open and covered with mesh until coagulation parameters can be corrected

7. A 75-year-old man slips and falls at home, hitting his right chest wall against the kitchen counter. He has an area of exquisite pain to direct palpation over the seventh rib, at the level of the anterior axillary line. A chest x-ray film confirms the presence of a rib fracture, with no other abnormal findings. Which of the following is the most appropriate initial step in management?

   (A) Supplemental oxygen to compensate for hypoventilation

   (B) Systemic narcotic analgesics

   (C) Binding of the chest to limit motion

   (D) Intercostal nerve block to minimize pain

   (E) Open reduction and internal fixation to accelerate healing

8. A 54-year-old woman is brought to the emergency department after a head-on automobile accident. On arrival, she is breathing well. She has multiple bruises over the chest and multiple sites of point tenderness over the ribs. X-ray films show multiple rib fractures on both sides, but the lung parenchyma is clear, and both lungs are expanded. Two days later she is in respiratory distress, and her lungs "white out" on repeat chest x-ray films. Which of the following is the most likely diagnosis?

   (A) Flail chest

   (B) Myocardial contusion

   (C) Pulmonary contusion

   (D) Tension pneumothorax

   (E) Traumatic rupture of the aorta

9. Renal ultrasound and intravenous pyelography (IVP) in a 65-year-old man evaluated for urinary incontinence reveal bilateral hydronephrosis. Which of the following is the most likely condition leading to this complication?

   (A) Age-associated detrusor overactivity

   (B) Alzheimer disease

   (C) Normal pressure hydrocephalus

   (D) Previous surgery

   (E) Prostatic hyperplasia

   (F) Stress incontinence

10. A 57-year-old man is undergoing a femoral-popliteal bypass of his right lower extremity because of severe peripheral vascular disease. This patient has a long-standing history of claudication and shortness of breath. He had a myocardial infarction 3 years ago and has had progressive limitation of his exercise capacity because of his peripheral vascular disease. He has not had any risk stratification after his infarction. Two weeks ago, he underwent a lower extremity arterial study that showed severe diffuse disease of his right leg arterial system. The patient is brought to the operating room, and, during the procedure, his right lower extremity is made bloodless by application of a thigh tourniquet for 1.5 hours. The surgeons complete their bypass and are preparing to restore blood flow. Which of the following is an expected consequence of this maneuver?

   (A) Decrease in blood pressure

   (B) Increase in cardiac output

   (C) Increase in preload

   (D) Increase in venous return

   (E) Sinus bradycardia

11. A 31-year-old man is brought to the emergency department after a motor vehicle accident. He sustained a severe head injury and, on arrival to the emergency department, has a Glasgow coma score of 8. His blood pressure is stable, and an urgent CT scan of the head reveals a large subdural bleed with evidence of a midline shift and cerebellar tonsillar compression. The patient is breathing spontaneously without any respiratory assistance and is not intubated. Which of the following is the most appropriate next step in management?

    (A) Obtain an urgent head MRI to evaluate for herniation

    (B) Administer IV mannitol

    (C) Perform endotracheal intubation and mild hyperventilation

    (D) Induce a barbiturate coma

    (E) Initiate immediate surgical decompression

12. A 40-year-old retired professional football player complains of the sudden onset of palpitations and shortness of breath 5 days after having knee replacement surgery. His pulse is 120/min and regular. Oxygen saturation is 90% on room air. An ECG reveals sinus tachycardia. A chest x-ray film is unremarkable. Which of the following is the most appropriate next step in management?

    (A) Obtain cardiac enzymes and troponin to evaluate for myocardial ischemia

    (B) Schedule a duplex Doppler examination of the lower extremities

    (C) Assure him that he likely just has postoperative pneumonia and empirically start him on Zithromax

    (D) Administer an intravenous beta blocker to slow his tachycardia

    (E) Administer oxygen and obtain an immediate CT angiogram of the patient's chest

13. A 19-year-old man is involved in a motorcycle accident in which he sustains a closed fracture of his right femur and a pelvic fracture. In addition to the obvious deformity in his leg, physical examination is remarkable for the presence of a scrotal hematoma and blood at the meatus. There is no blood in the rectal exam, but the prostate cannot be felt. The patient states that he feels the need to void, but cannot do it. Which of the following is the most appropriate next step in diagnosis?

    (A) CT scan of the pelvis

    (B) Scrotal sonogram

    (C) IV pyelogram (IVP)

    (D) Retrograde cystogram via Foley catheter

    (E) Retrograde urethrogram

14. A 25-year-old man is shot with a .22-caliber revolver. The entrance wound is in the anterior, lateral aspect of his thigh, and the bullet is seen on x-ray films to be embedded in the muscles posterolateral to the femur. The emergency department physician cleans the wound thoroughly. Which of the following is the most appropriate next step in management?

    (A) Tetanus prophylaxis, if needed

    (B) Doppler studies

    (C) Arteriogram

    (D) Surgical exploration of the femoral vessels

    (E) Surgical removal of the embedded bullet

15. A patient sustained third-degree burns on both his arms when his shirt caught on fire while he was lighting the backyard barbecue. The burned areas are dry, white, leathery, anesthetic, and circumferential all around the arms and forearms. Which of the following parameters should be very closely monitored?

    (A) Blood gases

    (B) Body weight

    (C) Carboxyhemoglobin levels

    (D) Myoglobinemia and myoglobinuria

    (E) Peripheral pulses and capillary filling

16. A previously healthy 60-year-old man is referred for urologic evaluation of macroscopic hematuria. Urinary cytology is positive for malignant cells, and cystoscopic examination reveals an exophytic multifocal tumor. A biopsy of the tumor demonstrates papillary fronds lined by cells similar to transitional epithelium but showing nuclear atypia, mitoses, and necrosis. Which of the following is the most important risk factor in the U.S. for the development of this type of tumor?

    (A) Aniline dyes

    (B) Cyclophosphamide

    (C) Phenacetin

    (D) Radiation

    (E) Recurrent cystitis

    (F) Schistosomiasis

    (G) Smoking

17. A 23-year-old man is admitted to the hospital after being struck by a motor vehicle. The patient sustained an open fracture of his left femur in the accident and has had moderate blood loss. He was admitted to the hospital, has been stabilized over the past few days, and is now preparing for physical therapy. His hematocrit is 24%. The man feels weak and fatigued and easily gets short of breath with mild exertion. Which of the following is the most appropriate next step in management?

    (A) Continue with physical therapy; no transfusion is indicated

    (B) Discontinue physical therapy until the patient recovers more of his strength

    (C) Transfuse fresh frozen plasma to a hematocrit goal of 30%

    (D) Transfuse packed red blood cells to a hematocrit goal of 30%

    (E) Transfuse whole blood to a goal hematocrit of 30%

18. A 24-year-old man comes to the physician 24 hours after sustaining an injury to the right knee while playing soccer. He can walk, but he limps on the right side. He reports that he was hit by another player on the lateral side of his right knee, but did not feel a snap or pop at the time of the accident. On examination, the right knee appears normal, but palpation elicits tenderness along the medial aspect of the joint line. Increased laxity is observed when a valgus stress is applied to the knee flexed at 30 degrees, but not when the knee is in full extension. Lachman's test and posterior drawer tests are negative. Which of the following is the most likely diagnosis?

    (A) Meniscus injury

    (B) Sprain of the lateral collateral ligament

    (C) Sprain of the medial collateral ligament

    (D) Tear of the anterior cruciate ligament

    (E) Tear of the posterior cruciate ligament

19. A 48-year-old man with alcoholic cirrhosis has several episodes of massive hematemesis. Upper gastrointestinal endoscopy confirms that he is bleeding from esophageal varices. Sclerosing injections fail to control the bleeding. After the patient has been transfused 7 units of packed red cells, he is subjected to an emergency side-to-side portacaval shunt. At the time of surgery he has a serum albumin level of 3.1 g/dL, a total bilirubin of 1.7 mg/dL, and a prothrombin time (PT) 2 seconds above the control. After surgery, the bleeding stops, and the patient wakes up briefly from the anesthetic but then lapses into a coma. The reason for his neurologic deterioration would most likely be revealed by a laboratory determination of which of the following?

    (A) Blood alcohol levels

    (B) Blood gases

    (C) Blood glucose

    (D) Serum ammonia

    (E) Serum sodium

20. A 57-year-old man is returned to the post-surgical recovery unit after an open cholecystectomy. The patient had an uneventful, but prolonged, operative course in a very cold operating room. His past medical history is unremarkable. The only attempt at patient warming was raising the ambient temperature of the room. His urine output since arrival in the post-anesthesia care unit (PACU) has been 5 mL/hr. Which of the following is most likely to confirm the diagnosis?

    (A) Low serum aldosterone

    (B) Serum BUN to creatinine ratio greater than 20

    (C) Urine osmolality of 280 mOsmol/kg

    (D) Urine sodium of 40 mEq/L

    (E) Urine specific gravity of less than 1.010

21. A 25-year-old man presents to the same day surgical center for repair of an old injury to his lateral collateral ligament. The anesthesiologist wants to perform an axillary block for local pain control. If the posterior wall of the axillary artery is pierced during placement of the block, which of the following nerves will most likely be affected?

    (A) Axillary

    (B) Median

    (C) Musculocutaneus

    (D) Radial

    (E) Ulnar

22. A 49-year-old woman seeks help for a vague, constant, epigastric distress that she began experiencing about 5 weeks after returning from a 10-day trip to Mexico. She relates that she drove to Mexico City and Guadalajara and was very careful with what she ate and drank. Nevertheless, she experienced acute diarrhea on the third day of her trip and was treated by a hotel physician with a pharmaceutical product that was said to contain "locally acting antibiotics." She had no further gastro-intestinal complaints, but on her drive home, she was involved in an automobile accident. She hit a cow that was crossing the road and suffered epigastric trauma when her upper abdomen hit against the steering wheel. She was kept overnight at a hospital in Monterrey for clinical observation and was discharged the next morning. She did not seek further medical help when she got to the United States because she was asymptomatic. On physical examination, she has a deep, large, ill-defined, epigastric mass that is not tender to palpation. She is afebrile, and her only other complaint is that she cannot eat a full meal because she feels "full" right away. After confirmation of the suspected diagnosis, the treatment of her condition may require which of the following?

    (A) Deployment of an intra-arterial stent
    (B) Endoscopic anastomosis
    (C) Laparoscopic repair of the injured structure
    (D) Long-term antibiotic therapy
    (E) Resection of the affected part of the liver

23. A 35-year-old man had a splenectomy 8 days ago, following a motor vehicle accident. He is now complaining of left shoulder pain. His temperature is 39.0° C (102.2° F), blood pressure is 110/80 mm Hg, pulse is 110/min, and respirations are 30/min and shallow. Physical examination shows clear lungs with equal breath sounds bilaterally and mild tenderness to palpation in the left upper quadrant with a well-healing midline laparotomy incision. Laboratory studies show:

Hemoglobin	15 g/dL
Hematocrit	45%
Leukocyte counts	15,000/mm^3

    A chest x-ray film shows no infiltrates or effusions. Which of the following is the most likely diagnosis?

    (A) Left clavicle fracture
    (B) Left lower lobe pneumonia
    (C) Post-splenectomy sepsis
    (D) Subphrenic abscess
    (E) Subphrenic hematoma

24. A 24-year-old woman is brought to the emergency department after being stabbed by her boyfriend. The examining physician notes a 1.5-cm puncture wound lateral to her sternum. She has a blood pressure of 70/palpable, distended neck veins, and muffled heart sounds. Which of the following is the most appropriate next step in management?

    (A) Cardiac surgery consult
    (B) Echocardiogram
    (C) CT scan of the chest
    (D) Chest tube placement
    (E) Pericardiocentesis

25. A 55-year-old woman of Asian descent goes to the emergency department because of vomiting and severe abdominal cramping of 3 days' duration. Her pain is centered on the umbilicus. She denies being exposed to a viral or bacterial illness. Her medical history includes a previous cholecystectomy and an appendectomy after which she developed an infection. Her abdomen is not tender, but hyperactive, high-pitched peristalsis with rushes coincides with palpable bowel cramping. Abdominal x-ray films taken in the supine and upright positions demonstrate a ladder-like series of distended small bowel loops. Which of the following is the most likely explanation for these findings?

    (A) Adhesions
    (B) *Ascaris* infection
    (C) Cancer
    (D) Intussusception
    (E) Volvulus

26. A young man is shot in the upper part of the neck with a .22 caliber revolver. Inspection of the entrance and exit wounds indicates that the trajectory of the bullet is all above the level of the angle of the mandible, but below the skull. He is fully conscious and neurologically intact. A steady trickle of blood flows from both wounds, and it does not seem to respond to local pressure. He is hemodynamically stable. Which of the following is the most appropriate next step in diagnosis?

    (A) Continued clinical observation
    (B) Barium swallow
    (C) Arteriogram
    (D) Endoscopy
    (E) Surgical exploration

27. A 60-year-old woman has a lumpectomy and a sentinel node biopsy performed for an infiltrating ductal carcinoma on the upper outer quadrant of her right breast. The surgical specimen measures 12 by 10 by 8 cm, and all of the surgical margins are reported as negative by the pathologist. The aggregate of the measurements and studies done on the specimen reveals that the size of the tumor was 3.8 by 3.5 by 2.8 cm. Two sentinel axillary nodes removed by the surgeon are negative for metastasis. The tumor is strongly positive for estrogen and progesterone receptors. Histologic grade was III/III, and prognostic studies of flow cytometric S phase, DNA index, ploidy, and Ki-67 antigen are all reported as unfavorable. Prior to surgery, the patient agrees to receive postoperative radiation therapy for the right breast. Which of the following would optimize her chances for a cure?

    (A) Chemotherapy and anastrozole

    (B) Chemotherapy and tamoxifen

    (C) Chemotherapy plus estrogens and progesterone

    (D) Completion of the operation to a radical mastectomy

    (E) Radiation therapy to the contralateral breast and the right axilla

28. A 62-year-old woman faints while waiting in line to get into a movie theater. When she is examined by her physician the next day, she is found to be pale, with yellowish sclera, and to have a hemoglobin level of 7 g/dL. Except for mild obesity, the rest of the physical examination is unremarkable, but her stool is strongly positive for occult blood. She is told that she will need a colonoscopy, but before the study is done, further laboratory results become available, showing that she has a total bilirubin of 3.5 mg/dL and an alkaline phosphatase of 850 U/L. The transaminases are minimally elevated. Her physician then orders a sonogram of the right upper quadrant, and the study shows dilated intrahepatic ducts, dilated extrahepatic ducts, and a large, distended, thin-walled gallbladder without stones. Which of the following should be the next diagnostic study performed?

    (A) Barium enema

    (B) CT scan of the liver

    (C) Liver biopsy

    (D) Percutaneous transhepatic cholangiogram

    (E) Upper gastrointestinal endoscopy

29. A 44-year-old woman has a 2-cm firm palpable mass in the upper outer quadrant of her right breast. The mass is freely movable, and her breast is of rather large size. There are no palpable axillary nodes. Mammogram shows no other lesions. A core biopsy establishes a diagnosis of infiltrating ductal carcinoma. She has no neurologic or skeletal symptoms, and a chest x-ray film and liver enzymes are normal. She understands that systemic therapy may eventually be needed once the full extent of her disease is known. Although she wants the best chance for cure, she is very concerned about cosmetic deformity and wants to know what can be done about the breast itself. Which of the following is the most appropriate management?

    (A) Radiation and chemotherapy without breast surgery

    (B) Lumpectomy, axillary sampling, and postoperative radiation

    (C) Simple total subcutaneous mastectomy with implants

    (D) Modified radical mastectomy with immediate rectus abdominis flap reconstruction

    (E) Radical mastectomy and postoperative radiation, with delayed reconstruction

30. In the first postoperative day after an open abdominal procedure, a patient develops a temperature of 38.9° C (102° F). He is encouraged to ambulate, cough, and breathe deeply, but he is noncompliant. On the second day, he is still febrile. Incentive spirometry and postural drainage are instituted, but his participation is less than enthusiastic. He lies in bed all day and hardly moves. By the third day, he is still spiking fevers in the same range. Although efforts to improve his ventilation continue, resolution of his problem will most likely require which of the following?

    (A) Doppler studies of deep leg and pelvic veins

    (B) Urinalysis, urinary cultures, and appropriate antibiotics

    (C) Chest x-ray, sputum cultures, and appropriate antibiotics

    (D) Cultures of his wound and wound opening if needed

    (E) CT scan of the abdomen and percutaneous drainage of abscess

31. A middle-aged man with symptomatic carotid stenosis underwent a carotid endarterectomy on the right side. The area of significant stenosis extended from the carotid bifurcation up into the internal carotid, requiring a very high dissection and clamping of the vessel. The endarterectomy was done with an in situ shunt and closed with a Dacron patch. In the postoperative period, the patient has persistent difficulty swallowing solids and even more difficulty swallowing liquids. Any attempt to do so results in violent coughing and aspiration. His lips look symmetric and move normally, he speaks in a normal tone of voice without tiring, and he has no trouble breathing. When he is asked to stick his tongue out, he does so without deviation to either side. His symptoms are due to intraoperative damage of which of the following nerves?

    (A) Main trunk of the tenth (vagus) nerve

    (B) Mandibular branch of the seventh (facial) nerve

    (C) Sensory fibers of the ninth (glossopharyngeal) nerve

    (D) Superior laryngeal branch of the tenth (vagus) nerve

    (E) Trunk of the twelfth (hypoglossal) nerve

32. A 52-year-old man has been impotent ever since he had an abdominoperineal resection for cancer of the rectum. The tumor was staged as T3, N0, M0. He gets no nocturnal erections, and his impotence extends to all situations, regardless of sexual partner, and includes inability to masturbate. His erectile dysfunction is most likely due to which of the following?

    (A) Arterial vascular insufficiency

    (B) Erectile nerve damage

    (C) Psychogenic factors

    (D) Tumor invasion of the urethra

    (E) Venous incompetence

33. A 62-year-old man who had a motorcycle accident has been in a coma for several weeks. He is on a respirator, has had pneumonia on and off, has been on pressors, and shows no signs of neurologic improvement. The family inquires about brain death and possible organ donation. An independent neurologic evaluation confirms that the patient is brain dead. What advice should be given to his family?

    (A) Anyone who has had pneumonia is excluded as a donor

    (B) He is not a suitable donor because of his age

    (C) Patients on respirators cannot donate organs

    (D) The harvesting team should evaluate him as a potential donor

    (E) The use of pressors precludes organ donation

34. A 22-year-old woman is taken to the emergency department after she injures her foot. She had been standing on a chair changing a light bulb, when she accidentally stepped off the chair backward. She heard a cracking sound when she fell and developed pain and swelling behind the ankle. Her symptoms worsened when she tried to descend the stairs in her house. Physical examination demonstrates marked swelling behind her ankle, and her pain is exacerbated by plantar flexion and dorsiflexion of the hallus. Which of the following is the most likely diagnoses?

    (A) Anterior Achilles tendon bursitis

    (B) Calcaneal spur syndrome

    (C) Epiphysitis of the calcaneus

    (D) Fracture of the posterolateral talar tubercle

    (E) Posterior tibial nerve neuralgia

35. A 26-year-old, drug-addicted man develops congestive heart failure over a period of a few days. He is febrile, has a loud, diastolic murmur at the right second intercostal space, and has a blood pressure of 120/20 mm Hg. A physical examination performed a few weeks ago, when he attempted to enroll in a detoxification program, was completely normal. His blood pressure at that time was 120/80 mm Hg, and no murmurs were noted. In addition to long-term antibiotic therapy, which of the following is the most appropriate next step in management?

    (A) Closure of the ventricular septal defect with a pericardial patch

    (B) Elective aortic valve repair if he develops a systolic gradient of 50 mm Hg

    (C) Emergency aortic valve replacement

    (D) Emergency mitral valve repair

    (E) Emergency pulmonic valve replacement

36. An 18-year-old man was traveling at a high speed when his car slammed into a wall. He is brought into the emergency department by ambulance. His blood pressure is 60/40 mm Hg, pulse is 115/min and weak, respirations are 18/min, and central venous pressure is 2 cm H_2O. He is responsive only to painful stimuli. Breath sounds are equal bilaterally, and cardiac auscultation reveals only tachycardia. The abdomen is soft, non-distended, and nontender with active bowel sounds. A chest x-ray film shows a widened mediastinum. Which of the following is the most likely diagnosis?

    (A) Cardiac contusion

    (B) Cardiac tamponade

    (C) Flail chest

    (D) Ruptured thoracic aorta

    (E) Tension pneumothorax

37. A 72-year-old chronic smoker with severe chronic obstructive pulmonary disease (COPD) is found to have a central hilar mass on chest x-ray. Bronchoscopy and biopsies establish a diagnosis of squamous cell carcinoma of the lung. Pulmonary function studies show that he has an FEV_1 of 1,100 mL, and a ventilation-perfusion scan indicates that 60% of his pulmonary function comes from the affected lung. Which of the following is the most appropriate next step in management?

    (A) CT scan of the upper abdomen to rule out liver metastasis

    (B) Mediastinoscopy to biopsy carinal nodes

    (C) Radiation and chemotherapy

    (D) Palliative pneumonectomy

    (E) Pneumonectomy with hope of cure

38. A 14-year-old boy presents in the emergency department with very severe pain of sudden onset in his right testicle. There is no history of either trauma or recent mumps. He is afebrile, and a urinalysis shows no pyuria. The testis is swollen, exquisitely painful, high in the scrotum, and riding in a horizontal position. The cord above the testis is not tender. Which of the following is the most appropriate next step in management?

    (A) Ice packs, analgesics, and careful observation

    (B) Sonogram of the testicle

    (C) IV antibiotics

    (D) Testicular biopsy

    (E) Emergency surgery

39. An 80-year-old man comes to the physician because of a slowly growing ulcerated mass on the glans penis. A biopsy is positive for squamous cell carcinoma. Which of the following conditions is usually present in association with this tumor?

    (A) Balanitis xerotica obliterans

    (B) Condyloma acuminatum due to human papillomavirus (HPV) type 6

    (C) Lack of circumcision

    (D) Peyronie disease

    (E) Syphilis

40. A 45-year-old woman with breast cancer undergoes a modified radical mastectomy with lymph node dissection. Six weeks later, she returns complaining of decreased mobility of her shoulder. On physical examination, the scapula protrudes from the body when pressing her outstretched arm on the wall. Which of the following nerves was most likely injured during the operation?

    (A) Intercostal
    (B) Lateral pectoral
    (C) Long thoracic
    (D) Medial pectoral
    (E) Thoracodorsal

41. A young man is brought to the emergency department following a head-on collision at 60 miles per hour. He is awake but confused. Other than forehead and chin lacerations, physical examination is normal and laboratory values are within normal limits. Chest x-ray films are unremarkable. Which of the following is the most appropriate next step in diagnosis?

    (A) CT scan of the head
    (B) CT scan of the head and cervical spine
    (C) CT scan of the abdomen
    (D) Immediate laparotomy
    (E) Peritoneal lavage

42. A 51-year-old man is undergoing abdominal surgery and becomes hypotensive while under general anesthesia. The patient had been doing well during most of the procedure but now has a blood pressure of 80/40 mm Hg. His past medical history is significant for coronary artery disease and diabetes mellitus. A pulmonary artery catheter placed prior to the procedure gives the following data:

Central venous pressure	10 mm Hg
Pulmonary artery pressure	60/30 mm Hg
Pulmonary capillary occlusion pressure	24 mm Hg
Cardiac output	2.3 L/min

Which of the following is the most likely diagnosis?

    (A) Acute left heart failure
    (B) Acute mitral regurgitation
    (C) Acute right heart failure
    (D) Hypoxic pulmonary vasoconstriction
    (E) Sepsis syndrome

43. An 18-year-old gang member is stabbed in the back, just to the right of the midline. Physical examination shows paralysis and loss of proprioception distal to the injury on the right side, and loss of pain perception distal to the injury on the left side. Which of the following is the most likely diagnosis?

    (A) Anterior cord syndrome
    (B) Central cord syndrome
    (C) Complete transection of the spinal cord
    (D) Hemisection of the spinal cord
    (E) Posterior cord syndrome

44. A 31-year-old man is brought by helicopter to the trauma center after a motor vehicle accident in which he sustained massive lower extremity crush injury. The patient is alert and awake but in tremendous pain. His blood pressure is 140/80 mm Hg, and his pulse is 110/min. There is copious ongoing blood loss from the sites of injury. Urgent laboratory data will most likely show which of the following electrolyte abnormalities?

    (A) Hyperkalemia

    (B) Hypernatremia

    (C) Hypocalcemia

    (D) Hypoglycemia

    (E) Hypophosphatemia

45. A 32-year-old woman has an episode of upper gastrointestinal bleeding after a night of heavy alcoholic intake followed by ingestion of multiple aspirin tablets for the hangover. There was no prior vomiting until the time when she felt nauseated, went to the bathroom, and "filled the wash basin with vomiting of bright red bloody fluid." When she arrives in the emergency department, an upper gastrointestinal endoscopy is promptly performed, which confirms a diagnosis of acute erosive gastritis. She has no duodenal ulcer and no esophageal varices. Gastric lavage with ice-cold saline is performed and the bleeding stops. Laser photocoagulation or electrocautery are not used, neither is pitressin infused. She remains hemodynamically stable throughout the procedure, and she has a normal hemoglobin. She is sent home 2 hours later. Four hours after discharge, she returns complaining of severe, constant chest pain. She is in acute distress, has a temperature of 39.0° C (102.2° F), is having chills, and looks quite ill. Physical examination is remarkable for the presence of crepitation to palpation in the upper chest and lower neck, and chest x-rays confirm the presence of air in the mediastinum and the subcutaneous tissues. Which of the following is the most likely diagnosis?

    (A) Boerhaave syndrome

    (B) Dissecting thoracic aortic aneurysm

    (C) Gastric perforation

    (D) Iatrogenic esophageal perforation

    (E) Myocardial infarction

46. A 45-year-old man comes to the emergency department because of severe right flank pain that began abruptly 3 hours ago. The pain comes in waves and radiates down to the ipsilateral testis. The patient is nauseated and extremely restless. His temperature is 37.0° C (98.6° F). Dipstick examination of urine is positive for hematuria. Urinary pH is 5.8. Which of the following is the most appropriate next step in diagnosis?

    (A) Intravenous pyelography (IVP)

    (B) Noncontrast CT of the abdomen and pelvis

    (C) Renal ultrasound examination

    (D) Serum calcium, phosphorus, electrolytes, and uric acid

    (E) Urine cultures

47. A 71-year-old man is involved in a minor automobile accident on the road between Guadalajara and Lake Chapala in Mexico. The man is an American citizen who at the age of 65 years retired to a lakeside home in that area. Although he is asymptomatic, he decides to return to the United States to be "thoroughly checked." He is admitted to a veteran's hospital in south Texas, where he undergoes a CT scan of his abdomen. There are no signs of traumatic injuries, but the scan reveals the presence of four simple, thin-walled cystic structures, approximately 1 cm in diameter, scattered throughout both lobes of his liver. They have no septations. There are no cysts in the kidneys or pancreas. The man is completely asymptomatic and afebrile. Liver function tests are normal, as is his white blood count and differential. Which of the following is the most likely diagnosis?

    (A) Amebic abscesses

    (B) Cystadenocarcinoma of the liver

    (C) Hydatid cysts

    (D) Polycystic liver disease

    (E) Simple liver cysts

The response options for items 48-50 are the same. You will be required to select one answer for each item in the set.

(A)   Acute postinfectious glomerulonephritis

(B)   Autosomal dominant polycystic kidney disease

(C)   Bacterial cystitis

(D)   Berger disease

(E)   Bladder transitional cell carcinoma

(F)   Hemorrhagic cystitis

(G)   Prostatic carcinoma

(H)   Testicular cancer

(I)   Transitional cell carcinoma of the pelvis

(J)   Tuberculosis

(K)   Ureteral stone

(L)   Urethral carcinoma

(M)   von Hippel-Lindau syndrome

For each patient with hematuria, select the most likely diagnosis.

48.   A 27-year-old woman who moved to the U.S. from Southeast Asia at the age of 10 presents with gross hematuria. She reports chronic low-grade fever and weight loss for over 1 year. Urinalysis also shows pyuria, but urinary cultures are negative for bacteria. Intravenous pyelography (IVP) reveals diminished contrast excretion in the right kidney and cavitary lesions in the right kidney.

49.   A 35-year-old woman with corticosteroid-resistant systemic lupus erythematosus is being treated with cyclophosphamide. She presents with increased frequency of urination and gross hematuria. Urinalysis is negative for pyuria or bacteriuria.

50.   A 35-year-old man with prior history of cerebellar hemangioblastoma and multiple cysts in the pancreas is found to have microhematuria on a routine check-up. One of his siblings developed hemangioblastomas and renal cell carcinoma in his youth, and similar cases are traceable on his father's side of the family. Renal ultrasonography reveals a 4-cm partially cystic mass in the right kidney, and a similar smaller lesion in the left kidney.

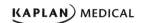

Surgery Test One:
Answers and Explanations

ANSWER KEY

1.	D	26.	C
2.	D	27.	A
3.	C	28.	E
4.	E	29.	B
5.	E	30.	C
6.	C	31.	C
7.	D	32.	B
8.	C	33.	D
9.	E	34.	D
10.	A	35.	C
11.	C	36.	D
12.	E	37.	C
13.	E	38.	E
14.	A	39.	C
15.	E	40.	C
16.	G	41.	B
17.	D	42.	A
18.	C	43.	D
19.	D	44.	A
20.	B	45.	D
21.	E	46.	B
22.	B	47.	E
23.	D	48.	J
24.	E	49.	F
25.	A	50.	M

1. **The correct answer is D.** A penetrating wound to the chest will produce either a pneumothorax, a hemothorax, or both. The absence of breath sounds confirms that one of those has occurred, and the hyperresonance to percussion indicates that air is present. The patient's good vital signs indicate that there is time to do the proper diagnostic study (chest x-ray). The appropriate treatment for a pneumothorax is placement of a chest tube.

    Infusion of 2 L Ringer lactate (**choice A**) would have been appropriate if the findings had suggested hemothorax (as evidenced by dullness to percussion), and he had been bleeding (as evidenced by low blood pressure and a fast pulse).

    A patient who is fully awake and alert, and who is speaking in a normal tone of voice, has an airway and can maintain it (compare with **choice B**).

    Immediate insertion of a needle into the right pleural space (**choice C**) would be appropriate management for a tension pneumothorax. If the patient had a tension pneumothorax, he would have been in shock and severe respiratory distress, and the mediastinum would have been shifted (evidenced by tracheal deviation).

    Sonographically guided evacuation of the pericardial sac (**choice E**) would be appropriate management for pericardial tamponade, which is not present in this patient. If the patient had developed tamponade, he would have been in shock, with a high central venous pressure (or distended veins).

2. **The correct answer is D.** Chronic nonbacterial prostatitis is characterized by persistent irritative voiding symptoms, such as dysuria and perineal discomfort, and leukocytes (especially foamy macrophages) in expressed prostatic secretion. No bacteria, however, are isolated from cultures of urine or prostatic secretions. This condition is believed to be of a noninfectious nature and possibly autoimmune-mediated. Treatment is based on symptomatic relief with sitz baths and anti-inflammatory agents. However, some authors recommend a trial with erythromycin.

    Acute cystitis (**choice A**) is usually infectious, so that irritative voiding symptoms are associated with positive urine cultures. Coliform bacteria are the usual pathogens. In men, prostatic hyperplasia is the most common predisposing factor.

    Acute prostatitis (**choice B**) is due to bacterial infection. Perineal pain, irritative voiding symptoms, extreme tenderness on digital rectal examination, and fever are the presenting symptoms. Urine cultures are positive for the offending agents, which are gram-negative rods (*Escherichia coli* and *Pseudomonas aeruginosa*).

    Chronic nonbacterial prostatitis must be differentiated from chronic bacterial prostatitis (**choice C**). Both disor-

ders present with similar symptomatology, but chronic bacterial prostatitis is associated with positive bacterial cultures of expressed prostatic secretions. Gram-negative rods are the most common pathogens. Treatment is based on antibiotic therapy as determined by susceptibility tests on the isolated organisms.

Prostatodynia (**choice E**) is an obscure entity characterized by dull perineal discomfort and pain mimicking chronic prostatitis. Microscopic examination and cultures of prostatic secretions, however, are negative for leukocytes and bacteria. The designation itself is a misnomer, since the prostate is entirely normal. The disease seems to be related to dysfunctional contractility of the bladder detrusor muscle, the sphincter, and/or the urethra. The treatment is symptomatic and includes alpha-blocking agents, diazepam (as a myorelaxant), biofeedback techniques, and sitz baths.

3. **The correct answer is C.** Ultrasonography is the most sensitive and least expensive method to discriminate between testicular and extratesticular masses. However, a physician should remember to first use a simple transillumination test for such a differential diagnosis. Fluid collections within the vaginal sac transilluminate, whereas testicular masses do not.

    CT scanning (**choice A**) is used to determine the spread of testicular tumors within the abdominal and thoracic cavity, but is of no use in the initial diagnosis of scrotal masses.

    Serum levels of hCG, alpha-fetoprotein, and LDH (**choice B**) are important adjunct parameters in the diagnosis and subsequent management of testicular neoplasms. LDH may be elevated in seminomas and nonseminomas, alpha-fetoprotein is elevated in nonseminomas (especially yolk sac tumors), and hCG is elevated in nonseminomas (especially choriocarcinomas).

    Needle biopsy (**choice D**) is not an adequate diagnostic tool in this case. It may be used in the evaluation of azoospermia related to infertility problems.

    Inguinal orchiectomy (**choice E**) is performed once ultrasonography has established that scrotal enlargement is caused by an intratesticular tumor. This allows the most accurate pathologic diagnosis and appropriate management.

4. **The correct answer is E.** A crescent-shaped hematoma is seen in acute subdural hematoma, whereas acute epidural hematoma produces a biconvex, lens-shaped collection. The diagnosis is therefore acute subdural hematoma as the hematoma is displacing midline structures. Evacuation is the first priority. The neurologic damage resulted from the initial blow and could be compounded by a subsequent increase in intracranial pressure.

High dose steroids (**choice A**) were once thought to have a beneficial impact on long-term outcome in patients with blunt spinal cord injuries. Over time, this has been proven to be incorrect and high-dose steroids are no longer used commonly for this indication. Steroids do lower the elevated intracranial pressure caused by brain tumors; however, for reasons that we do not understand, these agents do not do so in cases of increased intracranial pressure caused by trauma.

Hyperventilation (which is controversial), diuretics, and fluid restriction (**choice B**) can all help to decrease intracranial pressure; however, in the setting of acute intracranial hemorrhage with shift, only immediate neurosurgical intervention will significantly improve the outcome.

Vasodilators would increase intracranial pressure, whereas alpha blockers (**choice C**) would produce systemic hypotension and further reduce brain perfusion.

The patient does not have an epidural hematoma (**choice D**) as evidenced by the lack of a biconvex, lens-shaped collection on CT.

5. **The correct answer is E.** The abdomen is full of important structures that should not have holes in them: solid organs that can bleed, and hollow viscera that will spill "evil fluids" into the peritoneal cavity. Thus, the rule for abdominal gunshot wounds is simple: an exploratory laparotomy should be done in every case, before there are obvious signs of either bleeding or peritonitis.

Clinical observation alone (**choice A**) is not wise, since the risk of complications will increase the longer one waits.

Ultrasound (**choice B**), CT of the abdomen (**choice C**), and diagnostic peritoneal lavage (**choice D**) are used to assess the extent of internal damage in blunt abdominal trauma. They would be of little benefit in an abdominal gunshot wound.

6. **The correct answer is C.** In the setting of massive blood loss and multiple transfusions (more than 12 units of packed red cells), the development of coagulopathy is almost predictable. Packed red cells contain virtually no viable platelets and only a very small concentration of clotting factors. Prophylactic administration of clotting factors has not proven to be advantageous, but once the coagulopathy occurs, a shotgun approach to provide fresh frozen plasma and platelet packs is indicated.

Ignoring the coagulopathy and continuing to operate and transfuse (**choice A**) would be doomed to failure. Surgeons can ligate or cauterize big vessels but cannot do the same for capillaries. Proper clotting is indispensable in all surgical operations.

Although it would be more elegant to determine exactly what is missing, under these circumstances there is no time to do the detailed studies (**choice B**).

If hypothermia and acidosis had also developed, a more drastic approach would have been necessary: stop the operation and close the abdomen temporarily (**choice D**).

Closing with a mesh (**choice E**) is indicated when an abdominal compartment syndrome occurs—it has nothing to do with coagulopathy.

7. **The correct answer is D.** A rib fracture can be a serious injury in the elderly, because the pain prevents full inspiration, atelectasis ensues, and eventually pneumonia develops and may cause significant morbidity and mortality. The key to the treatment is to eliminate the pain without interfering with ventilation. An intercostal nerve block will accomplish this goal.

Although supplemental oxygen (**choice A**) would not be directly injurious, it would neither eliminate the pain nor preserve ventilation.

Systemic narcotic analgesics (**choice B**) would diminish the pain but would also increase the probability of complications by depressing the respiratory drive, thus reducing ventilation.

Binding the chest (**choice C**) diminishes the pain by limiting motion. In doing so, however, it limits ventilation.

Open reduction and internal fixation to accelerate healing (**choice E**) is totally unnecessary. The chest wall already is holding the rib in a good position for eventual healing. It will not happen faster if we intervene.

8. **The correct answer is C.** Severe blunt trauma to the chest can produce obvious injuries, such as broken ribs, but it can also lead to pathology that may not show up until later, such as pulmonary contusion or myocardial contusion. The former produces the classic "white-out" of the lung (contused lung is exquisitely sensitive to fluid overload, and the fluid leaks easily) along with respiratory distress.

Flail chest (**choice A**) is recognized by the paradoxical motion of a segment of the chest wall, which is not described here.

Myocardial contusion (**choice B**) shows up like an infarction, both clinically (arrhythmias) and on ECG. You would expect it in association with sternal fractures rather than with rib fractures.

Tension pneumothorax (**choice D**) produces shock and high central venous pressure (CVP), along with the respiratory distress, and air is seen in the x-ray.

The ultimate hidden injury in blunt chest trauma is traumatic rupture of the aorta (**choice E**). X-ray films would show widening of the mediastinum, and the eventual clinical manifestation would be exsanguinating hemorrhage.

9.   **The correct answer is E.** Prostatic hyperplasia results in partial obstruction of the proximal urethra, causing hesitancy and decreased force of stream. With increasing degrees of prostatic enlargement, the volume of urine remaining in the bladder after voiding increases progressively until complete urinary retention manifests with occasional overflow incontinence. Urinary retention leads to dilatation of the ureters and renal pelves (hydronephrosis).

Age-associated detrusor overactivity (**choice A**) is the most common cause of urinary incontinence in the elderly. It manifests with an uncontrollable urge to urinate not triggered by stress maneuvers. It seems to be related to a deficiency in the descending pathways that inhibit the voiding reflex triggered by bladder distension. This condition does not lead to urinary retention.

Urinary incontinence associated with Alzheimer disease (**choice B**) and normal pressure hydrocephalus (**choice C**) is similar to detrusor overactivity and results from failure to inhibit the contractions of the vesical detrusor muscle.

Previous surgery (**choice D**) may cause sphincteric damage, resulting in total incontinence, in which leakage of urine is continuous. Obviously, this condition will not result in hydronephrosis since there is no obstruction to urinary outflow.

Stress incontinence (**choice F**) is the second most common cause of urinary incontinence. It is frequent in women and rare in men. It manifests with instantaneous leakage during stress maneuvers, such as coughing. It does not lead to urinary obstruction or retention and thus is not associated with hydronephrosis.

10. **The correct answer is A.** Vascular surgical patients are often managed by the medical consult service because of the tremendous number of comorbidities. During vascular procedures, the use of cross-clamping and tourniquets produces localized or regional ischemia. The consequences of ischemia include the accumulation of metabolic waste products and acid load (so-called evil humors), which are freely available to wreak havoc on the systemic circulation once they gain access to it. The primary consequence of this is profound and dramatic systemic hypotension that can be prolonged for hours after a procedure. Such a phenomenon has obvious consequences for management of patients such as this man with coexisting cardiac disease.

A drop in systemic blood pressure from severe vasodilatation will lead to decreased preload (compare with **choice C**) and thus a decrease in stroke volume and cardiac output (**choice B**).

Restoration of circulation to the previously clamped limb opens an entirely new venous reservoir, thus dramatically reducing venous return (compare with **choice D**). In addition, the massive systemic vasodilatation would further decrease venous return. The result of these two events is a dramatic, and often profound, drop in systemic blood pressure.

Sinus bradycardia (**choice E**) is the opposite of the reflex tachycardia that is expected with profound hypotension.

11. **The correct answer is C.** This patient has an intracranial bleed, signs of increased intracranial pressure (ICP), and evidence on a CT scan of impending herniation. This patient requires rapid lowering of his ICP. The most rapid method available is mild hyperventilation to lower $PaCO_2$, which leads to decreased cerebral blood flow and ICP.

Obtaining an urgent head MRI to evaluate for herniation (**choice A**) is unnecessary since the head CT already showed clear signs of impending herniation. An MR scan adds nothing to the decision analysis and need for immediate therapy.

Administration of IV mannitol (**choice B**) is also an appropriate therapy in this case. However, mannitol has an onset of action approximately 90 minutes after dosing.

Induction of a barbiturate coma (**choice D**) is used as a last resort to dramatically lower ICP. In cases of severe emergency, patients are mechanically ventilated and placed in a barbiturate coma so that maximal lowering of ICP can be attained.

Initiating immediate surgical decompression (**choice E**) may be appropriate, but not until the airway has been secured. Like mannitol, surgical decompression (even as emergent surgery) is not immediate; therefore, therapy needs to be instituted during that interval.

12. **The correct answer is E.** This patient most likely has a pulmonary embolus. Pulmonary embolism occurs following general surgery in 1% to 2% of patients older than 40. The incidence is higher (5% to 10%) following orthopedic surgery of the hip or knee. Venous stasis due to immobilization is probably a major reason for venous thrombosis associated with surgery. However, other factors, such as increased blood fibrinolytic activity and vessel damage, may be involved as well. Hypoxia, as well as an increased alveolar-arterial oxygen difference (A-a gradient) seen on arterial blood gas (if obtained) supports the diagnosis, along with sinus tachycardia on ECG and a normal chest x-ray. The administration of oxygen to ALL hypoxic patients as a first step or most important step is always indicated.

Cardiac enzymes and troponin (**choice A**) are unlikely to be of any use in this scenario. This patient's problem is a clot in his lungs, not in his coronary arteries.

Duplex Doppler examination (**choice B**) will evaluate for the possible presence of a DVT; however, the lack of a DVT does not rule out a PE, so this would NOT be the most appropriate next step.

Postoperative pneumonia (**choice C**) does occur; however, one would expect that such a pneumonia would have positive x-ray findings. Empiric antibiotics are rarely a correct answer on the boards.

Intravenous beta blockers (**choice D**) are very good for lowering heart rate in primary tachycardia; however, in this situation the patient has a clear reason to be tachycardic (the PE), so simply slowing his rate will not help with his diagnosis or treatment.

13. **The correct answer is E.** The hallmark of a urologic injury is a trauma patient who has blood in the urine (or in the visible part of the urinary tract, as in this case). When a pelvic fracture is also present, we have to bet on the lower urinary tract: the bladder in either gender, or the bladder or urethra in the male. When the blood is visible at the meatus and you add the scrotal hematoma, the "vanishing" prostate, and the inability to void, the writing is on the wall: urethral injury. The last thing you want to do in this case is insert a Foley catheter; you might convert a partial urethral disruption into a complete transection. You want to inject the dye directly into the urethra (retrograde urethrogram).

A CT scan of the pelvis (**choice A**) might be needed to assess pelvic bleeding (if we had been told that this man was in shock), but it would not be the best way to detect a urethral leak.

A scrotal sonogram (**choice B**) can tell you whether the testicle is injured, but a ruptured testicle does not give you blood in the urinary tract.

The IV pyelogram (**choice C**) would be a round-about and unreliable way to get radiopaque material where you need it.

As pointed out above, inserting a Foley catheter to do a cystogram (**choice D**) would be absolutely contraindicated if the clinical picture suggests urethral injury.

14. **The correct answer is A.** All penetrating injuries require tetanus prophylaxis, an often overlooked detail when dealing with other more impressive problems. In this case, the key to the correct answer lies in the fact that the other options are not indicated. In gunshot wounds of the extremities, the main concern is the possibility of major vascular injuries. Such injuries can be evaluated with Doppler studies (**choice B**), arteriograms (**choice C**), or surgical exploration (**choice D**), but none of those are needed here. A rudimentary knowledge of anatomy allows the physician to skip all those expensive procedures: the femoral artery (with the femoral vein adjacent to it) is located anteromedial in the upper thigh and

eventually becomes centered on the axis of the extremity when it becomes the popliteal. It is never located on the lateral side of the thigh, where the bullet tract is located in this vignette. Removing the bullet (**choice E**), although obligatory in Western movies, is not necessary if it is not threatening to erode some vital structure.

15. **The correct answer is E.** Circumferential burns of the extremities pose a distinct hazard to peripheral circulation because the edema fluid resulting from the burn cannot expand under the unyielding envelope of the burn eschar. Compulsive monitoring of pulses and capillary filling is required; escharotomy also may be required.

Although flame burns can cause smoke inhalation and the so-called respiratory burn, they do so only when the victim is trapped in an enclosed space: a burning car, a plane, a building. In those situations you would monitor blood gases (**choice A**) and carboxyhemoglobin (**choice C**) levels. This fellow was burned in the backyard (a well-ventilated place), so these are not a valid concern.

Body weight (**choice B**) does not change much with the massive internal fluid shifts of a major burn. We guide our fluid therapy by urinary output and central venous pressure, not by monitoring body weight.

As for myoglobinemia and myoglobinuria (**choice D**), they are of paramount concern in high voltage electrical burns or crushing injuries, not in flame burns.

16. **The correct answer is G.** Transitional cell tumors represent 90% of the neoplasms arising from the urinary bladder. These tumors grow as exophytic, papillary masses, which most commonly present with gross or microscopic hematuria. Cigarette smoking is epidemiologically the most significant risk factor for transitional cell carcinoma and seems to account for more than two-thirds of cases. Formation of carcinogenic polycyclic aromatic hydrocarbons derived from tobacco smoke plays a key role in the pathogenesis.

Persons with a prolonged occupational exposure to aniline dyes (**choice A**), particularly beta-naphthylamine, exhibit a 50-fold increase in the incidence of bladder cancer of the transitional type compared with the general population. Currently, prior exposure to aniline dyes accounts for approximately 15% of the cases of bladder cancer.

The immunosuppressant drug cyclophosphamide (**choice B**) and the analgesic phenacetin (**choice C**) increase the likelihood of developing transitional cell carcinomas of the urinary tract, but cases related to these drugs are rare.

No relationship has been shown between transitional cell carcinoma of the bladder and radiation (**choice D**) or recurrent cystitis (**choice E**).

Urinary schistosomiasis (**choice F**), due to infestation with *Schistosoma hematobium*, is the most significant important risk factor for urinary bladder cancer in countries such as Egypt and Sudan, where schistosomiasis is endemic. Most of these tumors, however, are squamous (not transitional) cell carcinomas.

17. **The correct answer is D.** Transfusion of packed red cells (preparation of all the red cell mass from a pint of donated blood—it has no plasma or buffy coat and therefore no proteins [coagulation factors] or platelets) is one of the most frequent treatments executed by physicians. There exists in medicine a dogma of uncertain origin that states that anemic patients with a hematocrit less than 30% should be transfused with red cells until that value is attained. This rule is even more rigidly followed in patients with coexisting illness, such as cardiac or pulmonary disease. Although this "rule" is being called into question by recent publications, it is still generally accepted that patients with acute bleeds, such as the one in this vignette, merit repletion of red cells if they are symptomatic from such a bleed.

Continuing with physical therapy without transfusion (**choice A**) is a choice favored by many physicians. This is because many people believe that a 23-year-old man will replete his own red cells over time. In this case, however, the patient is clearly symptomatic with even minimal exertion. Therefore, his anemia is not benign and merits treatment. There is, of course, no reason to restore his pre-accident hematocrit, but he should be transfused to a level at which his symptoms would be lessened or abrogated (about 30%).

Discontinuing physical therapy until the patient recovers more of his strength (**choice B**) is not appropriate since the patient requires therapy to regain his strength, and the reason for his weakness likely relates to his acute anemia.

Transfusion of fresh frozen plasma (FFP) to a hematocrit goal of 30% (**choice C**) is incorrect. FFP is used to restore clotting factors. One unit generally increases plasma anticoagulation factors by 30%. Like all blood products, it is type-specific.

Transfusion of whole blood to a goal hematocrit of 30% (**choice E**) is not performed. Whole blood is the content of 1 pint of donated blood. It is unfiltered and contains plasma, platelets, white cells, and red cells. This product is usually processed so that each of these components are removed (except white cells) and used for transfusions in specific clinical situations.

18. **The correct answer is C.** The patient presents with the typical symptomatology associated with sprain of the medial collateral ligament. This ligament connects the distal femur to the proximal tibia on their medial aspects. Injuries to this ligament are the most frequent among traumatic knee injuries and typically result from a lateral blow to the joint. The injured knee is sometimes swollen, but often inspection reveals only walking difficulties. Physical examination should include maneuvers that assess ligamentous stability, comparing the injured and uninjured sites. A valgus stress test demonstrating increased laxity of the knee confirms sprain of the medial collateral ligament. These tests should be performed on both flexed and extended knees. Increased laxity of ligaments with the knee in full extension indicates concomitant capsular injury (absent in this case).

Meniscus injury (**choice A**) often results in a "locked-up" knee and is usually due to traumas that have a twisting component. Appropriate tests to evaluate meniscal integrity (such as the McMurray) should be part of the physical examination in case of knee injuries.

Sprain of the lateral collateral ligament (**choice B**) is usually due to blows to the medial aspect of the knee. The varus stress test would be positive.

Tears of the anterior cruciate ligament (**choice D**) and posterior cruciate ligament (**choice E**) will result in knee instability. Often, the patient reports feeling a snap or pop at the time of injury. Lachman's test is the most sensitive clinical maneuver to detect injuries to the anterior cruciate ligament. The examiner stabilizes the knee with one hand and pulls the tibia forward. Any forward movement of the tibia (compared with the uninjured side) is considered diagnostic of anterior cruciate ligament tear. The posterior drawer test is used to detect tears of the posterior cruciate ligament.

19. **The correct answer is D.** Portacaval shunts are very effective in decreasing the pressure in esophageal varices, and thus controlling bleeding from them. But the penalty paid for that diversion of blood flow is further impairment of liver function. One almost never sees cirrhotic patients come to surgery with normal liver function. And, if they are bleeding at the time, they also have a load of ammonia in the gut that has to be cleared by the liver. With the initial limited function, plus the trauma of surgery and the diversion of portal flow, ammonia (as well as other toxic substances) accumulates in the blood and leads to coma.

Blood alcohol levels (**choice A**) would be relevant in an alcoholic who has been drinking up to the time that some unexpected event necessitates emergency surgery. If the patient comes to the operating room with high levels of alcohol in the blood, one can predict that delirium tremens (DTs) will occur 2 or 3 days later.

Determination of blood gases (**choice B**) is always the first thing to do when unexplained mental deterioration occurs after surgery. Hypoxia is very likely to be the culprit. In this case, however, we do not have an unexplained occurrence, but one rather predictable problem.

Blood glucose (**choice C**) comes to mind for the diabetic patient known to use insulin who suddenly goes into coma, or for the unknown patient brought to the emergency department in coma and with no history of what happened to him. Although it is true that hypoglycemia is seen in liver failure, it occurs at the very end of the spectrum, when all other parameters of liver function are grossly deranged.

Rapid changes in serum sodium (**choice E**) can cause coma, such as in the precipitous hyponatremia seen in water intoxication or the hypernatremia of profound dehydration. Neither of those are likely to occur, however, in the setting of this vignette.

20. **The correct answer is B.** Post-surgical patients generally have moderate to severe derangement in fluid balance. They have been fasted before the procedure and then had a variety of sensible and insensible losses during the procedure. In this case, the idea of severe dehydration causing prerenal azotemia would be supported by an elevated BUN and creatinine, but in a ratio of greater than 20:1. This is due to the heightened reabsorption and retention of solute by the kidney that is reflected by the elevated BUN.

Low serum aldosterone (**choice A**) is incorrect. In conditions of volume depletion, the renin-angiotensin-aldosterone axis is activated with high levels of each hormone. In this case, aldosterone is acting on the distal tubules to affect sodium reabsorption.

Urine osmolality of 280 mOsmol/kg (**choice C**) is incorrect because in the case of volume depletion, the urine should be maximally or near maximally concentrated, reflecting retention of nearly all filtered water.

A urine sodium of 40 mEq/L (**choice D**) is not correct. With volume depletion, the urine sodium should be quite low (<20 mEq/L), reflecting retention of nearly all filtered water and sodium.

A urine specific gravity of less than 1.010 (**choice E**) is the opposite of what is expected. As with osmolality, this parameter should reflect maximal concentration of the urine, which is equivalent to minimal free water excretion.

21. **The correct answer is E.** This question simply requires a basic understanding of the anatomy of the brachial plexus. In every medical specialty, general medicine included, knowledge of key anatomic loci is crucial for patient care. Classic examples of this include placement of central venous lines or needle thoracentesis. In this case, the ulnar nerve, the end-terminal branch of the medial cord (posterior to the axillary artery) of the brachial plexus, is in jeopardy. Although the posterior cord is posterior to the axillary artery at lower levels, at this level the medial cord is interposed between the posterior cord and the artery. This is the so-called "region two of the axillary

artery (posterior to the pectoralis minor muscle)," where the axillary block is performed.

The axillary nerve (**choice A**) is a branch of the posterior cord, but arises very high in the plexus and immediately exits the axilla via the teres muscle groups.

The median nerve (**choice B**) is formed from the medial and the lateral cords, is very low in the brachium, and is not in danger from an axillary block.

The musculocutaneus nerve (**choice C**) is a branch of the lateral cord and is in no danger, as it is buried in muscle tissue from its origin.

The radial nerve (**choice D**), also a branch of the posterior cord, is in no danger of injury since it exits the axilla via the radial groove on the humerus, very deep to muscle. This nerve is most often injured during spiral fractures of the humerus.

22. **The correct answer is B.** Vague, epigastric distress, early satiety, and a large but ill-defined, epigastric mass developing 5 weeks after trauma to the upper abdomen is one of the classic presentations of a pancreatic pseudocyst (the other presentation would follow an episode of pancreatitis). Small, pancreatic pseudocysts may go away during clinical observation, but big, palpable pseudocysts probably will not. Thus, the patient will probably require either internal or external drainage. The most sophisticated way to achieve drainage is by performing an endoscopic cystogastrostomy. Two older treatments, radiologically guided external drainage and surgically constructed internal derivation, were not offered as options.

Intra-arterial stents (**choice A**) are used in conjunction with angioplasty for vascular stenosis, or as treatment for abdominal aortic aneurysms. This woman does not have an aneurysm. Aneurysms of the abdominal aorta are not produced by trauma, do not interfere with eating, and are sometimes palpable as a pulsatile mass.

Assuming that you had the correct diagnosis—a pancreatic injury that resulted in a pseudocyst—laparoscopic repair (**choice C**) is not the correct treatment. We do not attempt to repair the pancreas to treat this condition. We simply reroute the pancreatic secretions, and, eventually, the injury heals by itself.

The exposure to exotic bugs in Mexico and the brief episode of diarrhea might have led you into thinking of an infection that might require antibiotics (**choice D**). However, no such infection would produce a deep, epigastric mass, and the patient is afebrile. A brief episode of diarrhea is very common for travelers; it does not necessarily lead to further pathology. In this case, it is simply a red herring.

KAPLAN MEDICAL

At the same time, someone who becomes ill with diarrhea after visiting Mexico could be thought of as having an amebic abscess of the liver. But such patients are febrile, and their livers are tender. Their treatment starts with metronidazole and may require drainage but not resection of the affected part of the liver (**choice E**).

23. **The correct answer is D.** Subphrenic abscess is a common complication of splenectomy and is implied by the patient's elevated temperature and elevated WBC, pleuritic pain (which is the probable cause of his rapid and shallow respirations), and left upper quadrant tenderness. A subphrenic abscess would irritate the phrenic nerve (nerve root C3-C5), causing referred pain toward dermatome of the nerve root, which includes the left shoulder.

    Left clavicular fractures (**choice A**) appear erythematous at the site of fracture and may exhibit crepitus on palpation. The arm is usually held close to the body, and the ipsilateral shoulder appears lower than the opposite side.

    One would expect an abnormal chest x-ray or rales or rhonchi instead of clear lungs and equal breath sounds in a patient with left lower lobe pneumonia (**choice B**).

    Post-splenectomy sepsis (**choice C**) would not produce such localized symptoms.

    Subphrenic hematoma (**choice E**) is not consistent with the fever and leukocytosis observed in this patient.

24. **The correct answer is E.** The woman was stabbed in the heart, leading to cardiac tamponade (blood collecting in the pericardial sac). This causes impairment in heart function, leading to hypotension, distension of neck veins due to pump failure, and muffled heart sounds due to the collection of blood. The immediate concern is removing the blood from the pericardial sac by performing pericardiocentesis. All the other tests would lead to unnecessary delays in diagnosis and would result in death.

    A cardiac surgery consult (**choice A**) is necessary for this patient to ultimately repair the damaged heart; however, the first step in saving this woman before the specialist arrives is pericardiocentesis.

    Echocardiogram (**choice B**) could aid in the diagnosis of pericardial effusion but would take too long to perform in such an emergent situation.

    A CT scan (**choice C**) would show a pericardial effusion, but there already are enough data to support the diagnosis, so x-ray would cause unnecessary delay in therapy.

    Chest tube placement (**choice D**) is used for pneumothorax and hemothorax but would not be effective in the present scenario.

25. **The correct answer is A.** The clinical and radiologic findings are typical of small bowel (jejunoileal) obstruction. If the pain becomes continuous and bowel sounds vanish, suspect that strangulation has occurred. The most frequent causes of small bowel obstruction are adhesions and incarceration in hernias. To investigate adhesions, look for a history of peritonitis, Crohn disease, pelvic inflammations, or abdominal or pelvic surgery.

    Overwhelming *Ascaris* infection (**choice B**) can cause small bowel obstruction, most frequently in poorly developed, third-world tropical countries.

    Cancer (**choice C**) of the duodenum or pancreas is the most common cause of obstruction of the duodenum, but the ladder-like series of dilated bowel loops would not be seen because the obstruction would be proximal to the ileum.

    Intussusception (**choice D**) is relatively common in infants but is much rarer (and usually related to tumor) in adults.

    Volvulus (**choice E**) is rare in the midgut.

26. **The correct answer is C.** In gunshot wounds of the upper zone of the neck, the main concern is the possibility of significant vascular injuries. The area is too high to involve the aerodigestive tract, and it is also rather difficult to explore surgically. Arteriogram offers the best way to assess the extent of the injuries, and also provides a way for embolization of major arteries that might be bleeding significantly.

    Clinical observation (**choice A**) is the second best answer, but it would delay recognition of significant vascular injuries that the arteriogram might demonstrate. Clinical observation is often all we do in asymptomatic stab wounds, where serious damage is less likely to occur.

    Barium studies (**choice B**) are essential when one suspects esophageal injury that is not demonstrated by gastrografin swallow. As pointed out above, however, the area of injury here is well above where the esophagus begins.

    Endoscopy (**choice D**) is incorrect for the same reasons that barium studies have no role in this case: the trajectory of the bullet is too high to involve the aerodigestive tract.

    Surgical exploration (**choice E**) might be unavoidable in hemodynamically unstable patients whose vascular injuries cannot be controlled by arteriographic embolization. Surgery can be performed in this area if needed, but for technical reasons it is not our first choice of management.

27. **The correct answer is A.** There are two favorable findings in this patient: Her axillary lymph nodes do not have metastasis, and her tumor is strongly positive for hor-

monal receptors. However, everything else is unfavorable: The tumor is quite large, and the prognostic factors are all unfavorable. Clearly, the patient would benefit from chemotherapy, and she should be placed on hormonal therapy after chemotherapy and radiation therapy to take advantage of the positive hormonal receptors. The objective of the hormonal manipulations is to either block her receptors (with tamoxifen) or suppress the production of estrogens (with anastrozole). Randomized studies have shown that anastrozole is considerably more effective than tamoxifen in postmenopausal patients. Thus, it has become the drug of choice for that group.

Chemotherapy and tamoxifen (**choice B**) would be the best course of action for premenopausal patients, for whom anastrozole is not yet approved as the best drug. Chemotherapy and tamoxifen would have been the regimen for this patient before the advent of anastrozole.

Adding estrogens and progesterone to the chemotherapy (**choice C**) would be contraindicated. We want to deprive the tumor of the stimulation provided by those hormones.

Completion of the operation to a more radical form of resection (**choice D**) has no benefits. The patient has a very large margin of normal tissue around the tumor, all the margins are negative, and the patient has agreed to postoperative radiation. We do not cure breast cancer by cutting out more normal tissue. We do it by treating the systemic spread of the disease.

Radiation therapy (**choice E**) is focal in nature. It does not treat distant metastatic spread. The patient needs radiation to the breast that had the tumor to minimize the rate of local recurrence. Radiating the other breast and the axilla would not be helpful.

28. **The correct answer is E.** A woman of this age who is found to be anemic and have occult blood in the stool should be suspected of having a cancer on the right side of the colon. Thus, the colonoscopy that was initially planned was the appropriate study. However, the patient also has obstructive jaundice, which is most likely of malignant origin (she has the sonographic equivalent of a positive Courvoisier-Terrier sign). Good clinical thinking involves attempting to find one single disease that explains all of the concurrent findings. Therefore, assuming that the patient has colon cancer plus a cancer of the head of the pancreas is not a good bet. A single tumor that would bleed into the gastrointestinal lumen and obstruct the common duct is ampullary carcinoma, and upper gastrointestinal endoscopy should identify it.

If we insist in ruling out colon cancer, colonoscopy could be done during the session in which upper gastrointestinal endoscopy is performed. Barium enema (**choice A**) would be a less attractive alternative.

The problem is not in the liver and, thus, a CT scan (**choice B**) or a biopsy (**choice C**) of the organ is a misguided effort. Dilated intrahepatic ducts and dilated extrahepatic ducts point to a low obstruction of the biliary tree. They are not suggestive of liver metastasis or liver pathology. The laboratory findings are also suggestive of biliary obstruction rather than hepatocellular disease.

Further definition of the nature of biliary obstruction can be obtained with an endoscopic retrograde cholangiopancreatogram (ERCP) or a percutaneous transhepatic cholangiogram (PTC; **choice D**). However, if we suspect that the obstructing tumor grows out of the duodenal wall, performing the study via a liver puncture (i.e., PTC) will miss the pathology. ERCP would find it, but, in fact, the full study would not have to be completed: As soon as the endoscopist looks at the ampulla, the tumor will be discovered. Cannulation of the ducts and injection of dye would not be needed.

29. **The correct answer is B.** This is actually the ideal candidate for breast-sparing surgery: a patient with a small primary tumor in a large breast, located far away from the nipple and areola. Provided radiation is done afterward, the cure rates are identical to those for more mutilating procedures. The cosmetic outcome is excellent, and no reconstruction is needed (the void left by the lumpectomy fills in with body fluids and is eventually replaced by connective tissue).

No surgery at all (**choice A**) is not an option. As much as we want to preserve the breast, and as much as we rely on postoperative radiation to lower the local recurrence rates, leaving the primary tumor in place does not lead to cure.

Simple mastectomy (**choice C**) entails more surgery than needed for the tumor (for which a lumpectomy followed by radiation is sufficient in this case), but not enough to learn about the status of the axillary nodes. They have to be sampled (either by dissection or sentinel node biopsy). Physical examination is totally unreliable for that purpose.

Although modified radical mastectomy (**choice D**) may be unavoidable in patients with larger primary tumors in smaller breasts, or tumors located where the nipple and areola can't be preserved, this patient does not need that larger operation (no survival advantage) and shouldn't take the more complicated and less pleasing breast reconstruction.

Old-fashioned radical mastectomy (**choice E**) is unnecessarily aggressive and not justified unless the tumor is huge and invading the pectoralis muscle. Unless surgical margins are positive for tumor, postoperative radiation would be equally unnecessary if the whole breast is taken.

30. **The correct answer is C.** Fever on the first postoperative day is almost invariably from atelectasis, the treatment of which requires active participation and cooperation from the patient. If atelectasis does not resolve, it leads to the development of pneumonia, which can be identified in chest x-ray films and confirmed with sputum cultures. At that time the process is no longer purely mechanical, but is also infectious, thus requiring antibiotics.

Deep venous thrombosis (**choice A**) occurs about 5-7 days after surgery and is a "hidden" source of fever (i.e., nothing else seems to be wrong). This patient is clearly a candidate for thrombosis (he lies in bed doing nothing all day), but right now his problem is probably in the lung.

The urine (**choice B**) is a good possibility when the fever starts on day 3, but the persistence of fever since day 1 points to the lung.

Three days is too soon for a wound infection (**choice D**) to be the cause of the fever. Five to seven days is a more likely time frame.

Looking for an abdominal abscess (**choice E**) is a little premature on the third day after surgery. These typically take a week to 10 days to develop.

31. **The correct answer is C.** Sensory fibers of the ninth (glossopharyngeal) nerve are in the vicinity of the digastric muscle, and can be damaged by retraction and dissection in the area. The lack of sensory input at the base of the tongue prevents the normal protective reflex that closes the glottis when swallowing liquids.

Unilateral injury to the main trunk of the vagus (**choice A**) in the neck would produce symptoms from the recurrent fibers that innervate the larynx, producing a hoarse voice but no change in swallowing.

Injury to the mandibular branch of the facial nerve (**choice B**) would produce drooping of the corner of the mouth and leaking of fluid at that level. Soup running out of the corner of the mouth is annoying, but swallowing is not affected.

If the superior laryngeal branch of the vagus is damaged (**choice D**), the voice tires easily. Swallowing is not affected.

The twelfth nerve (**choice E**) is the most commonly damaged nerve during carotid endarterectomy because it crosses the internal and external carotids a short distance cephalad to the bifurcation. However, the outcome is deviation of the tongue to the affected side.

32. **The correct answer is B.** A well-known risk of abdominoperineal resection is damage to the erectile nerves, as the rectum is widely dissected away from the pelvic walls. A 50% incidence of postoperative impotence is commonly quoted. "Nerve sparing" surgery can be done if the dissection is closer to the rectal wall, but the extent of the tumor may preclude it. A T3 (which this man had) is a large, bulky, primary tumor.

Arterial insufficiency (**choice A**) will lead to impotence either of sudden onset after perineal trauma (motorcycle accident, for instance) or of very gradual development in chronic vascular disease.

Psychogenic impotence (**choice C**) has a sudden onset but is partner- or situation-specific. Typically, nocturnal erections are preserved, as is the ability to masturbate.

Tumor invasion (**choice D**), if it is into the pelvic tissues, may indeed require a dissection that damages the nerves, but the problem would not involve the urethra.

Venous incompetence (**choice E**) is a common source of organic impotence, which would have gradual onset and no connection with pelvic surgery.

33. **The correct answer is D.** Nowadays, when thousands of patients are awaiting transplants and many die before they get them, every potential donor should be evaluated by the experts. They may indeed reject some, but probably very few. For instance, corneas can be harvested even from people with cancer, and donors with chronic viral infections can be used for patients who have the same viral disease.

All the other options were at one time or another used to exclude donors. These situations still make solid organs less attractive, but not to the extent that evaluation should be precluded.

34. **The correct answer is D.** This is a typical history for fracture of the posterior lateral talar tubercle; this fracture also occurs in basketball and tennis players who come down hard after a jump. This type of fracture is a fairly common foot injury that you should be able to clinically recognize. The diagnosis can be confirmed with lateral x-ray films of the ankle. Treatment is with immobilization in a cast for 4-6 weeks.

Anterior Achilles tendon bursitis (**choice A**) would also cause pain behind the foot/ankle, but would develop more slowly.

Calcaneal spur syndrome (**choice B**) causes heel pain and usually develops slowly.

Epiphysitis of the calcaneus (**choice C**) is a painful cartilage break in the heel of young children in whom the two centers of ossification of the calcaneus have not yet fused.

Posterior tibial nerve neuralgia (**choice E**) causes pain (sometimes burning) around the ankle and sometimes extending to the toes; the pain is worse on walking.

35. **The correct answer is C.** You probably had no trouble discerning that bacterial endocarditis, triggered by the use of nonsterile IV drugs, damaged a heart valve in this man. Although we usually think of the right-sided valves

as the ones that are first in line to catch the bugs, any valve can become the seat of infection. The clinical presentation leaves no doubt that the aortic valve is the one that has been destroyed: the murmur is systolic, at the right base, and the very low diastolic pressure reveals the incompetence of the aortic valve. Furthermore, this was not a slow process allowing for compensation: he is in failure and close to death. He needs a new valve, pronto!

Closure of the ventricular septal defect with a pericardial patch (**choice A**) would have been more appropriate for a massive myocardial infarction producing a septal defect. The clinical presentation would have been different, with a systolic murmur and normal diastolic pressure.

Elective repair (**choice B**) is wrong for at least two reasons: it would not address an acute problem, and the criteria given were those for long-standing aortic stenosis (not insufficiency).

The mitral valve (**choice D**) does not produce the symptoms described.

The pulmonic valve (**choice E**) is not the culprit either. If it were destroyed, it would give few manifestations (it is almost a "disposable" valve).

36. **The correct answer is D.** This patient experienced a severe deceleration injury. He is hypotensive, tachycardic, and minimally responsive. He is in hemorrhagic shock. The chest x-ray reveals a widening mediastinum, suggesting a rupture of the thoracic aorta, which is a common catastrophic injury in deceleration accidents. This patient is in grave danger. After confirmation of the diagnosis by spiral CT scan, the treatment is immediate surgical repair of the injury with fluid and blood resuscitation.

Cardiac contusion (**choice A**) is common in blunt-force injuries in which the steering wheel has crushed the chest. Arrhythmias, bundle branch block, or ECG abnormalities mimicking infarction may occur. Pericardial effusion or rupture may develop.

Cardiac tamponade (**choice B**) is associated with hypotension and tachycardia. However, pulsus paradoxus (systolic blood pressure drops >10 mm Hg on respiration) and distant heart sounds might be discovered on physical examination, and his central venous pressure would be high. Chest x-ray films might show an enlarged cardiac silhouette. The ECG might exhibit low limb-lead voltage and variable QRS amplitude (electrical alternans). However, pericardiocentesis is both the diagnostic and therapeutic procedure of choice.

Flail chest (**choice C**) is diagnosed when a part of the chest wall bound by fractured ribs moves paradoxically during respiration. Ventilation is hampered.

Tension pneumothorax (**choice E**) occurs when air can enter but not leave the pleural space. The mediastinum appears to be shifted to the contralateral side on chest x-ray films. A region without peripheral lung markings outlined by a sharp pleural margin is characteristic. Breath sounds are depressed or absent on the affected side.

37. **The correct answer is C.** This man is not a surgical candidate, thus ruling out pneumonectomy (**choices D and E**). With a central lesion, he would require a pneumonectomy rather than a lobectomy. After resectional pulmonary surgery is done, however, a patient must be left with at least 800 mL in the FEV_1 to live a semi-decent life. Anything less than that would make him a pulmonary cripple, or outright kill him. Because of his COPD, this patient is already severely limited, with a total FEV_1 of 1,100 mL. Were the bad lung to be removed, he would be left with only 40% of 1,100 mL: 440 mL. The only option left is radiation and chemotherapy.

CT scan of the upper abdomen to rule out liver metastasis (**choice A**) and mediastinoscopy to biopsy carinal nodes (**choice B**) are necessary steps to establish curability. There is no point in doing a pneumonectomy if there are liver or carinal node metastases. But if a pneumonectomy cannot be done for reasons of poor function, there is no point in finding out whether the other limiting factors are present.

38. **The correct answer is E.** The child has testicular torsion, one of the very few true urologic emergencies. He needs immediate de-torsion if the testis is to be saved. No time should be wasted doing further studies.

Symptomatic care (**choice A**) is fine for testicular trauma with scrotal hematomas. In this case, it would amount to malpractice.

A sonogram (**choice B**) is always done when the clinical diagnosis is epididymitis, and we want to be sure that torsion is not being overlooked. But when the clinical diagnosis screams "torsion," as in this vignette, time wasted confirming the diagnosis with the sonogram could lead to loss of the testicle.

Antibiotics (**choice C**) are effective therapy for acute epididymitis, the condition with which testicular torsion may be confused. But the patient with epididymitis is usually somewhat older (sexually active) and has fever, pyuria, a very tender cord, and a normally positioned testicle.

Testicular biopsy (**choice D**) is done when we think that the diagnosis is cancer, but the scenario would be a painless mass in a young male.

39. **The correct answer is C.** Squamous cell carcinoma of the penis is admittedly a rare form of cancer in the U.S. (about 1% of all cancers in males). It is virtually unknown in nations that practice early (i.e., in infancy)

circumcision. It presents as a fungating or ulcerated mass on the glans penis or in the sulcus between the prepuce and the glans. Carcinogenic agents forming in the smegma are suspected to play a pathogenic role, which may be enhanced by lack of circumcision. Other risk factors include lesions (condyloma acuminatum) due to human papillomavirus (HPV) types 16 and 18. Genomic material from these HPV types has been demonstrated in numerous cases. No association has been observed between penile cancer or its precursors and other types of HPV, such as type 6 (**choice B**) or 11. Psoriasis is associated with a slightly increased risk.

Balanitis xerotica obliterans (**choice A**) results in fibrosis and thickening of the prepuce. This condition does not seem to confer a significantly increased risk of developing penile carcinoma.

Peyronie disease (**choice D**), which is a form of *fibromatosis* affecting the penis, results in induration, nodularity, and deformities. It causes severe functional deficits but is not associated with increased risk of cancer. This condition is akin to other forms of fibromatosis, such as Dupuytren contracture.

The primary stage of syphilis (**choice E**) manifests with a painless, sharply demarcated ulcer (*chancre*) often located in the glans. There is no association between syphilis and penile cancer.

40. **The correct answer is C.** This patient has scapular "winging," a protrusion of the scapula when the ipsilateral outstretched arm is pressed against a wall. Scapular winging results from paralysis of the serratus anterior muscle, which functions to carry the scapula forward and assist the deltoid in raising the arm. The serratus is innervated by the long thoracic nerve, which is derived from the fifth, sixth, and seventh cervical nerve roots. This woman had an axillary lymph node dissection that may have damaged the inferior part of the brachial plexus, leading to long thoracic nerve damage, paralysis of the serratus, and scapular winging.

The intercostal nerves (**choice A**) arise from the thoracic nerve roots and innervate the intercostal muscles of the chest wall.

The lateral pectoral (**choice B**) and medial pectoral (**choice D**) nerves innervate the pectoralis major and minor muscles.

The thoracodorsal nerve (**choice E**) innervates the latissimus dorsi muscle.

41. **The correct answer is B.** In patients sustaining trauma, there is a chance of bony cervical spine injury. Iatrogenic injury is to be avoided by immobilization of the cervical spine until bony injury is ruled out. In this scenario, the patient has sustained significant trauma about the head.

Because he has altered mental status, it is impossible to use clinical decision rules (such as NEXUS) to clear his cervical spine. Since he will require CT scanning of his head, continuing the scan to include his cervical spine is both cost effective and medically appropriate.

A CT scan of the head (**choice A**) is certainly indicated in a trauma patient with facial/head trauma and altered mental status. This is not the most appropriate answer, however.

CT scan of the abdomen (**choice C**) or peritoneal lavage (**choice E**) are useful for evaluating the degree of abdominal injury when abdominal examination is inadequate, especially in an unconscious trauma patient.

Immediate laparotomy (**choice D**) is not indicated in a hemodynamically stable patient with no outward evidence of chest or abdominal trauma.

42. **The correct answer is A.** Pulmonary artery (Swan-Ganz) catheters are ubiquitous in critical care settings; a basic ability to interpret data from them is vital to the practice of inpatient hospital medicine. This patient has a low cardiac output and a high filling pressure (>18 mm Hg) and is hypotensive. Therefore, this patient's shock syndrome is cardiogenic. Cardiogenic shock is caused by a number of underlying problems, but the end result is left ventricular failure. This also accounts for the secondarily high right-sided pressures and filling pressures (left heart failure causes right heart failure).

Acute mitral regurgitation (MR; **choice B**) is a possibility in this case. At first glance, acute MR could account for all of the patient's findings, both on physical examination and pulmonary artery catheter. However, unless the acute MR occurred in the setting of acute ischemia, there is no way to account for the severely depressed cardiac output (LV function). Therefore, isolated acute MR from a papillary muscle rupture or chordae rupture could not alone account for all of this patient's findings.

Acute right heart failure (**choice C**) is incorrect because it fails to explain the elevated left-sided filling pressures.

Hypoxic pulmonary vasoconstriction (**choice D**) would acutely produce elevated pulmonary artery pressures and possibly right heart failure over the long term, but not in an acute manner.

Sepsis syndrome (**choice E**) is defined as hyperdynamic cardiac output (supraphysiologic) with systemic hypotension. This patient has a depressed output, not compatible with sepsis.

43. **The correct answer is D.** Even if you do not remember all the spinal cord tracts and pathways, you should recognize that deficits in one set of functions below the injury on one side, combined with deficits in a different group of functions on the other side, spells out hemisec-

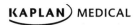

tion. Furthermore, such clean-cut division of one side of the spinal cord can happen only with a knife or a bullet, which is the setting in this vignette.

Anterior cord syndrome (**choice A**) is characterized by sparing of the posterior columns, with preservation of vibration and position sense. The etiology is typically vascular.

Central cord syndrome (**choice B**) is seen in whiplash injuries, in which it produces severe deficits in the upper extremities, with relative sparing of the lower extremities. Sensory loss consists of loss of pain and temperature sense in a "cape" distribution over the shoulders, lower neck, and upper trunk with posterior column function (light touch, vibration, conscious proprioception) relatively preserved.

Complete transection (**choice C**) would result in spastic paralysis below the level of the injury with flaccid paralysis at the level of the injury. Ascending sensory fibers would also be interrupted, producing a total sensory deficit below the level of the lesion.

Posterior cord syndrome (**choice E**) would result in selective loss of conscious proprioception, vibratory sense, stereognosis, graphesthesia, and two point discrimination. It is fairly rare.

44. **The correct answer is A.** Crush injury results in massive tissue damage. There are obvious organ-specific consequences of such injury, but it is the musculoskeletal system that is the focus of this question. Massive necrosis and lysis of muscle releases intracellular myoplasm components that are toxic in high concentrations. Examples of such constituents include potassium, creatine kinase, and protein. It can be generally assumed that any patient with significant crush injuries will have autoinfusion of hundreds of milliequivalents of potassium into the blood.

There is no significant derangement in sodium levels, such as hypernatremia (**choice B**), after a crush injury.

Cells in general, and myocytes in particular, are storehouses of calcium. With significant myonecrosis, serum calcium can rise to dangerous levels, producing hypercalcemia, rather than hypocalcemia (**choice C**).

Hypoglycemia (**choice D**) would not be seen in this patient. Because of the stress of his injuries and the elevated levels of cortisol and epinephrine in his blood, massive amounts of glucose would be mobilized. Thus, if any derangement in glucose homeostasis were present, it would likely be hyperglycemia.

Hyperphosphatemia, rather than hypophosphatemia (**choice E**), is observed with a crush injury. Phosphate is an intracellular buffer that is also released from cells after necrosis and lysis.

45. **The correct answer is D.** Acute mediastinitis with air in the tissues that occurs within a few hours of an upper gastrointestinal endoscopy is virtually diagnostic of instrumental, iatrogenic esophageal perforation.

Boerhaave syndrome (**choice A**) is also a form of esophageal perforation, but it is caused by protracted, forceful vomiting, which this patient did not have.

A dissecting aneurysm of the thoracic aorta (**choice B**) can mimic a myocardial infarction, but it would not fill the mediastinum with air.

In upper gastrointestinal endoscopy, the esophagus, which has narrow lumen and a flimsy wall, can be perforated easily, but the stomach (**choice C**), which has ample lumen and a thick, strong wall, almost never is. Furthermore, other than looking, nothing was done that could damage the stomach (laser or electrocoagulation). Finally, a hole in the stomach gives an acute abdomen with free air under the diaphragm, rather than mediastinitis with air in the mediastinum.

A real myocardial infarction (**choice E**) is rare in a 32-year-old, and like the previous option, it produces pain but not mediastinitis with air.

46. **The correct answer is B.** A noncontrast CT is most likely to detect a stone in this patient, who manifests the typical symptomatology of renal colic, most commonly due to a urinary stone impacted in the ureter. Usually, gross or microscopic hematuria is present. Absence of fever and bacteriuria is an important negative sign excluding coexistence of urinary tract infection.

Intravenous pyelography (IVP; **choice A**) is rarely necessary in patients with the typical presentation of renal colic. Frequently, this investigation will demonstrate dilatation of the ureter proximal to the site of stone blockage.

Renal ultrasound examination (**choice C**) may show hydronephrosis or stones in the kidney, supporting but not confirming urethral stones.

Serum calcium, phosphorus, electrolytes, and uric acid (**choice D**) should be evaluated in patients experiencing a recurrent urinary tract stone, but serum chemistry studies are not necessary as initial diagnostic investigations.

Urine cultures (**choice E**) are not necessary for uncomplicated urinary stone disease without clinical evidence of urinary tract infection. However, abnormal urinary pH should suggest participation of infectious agents in stone formation. *Proteus* infections result in alkaline pH because of urease production. On the other hand, a pH lower than 5.0 suggests urate or cystine stones.

47. **The correct answer is E.** The description is perfect for simple liver cysts, which occur in roughly 10% of the population at large. Nothing needs to be done about this.

KAPLAN) MEDICAL

The "Mexico connection" is the tip-off to suspect amebic abscess (**choice A**) in a patient who lives there and who presents with fever, leukocytosis, a tender liver, and elevated alkaline phosphatase. That is not the clinical picture this patient has, however.

Cystadenocarcinomas (**choice B**) have thick walls with multiple septations. Calcifications in the cyst wall also may be present, and usually the affected patient is a middle-aged woman.

Hydatid cysts (**choice C**) can occur but are not particularly prevalent in Mexico, a little geographic detail unknown to most American physicians. High plains in the Andes or a Mediterranean country would be a better location. In any event, however, the hydatid cyst is characteristic, with a large mother cyst containing daughter cysts around the periphery.

The cysts of polycystic liver disease (**choice D**) occur in much larger numbers, tend to enlarge over the years, and often are accompanied by renal cysts.

48. **The correct answer is J.** Secondary tuberculosis commonly affects the kidneys by hematogenous dissemination. Cavitary lesions may be demonstrated by intravenous pyelography (IVP). The patient frequently gives a history of weight loss and low-grade fever. The infection spreads with the urinary flow down into the bladder, frequently involving the epididymis and prostate in men. Sometimes, the first clinical manifestation of urinary tract tuberculosis is hematuria. Urine cultures are often negative, but the urine contains large numbers of leukocytes (so-called *sterile pyuria*).

49. **The correct answer is F.** Hemorrhagic cystitis is characterized by marked hematuria, resulting from extensive erosions of the urinary bladder mucosa. Cyclophosphamide is one of the most common etiologic agents of this form of cystitis. Another cause of hemorrhagic cystitis is radiation.

50. **The correct answer is M.** Von Hippel-Lindau syndrome is a hereditary autosomal dominant disease characterized by hemangioblastomas of the CNS (most frequently in the cerebellum and retina), cysts of the pancreas and kidneys, and renal cell carcinoma. The patient's family history is perfectly compatible with this diagnosis. Thus, the presence of hematuria, along with coexistent renal lesions detected on ultrasonography, indicates that renal cell carcinoma has also developed in this patient. Renal cell carcinoma associated with von Hippel-Lindau syndrome is often multicentric and cystic. Recall that the gene involved in this disease (VHL gene) has been found mutated in most cases of the more common sporadic renal cell carcinoma.

Acute postinfectious glomerulonephritis (**choice A**) manifests with nephritic syndrome, characterized by hematuria, hypertension, proteinuria less than 3 g/day, and mild edema (periorbital and pedal). It usually occurs in children 1-3 weeks following group A *Streptococcus* pharyngitis or impetigo.

Autosomal dominant polycystic kidney disease (**choice B**) manifests in middle-aged or elderly individuals with hematuria and *hypertension*. Usually, palpable enlarged kidneys are found on physical examination.

Bacterial cystitis (**choice C**) is commonly due to *Escherichia coli*. Dysuria, frequency of urination, and suprapubic discomfort are the principal symptoms. Hematuria, gross or microscopic, is frequently seen on dipstick urinalysis.

Berger disease (**choice D**) is the most frequent cause of glomerulonephritis, manifesting with hematuria and/or proteinuria. It is often discovered incidentally. *IgA deposition* in the mesangium and high serum IgA levels are the defining features.

Bladder transitional cell carcinoma (**choice E**) is associated with hematuria, but usually not with other symptoms. Intravenous pyelography (IVP) is not sensitive enough to detect this type of cancer. *Urinary cytology* and cystoscopy are necessary for diagnosis.

Prostatic carcinoma (**choice G**) rarely manifests with hematuria as its first presenting sign. The most common mode of presentation nowadays is by *elevated prostatic-specific antigen* (PSA) and/or abnormal findings on digital rectal examination.

Testicular cancer (**choice H**) is not associated with hematuria. Its most common first sign is *painless testicular enlargement*, associated with a sensation of heaviness. Frequently, patients come to the physician many months after the initial onset of these signs.

Transitional cell carcinoma of the pelvis (**choice I**) is relatively rare compared with renal cell carcinoma and urinary bladder transitional carcinoma. Its most common presentation is hematuria, but IVP demonstrates these tumors as filling defects in the pelvicaliceal system.

A ureteral stone (**choice K**) most commonly presents with *renal colic*, a paroxysmal form of flank pain associated with extreme restlessness that results from ureteral obstruction. Hematuria is present during colicky episodes and sometimes in asymptomatic periods. IVP would show dilatation of the ureter proximal to the impacted stone.

Urethral carcinoma (**choice L**) usually comes to medical attention because of bloody urethral discharge in an elderly patient. If hematuria is present, it is detected in the first few milliliters of urine (*initial hematuria*) when urine is collected in separate aliquots.

Surgery: **Test Two**

1. A neonate does not pass any meconium during the first day of life. On day 2 he is brought for evaluation because of repeated green vomiting and progressive abdominal distention. X-ray films of the abdomen show multiple dilated loops of small bowel and no gas in the colon. A contrast enema shows a normally positioned microcolon, and the contrast material refluxes freely into the small bowel, filling some of the more distal distended loops. Exploratory laparotomy is done. There is no malrotation, the small bowel does not have any atretic or obstructed segments, and there is no inspissated meconium in it. Which of the following is most appropriate next step in management?

    (A) Diverting ileostomy

    (B) Diverting ileostomy and appendectomy

    (C) Transverse loop colostomy

    (D) Total colectomy

    (E) Total proctocolectomy and permanent ileostomy

2. A 24-year-old woman develops moderate, generalized abdominal pain of sudden onset and shortly thereafter faints. At the time of evaluation in the emergency department, she has regained consciousness, is pale, and has a blood pressure of 95/70 mm Hg and a faint pulse rate of 90/min. The abdomen is mildly distended and tender, with normal bowel sounds. Her hemoglobin is 7 g/dL. There is no history of trauma, but it is suspected that she might be bleeding into her abdomen, and a bedside fast ultrasound is performed. The study shows that there is free blood in the peritoneal cavity. She denies the possibility of pregnancy because she has been on birth control pills since the age of 14 and has never missed taking them. Pelvic examination is normal, and a pregnancy test is negative. At laparotomy, the surgeons are likely to find which of the following?

    (A) Bleeding ovarian follicle

    (B) Ruptured abdominal aortic aneurysm

    (C) Ruptured ectopic pregnancy

    (D) Ruptured hepatic adenoma

    (E) Ruptured hepatic artery aneurysm

3. A 56-year-old man presents to his urologist for continued evaluation of hypertension and hematuria. The patient has a 10-year history of hypertension and recent onset of painless hematuria for which he sought the attention of an urologist 3 months ago. On detailed questioning, the man states that he has been having severe headaches that are refractory to narcotic analgesics. Three days ago, a renal ultrasound was obtained that demonstrated bilaterally enlarged kidneys with multiple cysts. Which of the following is the most appropriate next step in diagnosis?

    (A) CT scan of the pelvis

    (B) CT scan of the thorax

    (C) MRI of the brain

    (D) Intravenous pyelography (IVP)

    (E) Magnetic resonance angiogram (MRA) of the brain

4. A patient involved in a high-speed automobile collision arrives in the emergency department unconscious, with multiple facial fractures; brisk bleeding into his nose, mouth, and throat; and gurgly, irregular, noisy breathing. Which of the following would be the best method to secure an airway in this patient?

    (A) Nasotracheal intubation with visualization of the cords

    (B) Orotracheal intubation with rapid anesthetic induction

    (C) Percutaneous transtracheal ventilation

    (D) Cricothyroidotomy done in the emergency department

    (E) Emergency tracheostomy done in the emergency department

5. A 25-year-old man presents with a painless, hard, 3-cm testicular mass that he discovered serendipitously while taking a shower. Physical examination confirms that the mass arises from the testicle itself, is not part of the epididymis, and is solid rather than a fluid collection. The rest of the physical examination is unremarkable. Which of the following would be the most appropriate next step?

   (A) Serum levels of alpha-fetoprotein and beta human chorionic gonadotropin
   (B) Trans-scrotal needle biopsy of the mass
   (C) Trans-scrotal incisional biopsy at the edge of the mass
   (D) Trans-scrotal orchiectomy
   (E) Radical inguinal orchiectomy

6. A 72-year-old man has a 4-cm hard mass in the left supraclavicular area. The mass is movable and non-tender and has been present and steadily growing for the past 3 months. On direct questioning the only additional findings include a 20-pound weight loss and a vague feeling of epigastric discomfort over the past 2 months. Physical examination shows evidence of the weight loss but no other significant findings in the abdominal examination. The supraclavicular mass is obvious, but no other masses can be felt anywhere else in the neck, axillas, or groins. There is occult blood in the stool, and his hemoglobin is 10.5 g/dL. Which of the following would a biopsy of the supraclavicular mass most likely reveal?

   (A) Chronic inflammation
   (B) Lymphoma
   (C) Metastatic gastric cancer
   (D) Metastatic squamous cell carcinoma
   (E) Metastatic thyroid cancer

7. A 65-year-old man comes to the physician for a health maintenance examination. Which of the following screening methods would allow the highest detection rate of prostatic carcinoma in early stages?

   (A) Cytologic examination of prostatic secretion
   (B) Digital rectal examination alone
   (C) Serum PSA determination alone
   (D) Serum PSA and digital rectal examination
   (E) Transrectal ultrasonography

8. A 62-year-old, right-handed man who has no medical problems and takes no medications has a sudden onset of neurologic deficits. While he was watching the news on television, he suddenly could not move his right upper extremity or speak. His family promptly transported him to the nearest emergency room, where he arrived about 20 minutes after the onset of symptoms. He is found to be normotensive, awake, and alert with a normal fingerstick glucose but unable to move his right arm or articulate his speech. He can understand what is said to him but can only respond by nodding his head or motioning his left arm. He denies the presence of any headache when his symptoms developed. He is rapidly moved to the CT scan machine, and a CT scan of his head is completed within the next 20 minutes. The scan shows a small area of cortical ischemia on the left side, affecting the motor strip and the speech center. There are no radiologic signs of intracranial bleeding. By the time he returns from the scanner, approximately 50 minutes have elapsed since his symptoms began. His neurologic deficits have not changed. Which of the following should be the next step in management?

   (A) Continued clinical observation for 3 hours
   (B) Duplex scanning of his carotid arteries
   (C) Emergency left carotid endarterectomy
   (D) Intravenous heparin and loading dose of oral warfarin
   (E) Intravenous infusion of tissue-type plasminogen activator after consultation with a neurologist and appropriate consent

9. A 78-year-old man comes to the physician because of a bloody urethral discharge for 3 days. He has had increasing frequency of urination and hesitancy for the past 2 years, but these symptoms have never been severe enough to require medical attention. Digital rectal examination reveals a slightly enlarged and firm prostate. Expressed prostatic secretions are negative for bacteria and leukocytes. Collection of a clean-catch urine in separate aliquots reveals initial hematuria, with blood present in the first 5 mL. Which of the following is the most likely diagnosis?

   (A) Gonococcal infection
   (B) Nonbacterial prostatitis
   (C) Prostatic carcinoma
   (D) Testicular cancer
   (E) Urethral carcinoma

10. While playing football, a college student injures his shoulder. He comes in with his arm held close to his body, complaining of pain over the clavicle, rather than the shoulder joint. Physical examination shows a normal shoulder, but there is point tenderness at the junction of the middle and distal thirds of the clavicle. Gentle pressure elicits a gritty feeling of bone crunching on bone. He has normal pulses on that arm. After appropriate x-ray studies are performed, which of the following is the most appropriate initial step in management?

    (A) Analgesics only

    (B) Immobilization by a figure-eight device

    (C) Immobilization by hanging cast

    (D) Arteriogram of the subclavian vessels

    (E) Open reduction and internal fixation

11. A 38-year-old immigrant from Latin America sustained a third-degree burn in the lateral aspect of her lower leg when she was 14. The burn was untreated. Ever since the incident, she has had shallow ulcerations at the scar site that heal and break down all the time. In the past few months she has developed an indolent, dirty-looking, deeper ulcer at the site, with "heaped up" tissue growth around the edges. The ulcer is steadily growing and showing no signs of healing. Which of the following is the most appropriate next step in diagnosis?

    (A) Doppler studies

    (B) Venous pressure tracings

    (C) Culture of the ulcer base

    (D) Biopsy of the ulcer edge

    (E) Arteriogram

12. A 67-year-old woman of Asian descent presents at the emergency room at 9 P.M. complaining of an extremely severe right frontal headache. The pain started while she was at the movies, watching the second film of a double-feature program. The pain forced her to leave the movie theater, and her husband had to drive her to the emergency room because in addition to her very severe headache, she saw halos around all of the streetlights and headlights of oncoming traffic. During the drive, she suffered from severe nausea and tried to vomit twice, but "nothing came up." On physical examination, her right eye is red and tearing, the cornea has a greenish, steamy look, and the right pupil is fixed in mid-dilation. She has decreased vision in that eye, and when she is questioned about it, she admits that it is her eye, not her head, that hurts terribly. Palpation suggests that the right eye is "hard as a rock." Which of the following should be started as emergency treatment while awaiting ophthalmologic consultation?

    (A) Copious irrigation of the eye with sterile saline

    (B) Intravenous carbonic anhydrase inhibitor

    (C) Ophthalmologic atropine drops

    (D) Topical antihistamines or mast cell inhibitors

    (E) Topical corticosteroid-antibiotic combination

13. A window cleaner falls from a third-story scaffold and lands on his feet. Physical examination and x-rays show comminuted fractures of both calcaneus. He is tender to palpation over multiple bruises and abrasions in other parts of his trunk and extremities, but he has normal vital signs and a normal neurologic exam. Given the mechanism of injury, which of the following is the most appropriate next step in diagnosis?

    (A) Abdominal CT scan

    (B) Cervical spine x-ray films

    (C) X-ray films of thoracic and lumbar spine

    (D) Appropriate arteriograms

    (E) Retrograde urethrogram

14. A 22-year-old woman is brought to the emergency department after a motorcycle accident in which she sustained severe crush injuries of her lower extremities. In the field, her Glasgow Coma Score was 14. She is awake and alert on arrival after having been given morphine for pain control. Details of her past medical history are unknown. Initial examination shows a blood pressure of 140/80 mm Hg and pulse of 100/min. Her oxygen saturation on room air is 95% by pulse oximeter. An ECG is obtained and shows very large, peaked T-waves in leads V1 to V6. Which of the following is the most appropriate initial step in patient care?

   (A) Administer oral sodium polystyrene sulfonate (Kayexalate)

   (B) Administer IV calcium gluconate

   (C) Administer IV bicarbonate

   (D) Administer IV insulin and dextrose

   (E) Initiate urgent hemodialysis

15. Eight days after a difficult hemigastrectomy and gastroduodenostomy for gastric ulcer, a patient begins to leak 2 to 3 L of greenish fluid per day through the right corner of his bilateral subcostal surgical incision. He is afebrile and has no clinical signs of an acute abdomen. At surgery, a feeding catheter jejunostomy was placed, through which the patient has been receiving 3 L/day of elemental diet with a caloric content of 1 cal per mL, and 1 g nitrogen per 100 cal. The nursing staff has rigged a very effective collection device for the fluid that is leaking through the wound, and the skin around the site is well protected. Which of the following is the most appropriate next step in management?

   (A) No changes in the present therapeutic plan

   (B) Addition of 2 to 3 L per day of IV Ringer's lactate

   (C) Immediate discontinuation of the jejunal feeding, and replacement by 5 L/day of IV 5% dextrose-half normal saline

   (D) Surgical drainage of the operative area

   (E) Surgical reconstruction of the gastroduodenostomy

16. A pedestrian is hit by a car. Physical examination shows the leg to be angulated midpoint between the knee and the ankle. X-ray films confirm fractures of the shaft of the tibia and fibula. Satisfactory alignment is achieved by external manipulation, and a long leg cast applied. In the ensuing 8 hours, the patient complains of increasing pain. When the cast is removed, the pain persists, the muscle compartments feel tight, and there is excruciating pain with passive extension of the toes. Which of the following is the most appropriate next step in management?

   (A) Re-casting with a looser cast

   (B) Nerve block prior to re-casting

   (C) Arteriogram

   (D) Fasciotomy

   (E) Open reduction and internal fixation

17. A 27-year-old man is shot point blank with a .22-caliber revolver. The entrance wound is in the anterior chest wall, just to the left of the sternal border, at the level of the 4th intercostal space. There is no exit wound. He is diaphoretic, cold, shivering, and anxious, and is asking for a blanket and a drink of water. His blood pressure is 65/40 mm Hg, and his pulse is 145/min and barely perceptible. He has large, distended veins in his neck and forehead. He is breathing adequately and has bilateral breath sounds. He is neurologically intact. Which of the following is the most likely diagnosis?

   (A) Extrinsic cardiogenic shock due to pericardial tamponade

   (B) Extrinsic cardiogenic shock due to tension pneumothorax

   (C) Hemorrhagic shock

   (D) Intrinsic cardiogenic shock due to myocardial damage

   (E) Vasomotor shock

18. A college student is tackled while playing football and develops severe knee pain. When examined shortly thereafter, the knee is swollen and the patient has pain on direct palpation over the lateral aspect of the knee. With the knee flexed 30 degrees, passive adduction elicits pain on the same area, and the leg can be adducted further than in the normal contralateral leg (varus stress test). The anterior drawer test, posterior drawer test, and Lachman test are negative. Which of the following is the most likely site of injury?

    (A) Anterior cruciate ligament
    (B) Lateral collateral ligament
    (C) Lateral meniscus
    (D) Medial collateral ligament
    (E) Posterior cruciate ligament

19. Six hours after undergoing laparoscopic bilateral inguinal hernia repairs, a 62-year-old man complains of suprapubic discomfort and fullness. He feels the need to void but has not been able to do so since the operation. There is a palpable suprapubic mass that is dull to percussion. Palpation of that mass exacerbates the symptoms. Which of the following is the most appropriate next step in management?

    (A) Abdominal x-ray films to ascertain the nature of the mass
    (B) Increased rate of IV fluid administration
    (C) Loop diuretics
    (D) In and out bladder catheterization
    (E) Placement of indwelling Foley catheter

20. A 49-year-old man crashes his car against a bridge abutment at high speed. On arrival at the emergency department, he is breathing well, but he has multiple bruises over the chest, and there is a specific spot at about the middle of the sternum that is exquisitely painful to touch. Gentle palpation of that area elicits a gritty feeling of bone grating on bone. He distinctly recalls hitting the steering wheel with his chest and is certain that he hurt that particular spot in that manner. Anteroposterior and lateral chest x-ray films confirm that he has a sternal fracture. The films do not show any mediastinal widening or mediastinal air, and both lung fields are clear. His vital signs are normal, and he does not have subcutaneous emphysema. Which of the following studies is most likely to show evidence of additional injuries?

    (A) Serial ECGs
    (B) Abdominal x-ray films
    (C) Gastrografin swallow
    (D) Bronchoscopy
    (E) Esophagoscopy

21. A 60-year-old man complains of anal itching and discomfort, particularly toward the end of the day. He works as a salesman in a department store, where he has to be on his feet all day. When he goes home in the evening, he finds himself sitting sideways to avoid the discomfort. He has no fever, rectal bleeding, or soiling of his underwear, and he has never had surgery in that area. Which of the following is the most likely diagnosis?

    (A) Anal fissure
    (B) External hemorrhoids
    (C) Fistula in ano
    (D) Internal hemorrhoids
    (E) Perirectal abscess

22. A 45-year-old man shows up in the emergency department with a pale, pulseless, paresthetic, painful, and paralytic right lower extremity. The process began suddenly 2 hours ago. On examination, no pulses are apparent in the right lower extremity. Pulse at the wrist is 95/min and grossly irregular. Treatment would likely be based on which of the following?

    (A) Dacron prosthetic vascular conduits

    (B) Fogarty balloon tipped catheters

    (C) Heparin and dicumarol

    (D) Saphenous vein bypasses

    (E) Selective sympathetic blocks

23. A 62-year-old, right-handed man has transient episodes of paralysis of the right arm and inability to express himself. There is no associated headache. The episodes have sudden onset, last about 5 to 10 minutes, and leave no neurologic sequela. The patient is overweight and sedentary. He smokes one pack of cigarettes per day and has high cholesterol, but he is not hypertensive. The only abnormality in the physical examination is a bruit over the left carotid bifurcation. Which of the following is the most appropriate initial step in diagnosis?

    (A) CT scan of the head

    (B) Duplex scanning of the carotids

    (C) Echocardiogram

    (D) MRI of the brain

    (E) Aortic arch arteriogram

24. Eight hours after undergoing a transnasal, transsphenoidal resection of a prolactinoma, a young lady becomes lethargic, confused, and eventually comatose. Review of the record shows that her urinary output since surgery has averaged 600 mL/hr, while her intake of IV fluids (5% dextrose in 0.45% saline) has been 100 mL/hr. Her blood pressure is 110/75 mm Hg, and her pulse is 88/min. Which of the following would most likely yield the correct diagnosis?

    (A) Blood glucose determination

    (B) CT scan of the head

    (C) Creatinine clearance

    (D) Serum levels of ACTH

    (E) Serum sodium determination

25. A 69-year-old man, who smokes and drinks heavily, complains of an earache on his left side. The earache has been present for 6 weeks and is not getting any better despite systemic antibiotics and ear drops. On physical examination, he is found to have very poor oral hygiene, only a few remaining stumps of rotten teeth, and big tonsils that are hard to see because he gags easily. Otoscopic examination shows a perfectly normal right tympanic membrane, although the left is distorted by what appears to be a serous otitis media. Tuning fork testing shows conductive hearing loss on the left but equal bone conduction on both sides. He is afebrile. Which of the following will most likely confirm the diagnosis?

    (A) Audiometry

    (B) MRI studies of the eighth nerve

    (C) Culture of fluid aspirated from the left ear

    (D) Biopsies of the tympanic membrane and ear canal

    (E) Panendoscopy and biopsies

26. A 53-year-old woman sustains multiple injuries in a head-on automobile collision. She was driving the car and wearing a seat belt. At the moment of impact, she was held in place by the belt, but she hit the windshield with her face, the dashboard with her arms, and the steering wheel with her abdomen. Initial survey reveals closed fractures in both upper extremities, facial lacerations, and abdominal bruises. She is breathing well and is neurologically intact, but she is complaining of severe abdominal pain. Her blood pressure is 75/55 mm Hg, pulse is 110/min, and central venous pressure is zero. Physical examination of the abdomen shows tenderness, guarding, and rebound tenderness on all quadrants. There is no evidence of pelvic fracture. Which of the following would be the most appropriate study to evaluate her abdominal injuries?

    (A) Sonogram of the abdomen

    (B) Flat and upright x-ray films of the abdomen

    (C) CT scan of the abdomen

    (D) Diagnostic peritoneal lavage

    (E) Exploratory laparotomy

27. A 40-year-old obese woman, mother of five children, presents with progressive jaundice that she first noticed 4 weeks ago. She has a total bilirubin of 22 mg/dL, with 16 mg/dL direct (conjugated) and 6 mg/dL indirect (unconjugated). Her transaminases (AST and ALT) are minimally elevated, but her alkaline phosphatase is about six times the upper limit of normal. She has no anemia or occult blood in the stools. She has a history of multiple episodes of colicky right upper quadrant abdominal pain, brought about by the ingestion of fatty food; the last episode occurred a few days before her jaundice was first noted. She currently has no pain and is afebrile. A sonogram of her upper abdomen shows a contracted gallbladder full of stones, as well as dilated intrahepatic and extrahepatic biliary ducts; however, no stone can be identified in the common duct. Which of the following is the most appropriate next step in diagnosis?

    (A) Serology to determine presence and type of hepatitis

    (B) Endoscopic retrograde cholangiopancreatography (ERCP)

    (C) Upper gastrointestinal endoscopy and biopsy of ampullary area

    (D) Percutaneous needle biopsy of the liver

    (E) Percutaneous needle biopsy of the pancreatic head guided by CT scan

28. A 62-year-old woman has an eczematoid lesion in the areola of her right breast that has been present for 3 months. She has self-medicated with skin lotions and over-the-counter steroid ointments, but the area has not improved. On physical examination, the nipple is inverted, the skin of the areola is reddish and desquamated, and the entire area feels firm, with no discrete mass demarcated from the rest of the breast. Which of the following is the most appropriate next step in management?

    (A) Estrogen cream and systemic estrogen replacement

    (B) Mammogram and galactogram

    (C) Mammogram and punch biopsies

    (D) Serum levels of glucagon and CT of the pancreas

    (E) Skin scrapings, culture, and appropriate topical antibiotic

29. A 35-year-old woman has dyspnea on exertion, orthopnea, paroxysmal nocturnal dyspnea, cough, and hemoptysis. The symptoms have been slowly progressive for about 5 years. She looks thin and cachectic, and has atrial fibrillation and a low-pitched, rumbling diastolic apical heart murmur. At age 15, she had rheumatic fever. Surgery has been recommended. Which of the following is the most appropriate management?

    (A) Closure of the ventricular septal defect

    (B) Mitral annuloplasty to tighten an incompetent mitral valve

    (C) Mitral commissurotomy to open a stenotic mitral valve

    (D) Prosthetic replacement of the aortic valve

    (E) Prosthetic replacement of the mitral valve

30. A 62-year-old chronic smoker has an episode of hemoptysis. Other than a barrel chest suggestive of chronic obstructive pulmonary disease, his physical examination is unremarkable. A chest x-ray film shows a central hilar mass. Bronchoscopy and biopsy establish a diagnosis of squamous cell carcinoma of the lung. Pulmonary function studies show that he has a forced expiratory volume at 1 second (FEV_1) of 2,200 mL, and a ventilation perfusion scan shows that 30% of his pulmonary function comes from the affected lung. Which of the following is the most appropriate next step in management?

    (A) CT scan of the chest and upper abdomen

    (B) Radiation and chemotherapy

    (C) Random sampling of supraclavicular nodes

    (D) Lobectomy

    (E) Pneumonectomy

31. A 74-year-old man presents with sudden onset of extremely severe, tearing precordial chest pain that radiates to the back and migrates downward shortly after its onset. As far as the man can tell, there was no precipitating event. He is seen within an hour and is in obvious distress. He is afebrile, but his blood pressure is 220/110 mm Hg and his pulses in the upper extremities are unequal at 102/min. Chest x-ray shows a wide mediastinum. Which of the following could best establish the diagnosis?

    (A) ECG and cardiac enzymes

    (B) Gastrografin swallow, followed by barium if negative

    (C) Spiral CT scan or MRI angiogram

    (D) Ventilation-perfusion scan

    (E) Pulmonary angiogram

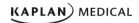

32. An otherwise healthy 24-year-old man presents in the emergency department with very severe pain of recent onset in his right scrotum. The pain is constant and began about 3 hours prior to his arrival. Physical examination shows a temperature of 39.4° C (103.0° F) but is otherwise unremarkable, except for the scrotal area. The testis on the affected side is in the normal position; however, it appears to be swollen and is exquisitely tender to palpation. The cord above the testis is equally painful and tender. Urinalysis shows pyuria. Which of the following is the most appropriate next step in management?

    (A) Antiviral medication started within the hour
    (B) Scrotal sonogram and antibiotics
    (C) Cystoscopy and bladder irrigation
    (D) Trans-scrotal biopsy and appropriate resection
    (E) Emergency surgery and bilateral orchiopexy

33. A 16-year-old boy is persuaded by his older brother to accompany him and his friends on a beer-drinking binge. This is the first such experience for the boy, and it leads to the development of severe colicky left flank pain. When rescued by his parents, he is diaphoretic and doubled up in pain. He relates that he began to urinate frequently and profusely after the third or fourth beer and that the pain seized him shortly thereafter. He is tender to fist percussion over the left costovertebral angle but is afebrile. Which of the following is the most likely diagnosis?

    (A) Bladder calculi
    (B) Low implantation of one ureter
    (C) Ureteral stone
    (D) Ureteropelvic junction obstruction
    (E) Vesicoureteral reflux

34. A 25-year-old man is found on a pre-employment chest x-ray film to have a 3-cm peripheral coin lesion. The patient has never smoked, and a chest x-ray film that he had 2 years ago when he enrolled in graduate school had been normal. Prompted by this finding, he undergoes a more thorough physical examination, which discloses the presence of a firm, 2-cm testicular mass of which he was not previously aware. There are also palpable inguinal nodes on the same side. Which of the following is the most appropriate next step in management?

    (A) Supportive symptomatic palliative care
    (B) Bronchoscopy and biopsy of the lung mass
    (C) Trans-scrotal incisional biopsy of the testicular mass
    (D) Trans-scrotal orchiectomy and sampling of inguinal nodes
    (E) Radical orchiectomy by the inguinal route

35. A 53-year-old man is brought to the emergency department by his wife because of headache and visual changes. Approximately 3 hours ago, he had the acute onset of an extremely severe posterior headache that was nonradiating but was associated with nausea and vomiting. This headache subsided, but over the past hour he has developed mild neck stiffness and pain on flexion of his neck. The patient is not cooperative, so no additional history is known; however, his wife states that he was feeling well until recently and has no allergies. The patient appears moderately uncomfortable and is complaining of the worst headache he has ever experienced. Which of the following is the most likely cause for his symptoms?

    (A) Arteriovenous malformation
    (B) Cerebellar bleed
    (C) Putamenal bleed
    (D) Ruptured berry aneurysm
    (E) Thalamic bleed

36. A 25-year-old man is shot with a .22-caliber revolver. The entrance wound is in the anteromedial aspect of his upper thigh, 5 cm below the groin crease. The exit wound is in the posterolateral aspect of the thigh, halfway between the greater trochanter and the knee. He has palpable pulses in the dorsum of his foot and in the posterior tibial artery behind the malleolus. The popliteal pulse is reported as normal by one examiner, but cannot be felt by another. There is no hematoma under the entrance wound, and blood is oozing from both wounds but not at an alarming rate. He is hemodynamically stable. Neurologic examination of the leg is normal. X-ray films show the femur to be intact. In addition to local wound care and the appropriate tetanus prophylaxis, which of the following is the most appropriate next step in management?

   (A) Digital exploration of the wounds in the emergency department
   (B) Discharge home
   (C) Doppler studies or arteriogram
   (D) Formal surgical exploration of the area in the operating room
   (E) Hospitalization to observe for development of complications

37. A 62-year-old man with alcoholic cirrhosis of the liver and ascites presents with generalized abdominal pain that started 12 hours ago. He now has moderate tenderness over the entire abdomen, with minimal guarding and equivocal rebound. Bowel sounds are diminished but present. He has a temperature of 38.4° C (101.2° F) and a leukocyte count of 11,000/mm³. Although he used to be a heavy drinker, he has not touched a drop of alcohol for the past 7 years. Except for the presence of ascites, upright and flat x-ray films of the abdomen are unremarkable. Which of the following is the most appropriate next step in diagnosis?

   (A) CT scan of the abdomen
   (B) Serum amylase determinations
   (C) Sonogram of the right upper quadrant
   (D) Culture of the ascitic fluid
   (E) Laparoscopy

38. A 56-year-old man presents with progressive jaundice that he first noted 6 weeks ago. The patient has lost about 20 pounds over the past 2 months and he has persistent, nagging pain deep into his epigastrium and upper back. Except for the obvious jaundice and the signs of weight loss, physical examination is remarkable only for the presence of a vaguely palpable, nontender mass under the liver edge. His hemoglobin is 14 g/dL, and there is no occult blood in the stool. Total bilirubin is 22 mg/dL, with 16 mg/dL direct (conjugated) fraction. The transaminases are minimally elevated, whereas the alkaline phosphatase is about eight times the upper limit of normal. A sonogram shows dilated intrahepatic ducts, dilated extrahepatic ducts, and a very distended, thin-walled gallbladder without stones. Which of the following is the most appropriate next step in diagnosis?

   (A) CT scan of the abdomen
   (B) Serologies
   (C) Duodenal endoscopy and biopsies
   (D) Endoscopic retrograde cholangiopancreatography (ERCP)
   (E) Percutaneous transhepatic cholangiogram (PTC)

39. A 31-year-old accounting student presents with a persistent headache that began approximately 4 months ago. The headache has been gradually increasing in intensity, and is worse in the mornings. Thinking that she might need new glasses, she sought help from her optometrist, who discovered that she has bilateral papilledema and sent her in for medical evaluation. On direct questioning, she admits to repeated vomiting for the past 3 weeks, with no heaving, straining, or preceding nausea. "I would just open my mouth, and the stuff would hit the wall," she explains. She denies any other neurological symptoms. Which of the following is the most likely diagnosis?

   (A) Brain abscess
   (B) Brain tumor
   (C) Chronic subdural hematoma
   (D) Multiple sclerosis
   (E) Subarachnoid bleeding

40. An 82-year-old man develops severe abdominal distention, nausea, vomiting, and colicky abdominal pain. He
has not passed any gas or stools for the past 12 hours. His
vital signs are normal, and his pulse is regular. He has a
distended, tympanitic abdomen, with hyperactive, high-
pitched bowel sounds. There are no signs of peritoneal
irritation. Rectal examination is negative for masses or
occult blood, and the rectal vault is empty. Abdominal
x-ray films show distended loops of small and large
bowel, as well as a very large round gas shadow that is
located in the right upper quadrant and tapers toward
the left lower quadrant in the shape of a parrot's beak.
The patient has never had any abdominal surgery, and he
does not have any palpable hernias. Which of the following is the most appropriate next step in management?

    (A) Nasogastric suction, IV fluids, and observation

    (B) Repeated enemas and laxatives

    (C) Emergency celiac and mesenteric arteriogram

    (D) Proctosigmoidoscopy

    (E) Emergency exploratory laparotomy

41. A 42-year-old woman drops a hot iron on her lap while
doing the laundry. She comes in with the shape of the
iron clearly delineated on her upper thigh. The area is
white, dry, leathery, and anesthetic. Which of the following is the most appropriate next step in management?

    (A) Application of mafenide acetate

    (B) Application of silver sulfadiazine

    (C) Use of triple antibiotic ointment

    (D) Repeated debridement and wet to dry dressings

    (E) Immediate excision and grafting

42. A patient involved in a car accident sustains burst fractures of several thoracic vertebral bodies. At the time of
admission, he has no neurologic function at all below
the level of the injury and he has flaccid sphincters.
After a few days, there is partial recovery of function;
the remaining deficits are loss of motor function and
loss of pain and temperature sensation on both sides
distal to the injury, with preservation of vibratory and
positional senses. Which of the following is the most
likely diagnosis?

    (A) Anterior cord syndrome

    (B) Central cord syndrome

    (C) Complete cord transection

    (D) Cord hemisection

    (E) Spinal shock

43. A 6-year-old boy has insidious development of limp-
ing with decreased motion in one hip. He complains
occasionally of knee pain on that side. He walks into
the office with an antalgic gait. Examination of the knee
is normal, but passive motion of the hip is guarded.
The child is afebrile, and the parents indicate that his
gait and level of activity were completely normal all his
life until this recent problem. He has not had a recent
febrile illness. Which of the following is the most likely
diagnosis?

    (A) Avascular necrosis of the capital femoral epiphysis

    (B) Developmental dysplasia of the hip

    (C) Hematogenous osteomyelitis of the femoral head

    (D) Septic hip

    (E) Slipped capital femoral epiphysis

44. A 39-year-old woman is involved in a head-on, high-speed automobile collision. She arrives at the emergency department in a deep coma, with bilaterally fixed dilated pupils. She has normal blood pressure and pulse rate. CT scan of the head shows diffuse blurring of the gray-white interface and multiple small punctate hemorrhages. There is no single large hematoma or displacement of the midline structures. Extension of the CT to include the neck shows no cervical spine fractures. Which of the following is the most appropriate initial step in management?

    (A) Improvement of cerebral perfusion by infusion of large amounts of IV fluids

    (B) Improvement of cerebral perfusion by the use of systemic vasodilators

    (C) Preservation of neurologic function by the use of hyperbaric oxygen

    (D) Prevention of further damage due to development of increased intracranial pressure

    (E) Surgical evacuation of the multiple punctate hemorrhages

45. On the second postoperative day after an abdomino-perineal resection for cancer of the rectum, a 72-year-old man complains of severe retrosternal pain. The pain is crushing in nature and radiates to the left arm. He also becomes short of breath and tachycardic. Except for his fresh surgical wounds and postoperative discomfort, physical examination is unremarkable. He does not have distended neck veins. Which of the following is the most appropriate next step in diagnosis?

    (A) Blood gases

    (B) Chest x-ray film

    (C) Pulmonary angiogram

    (D) Transaminase levels (ALT, AST)

    (E) EKG

46. A 14-year-old girl has a firm, movable, rubbery mass in her left breast. The mass was first noticed 6 months ago and has since grown to about 6 cm in diameter. Which of the following is the most likely diagnosis?

    (A) Cancer of the breast

    (B) Cystosarcoma phyllodes

    (C) Fibrocystic disease (mammary dysplasia)

    (D) Giant juvenile fibroadenoma

    (E) Intraductal papilloma

47. A 3-week-old infant is brought in because of 2 days of protracted bilious vomiting. He looks acutely ill, and plain x-rays show two large air fluid levels in the upper abdomen, the larger one on the left side and a smaller one on the right side. The radiologist describes the finding as a "double bubble sign." He also reports that there is intraluminal gas distal to those two air fluid levels, but that it is sparse and does not outline distended loops. Which of the following is the most likely tentative clinical diagnosis?

    (A) Hypertrophic pyloric stenosis

    (B) Intestinal atresia

    (C) Malrotation

    (D) Meconium ileus

    (E) Necrotizing enterocolitis

48. A 30-year-old woman comes to the physician 6 hours after falling on her outstretched right hand. She has pain and limitation of movement in her wrist, but denies sensations of tingling or numbness. The right wrist is mildly swollen, and its range of passive motion is limited compared with the left side. Palpation elicits maximal tenderness in the area of the anatomic snuffbox, between the tendons of the extensor pollicis longus and abductor pollicis muscles. Ulnar and radial pulses are normal, and Tinel's and Phalen's tests are negative. Further examination rules out signs of nerve or vascular damage. Plain x-ray films performed in the antero-posterior, lateral, and oblique views fail to show any evidence of fractures. At this time, which of the following is the most appropriate next step in management?

    (A) Bone scanning

    (B) MRI examination of the wrist

    (C) Treatment for wrist sprain

    (D) Treatment for scaphoid fracture

49. A 72-year-old woman undergoes a partial colectomy for adenocarcinoma of the sigmoid colon. She receives appropriate antibiotic coverage and low-dose heparin prophylaxis. On the fifth hospital day, the patient begins complaining of right chest pain, difficulty in breathing, and a dry cough. Her temperature is 37.9° C (100.2° F), blood pressure is 134/78 mm Hg, pulse is 115/min and regular, and respirations are 20/min. Examination shows crackles in the right chest, but no tenderness or edema in the legs. A chest x-ray shows several areas of atelectasis, as well as patchy pneumonic infiltrates, on both lungs. ECG reveals sinus tachycardia with nonspecific ST changes. Laboratory studies show:

Arterial blood gas analysis

PaO_2	74 mm Hg
$PaCO_2$	37 mm Hg
pH	7.35

Blood/serum

Hematocrit	40%
Leukocytes	8,300/mm^3
Lactate dehydrogenase	350 U/L
Fibrin D-dimer	600 ng/mL
(normal upper limit 500 ng/mL)	

Which of the following is the most appropriate step in diagnosis?

(A) Bronchoalveolar lavage

(B) Contrast venography

(C) Pulmonary angiography

(D) Spiral CT scan of the chest

(E) Ultrasonography of the lower extremities

(F) Ventilation-perfusion lung scanning

50. A 65-year-old man reports episodes of gross, total, painless hematuria that have been on and off for about the past 2 months. He also has vague, mild, irritative voiding symptoms, but he reports no fever or outright pain on urination. He is obese, has a sedentary lifestyle, drinks alcohol in moderation, and has been smoking two packs of cigarettes per day since age 18. He denies a history of trauma to his abdomen or flanks, and other than moderate emphysema and his current complaint, he considers himself to be in good general health. The physical examination is noncontributory. Rectal examination shows a large, soft, boggy prostate with no nodules, and his prostate-specific antigen is normal for his age. Urinalysis reveals packed red cells, a few white cells, and no casts. An intravenous pyelogram is obtained, and the study is reported as normal. Which of the following should be the next step in management?

(A) CT scan of both kidneys

(B) Cystoscopy

(C) Prescribe levofloxacin

(D) Prostatic biopsy

(E) Retrograde cystogram

Surgery Test Two:
Answers and Explanations

ANSWER KEY

1.	B		26.	E
2.	D		27.	B
3.	E		28.	C
4.	D		29.	C
5.	E		30.	A
6.	C		31.	C
7.	D		32.	B
8.	E		33.	D
9.	E		34.	E
10.	B		35.	D
11.	D		36.	C
12.	B		37.	D
13.	C		38.	A
14.	B		39.	B
15.	B		40.	D
16.	D		41.	E
17.	A		42.	A
18.	B		43.	A
19.	D		44.	D
20.	A		45.	E
21.	B		46.	D
22.	B		47.	C
23.	B		48.	D
24.	E		49.	D
25.	E		50.	B

1. **The correct answer is B.** The diagnosis is one of exclusion: the multiple dilated loops of small bowel rule out duodenal atresia or annular pancreas, leaving malrotation as a possibility. That was ruled out by the contrast enema, and the operative findings. The microcolon is the sign of an "unused" colon (i.e., nothing has been getting to it) which brings to mind intestinal atresia or meconium ileus, both of which have been ruled out as well. That leaves us with aganglionic colon (Hirschsprung disease), the extent of which can vary tremendously. If the entire colon is aganglionic, this exact clinical picture will result. The diverting ileostomy will take care of the functional obstruction, whereas the appendix provides the safest way to obtain tissue for the pathologist to confirm the absence of ganglia. Definitive repair will be done when the child is a little older.

A diverting ileostomy alone (**choice A**) would take care of the immediate problem, but would not help establish the diagnosis.

Diversion at the transverse colon (**choice C**) would leave a functionally obstructed segment in the circuit.

Total colectomy (**choice D**) will eventually be done, but not before establishing a diagnosis.

Total proctocolectomy (**choice E**) is not done for aganglionic megacolon. The denervated segment is removed, but the normal gut is then brought down to the anus or a portion of the distal rectum.

2. **The correct answer is D.** A known complication of long-standing use of birth control pills is the development of hepatic adenomas that may rupture and bleed.

A bleeding ovarian follicle (**choice A**) can give mild abdominal pain right at the midpoint of the menstrual cycle, but it would not produce bleeding of this magnitude.

An abdominal aortic aneurysm (**choice B**) would be very rare at this age, and bleeding typically begins retroperitoneally with excruciating back pain. Once the aneurysm ruptures into the peritoneal cavity, complete vascular collapse ensues.

An ectopic pregnancy (**choice C**) is the first thought when a sexually active young woman has spontaneous intra-abdominal bleeding, but in this case it has been ruled out by the history, the pelvic examination, and the pregnancy test.

Other visceral aneurysms (**choice E**) can indeed bleed, and have a tendency to do so during pregnancy. They are very rare and favor the splenic artery. They can also occur in the hepatic artery, but the odds are extremely low.

3. **The correct answer is E.** This patient has adult onset polycystic kidney disease (APKD). APKD is an autoso-mal dominant disease that presents with hypertension, renal cysts, hematuria, and possible renal failure, usually after age 30. There is a 10% to 20% incidence of berry aneurysms in these patients, and they need to be screened with angiography to determine the presence or absence of these malformations. A magnetic resonance angiogram (MRA) of the brain is the standard option for such imaging in most medical centers.

CT scan of the pelvis (**choice A**) is not indicated since clinical history and renal ultrasound alone can make the diagnosis of APKD. The concern here is to screen for the concomitant presence of intracranial pathology.

CT scan of the thorax (**choice B**) is incorrect. Unless these lesions were mistaken for renal cell carcinoma, there is no indication to scan a distant site like the lungs as this disease has no malignant potential.

MRI of the brain (**choice C**) is not useful for detecting circulatory malformations without the aid of angiographic contrast material.

Intravenous pyelography (IVP; **choice D**) is used to evaluate the collecting system of the urinary tract and is not indicated in this case, as the diagnosis of APKD is almost certainly based on the ultrasound and clinical presentation. This study adds no diagnostic information to the results of the ultrasound already obtained.

4. **The correct answer is D.** The profuse bleeding into the upper airway makes any approach through the mouth or nose doomed to failure, and will likely worsen the existing injuries. A direct route to the airway lower in the neck is needed, and the best option for quick use in the emergency department is a cricothyroidotomy.

As pointed out above, attempted nasotracheal intubation (**choice A**) would worsen existing nasal injuries, and visualization of the cords would not be possible with all the blood in the field.

The same is true of orotracheal intubation (**choice B**): only blood would be seen as attempts are made to visualize the cords. Furthermore, rapid induction anesthesia would be quite redundant in an unconscious patient.

Percutaneous transtracheal ventilation (**choice C**) is the best alternate option but is not as good as the cricothyroidotomy. Contrary to what the name implies, one can oxygenate a patient through a small diameter catheter placed percutaneously into the trachea, but ventilation cannot be done very well by that route. In an unconscious patient, one may need better ventilation to help lower intracranial pressure.

Emergency tracheostomy done in the emergency department (**choice E**) is an absolute no-no. Tracheostomy is a formal operative procedure that should be done in the operating room, with all the help, light, instruments, and exposure appropriate for such an undertaking. To do so, an airway must have been previously secured in some other way. Attempting to operate in the neck without a secure airway, and in less than ideal conditions, can very quickly turn into a horror show.

5. **The correct answer is E.** To the uninitiated, this is a drastic step that smacks of "shoot first, ask questions later." However, virtually all solid testicular masses are malignant tumors. The best way to avoid dissemination is to open the inguinal canal, do a high ligation of the cord, and pull the testicle out.

Serum markers (**choice A**) are indeed taken prior to surgery, but it is done primarily to facilitate follow up. It is true that elevated levels confirm the presence of tumor, but they do not provide precise information as to the exact cellular mix of the tumor, which is essential to plan therapy. The exact cellular mix will also not be determined with a fine needle aspiration (**choice B**).

The trans-scrotal approach, regardless of how minor (**choice B**), intermediate (**choice C**), or complete (**choice D**), is universally condemned because it spreads the tumor even as one is sampling it.

6. **The correct answer is C.** The rule is that lymph nodes that progressively enlarge over several months are malignant. Furthermore, when they are in the supraclavicular area, they typically harbor metastasis from a primary tumor below the clavicles (i.e., not in the head and neck). In this case, gastric cancer was the only choice offered that fit the rule, and the rest of the vignette is actually suggestive of that particular malignancy. Don't be put off by the inability to feel it by palpation; gastric cancers are seldom palpable.

Inflammatory nodes (**choice A**) typically have a time-table of weeks rather than months, and they would not explain weight loss, epigastric discomfort, and occult blood in the gastrointestinal tract.

Lymphoma (**choice B**) would have been an excellent choice in a young person with fever, night sweats, and multiple enlarged lymph nodes at several locations.

Squamous cell carcinoma (**choice D**) would have been perfect for an old man who smokes and drinks and has rotten teeth, if the node had been higher up in the neck.

Thyroid cancer (**choice E**) would likewise metastasize to the jugular nodes before it would involve the supraclavicular area.

7. **The correct answer is D.** Intense clinical investigations have been conducted to identify the most effective screening approach to prostatic cancer detection. The aim of an effective screening program is to detect prostatic cancer in the earliest stages, when surgery results in high cure rates. Digital rectal examination (DRE) alone (**choice B**) is a specific but not sensitive method; 1.5% of men older than 50 are found to have prostatic neoplasia on DRE alone. In contrast, because of the considerable overlap between the values due to prostatic hyperplasia and those resulting from prostatic cancer, serum PSA alone (**choice C**) is sensitive but not specific. Approximately 2% of men older than 50 are found to have prostatic neoplasia by serum PSA measurements without DRE. The combination of abnormal DRE and elevated PSA affords the highest positive predictive value. The issue, however, is still under active scrutiny. Increasingly more centers are using age-specific reference ranges of serum PSA, along with ratios between free and protein-bound PSA, to improve sensitivity and specificity of this test.

Cytologic examination of prostatic secretion (**choice A**) has proved ineffective in detecting prostatic cancer.

Transrectal ultrasonography (**choice E**) is too expensive as a screening test and it does not significantly improve the detection rate when compared with combined DRE and serum PSA. Transrectal ultrasonography should be reserved mainly for staging purposes and to guide prostatic biopsies.

8. **The correct answer is E.** When this man first arrived at the emergency room, he might have been suffering from a transient ischemic attack, from which he might have spontaneously recovered. But in the time taken to do a quick neurologic evaluation and scan of the patient's head, there has been no resolution of his neurologic deficits. He may, in fact, be having the onset of an ischemic stroke. The scan shows no bleeding and no extensive infarction, making him an ideal candidate for thrombolytics. These are best when used within the first 90 minutes of symptoms, and, in this case, that window of opportunity is about to run out. Infusion of tissue-type plasminogen activator should be started.

The absolute time constraint for using clot busters for ongoing ischemic stroke is 3 hours, and the results are slightly better if the treatment is started within the first 90 minutes. Continued clinical observation for 3 additional hours (**choice A**) would waste that time window and preclude their use. It is true that the patient might spontaneously recover neurologic function during that time, proving that he had a transient ischemic attack instead of a stroke, but gambling on that outcome would be irresponsible.

Duplex scanning of the carotids (**choice B**) and subsequent carotid endarterectomy (**choice C**) are used in patients who have had transient ischemic attacks, have recovered neurologic function, and have to be protected from a future stroke. Once this man has been effectively treated for his current problem, he will need the carotid study and probably an endarterectomy. However, these steps would not correct the current situation, if he is indeed having a stroke.

Anticoagulants are not the same as clot busters. Heparin and warfarin (**choice D**) would not affect the existing clot that is blocking the patient's cerebrovascular circulation. Tissue-type plasminogen activator, on the other hand, will dissolve the existing clot.

9. **The correct answer is E.** Bloody urethral discharge in an old man is highly suspicious of urethral carcinoma. This is a rare cancer, but an early diagnosis allows a good chance of cure. If gross hematuria is the initial presentation, discrimination between upper tract, lower tract (vesical), and urethral sources may be obtained by evaluation of the *timing* of hematuria. A clean-catch urine is collected in separate aliquots. The last few milliliters are collected after performing prostatic massage to obtain prostatic secretions. Initial hematuria is characteristic of urethral lesions, midstream or total hematuria results from upper urinary tract and vesical sources, and terminal hematuria reflects prostatic disease.

Gonococcal infection (**choice A**) manifests with a yellow (purulent) discharge, which is most abundant in the early morning. The discharge contains numerous neutrophils with gram-negative diplococci.

Nonbacterial prostatitis (**choice B**) results in chronic suprapubic pain or discomfort. Hematuria is usually absent. Microscopic examination of prostatic secretions reveals more than 10 leukocytes per high power field, but cultures are negative. The pathogenesis of this condition is probably noninfectious.

Prostatic carcinoma (**choice C**) is most commonly detected by digital rectal examination and/or abnormally elevated serum prostatic-specific antigen (PSA). If hematuria is present, it is of the *terminal* type (i.e., present in the last aliquot of a fractionated urine collection).

Testicular cancer (**choice D**) does not manifest with bloody urethral discharge or hematuria. Its most frequent presenting sign is *painless enlargement* of the testis.

10. **The correct answer is B.** Clinically, this a classic presentation for fracture of the clavicle, at the point at which they usually occur. As with most fractures, some kind of immobilization is required, and this is achieved with a figure-eight device.

Analgesics with no immobilization of any kind (**choice A**) would be painful and disruptive to the healing process, an obviously incorrect choice for the clavicle (but a reasonable option in bones that are more-or-less kept in place by other anatomic structures, such as the ribs).

Hanging casts (**choice C**) are used when the arm has to be kept pulled down, a position that would not help this broken clavicle.

The subclavian vessels are at risk in sternoclavicular dislocations with posterior displacement, which is not the injury here, so an arteriogram (**choice D**) is not necessary.

As a general rule, open reduction and internal fixation (**choice E**) are required only when very precise alignment of bone fragments is required, or when proper reduction and immobilization cannot be achieved by more conservative means.

11. **The correct answer is D.** A long-standing cycle of repeated healing and breaking down may eventually give rise to a squamous cell carcinoma of the skin, known as a Marjolin ulcer. The history and the heaped up edges are the clues. Obviously, biopsy is needed for diagnosis.

Doppler studies (**choice A**) would be appropriate in a vascular work-up.

Venous pressure tracings (**choice B**) might be useful if the ulcers were due to venous disease. Such ulcers are usually located above the medial malleolus, in hyperpigmented, edematous skin.

If you saw a connection between Latin America and "strange bugs" that you wanted to culture (**choice C**), you got the wrong clue. The personal history explains why her third-degree burn was never treated.

Ulcers due to arterial insufficiency are found distally, at the tip of the toes, in patients with other manifestations of the disease. After Doppler studies are done, an arteriogram (**choice E**) would be indicated.

12. **The correct answer is B.** The clinical picture is that of acute-angle closure glaucoma. Treatment is urgent and consists of oral or intravenous carbonic anhydrase inhibitors, topical beta blockers, and alpha-2-selective adrenergic agonists. Osmotic diuretics may also be needed, and the definitive treatment is laser peripheral iridotomy.

Copious irrigation (**choice A**) is the emergency treatment for caustic burns of the eyes. It would not help in this case.

Atropine drops (**choice C**) would lead to mydriasis, which, as a rule, impedes, rather than enhances, aqueous outflow. The patient needs aqueous production to be diminished (which the carbonic anhydrase inhibitors do) and outflow to be improved.

Topical antihistamines or mast cell inhibitors (**choice D**) and topical corticosteroid-antibiotics (**choice E**) are indicated in other ophthalmologic conditions, not in the treatment of glaucoma.

13. **The correct answer is C.** The direction of force that produces a fracture often predicts the possibility of other less obvious injuries. The vertical fall depicted in this vignette classically results in compression fractures of thoracic and lumbar vertebral bodies. The patient is distracted by the pain in his feet, but the physician must look for those additional injuries. Alternative answers would have been appropriate under different circumstances.

    CT scan of the abdomen (**choice A**) is used to assess intra-abdominal injuries in a patient with blunt abdominal trauma who has signs of bleeding but is hemodynamically stable.

    Cervical spine x-ray films (**choice B**) are always a top priority in multiple injury patients, but the triggering findings are head or facial injuries and a tender neck, none of which are present here.

    An arteriogram (**choice D**) is needed in posterior dislocation of the knee.

    A retrograde urethrogram (**choice E**) is an appropriate study in a patient with a pelvic fracture and blood at the meatus.

14. **The correct answer is B.** Crush injuries produce massive necrosis, and lysis of muscle releases potassium, creatine kinase, and protein in large amounts. All the listed choices are options for managing the resultant hyperkalemia, but only administration of calcium is absolutely mandatory in the presence of hyperkalemia accompanied by ECG changes. Calcium acts as a membrane-stabilizing agent to balance against the imminent hyperkalemia-induced global depolarization of the myocardium.

    Administering oral sodium polystyrene sulfonate (Kayexalate; **choice A**) is an effective way of permanently removing potassium from the body over a period of 4-10 hours. Its action is not acute, and it has no value in acute situations.

    Administering IV bicarbonate (**choice C**) is also only a temporizing measure that acts in a similar manner to insulin by causing a transcellular shift of potassium from extracellular to intracellular spaces.

    Administering IV insulin and dextrose (**choice D**) is a temporizing measure that acts to force a transcellular shift of potassium from outside to in. This will afford only brief protection against rapidly rising serum potassium.

    Initiating urgent hemodialysis (**choice E**) is indicated only if the medical management of the hyperkalemia fails.

15. **The correct answer is B.** The patient obviously has developed a fistula at the operative site, but there are no signs that the gastrointestinal contents are spilling into the abdomen (no signs of an acute abdomen) or collecting inside a pocket (no fever). Thus, we can provide general support and wait for the fistula to close. He is already getting two of the essential components of therapy: the skin is well protected, and he is getting good nutritional support distal to the fistula, with a feeding solution that does not stir up enzymatic activity (elemental diet) and that is rich in protein (a calorie-nitrogen ratio lower than 150). But he needs replacement of the fluids and electrolytes pouring out through the fistula. The green fluid indicates a duodenal origin (alkaline fluid), so Ringer's lactate is a suitable replacement fluid. Cramming 6 L a day via the jejunostomy might be too much; thus, the IV route is better for the additional fluid.

    No change in therapy (**choice A**) would lead to prompt dehydration and electrolyte depletion. He needs the 3 L per day of jejunal feeding for his own needs. The fistula losses have to be replaced separately.

    Stopping the nutritional support (**choice C**) would not help the fistula to close. If he had been eating meat and potatoes by mouth, they would have had to be stopped. As he is, however, the feeding does not disturb the fistula. Furthermore, 5% dextrose (D5)-half normal saline would be a poor choice of IV fluid to replace alkaline loses from the duodenum.

    Surgical drainage (**choice D**) addresses a nonexistent problem. The gastrointestinal fluid is already coming out, not pooling inside.

    As for surgical reconstruction (**choice E**), it might have to be done if conservative management does not lead to fistula closure. But one does not begin with such a high-risk, technically difficult step. Most fistulas close if there is no foreign body, epithelialization, tumor, infection, or distal obstruction to prevent it.

16. **The correct answer is D.** Two locations in the body have the highest risk for development of the dreaded compartment syndrome: the forearm and the lower leg. Although long-standing ischemia followed by reperfusion might be the most common cause, any injury with subsequent swelling can do it, as it did here. The classic findings are all there, including the most reliable one: excruciating pain on passive extension. Fasciotomy is the only effective therapy.

    Re-casting, with or without nerve blocks (**choices A and B**), would not address the problem of the compartment syndrome and would lead to permanent disability.

    An arteriogram (**choice C**) is not needed to make the diagnosis. Time would be wasted, and a normal study would not exclude the diagnosis. In fact, there may even be normal palpable pulses in the presence of a compartment syndrome (pressure above 30 mm Hg in the compartment is all it takes to kill the muscles).

As for open reduction and internal fixation (**choice E**), the problem in this case is not the position of the bones (it might have been if reduction couldn't be achieved). Further, the incision needed for that operation would not necessarily open all the affected compartments widely enough. The only correct answer is fasciotomy.

17. **The correct answer is A.** It is obvious that the patient is in shock, and the distended veins identify the type as cardiogenic. Given the location of the injury, pericardial tamponade is the obvious mechanism. Other possibilities are excluded as noted below.

    Tension pneumothorax (**choice B**) is another form of extrinsic cardiogenic shock that can be seen with penetrating injuries of the chest. However, there would be respiratory distress and absent breath sounds on the affected hemithorax.

    Hemorrhagic shock (**choice C**) is by far the most common reason for shock in the trauma victim, and thus it always has to be a consideration. However, his veins would have been empty rather than bulging.

    Intrinsic cardiogenic shock (**choice D**) is seen with massive myocardial infarctions or fulminating myocarditis. The large distended veins would be there, but the setting would not be that of a penetrating injury.

    Vasomotor shock (**choice E**) should not be overlooked, since a high spinal cord transection can produce it. But the patient would be pink and warm rather then pale and cold. Furthermore, this patient was neurologically intact.

18. **The correct answer is B.** The lateral collateral ligament is the location of the pain on direct palpation, and the function of that ligament is to prevent the leg from being bent inward (adducted, assuming the varus position). The damage allows that motion to go beyond the normal limits. Incidentally, we can infer that he was hit from the inside, and the knee was forcefully bent outward.

    Anterior cruciate ligament injuries (**choice A**) are manifested by the positive anterior drawer and Lachman test, which are negative in this case.

    Injuries to the meniscus (**choice C**) produce limitations in the mobility of the knee and "catching" on loose intra-articular fragments.

    The medial collateral ligament (**choice D**) is also a good candidate for tackling injuries when the blow is from the outside and the knee is forcefully bent inward; however, the findings on physical examination would be the exact opposite (mirror image) of those described here.

    Although anything can happen to the knees of football players, injuries to the posterior cruciate ligament (**choice E**) are rare. When they do occur, the unstable knee shows a positive posterior drawer test (which was not present here).

19. **The correct answer is D.** The problem is urinary retention, which is extremely common in the immediate postoperative period after lower abdominal, inguinal, or perineal surgery. The bladder must be emptied by catheterization and allowed to regain normal function with the passage of time.

    X-ray films (**choice A**) are not needed. The nature of the mass is clear from the physical examination and the circumstances of the case.

    Increasing the rate of fluid administration (**choice B**) would simply compound the problem. The patient is not voiding because of a functional problem at the bladder neck, not because he is not making enough urine.

    Loop diuretics (**choice C**) are wrong for the same reasons that more fluids would be wrong.

    An indwelling Foley catheter (**choice E**) would indeed solve the problem, but it would be too aggressive a step. No one advocates leaving a catheter in place at the first catheterization. If it needs to be repeated once (and some say if it needs to be repeated twice), then an indwelling catheter is needed.

20. **The correct answer is A.** A sternal fracture is very likely to be complicated by myocardial contusion, which may not be evident immediately but will show up in serial ECGs with signs very similar to those of a myocardial infarction.

    Abdominal x-ray films (**choice B**) would not add to our present information. If he had free air under the diaphragms, or had a diaphragmatic rupture with bowel in the chest, both would be seen in his chest x-ray films.

    An injury of the tracheobronchial tree would produce pneumothorax, mediastinal air, or subcutaneous emphysema, so bronchoscopy (**choice D**) would not be warranted.

    The esophagus typically gets injured during instrumentation or by penetrating injuries. Blunt trauma does not disrupt it, so a Gastrografin swallow (**choice C**) or esophagoscopy (**choice E**) would not be necessary.

21. **The correct answer is B.** As a rule, internal hemorrhoids bleed but do not hurt, whereas external hemorrhoids hurt but do not bleed. This is the typical symptomatology of external hemorrhoids.

    Anal fissure (**choice A**) occurs in young women and babies, who have excruciating pain when they have a bowel movement and blood streaks on the toilet paper.

    Fistula in ano (**choice C**) occurs in people who have had a perirectal abscess drained. The typical complaint is soiling of the underwear from the drainage of the fistula.

As pointed out above, internal hemorrhoids (**choice D**) tend to bleed, but they have no innervation for pain.

Perirectal abscess (**choice E**) would cause very intense pain, along with fever, and would have a short clinical course ending with spontaneous drainage of pus, if not surgically drained first.

22. **The correct answer is B.** The clinical picture is that of embolic occlusion of the right common iliac at the aortic bifurcation (or possibly a similar process at the bifurcation of the common iliac into internal and external branches). The source is also obvious in the vignette: atrial fibrillation (manifested by the grossly irregular pulse). He needs an emergency embolectomy, which is done with the balloon tipped catheters invented by Fogarty. If he had been ischemic for a longer period of time, he might have required a fasciotomy of the lower leg as well. Thrombolytics were not offered as an option. They can be used in highly selected cases, but the question did not offer all the necessary details that would have enabled a very experienced vascular surgeon to choose this approach. Of the choices offered, only the embolectomy is correct.

Dacron prosthetic vascular conduits (**choice A**) are appropriate for cases of arteriosclerotic occlusive disease blocking the iliacs, in which the native vessel cannot be opened and a graft has to go from the aorta to the femorals.

Anticoagulants (**choice C**) are an adjunct to vascular procedures, but are not the primary treatment for a clot that has already traveled from the atrial appendage to the lower extremity. Anticoagulants cannot dissolve existing clots.

Saphenous vein bypass (**choice D**) is the preferred way to deal with chronically occluded common femoral arteries, but it is not a choice when the native vessel is fine and can be unplugged.

Sympathetic blocks (**choice E**) are rarely used in vascular surgery. They are more appropriate for functional problems than for mechanical obstructions.

23. **The correct answer is B.** The history is that of transient ischemic attacks (TIAs), which are most commonly due to an ulcerated plaque at the carotid bifurcation or a stenosis greater than 70% of the lumen. For many years, an arteriogram was the only way to diagnose such lesions, but this invasive study sometimes can precipitate the very same stroke that carotid surgery was designed to prevent. Duplex scanning, a noninvasive alternative, is now available. Many patients can be fully diagnosed and operated on without ever needing an arteriogram. For those in whom the study is inconclusive, an arteriogram is the next step.

CT scan (**choice A**) is our best tool when intracranial bleeding is suspected, but the hallmark of such an event is extremely severe headache heralding the neurologic deficits.

Echocardiogram (**choice C**) is indicated if the heart is suspected as the source of emboli. The left carotid (where the bruit is) is the likely source of the problem in this vignette.

MRI (**choice D**) is our choice when brain tumor is suspected. The history would be one of several months of increasingly severe headaches that are worse in the mornings, along with eventual development of projectile vomiting and blurred vision.

Aortic arch arteriogram (**choice E**) is required if there is evidence of involvement of the vertebral arteries (neurologic deficits involving visual cortex and cerebellum), or if less invasive studies do not provide a satisfactory explanation of the symptoms. It would not be the first test performed.

24. **The correct answer is E.** The obvious clinical finding is a very large urinary output, which is neither in response to nor being matched by her fluid intake. With a history of surgery in the area of the pituitary gland, we have to suspect that damage to the posterior pituitary gland, or to the stalk, may have occurred and that diabetes insipidus has developed. If that is the case, we will see a significant increase in the serum sodium concentration, explaining the neurologic findings.

Blood glucose (**choice A**) would not be increased by the fluids she is getting. It could be decreased if pituitary insufficiency and secondary adrenal insufficiency had developed, but in that case the presentation would have been one of otherwise unexplained shock.

CT scan of the head (**choice B**) would have been a good idea if she had a normal urinary output but had reported a horrible headache, followed by neurologic deterioration, suggesting intracranial bleeding.

Creatinine clearance (**choice C**) assumes that something is intrinsically wrong with the kidneys. Her kidneys are fine; they simply are not getting ADH and therefore are excreting high volumes of very diluted urine.

Serum levels of ACTH (**choice D**) follows the same line of reasoning as **choice A**. Secondary adrenal insufficiency would have produced shock, hypoglycemia, and hyperkalemia in a patient who would be awake and without significantly increased urinary output.

25. **The correct answer is E.** An old man who smokes, drinks, and has rotten teeth is the perfect candidate to develop squamous cell carcinoma of the mucosa of the head and neck. An unhealing ulcer in the floor of the mouth, a big lymph node on the side of the neck, hoarseness that

does not go away, and unilateral ear ache are the classic presentations. In this case, the tumor is probably occluding the Eustachian tube and leading to the accumulation of fluid in the middle ear. Systematic examination of the entire mucosa, with biopsies, will demonstrate the primary tumor.

Audiometry (**choice A**) would document the conductive hearing loss but will do nothing to find the tumor.

A tumor of the acoustic nerve (**choice B**) would lead to gradual unilateral hearing loss, but it would be sensory, not conductive.

Culture (**choice C**) mistakenly assumes the problem to be infectious in origin.

Biopsies of the ear itself (**choice D**) are misplaced. The tumor is not there; it is inside the mouth.

26. **The correct answer is E.** Indications for exploratory laparotomy in trauma patients include those with intra-abdominal bleeding that has been demonstrated by appropriate tests, but also those with an acute abdomen (severe pain, tenderness, guarding, and rebound tenderness) following abdominal trauma. This woman is probably bleeding into her abdomen (she has no other obvious source). Even if that were not the case, however, she needs an exploratory laparotomy to deal with the source of the acute abdomen, which is bound to be injuries of hollow viscera.

Sonogram (**choice A**) is used extensively to diagnose intra-abdominal bleeding, but it does not tell us what to do, or not to do, for the acute abdomen.

X-ray films (**choice B**) would add little to our decision. Free air under the diaphragm would prove visceral disruption, but the absence of such a finding would not exclude it.

CT scan (**choice C**) is excellent in the hemodynamically stable patient in whom the only question is intra-abdominal bleeding. In this case, we are also contending with the acute abdomen. Furthermore, with a systolic blood pressure of 75 mm Hg, this woman cannot afford a trip to the CT scanner.

Diagnostic peritoneal lavage (**choice D**) is excellent to prove intra-abdominal injury, and is also extensively used to diagnose peritoneal contamination from ruptured hollow viscera. However, the latter is required only when the abdomen cannot be examined reliably (e.g., the drunk or the unconscious patient). This woman is telling us that her belly hurts, and our physical exam is diagnostic.

27. **The correct answer is B.** All the findings indicate obstructive jaundice (high alkaline phosphatase, dilated ducts), with gallstones as the source. The fact that no stone can be seen impacted within the common duct is meaningless, since only about 50% of those can be seen by sonogram (the air in the duodenal loop interferes with the study). Endoscopic retrograde cholangiopancreatography (ERCP) can outline the stone and even allow extraction, limiting subsequent surgery to cholecystectomy.

Serology (**choice A**) would have been a splendid idea if she had very high transaminases and minimal elevation of the alkaline phosphatase, and if the sonogram had shown normal size ducts.

Ampullary cancer (**choice C**) should be suspected in the patient with obstructive jaundice, along with anemia and occult blood in the stool; this is not the case here.

Liver biopsy (**choice D**) assumes that we expect intrinsic liver disease, which is not the case here.

Neither should we suspect cancer of the pancreatic head (**choice E**) when the gallbladder is contracted rather than dilated and all the signs point to stones as the problem. ERCP will also give us the diagnosis in the case of the rare patient with two diseases (stones plus an unrelated cancer).

28. **The correct answer is C.** This is the classic description of Paget disease, an infiltrating cancer of the breast directly underneath the areola that is permeating the skin lymphatics and the skin itself. Although it is true that the areola is not immune to other benign skin conditions, missing the cancer would be lethal. Thus, any other answer that does not seek to rule out cancer first is wrong.

Treatment with estrogens (**choice A**) assumes a benign, age-related atrophy, which is common in the vagina but not in the areola.

A mammogram and galactogram (**choice B**) are indicated to find intraductal papilloma, the presentation of which is bloody nipple discharge in a younger woman.

Looking for a glucagonoma (**choice D**) is a distracter that might appeal to those who are convinced that the USMLE emphasizes bizarre, rare diseases. Indeed glucagonoma shows up as an intractable skin condition, but it is migratory, necrolytic, and exfoliative. It occurs in anemic diabetic patients with glossitis, and shows no preference for the areola.

Culture and topical antibiotics (**choice E**) is the intuitive answer if you assume that this is a nasty skin infection, but never make that your first diagnosis in this setting!

29. **The correct answer is C.** The clinical picture is that of mitral stenosis, with the apical diastolic murmur plus all the typical symptoms for that condition. As a rule, cardiovascular surgeons prefer to repair the patient's own mitral valve, rather than replacing it. Stenosis is due to fusion at the commissures, which commissurotomy can correct.

A ventricular septal defect (**choice A**) would produce a systolic murmur and, if uncorrected by age 35, would have produced pulmonary vascular damage, with a potential reversal of the shunt and even cyanosis.

Although mitral annuloplasty (**choice B**) targets the correct valve, it assumes that the problem is insufficiency rather than stenosis. Had that been the case, the apical murmur would have been systolic, rather than diastolic.

Replacement of the aortic valve (**choice D**) would be correct if the patient had a deformed aortic valve, as these cannot be easily repaired. In this case, however, the sick valve is the mitral (with an apical murmur) rather than the aortic, which would have produced a murmur best heard at the base.

Replacement of the mitral valve (**choice E**) can be done, and is indeed done, but not as the first choice if repair is possible.

30. **The correct answer is A.** Pneumonectomy is the preferred treatment for centrally located non-small cell cancers of the lung. The patient's pulmonary function studies (prompted by the suggestion of COPD) show that he can tolerate the removal of one third of his current lung capacity, as it would leave him with more than 800 mL forced expiratory volume at 1 second (FEV_1). However, there is no point in undertaking surgical therapy unless cure is possible, which would not be the case if he has liver metastasis, metastasis on the other lung, or involved mediastinal nodes at or above the carina. CT scan is the first step to answer those questions, before the pneumonectomy is considered.

Radiation and chemotherapy (**choice B**) would have been the chosen palliative therapy if metastatic spread had contraindicated surgery. It would also have been the correct answer if the tumor had been small cell, rather than squamous cell, carcinoma.

The supraclavicular nodes (**choice C**) can be involved in lung cancer, but they are not the first level. Thus, a negative biopsy would not have given the green light for surgery. If a CT scan does not give a satisfactory answer as to the status of mediastinal nodes, a cervical mediastinal exploration would be the procedure of choice to sample carinal nodes.

Lobectomy (**choice D**) is not suitable for central lesions, but it might have been the operation of choice for a peripheral tumor.

Pneumonectomy (**choice E**) is indeed our goal, but one would not do it without first making sure that extensive metastases are not present.

31. **The correct answer is C.** The clinical picture is classic for a dissecting aneurysm of the thoracic aorta. The presentation resembles that of a myocardial infarction, but it happens in hypertensive patients who develop a wide mediastinum. At one time, only an arteriogram could establish the diagnosis (at considerable risk), but noninvasive imaging is currently preferred.

ECG and cardiac enzymes (**choice A**) are usually done on anyone with chest pain, but the results would have been negative here. They would have ruled out infarction but would not establish the alternate diagnosis.

Studying the esophagus with Gastrografin swallow, followed by barium if negative (**choice B**), would have been a good idea if the patient had vomited repeatedly before developing the chest pain and if the x-ray film had shown mediastinal air rather than a wide mediastinum.

Ventilation-perfusion scan (**choice D**) would actually have been the best choice if a pulmonary embolus had been suspected.

Pulmonary angiogram (**choice E**) might have come to mind if he had been immobilized by recent surgery and had then developed signs suggestive of pulmonary embolus: pleuritic pain, shortness of breath, hemoptysis, and distended head and neck veins. Actually, although the angiogram is supposed to be the gold standard in such cases, it is seldom done. Less invasive diagnostic means, as suggested in **choice C**, are preferred.

32. **The correct answer is B.** The clinical picture is that of acute epididymitis, which is treated with antibiotics. The differential diagnosis includes testicular torsion. Although all the details in this case point to epididymitis, the consequences of missing a diagnosis of testicular torsion are so dire that sonogram is always done to rule it out with certainty.

Orchitis secondary to mumps could produce a painful testicle, and you might think of treating it with antivirals (**choice A**). In this patient, however, neither the history nor physical examination indicates that the parotids are swollen.

Cystoscopy (**choice C**) is included as a distracter to emphasize the point that instrumentation of the urinary tract should never be done when there are signs of current urinary tract infection.

Testicular tumors (hinted at in **choice D**) are typically painless. If one were thought to be present, however, the correct way to biopsy it would be by inguinal orchiectomy, never by the trans-scrotal route.

Surgery and orchiopexy (**choice E**) would be the correct answer for testicular torsion, in which case the testicle would have been high and in a horizontal position, the cord would have been nontender, and neither fever nor pyuria would have been present.

KAPLAN) MEDICAL

33. **The correct answer is D.** The correlation between ureteropelvic junction obstruction and profuse diuresis is classic. A congenital narrowing at the ureteropelvic junction allows normal passage of urine at a normal flow rate, but the lumen cannot accommodate a suddenly increased flow rate. Beer is a wonderful diuretic; if he had never been exposed to it, his congenital anomaly could have remained hidden.

    Bladder calculi (**choice A**) would give suprapubic pain and symptoms of an irritative bladder.

    Low implanted ureter (**choice B**) is typically asymptomatic in the male but could lead to incontinence in the female.

    Ureteral stone (**choice C**) is a good second choice, and it could cause flank pain radiating to the inner thigh and scrotum. However, the youngster who develops colicky flank pain when first exposed to beer is so classic for ureteropelvic junction obstruction that urologists can make the correct diagnosis over the telephone.

    Vesicoureteral reflux (**choice E**) gives a febrile picture along with flank pain. It is typically seen in younger children, who eventually outgrow their problem.

34. **The correct answer is E.** His age and status as a non-smoker make a primary testicular cancer with lung metastasis far more likely than the opposite combination, or the existence of two unrelated lesions. The fact that the tumor has spread should not preclude attempts at diagnosis and treatment, since most testicular cancers are exquisitely radio- and chemosensitive and may be cured even when they have metastasized. The correct way to diagnose a testicular cancer is by radical orchiectomy via the inguinal route.

    Palliative care only (**choice A**) is often the best thing to do for far advanced, very aggressive tumors, for which there is no effective treatment anyway. This is not the case for testicular cancer. Do not give up in this case. Cure is still possible.

    Going after the metastasis first, rather than the assumed primary tumor (**choice B**), makes sense if the metastasis is more accessible, which is not the case here. Furthermore, bronchoscopy is not likely to provide access to a peripheral metastatic lesion.

    Urologists cringe at the thought of trans-scrotal approaches for testicular cancer, whether for biopsy or excision (**choices C and D**). The tumor is spread to the incision site, complicating further management. The only acceptable biopsy for a testicular mass is a formal orchiectomy by the inguinal route, with high ligation of the cord ("radical orchiectomy").

35. **The correct answer is D.** This is a classic presentation of a ruptured berry aneurysm. There must be a high suspicion for this diagnosis, since failure to make it will likely result in the death of the patient. Although the diagnosis of headache is quite common, the classic pattern is that of a sentinel bleed followed by meningismus and agitation that herald a rebleed in more than 70% of subarachnoid hemorrhage (SAH) patients within 48 hours. Once the SAH is identified (usually with a CT scan), neurosurgical intervention to stop the bleeding can be begun, and the patient thereafter has a normal life expectancy. The most common nontraumatic cause for SAH is a berry aneurysm in the anterior portion of the circle of Willis.

    Arteriovenous malformation (**choice A**) is a rare cause of a SAH and intracranial bleeds in general.

    The cerebellum (**choice B**) is an uncommon site for bleeds. When they do occur, they are generally due to severe hypertension. Such bleeds are urgent because they can cause brain stem compression or obstructive hydrocephalus if not promptly evacuated.

    The putamen (**choice C**) and thalamus (**choice E**) are the most common sites for hypertensive bleeds. Such bleeds do not produce meningismus, only mental status changes and focal neurologic deficits.

36. **The correct answer is C.** Anatomic proximity to major vessels is the main criterion to suspect vascular injury in gunshot wounds of the extremities. Although absent pulses and an expanding hematoma make such an injury virtually certain (and dictate the need for surgical exploration), the presence of normal pulses and the absence of a hematoma do not rule out vascular injury. Noninvasive Doppler studies or, if necessary, an arteriogram can provide the necessary reassurance.

    Massive external bleeding might be currently prevented by clots. Disturbing them in the emergency department (**choice A**) could lead to a lot of unnecessary excitement in a place ill-equipped to deal with the problem. When vascular injuries are explored in the operating room, proximal and distal control are obtained first, before the wound itself is probed.

    If his vessels are indeed injured, sending him home (**choice B**) would risk the development of complications, such as late bleeding, vascular occlusion from intimal flaps, or development of an AV fistula.

    Formal surgical exploration (**choice D**) would be mandatory if he were exsanguinating, had no distal pulses, or had an expanding hematoma. When the only reason to suspect vascular injury is anatomic proximity, a less aggressive approach is indicated.

    Waiting for complications to develop (**choice E**) would be expensive and lead to higher morbidity.

37. **The correct answer is D.** Cirrhotic patients with ascites may develop spontaneous primary bacterial peritonitis,

which gives a "mild picture of acute abdomen," and is identified by growing a single organism out of the ascitic fluid.

CT scan (**choice A**) is an excellent way to rule out common intra-abdominal conditions that may be suggested by equivocal clinical presentations (e.g., appendicitis, pancreatitis, and diverticulitis). In this case, it would simply show the ascites and nothing else. Thus, it would rule out other things but would not establish the diagnosis.

Serum amylase (**choice B**) ought to be the first thought in an alcoholic who develops an acute abdomen, but not if he has not drunk anything for 7 years. This is not the clinical picture of pancreatitis, either.

The biliary tract, which a sonogram (**choice C**) would check, can be the source of abdominal pain in a cirrhotic, but it would have the typical clinical presentation of right upper quadrant pain.

Laparoscopy (**choice E**) is being used in lieu of exploratory laparotomy when "taking a peek in the abdomen" would establish a diagnosis. It would be a rather invasive way to show that this man has nothing other than ascitic fluid in his abdomen. Furthermore, there would be a risk of prolonged postoperative leak of ascitic fluid through the incision sites.

38. **The correct answer is A.** The clinical diagnosis is obstructive jaundice (high alkaline phosphatase, dilated biliary ducts), which is malignant in nature (thin walled, distended, palpable gallbladder) and probably due to cancer of the head of the pancreas (bulky tumor producing weight loss and back pain). The tumor can probably be seen in the CT scan, which is the least invasive of the proposed imaging studies.

Serologies (**choice B**) would be in order if we suspected hepatitis, which would be the case if the transaminases were very high, the alkaline phosphatase only modestly altered, and the ducts not dilated in the sonogram.

Duodenal endoscopy and biopsies (**choice C**) would be the first choice if we suspected cancer of the ampulla of Vater, in which case there would be no pain and probably no weight loss, but there would be anemia and occult blood in the stools.

ERCP (**choice D**) is the first choice if stones are suspected. In that case, however, there would be a nondistended gallbladder with stones in it. When pancreatic cancer is suspected, ERCP is the next test to do if the CT scan is negative and we therefore assume either that the pancreatic cancer is very small or that there is common duct cancer.

Percutaneous transhepatic cholangiogram (PTC) (**choice E**) does the same as ERCP (put dye directly into the ducts) and is also invasive. If we elected to do PTC

instead of ERCP, it would still be preceded in this case by the CT scan, which might render either test unnecessary.

39. **The correct answer is B.** Progressive headache that is worse in the mornings and present for several months indicates a brain tumor. Furthermore, the papilledema and projectile vomiting leave no doubt about the presence of increased intracranial pressure, something that a brain tumor eventually will produce. Do not be fooled by the absence of other neurologic symptoms; that can happen when tumors press on a "silent area" of the brain.

Brain abscess (**choice A**) is also an intracranial mass that can do the same things described here, but the timetable would be shorter (days or weeks) and the source of infection would be described in the vignette (mastoiditis or frontal sinusitis, for instance).

Chronic subdural hematoma (**choice C**) affects very old or alcoholic patients, who gradually lose their mental capacity after trivial trauma to the head.

Degenerative diseases, like multiple sclerosis (**choice D**), typically have on and off neurologic deficits for years before they are diagnosed.

Subarachnoid bleeding from an intracranial aneurysm (**choice E**) can indeed strike a young person, but the presentation is an extremely intense headache of sudden onset, "like a thunderclap."

40. **The correct answer is D.** The clinical picture and the radiographic description are those of a sigmoid volvulus, a common condition in elderly patients. The endoscopic instrument can untwist the bowel from the inside, relieve the obstruction, and allow placement of a long rectal tube. Repeated episodes may require corrective surgery.

The combination of nasogastric suction, IV fluids, and observation (**choice A**) is a conservative approach that is appropriate when adhesions are the suspected reason for obstruction affecting only the small bowel. This will occur in patients with a previous laparotomy.

Enemas and laxatives (**choice B**) are often needed in elderly patients who develop fecal impaction. However, an empty rectal vault in the physical exam excludes that diagnosis.

Arteriogram (**choice C**) comes to mind for the other common abdominal catastrophe in the elderly: mesenteric embolus. In that setting, however, one expects atrial fibrillation or a very recent myocardial infarction as the source of the clot. In addition, the patient is typically sicker and has a silent abdomen and blood in the stool. The x-ray film would show small bowel distention and distention of the colon up to the middle of the transverse, but no huge loop or parrot's beak.

Exploratory laparotomy (**choice E**) would be needed if the loop could not be straightened out and emptied endoscopically, or if the patient had signs of strangulation (e.g., fever, an acute abdomen).

41. **The correct answer is E.** At one time, all full thickness burns were allowed to heal by granulation over a period of 2 or 3 weeks, before skin grafting was done. The area was kept free of bacteria by the use of topical agents, such as the ones listed in the alternate answers. The process was expensive, painful, time-consuming, and prone to complications. The current preference is to do immediate excision and grafting of burned areas that appear to be full thickness, if they are not very extensive. This one is a perfect example.

If the extent of the burn precludes early excision and grafting, mafenide acetate (**choice A**) is used in areas where deep penetration is needed. Otherwise it is not a first choice because it hurts and can produce acidosis.

Silver sulfadiazine (**choice B**) is the "workhorse" of burn wound antibacterial therapy, but as pointed out, it would be a perfect choice only if we had to go the slow route of preparing the area for delayed skin grafts.

Triple antibiotic ointment (**choice C**) is preferred for burns around the eyes, as the other two topical agents are very irritating.

Debridement is often indicated in the long-term preparation of an area to be grafted, but wet-to-dry dressings (**choice D**) would be less effective than antibacterial agents. In any event, we want immediate excision and grafting for this patient.

42. **The correct answer is A.** The mechanism of injury suggests anterior cord syndrome, because the burst vertebral bodies are more likely to damage the anterior part of the cord that lies right behind them. The final neurologic deficits confirm it, since the only preserved functions are those that travel in the posterior part of the cord.

Central cord syndrome (**choice B**) is seen with hyperextension injuries of the neck, resulting in severe deficits in the upper extremities but better preservation of function in the lower extremities.

Complete cord transection (**choice C**) would have no function at all below the level of the lesion.

Hemisection (**choice D**) would have the classic "split deficits"—below the lesion some functions are affected on one side and a different set of functions are affected on the other.

Spinal shock (**choice E**) was present in this patient right after the injury (nothing worked), but it is not the final lesion.

43. **The correct answer is A.** Hip pathology often presents with knee pain, and in this case the problem is clearly in the hip. Age is the next clue. Avascular necrosis (also known as idiopathic aseptic necrosis, or Legg-Calve-Perthes disease) occurs typically in this age group, with preference for boys rather than girls.

Developmental dysplasia (**choice B**) is present at birth (it used to be called congenital dislocation of the hip, a name that was changed for medicolegal reasons) and, if untreated, would have caused problems earlier.

Osteomyelitis (**choice C**) is usually seen in peripheral bones, following a febrile illness in toddlers. Fever is also usually seen at the time that the osteomyelitis has developed.

The same is true of a septic hip (**choice D**), which should be suspected when a toddler with a recent febrile illness suddenly refuses to move a hip and has so much pain that he does not allow anyone to examine it.

Slipped capital femoral epiphysis (**choice E**) should be suspected when a chubby, 12- to 14-year-old boy shows up with hip pain and inability to internally rotate the hip. Age, again, is the first clue.

44. **The correct answer is D.** The patient has already sustained the neurologic damage due to the initial blow and is not threatened by a single large hematoma displacing the midline structures. However, she is still vulnerable to further neurologic impairment resulting from the development of increased intracranial pressure. If the intracranial pressure is medically prevented or minimized (with fluid restriction, diuretics, and modest hyperventilation), her chances of recovery are somewhat better.

The patient has normal vital signs; therefore, infusing IV fluids (**choice A**) would not help. If she had been in shock, the brain would have suffered from inadequate perfusion, and restoring intravascular volume would have been a good idea. In this case, the additional fluid would simply compound the problem of increased intracranial pressure.

Systemic vasodilators (**choice B**) would decrease intravascular pressure and work against the local vasoconstriction that modest hyperventilation may have offered. The end result would be less cerebral perfusion.

Hyperbaric oxygen (**choice C**) has no role in the prevention or treatment of increased intracranial pressure.

Surgical evacuation (**choice E**) is indicated for hematomas that are displacing the midline structures.

45. **The correct answer is E.** The differential diagnosis of severe postoperative chest pain with tachycardia and shortness of breath is between myocardial infarction and pulmonary embolus. Timing offers the first clue:

Myocardial infarction typically occurs within the first 2 to 3 days, whereas pulmonary embolus is more commonly seen after 5 to 7 days. Although postoperative myocardial infarction often does not have the typical chest-pain pattern, this case presents with pain of a fairly typical nature and radiations. Both ECG and cardiac enzymes are used to confirm myocardial infarction; however, an EKG can be performed quickly and easily and may identify those individuals with an acute ST segment elevation MI that may require immediate transfer to the cath lab.

Blood gases (**choice A**) would be the first step to build a case for pulmonary embolus, in which case they would show hypoxia and hypocapnia. However, the timing does not suggest pulmonary embolus.

A chest x-ray film (**choice B**) is nonspecific for either of the two diagnoses under consideration. Other problems that could be diagnosed with a chest x-ray film in this setting, such as atelectasis, pneumonia, or pneumothorax, could account for shortness of breath and should remain on the differential.

Pulmonary angiogram (**choice C**) is the ultimate, "gold-standard" test for pulmonary embolus. It is seldom done clinically (ventilation-perfusion scan and CT angiogram are more commonly used), and, as noted above, it addresses a problem that clinically has already been excluded or made much less likely.

Transaminases (**choice D**) would be very helpful in the differential diagnosis of jaundice, but they have no role in identifying the source of chest pain.

46. **The correct answer is D.** Rubbery, movable breast masses in young women are fibroadenomas, and a rapidly growing variant is known to affect adolescents.

Cancer (**choice A**) is virtually unknown in this age group.

Cystosarcoma phyllodes (**choice B**) grows to very large size, but it does so over a period of several years. It starts in women in their early or mid twenties, and reaches large size by the time they are in their late twenties or early thirties.

Mammary dysplasia (**choice C**) is typically seen in women aged 20-40. It is characterized by painful breasts and recurrent formation of cysts.

Intraductal papilloma (**choice E**) is the least likely answer. Those tumors produce bloody nipple discharge, and their size is measured in millimeters.

47. **The correct answer is C.** The double bubble sign with a little gas beyond is highly suggestive. The diagnosis must be promptly confirmed (by barium enema or contrast study from above) so that emergency surgery can be performed before the bowel dies twisted on its vascular

pedicle. This condition can be present at birth or it can also show up later, as in this example.

Hypertrophic pyloric stenosis (**choice A**) is suggested by the age (it presents at 3 weeks). However, the vomiting would have been projectile and free of bile, and x-ray films would have shown only gastric distention.

Intestinal atresia (**choice B**) shows up at birth, and the x-ray films show multiple air fluid levels.

Meconium ileus (**choice D**) is also obvious earlier in life, but the infant would have cystic fibrosis, an unused microcolon, and inspissated meconium in the ileum giving a ground glass appearance in the x-ray films.

Necrotizing enterocolitis (**choice E**) occurs in the premature infant when first fed.

48. **The correct answer is D.** The mechanism of injury and symptomatology are consistent with fracture of the scaphoid bone. The most important clue to diagnosis is the presence of pain on pressure in the "anatomic snuffbox." Plain x-ray films in the first 24-48 hours usually fail to reveal evidence of fractures, and the patient may be mistakenly diagnosed as having a sprain. In the presence of the characteristic history and findings on physical examination, appropriate treatment for presumptive scaphoid fracture should be instituted, until proven otherwise.

Bone scanning (**choice A**) may be performed to confirm the presence of scaphoid fracture. It is more sensitive than plain x-rays, but it frequently gives false negative results in the first 48 hours following trauma.

MRI examination of the wrist (**choice B**), as well as CT scans, can be performed if there is a need for prompt confirmation of the clinical suspicion of scaphoid fractures. However, these radiologic investigations are not cost-effective.

Treatment for wrist sprain (**choice C**) is the most common mistake when dealing with scaphoid fractures, especially because plain x-ray films are often negative in the first day or two after the fracture occurs. Missed scaphoid fracture is among the top 10 reasons for malpractice suits.

49. **The correct answer is D.** Despite prophylactic treatment with low-dose heparin, this patient has developed signs and symptoms of pulmonary thromboembolism (PTE). This case highlights the diagnostic problems in the clinical approach to PTE, which is frequently encountered in a hospital setting. Ventilation-perfusion scan cannot be expected to be diagnostic in the presence of areas of atelectasis and pneumonic infiltrates. Therefore, spiral CT scan of the chest is a better diagnostic choice.

Bronchoalveolar lavage (**choice A**) has no role in the diagnosis of PTE. It is most useful in obtaining samples of lower respiratory tract secretions to determine the etiologic agent of pneumonia.

Contrast venography (**choice B**) is used to investigate the presence of deep venous thrombosis (DVT), but it should not be the first diagnostic method in the diagnostic workup of possible PTE.

Pulmonary angiography (**choice C**) is the definitive diagnostic method for PTE, but it should be used only after noninvasive procedures have failed.

Ultrasonography of the lower extremities (**choice E**) is a noninvasive method of diagnosing DVT. This procedure (as well as any other test for DVT) should also be carried out only if chest scanning gives equivocal or inconclusive results.

Ventilation-perfusion lung scanning (**choice F**) is frequently performed to diagnose pulmonary emboli. However, as is pointed out above, the test is not reliable if there are areas of atelectasis and pneumonic infiltrates in the chest x-ray.

50. **The correct answer is B.** The relationship between smoking and bladder cancer is even more significant than the well-known relationship between smoking and lung cancer. This man is a prime candidate for bladder cancer. His workup has been appropriate until now because the intravenous pyelogram (IVP) is often the first test done in patients with hematuria. This study diagnoses renal cell carcinomas and ureteral tumors, but it is notoriously inaccurate for early bladder cancers. Thus, the patient's workup has not been completed, and he now needs a cystoscopy.

CT scan of the kidneys (**choice A**) is also an excellent study for diagnosing renal cell carcinoma, but this diagnosis has already been excluded with the IVP, and the CT scan is not the best test to find early bladder cancers.

We are not ready to prescribe medications (**choice C**). Valuable time will be wasted if we assume that the patient has a urinary tract infection or prostatitis (for which we have no convincing findings) and we go for a trial of therapy. The patient will not respond to it, and, eventually, we will have to look into his bladder. A 65-year-old man with hematuria, a normal IVP, and a very strong history of smoking needs an immediate cystoscopy.

Hematuria is not the typical presentation for prostatic cancer. Prostatic cancer is found by discovering a hard nodule on rectal exam, or by being alerted by a high PSA, neither of which is present here. Thus, there is nothing to biopsy in that organ (**choice D**).

Retrograde cystogram (**choice E**) is used to rule out bladder injuries in trauma patients. It is not the best test for early bladder cancer. In fact, we have already injected radiopaque dye in this patient's bladder (as part of the IVP), and it failed to outline the tumor.

STANDARD REFERENCE LABORATORY VALUES

	REFERENCE RANGE	SI REFERENCE INTERVALS
BLOOD, PLASMA, SERUM		
* Alanine aminotransferase (ALT, GPT at 30C)	8-20 U/L	8-20 U/L
Amylase, serum	25-125 U/L	25-125 U/L
* Aspartate aminotransferase (AST, GOT at 30C)	8-20 U/L	8-20 U/L
Bilirubin, serum (adult) Total // Direct	0.1-1.0 mg/dL // 0.0-0.3 mg/dL	2-17 mol/L // 0-5 mol/L
* Calcium, serum (Total)	8.4-10.2 mg/dL	2.1-2.8 mmol/L
* Cholesterol, serum	140-250 mg/dL	3.6-6.5 mmol/L
Cortisol, serum	0800 h: 5-23 g/dL // 1600 h: 3-15 g/dL	138-635 nmol/L // 82-413 nmol/L
	2000 h: 50% of 0800 h	Fraction of 0800 h: 0.50
Creatine kinase, serum (at 30C) ambulatory	Male: 25-90 U/L	25-90 U/L
	Female: 10-70 U/L	10-70 U/L
* Creatinine, serum	0.6-1.2 mg/dL	53-106 mol/L
Electrolytes, serum		
Sodium	135-147 mEq/L	135-147 mmol/L
Chloride	95-105 mEq/L	95-105 mmol/L
* Potassium	3.5-5.0 mEq/L	3.5-5.0 mmol/L
Bicarbonate	22-28 mEq/L	22-28 mmol/L
Estriol (E_3) total, serum (in pregnancy)		
24-28 weeks // 32-36 weeks	30-170 ng/mL // 60-280 ng/mL	104-590 // 208-970 nmol/L
28-32 weeks // 36-40 weeks	40-220 ng/mL // 80-350 ng/mL	140-760 // 280-1,210 nmol/L
Ferritin, serum	Male: 15-200 ng/mL	15-200 g/L
	Female: 12-150 ng/mL	12-150 g/L
Follicle-stimulating hormone, serum/plasma	Male: 4-25 mIU/mL	4-25 U/L
	Female: premenopause 4-30 mIU/mL	4-30 U/L
	midcycle peak 10-90 mIU/mL	10-90 U/L
	ostmenopause 40-250 mIU/mL	40-250 U/L
Gases, arterial blood (room air)		
pO_2	75-105 mm Hg	10.0-14.0 kPa
pCO_2	33-44 mm Hg	4.4-5.9 kPa
pH	7.35-7.45	[H^+] 36-44 nmol/L
Glucose, serum	Fasting: 70-110 mg/dL	3.8-6.1 mmol/L
	2-h postprandial: <120 mg/dL	<6.6 mmol/L
Growth hormone – arginine stimulation	Fasting: <5 ng/mL	<5 g/L
	provocative stimuli: >7 ng/mL	>7 g/L
Immunoglobulins, serum		
IgA	76-390 mg/dL	0.76-3.90 g/L
IgE	0-380 IU/mL	0-380 kIU/mL
IgG	650-1,500 mg/dL	6.5-15 g/L
IgM	40-345 mg/dL	0.4-3.45 g/L
Iron	50-170 g/dL	9-30 mol/L
Lactate dehydrogenase (L → P, 30C)	45-90 U/L	45-90 U/L
Luteinizing hormone, serum/plasma	Male: 6-23 mIU/mL	6-23 U/L
	Female: follicular phase 5-30 mIU/mL	5-30 U/L
	midcycle 75-150 mIU/mL	75-150 U/L
	postmenopause 30-200 mIU/mL	30-200 U/L
Osmolality, serum	275-295 mOsmol/kg	275-295 mOsmol/kg
Parathyroid hormone, serum, N-terminal	230-630 pg/mL	230-630 ng/L
* Phosphatase (alkaline), serum (p-NPP at 30C)	20-70 U/L	20-70 U/L
* Phosphorus (inorganic), serum	3.0-4.5 mg/dL	1.0-1.5 mmol/L
Prolactin, serum (hPRL)	<20 ng/mL	<20 g/L
* Proteins, serum		
Total (recumbent)	6.0-7.8 g/dL	60-78 g/L
Albumin	3.5-5.5 g/dL	35-55 g/L
Globulins	2.3-3.5 g/dL	23-35 g/L
Thyroid-stimulating hormone, serum or plasma	0.5-5.0 U/mL	0.5-5.0 mU/L
Thyroidal iodine (^{123}I) uptake	8%-30% of administered dose/24 h	0.08-0.30/24 h
Thyroxine (T_4), serum	5-12 g/dL	64-155 nmol/L
Triglycerides, serum	35-160 mg/dL	0.4-1.81 mmol/L
Triiodothyronine (T_3), serum (RIA)	115-190 ng/dL	1.8-2.9 nmol/L
Triiodothyronine (T_3), resin uptake	25%-35%	0.25-0.35
* Urea nitrogen, serum (BUN)	7-18 mg/dL	1.2-3.0 mmol urea/L
* Uric acid, serum	3.0-8.2 mg/dL	0.18-0.48 mmol/L

(*) Included in the Biochemical Profile (SMA-12)

	REFERENCE RANGE	SI REFERENCE INTERVALS
CEREBROSPINAL FLUID		
Cell count	0-5 cells/mm^3	0-5 x 10^6/L
Chloride	118-132 mmol/L	118-132 mmol/L
Gamma globulin	3%-12% total proteins	0.03-0.12
Glucose	40-70 mg/dL	2.2-3.9 mmol/L
Pressure	70-180 mm H$_2$O	70-180 mm H$_2$O
Proteins, total	<40 mg/dL	<0.40 g/L
HEMATOLOGIC		
Bleeding time (template)	2-7 minutes	2-7 minutes
Erythrocyte count	Male: 4.3-5.9 million/mm^3	4.3-5.9 x 10^{12}/L
	Female: 3.5-5.5 million/mm^3	3.5-5.5 x 10^{12}/L
Hematocrit	Male: 41%-53%	0.41-0.53
	Female: 36%-46%	0.36-0.46
Hemoglobin, blood	Male: 13.5-17.5 g/dL	2.09-2.71 mmol/L
	Female: 12.0-16.0 g/dL	1.86-2.48 mmol/L
Hemoglobin, plasma	1-4 mg/dL	0.16-0.62 mol/L
Leukocyte count and differential		
Leukocyte count	4,500-11,000/mm^3	4.5-11.0 x 10^9/L
Segmented neutrophils	54%-62%	0.54-0.62
Band forms	3%-5%	0.03-0.05
Eosinophils	1%-3%	0.01-0.03
Basophils	0%-0.75%	0-0.0075
Lymphocytes	25%-33%	0.25-0.33
Monocytes	3%-7%	0.03-0.07
Mean corpuscular hemoglobin	25.4-34.6 pg/cell	0.39-0.54 fmol/cell
Mean corpuscular hemoglobin concentration	31%-36% Hb/cell	4.81-5.58 mmol Hb/L
Mean corpuscular volume	80-100 μm^3	80-100 fl
Partial thromboplastin time (nonactivated)	60-85 seconds	60-85 seconds
Platelet count	150,000-400,000/mm^3	150-400 x 10^9/L
Prothrombin time	11-15 seconds	11-15 seconds
Reticulocyte count	0.5%-1.5% of red cells	0.005-0.015
Sedimentation rate, erythrocyte (Westergren)	Male: 0-15 mm/h	0-15 mm/h
	Female: 0-20 mm/h	0-20 mm/h
Thrombin time	<2 seconds deviation from control	<2 seconds deviation from control
Volume		
Plasma	Male: 25-43 mL/kg	0.025-0.043 L/kg
	Female: 28-45 mL/kg	0.028-0.045 L/kg
Red cell	Male: 20-36 mL/kg	0.020-0.036 L/kg
	Female: 19-31 mL/kg	0.019-0.031 L/kg
SWEAT		
Chloride	0-35 mmol/L	0-35 mmol/L
URINE		
Calcium	100-300 mg/24 h	2.5-7.5 mmol/24 h
Chloride	Varies with intake	Varies with intake
Creatinine clearance	Male: 97-137 mL/min	
	Female: 88-128 mL/min	
Estriol, total (in pregnancy)		
30 weeks	6-18 mg/24 h	21-62 μmol/24 h
35 weeks	9-28 mg/24 h	31-97 μmol/24 h
40 weeks	13-42 mg/24 h	45-146 μmol/24 h
17-Hydroxycorticosteroids	Male: 3.0-10.0 mg/24 h	8.2-27.6 μmol/24 h
	Female: 2.0-8.0 mg/24 h	5.5-22.0 μmol/24 h
17-Ketosteroids, total	Male: 8-20 mg/24 h	28-70 μmol/24 h
	Female: 6-15 mg/24 h	21-52 μmol/24 h
Osmolality	50-1400 mOsmol/kg	
Oxalate	8-40 μg/mL	90-445 μmol/L
Potassium	Varies with diet	Varies with diet
Proteins, total	<150 mg/24 h	<0.15 g/24 h
Sodium	Varies with diet	Varies with diet
Uric acid	Varies with diet	Varies with diet